Clinical Management of Sensorimotor Speech Disorders

Second Edition

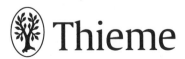

Clinical Management of Sensorimotor Speech Disorders

Second Edition

Malcolm R. McNeil, PhD, CCC-SLP, BC-ANCDS
Distinguished Service Professor and Chair
Department of Communication Science and Disorders
University of Pittsburgh
Research Career Scientist
Veterans Administration Pittsburgh Healthcare System
Geriatrics Research Education and Clinical Center
Pittsburgh, Pennsylvania

Thieme
New York · Stuttgart

Thieme Medical Publishers, Inc.
333 Seventh Ave.
New York, NY 10001

Editor: Timothy Y. Hiscock
Editorial Assistant: David Price
Vice President, Production and Electronic Publishing: Anne T. Vinnicombe
Production Editor: Kenneth L. Chumbley, Publication Services
Vice President, International Marketing and Sales: Cornelia Schulze
Chief Financial Officer: Peter van Woerden
President: Brian D. Scanlan
Compositor: Thomson Digital
Printer: Maple-Vail Book Manufacturing Group

Library of Congress Cataloging-in-Publication Data

Clinical management of sensorimotor speech disorders / [edited by] Malcolm R. McNeil. — 2nd ed.
   p. ; cm.
 Includes bibliographical references and index.
 ISBN 978-1-58890-514-7
 1. Articulation disorders. 2. Speech disorders. 3. Sensorimotor integration. I. McNeil, Malcolm Ray, 1947-
 [DNLM: 1. Speech Disorders—therapy. 2. Dysarthria. 3. Speech—physiology. 4. Speech Disorders—diagnosis. WL 340.2 C641 2009]
 RC424.7.C576 2009
 616.85'5—dc22

                                        2008007806

Important note: Medical knowledge is ever-changing. As new research and clinical experience broaden our knowledge, changes in treatment and drug therapy may be required. The authors and editors of the material herein have consulted sources believed to be reliable in their efforts to provide information that is complete and in accord with the standards accepted at the time of publication. However, in view of the possibility of human error by the authors, editors, or publisher of the work herein or changes in medical knowledge, neither the authors, editors, nor publisher, nor any other party who has been involved in the preparation of this work, warrants that the information contained herein is in every respect accurate or complete, and they are not responsible for any errors or omissions or for the results obtained from use of such information. Readers are encouraged to confirm the information contained herein with other sources. For example, readers are advised to check the product information sheet included in the package of each drug they plan to administer to be certain that the information contained in this publication is accurate and that changes have not been made in the recommended dose or in the contraindications for administration. This recommendation is of particular importance in connection with new or infrequently used drugs. Some of the product names, patents, and registered designs referred to in this book are in fact registered trademarks or proprietary names even though specific reference to this fact is not always made in the text. Therefore, the appearance of a name without designation as proprietary is not
to be construed as a representation by the publisher that it is in the public domain.

Printed in the United States of America

5 4 3 2 1

ISBN: 978-1-58890-514-7

Contents

Part II. Pathology

Foreword

When the first edition of *Clinical Management of Sensorimotor Speech Disorders* appeared more than 10 years ago, the "decade of the brain" was in full swing. That decade was aptly named because it was marked by an explosion of new knowledge in the neurosciences and in our understanding and management of neurologic disease. The decade saw a similar acceleration of efforts to understand, assess, and manage sensorimotor speech disorders, which has continued unabated into this new century. As a result, a second edition of *Clinical Management of Sensorimotor Speech Disorders* is justified, necessary, and important.

Dr. McNeil has wisely decided to retain the Darley, Aronson, and Brown paradigm as the foundation for this edition, because it continues to guide much of our thinking about sensorimotor speech disorders. Although there has been no paradigm shift—such shifts are rare—growth and perturbations are evident. The volume's contributing researchers and clinicians have been well-chosen to critically address the changes and refinements in theory, methods of study, experimental findings, and clinical observations that make up our current understanding of these disorders.

As was true for the first edition, this volume contains a very appropriate blend of gestalt overview and depth of detail. There is a wealth of useful information for both generalists and specialists, be they students, clinicians, or researchers. The addition of numerous brief chapters on many not-so-common disorders (or treatments, as in the case of pallidotomy) that represent or can be associated with sensorimotor speech disorders is welcome. These chapters provide fundamental information that may not be familiar even to many experienced clinicians and researchers. They will certainly help the busy clinician in need of a concise overview of a newly encountered disorder. Many of them also serve to establish that there are numerous diseases and conditions whose effects on speech and communication we know little about. From that standpoint, they point the way to some of the descriptive work and in-depth study that needs to be done in the future. Viewed broadly, this new edition of *Clinical Management of Sensorimotor Speech Disorders* reflects the state of the art and science. It also provides a compass for future research and clinical work that will improve our understanding, diagnosis, and management of these disorders, which can so profoundly affect the ability to speak.

Joseph R. Duffy, PhD, BC-NCD
Head
Division of Speech Pathology
Department of Neurology
Mayo Clinic
Professor of Speech Pathology
Mayo Clinic College of Medicine
Rochester, Minnesota

Preface

The influence of the Darley, Aronson, and Brown's (1969a,b) theoretical and diagnostic classification of sensorimotor speech disorders remains as pertinent today as it was at the time of the publication of the first edition of this book. It represents the prevailing scientific paradigm in sensorimotor speech disorders, in the Kuhnian sense (Kuhn, 1970), and has retained its influence on both the diagnosis and treatment of these disorders. In spite of a challenge to the basic division of the programming and execution levels of sensorimotor organization underlying this paradigm's classification of disorders, offered by van der Merwe (1997) in the first edition, there does not seem to have been a shift in thinking or practice among a majority of practitioners in this science. As such, the Darley, Aronson, and Brown (1969a,b) paradigm again forms the basic organization of this second edition of *Clinical Management of Sensorimotor Speech Disorders.*

Content from the first edition that has stood the test of time and continues to contribute unique information to basic understanding and clinical practice has been preserved. Where information has changed, those changes are reflected in this new edition. In most cases, the changes have required the addition of information rather than the correction of inaccuracies. To maintain a reasonable length and content coherence for this edition, this growth of information has required difficult decisions about what to include and what to leave out, and in some cases, what to delete from the content of the first edition. Most notably, this edition does not contain a chapter on ultrasound measurement of speech movements. This measurement technology, however, produces kinematic and morphological data that are addressed in other chapters. Likewise, the review of treatment in the apraxia of speech chapter has been sacrificed for a more detailed account of evidence relevant to the nature and diagnosis of the disorder. Two new chapters have been added, one by DeNil, Rochon, and Jokel on sensorimotor fluency disorders, and one by Rosenbek and Jones on principles of treatment for sensorimotor speech disorders. Both chapters make unique and important contributions to this second edition.

The second edition of *Clinical Management of Sensorimotor Speech Disorders* starts, as it did in the first edition, with an initial chapter detailing a model of speech motor control that proposes a unique and coherent conceptual framework for the differentiation and classification of sensorimotor speech disorders, authored by Anita van der Merwe. Following this initial chapter are six chapters that provide the theoretical underpinnings, strategies, and tactics for the assessment of sensorimotor speech disorders from the premier experts in the discipline. Ray Kent outlines the perceptual sensorimotor examination for motor speech disorders; Kirrie Ballard, Nancy Solomon, Donald Robin, Jerry Moon, and John Folkins address the theoretical and clinical issues surrounding the nonspeech assessment of the speech production mechanism; Karen Forrest and Gary Weismer present the acoustic analysis of motor speech disorders; David Zajac, Donald Warren, and Virginia Hinton discuss the aerodynamic assessment of motor speech disorders; Steven Barlow, Donald Finan, Richard Andreatta, and Carol Boliek discuss the theoretical underpinnings and the techniques used in the kinematic measurement of speech and early orofacial movement; and Erich Luschei and Eileen Finnegan present a clear and concise tutorial on the electromyographic techniques for the assessment of motor speech disorders.

Each of the next eight chapters is dedicated to a unique class of sensorimotor speech disorder and describes clearly and in detail the underlying mechanisms and presenting signs and symptom of that class of speech pathology. Carlin Hageman discusses flaccid dysarthria; Michael Cannito and Thomas Marquardt, ataxic dysarthria; Richard Zraick and Leonard LaPointe, hyperkinetic dysarthria; Scott Adams and Allyson Dykstra, hypokinetic dysarthria; Bruce Murdoch, Elizabeth Ward, and Deborah Theodoros, spastic dysarthria; Sheila Pratt and Nancy Tye-Murray, speech impairment secondary to hearing loss; Luc De Nil, Elizabeth Rochon, and Regina Jokel, sensorimotor fluency disorders; and Malcolm McNeil, Donald Robin, and Richard Schmidt, apraxia of speech. The final chapter in this section of the book presents a unique treatise on the principles of treatment for sensorimotor speech disorders by John Rosenbek and Harrison Jones.

Finally the greatest change in the second edition is the inclusion of forty-six epigrammatic chapters on pathologies that create or are accompanied by sensorimotor speech disorders. These chapters are in alphabetical order by disease, disorder, syndrome, or pathology or by the speech diagnosis that would be noted during a clinical evaluation. Both common and infrequently occurring disorders are included. Each chapters describes general information about the disorder including clinical medical presentation, diagnostic signs/symptoms, neuropathology, epidemiology, and genetics and follows with coverage of the speech impairment associated with the disorder including the diagnostic signs and symptoms, etiology, neuropathology, associated cognitive, linguistic, and communicative signs and symptoms, and special diagnostic considerations and treatment.

Carefully selected references in these chapters serve as a quick reference-overview and beginning reading on these disorders, which speech–language pathologists, physicians, and other health-care professionals are likely to encounter in contemporary clinical practice. We hope that the lack of information about the speech production mechanisms underlying some of these sensory motor speech disorders will serve to encourage research into these disorders and many that are not included in this edition.

It is the goal of these chapters to provide an otherwise unavailable resource of state-of-the-science information on these disorders from which an initial assessment and treatment plan could be constructed.

Ultimately, it is the goal of this volume to provide an advanced understanding of the nature, assessment, and management of sensorimotor speech disorders for the improved care of individuals with these disorders.

Malcolm R. McNeil, PhD
Pittsburgh, Pennsylvania
2008

References

Darley, F.L., Aronson, A.E., & Brown, J.R. (1969a). Differential diagnostic patterns of dysarthria. *Journal of Speech and Hearing Research, 12,* 249–269

Darley, F.L., Aronson, A.E., & Brown, J.R. (1969b). Clusters of deviant speech dimensions in the dysarthrias. *Journal of Speech and Hearing Research, 12,* 462–496

Kuhn, T.S. *The structure of scientific revolutions.* (2nd. Ed.). (1970). Chicago: University of Chicago Press. 1970

van der Merwe, A. (1997). A theoretical framework for the characterization of pathological speech sensorimotor control. In: M.R. McNeil (Ed.), *Clinical Management of Sensorimotor Speech Disorders,* (1–25). New York: Thieme Medical Publishers

List of Contributors

Scott G. Adams, PhD
Associate Professor
School of Communication Sciences
    and Disorders
University of Western Ontario
London, Ontario, Canada

Robin L Alvares, PhD, CCC-SLP
Scientific and Editorial Board Member
Augmentative and Alternative
    Communication Institute
Pittsburgh, Pennsylvania

Richard D. Andreatta, PhD
Associate Professor
Department of Rehabilitation
    Sciences
Division of Communication Disorders
    and Sciences
University of Kentucky
Lexington, Kentucky

Joan C. Arvedson, PhD, BC-NCD
Program Coordinator
Feeding and Swallowing Services
Children's Hospital of
    Wisconsin-Milwaukee
Clinical Professor
Department of Pediatrics
Medical College of
    Wisconsin-Milwaukee
Milwaukee, Wisconsin

Kirrie J. Ballard, PhD
Senior Lecturer
Department of Speech Pathology
University of Sydney
Lidcombe, NSW, Australia

Steven M. Barlow, PhD
Professor
Department of Speech-Language-
    Hearing, Neuroscience
University of Kansas
Lawrence, Kansas

Jared Bennett, MS
Speech Pathologist
Department of Communication
    Sciences and Disorders
University of Utah
Salt Lake City, Utah

Carol Boliek, PhD
Associate Professor
Department of Speech Pathology
    and Audiology
University of Alberta
Edmonton, Alberta, Canada

Ryan C. Branski, PhD
Assistant Attending Scientist and
    Associate Professor
Department of Head and Neck
    Surgery
Memorial Sloan-Kettering
    Cancer Center
New York, New York

Thomas Campbell, PhD, BC-NCD
Professor
School of Behavioral and
    Brain Sciences
Executive Director
Callier Center for Communication
    Disorders
University of Texas at Dallas
Dallas, Texas

Michael P. Cannito, PhD, CCC-SLP
Professor
School of Audiology and Speech-
    Language Pathology
University of Memphis
Memphis, Tennessee

Chris Code, PhD, FRCSLT, FBPsS
Professor
Department of Psychology
University of Exeter
Exeter, England

James L. Coyle, PhD, CCC-SLP
Clinical Instructor
Department of Communication
    Science and Disorders
University of Pittsburgh
Pittsburgh, Pennsylvania

Luc F. De Nil, PhD
Associate Professor and Chair
Department of Speech-Language
    Pathology
University of Toronto
Toronto, Ontario, Canada

Nayan P. Desai, MD
Assistant Professor
Department of Neurosciences
University of California–San Diego
San Diego, California

Kimberley M. Docking, PhD
Research Fellow
Department of Speech Pathology
University of Queensland
Brisbane, Queensland, Australia

Neila J. Donovan, PhD, CCC-SLP
Assistant Professor
Department of Communication
    Sciences and Disorders
Louisiana State University
Baton Rouge, Louisiana

Sakina S. Drummond, PhD, CCC-SLP
Professor and Chairperson
Department of Communication Disorders
Southeast Missouri State University
Cape Girardeau, Missouri

Joseph R. Duffy, PhD, BC-NCD
Head
Division of Speech Pathology
Department of Neurology
Mayo Clinic
Professor
Mayo Clinic College of Medicine
Rochester, Minnesota

Allyson Dykstra, PhD
Research Associate
School of Communication Sciences
    and Disorders
University of Western Ontario
London, Ontario, Canada

Cynthia A. Eberwein, MS
Senior Research Program Supervisor
Department of Medicine
John Hopkins University
Baltimore, Maryland

John Ellul, MD, DM
Lecturer of Neurology
Department of Neurology
Regional University Hospital of Patras
Rio, Patras, Greece

Pam Enderby, DSc, PhD, FRCSLT
Professor
School of Health and Related Research
University of Sheffield
Sheffield, England

Donald S. Finan, PhD
Assistant Professor
Department of Speech, Language,
    and Hearing Sciences
University of Colorado
Boulder, Colorado

Eileen M. Finnegan, PhD
Associate Professor
Department of Speech Pathology
    and Audiology
University of Iowa
Iowa City, Iowa

John W. Folkins, PhD
Chief Executive Officer
Bowling Green State University
    Research Institute
Bowling Green State University
Bowling Green, Ohio

Karen Forrest, PhD
Professor
Department of Speech and Hearing
    Sciences
Indiana University
Bloomington, Indiana

Damirez T. Fossett, MD, FACS
Assistant Professor
Department of Neurosurgery
George Washington University
Washington, DC

Tepanta R. D. Fossett, PhD
Department of Communication
    Science and Disorders
University of Pittsburgh
Research Associate
Department of Audiology and Speech
    Pathology
Veterans Administration Pittsburgh
    Healthcare System
Pittsburgh, Pennsylvania

Geoffrey V. Fredericks, PhD, CCC-SLP
Assistant Professor
Department of Communication
    Science and Disorders
University of Pittsburgh
Pittsburgh, Pennsylvania

Skott E. Freedman, MA, CCC-SLP
Predoctoral Fellow
School of Speech, Language, and
    Hearing Sciences
San Diego State University
San Diego, California

Justine V. Goozée, PhD
Senior Research Officer
School of Health and Rehabilitation
    Sciences
University of Queensland
Brisbane, Queensland, Australia

Sharon A. Gretz, MEd
Doctoral student
Department of Communication
    Science and Disorders
University of Pittsburgh
Pittsburgh, Pennsylvania

Carlin F. Hageman, PhD, CCC-SLP
Professor
Department of Communication
    Sciences and Disorders
University of Northern Iowa
Cedar Falls, Iowa

Michael J. Hammer, PhD, CCC-SLP
School of Medicine and Public Health
University of Wisconsin
Madison, Wisconsin

Bonnie Heintskill, MS, CCC-SLP
Home Care and Private Practice
Thiensville, Wisconsin

Virginia A. Hinton, PhD, CCC-SLP
Associate Professor
Department of Communication
    Sciences and Disorders
University of North Carolina–Greensboro
Greensboro, North Carolina

Shannon N. Austermann Hula, MS, CCC-SLP
Doctoral Candidate
Joint Doctororal Program in Language
    and Communicative Disorders
San Diego State University/University
    of California–San Diego
San Diego, California
Predoctoral Research Fellow
Veterans Administration Pittsburgh
    Healthcare System
Pittsburgh, Pennsylvania

William D. Hula, PhD
Adjunct Assistant Professor
Department of Communication
    Science and Disorders
University of Pittsburgh
Speech Pathologist
Audiology and Speech Pathology
    Program
Veterans Administration Pittsburgh
    Healthcare System
Pittsburgh, Pennsylvania

Mary E. Jenkins, MD, FRCPC
Assistant Professor
Department of Clinical Neurological
    Sciences
University of Western Ontario
London, Ontario, Canada

Mandar Jog, MD
Professor of Neurology
University of Western Ontario
Director
Movement Disorders Program
London Health Sciences Centre
London, Ontario, Canada

Regina Jokel, PhD
Fellow
Kunin-Lunenfeld Applied Research
    Unit
University of Toronto
Toronto, Ontario, Canada

Harrison N. Jones, PhD
Assistant Professor
Division of Speech Pathology and
    Audiology
Duke University
Durham, North Carolina

Amy H. Kao, MD, MPH
Assistant Professor
Division of Rheumatology and Clinical
    Immunology
University of Pittsburgh
Pittsburgh, Pennsylvania

Ray D. Kent, PhD
Professor Emeritus
Waisman Center
University of Wisconsin
Madison, Wisconsin

Leonard L. LaPointe, PhD, CCC-SLP
Francis Eppes Professor of
 Communication Disorders
Deparment of Communication
 Disorders
College of Medicine
Florida State University
Tallahassee, Florida

Erich S. Luschei, PhD
Professor Emeritus
Department of Speech Pathology
 and Audiology
University of Iowa
Iowa City, Iowa

Edwin Maas, PhD
University Associate
Department of Speech, Language,
 and Hearing
University of Arizona
Tucson, Arizona

Thomas P. Marquardt, PhD, CCC-SLP
Ben F. Love Regents Professor
Department of Communication
 Sciences and Disorders
University of Texas
Austin, Texas

Christine T. Matthews, MS
Adjunct Clinical Instructor
Department of Communication
 Science and Disorders
University of Pittsburgh
Pittsburgh, Pennsylvania

**Shannon Cook Mauszycki, PhD,
CCC-SLP**
Speech Language Pathologist
Aphasia and Apraxia of Speech
 Research Program
Veterans Administration Salt Lake
 City Healthcare System
Salt Lake City, Utah

**Malcolm R. McNeil, PhD, CCC-SLP,
BC-ANCDS**
Distinguished Service Professor
 and Chair
Department of Communication
 Science and Disorders
University of Pittsburgh
Research Career Scientist

Veterans Administration Pittsburgh
 Healthcare System
Geriatrics Research Education
 and Clinical Center
Pittsburgh, Pennsylvania

Jerald B. Moon, PhD
Associate Professor
Department of Speech Pathology
 and Audiology
University of Iowa
Iowa City, Iowa

Bruce E. Murdoch, PhD, DSc
Professor
Department of Health and
 Rehabilitation
University of Queensland
Brisbane, Queensland, Australia

**Ilias Papathanasiou PhD, MRCSLT
MCSP**
Clinical Assistant Professor
Department of Speech and Language
 Therapy
Technological Educational Institute
 of Patras
Patras, Greece

Stacey L Pavelko, MA, CCC-SLP
Graduate Assistant
Department of Communication
 Science and Disorders
University of Pittsburgh
Pittsburgh, Pennsylvania

Richard K. Peach, PhD, BC-ANCDS
Professor
Department of Communication
 Disorders and Sciences
Rush University Medical Center
Chicago, Illinois

Sheila R. Pratt, PhD
Associate Professor
Department of Communication
 Science and Disorders
School of Health and Rehabilitation
 Sciences
University of Pittsburgh
Research Scientist
Veterans Administration Pittsburgh
 Healthcare System
Pittsburgh, Pennsylvania

Donald A. Robin, PhD
Professor
Research Imaging Center
Departments of Otolaryngology–Head
 and Neck Surgery, Physical Therapy,

Radiology, and Program in
 Biomedical Engineering
Chief
Speech and Language Sciences Program
Research Imaging Center
University of Texas–San Antonio
 Health Science Center
San Antonio, Texas

Elizabeth Rochon, PhD, S-LP(C)
Associate Professor
Department of Speech-Language
 Pathology
University of Toronto
Toronto, Ontario, Canada

John C. Rosenbek, PhD
Professor and Chair
Department of Communicative
 Disorders
College of Health Professions
University of Florida
Gainesville, Florida

Richard A. Schmidt, PhD
Professor
Department of Psychology
University of California–Los Angeles
Los Angeles, California

Nancy Pearl Solomon, PhD, CCC-SLP
Research Speech-Language Pathologist
Army Audiology and Speech Center
Walter Reed Army Medical Center
Washington, DC

**Edythe A. Strand, PhD, CCC-SLP,
BC-NCD**
Consultant
Division of Speech Pathology
Department of Neurology
Mayo Clinic
Associate Professor
Mayo College of Medicine
Rochester, Minnesota

Debra M. Suiter, PhD
Assistant Professor
School of Audiology and
 Speech-Language Pathology
University of Memphis
Memphis, Tennessee

Deborah G. Theodoros, Ph.D.
Associate Professor, Division Head
Division of Speech Pathology
School of Health and Rehabilitation
 Sciences
University of Queensland
Brisbane, Queensland, Australia

Nancy Tye-Murray, PhD, CCC-A
Research Professor
Department of Otolaryngology
Washington University School
    of Medicine
St. Louis, Missouri

Anita van der Merwe, PhD
Professor
Department of Communication
    Pathology
University of Pretoria
Pretoria, South Africa

Vaia Varsami, MA, MRCSLT
Private Practice
Athens, Greece

Julie L. Wambaugh, PhD, CCC-SLP
Associate Professor
Department of Communication
    Sciences and Disorders
University of Utah
Research Career Scientist
Veterans Administration Salt Lake
    City Healthcare System
Salt Lake City, Utah

Elizabeth C. Ward, PhD
Senior Lecturer
Division of Speech Pathology
School of Health and Rehabilitation
    Sciences
University of Queensland
Brisbane, Queensland, Australia

Donald W. Warren, DDS, PhD
Kenan Professor and Director Emeritus
University of North Carolina Cranial
    Facial Center
University of North Carolina
Chapel Hill, North Carolina

Gary Weismer, PhD
Professor
Department of Communicative Disorders
University of Wisconsin
Madison, Wisconsin

Brooke-Mai Whelan, PhD
Research Fellow
Department of Speech Pathology
School of Health and Rehabilitation
    Sciences
University of Queensland
Brisbane, Queensland, Australia

Tara L. Whitehill, PhD, CCC-SLP
Professor
Division of Speech and Hearing Sciences
University of Hong Kong
Hong Kong, China

Gail Woodyatt, PhD
Senior Lecturer
Division of Speech Pathology
School of Health and Rehabilitation
    Sciences
University of Queensland
Brisbane, Queensland, Australia

David J. Zajac, PhD
Associate Professor
Department of Dental Ecology
School of Dentistry
University of North Carolina
Chapel Hill, North Carolina

Saša A. Živković, MD
Assistant Professor of Neurology
Department of Neurology
University of Pittsburgh School
    of Medicine
Pittsburgh, Pennsylvania

Richard I. Zraick, PhD, CCC-SLP
Associate Professor
Department of Audiology and
    Speech Pathology
University of Arkansas–Little Rock
University of Arkansas for Medical
    Sciences
Little Rock, Arkansas

Part I

Primary Topics

Chapter 1

A Theoretical Framework for the Characterization of Pathological Speech Sensorimotor Control

Anita van der Merwe

The need to work from a sound theoretical framework based on the normal process of speech and language production for both research and management of communication disorders has long been proclaimed by speech-language pathologists (Ballard, 2001; Kent & McNeil, 1987; McNeil & Kent, 1990). The almost overwhelming corpus of ever-increasing data on the intricate details of the speech production process and the neurophysiology of motor control and unresolved issues concerning the nature of neurogenic speech disorders (Kent, Duffy, Slama, Kent, & Clift, 2001; McNeil & Kent, 1990) underscore the necessity of a comprehensive explanatory framework. Phenomenological models have great explanatory power (Scully & Guerin, 1991), and the practicing clinician can use a coherent model to put diagnosis, differential diagnosis, and management on a sound theoretical basis.

A functional model applicable to neurogenic speech disorders should explain the speech production process as a fine sensorimotor skill (Netsell, 1982). Such a model should also be in line with current concepts, developments, and terminology in neuroscience. The neural basis of sensorimotor control is "a field in a wild flux of rapid evolution" (Brooks, 1986, p. ix), and the ever-expanding theoretical framework based on animal movement studies, in particular, should be explored to enhance as far as possible our own insight into speech movements and movement disorders. Direct access to the human brain (which can produce speech) is for obvious reasons not possible. To draw from this knowledge base, an important prerequisite, however, would be correspondence in terminology. Clinical intervention and interdisciplinary teamwork can only benefit as an additional advantage.

The theoretical framework proposed here portrays the transformation of the speech code from one form to another as seen from a brain-behavior perspective. This framework poses a novel view of the phases involved during the transformation, and stresses the importance of the sensorimotor interface. This proposal represents a paradigm shift from the traditional three-level speech production model (Itoh & Sasanuma, 1984) consisting of linguistic encoding, programming, and execution to one of four levels based on current neurophysiological data on sensorimotor control. McNeil and Kent (1990) state that assumptions underlying neurogenic pathological populations need to be seriously reconsidered and that particular attention should be given to the motoric aspects of speech production. The

proposed four-level framework could be a step toward this goal. Before the different phases or levels of the proposed framework are fully explained, it is necessary to justify the entries and to delineate the theoretical context within which it functions.

◆ Background

Speech is the externalized expression of language, and speech sensorimotor control can be defined as "the motor-afferent mechanisms that direct and regulate speech movements" (Netsell, 1982, p. 247). As a motor skill, speech is "goal-directed" and "afferent-guided"; it "meets the general requirements of a fine motor skill, it (1) is performed with accuracy and speed, (2) uses knowledge of results, (3) is improved by practice, (4) demonstrates motor flexibility in achieving goals and (5) relegates all of this to automatic control, where 'consciousness' is freed from the details of action plans" (Netsell, 1982, p. 250).

To appreciate the complexity of the speech production process, one only has to study the summary charts of events in respiration, voicing, and articulation during production of a short sentence, as summarized by Borden, Harris, and Raphael (2003). All of these motor events have to be coordinated and produced in such a way that the desired acoustic result is achieved. This process seems to occur in phases of processing.

Phases in the Transformation of the Speech Code

During the production of speech, the intended message has to be changed from an abstract idea to meaningful language symbols and then to a code amenable to a motor system. There is, in other words, a gradual appearance of new formations out of preexisting ones. The evolutionary change renders the code compatible with every level of processing. The phases involved in this process, however, remain problematic and debatable.

Most neurophysiologists recognize that the overall motor control process involves several phases or hierarchical levels of organization (Jakobson & Goodale, 1991; Lacquaniti, 1989; Nolte 1999). The phases are identified as planning, programming, and execution (Brooks, 1986; Marsden, 1984;

Rose, 1997; Schmidt, 1978). The control of movements is exerted through a command (or sensorimotor) hierarchy that can be portrayed as highest, middle, and lowest levels. The highest level is mediated by the association cortex (e.g., prefrontal, parietal, and temporal lobes), that generates overall invariant motor plans. Motor plans are converted into motor programs at the middle level, which consists of the sensorimotor cortex, the cerebellum, and the putamen loop of the basal ganglia. At this level the specific parameters of the movement (e.g., velocity) are defined. At the lowest level programs are translated into muscular activity and motor execution occurs (Brooks, 1986; Lacquaniti, 1989; Marsden, 1984; Nolte, 1999; Schmidt, 1978).

In the literature on speech production, the deduction is usually made that the stage of motor planning referred to by neurophysiologists is equivalent to linguistic-symbolic planning. For example, Darley, Aronson, and Brown (1975) suggest that the phase of spatial-temporal planning of movement corresponds to syntactic planning during speech production. More often, however, the motor planning stage is equated to phonological planning during speech production. The true nature of motor planning of speech movements is therefore not adequately contemplated and not differentiated from phonological planning.

The inadequate formulation of the process of speech motor planning is perhaps partially due to the impact of linguistic terminology within which the speech pathologist traditionally functions. Phonology as a linguistic term includes both the phonological and phonetic components (also referred to as covert and overt speech [Edwards & Shriberg, 1983]), and, based on this premise, phonetic or motor planning of speech is assumed to be a linguistic function. It is true that speech needs to be "viewed within the superordinate behavior of language" (McNeil & Kent, 1990, p. 352), but it is also imperative to view speech as a sensorimotor function of the human brain. A motor plan (not an abstract linguistic choice of a phoneme to be uttered) is necessary to guide speech movements. Motor planning of speech is a discernible process aimed at defining motor goals. In the formulation of a comprehensive theory on motor planning of speech, certain well-known speech phenomena may prove to be central. Data on the invariant and variant aspects of the spatial and temporal features of speech movements are particularly important, as will be explained later in the text.

An important consequence of the deduction that motor planning is a linguistic process and can be referred to as phonological planning is that the terms *motor planning* and *programming* are used interchangeably as if they constitute more or less the same process. A consequence of this line of reasoning is that programming is regarded as the highest level of motor control of speech. From a neurophysiological viewpoint, however, motor planning and programming should be differentiated. During the planning stage general decisions are made, which in the case of speech will probably be guided by phonologically based specifications such as manner and place of articulation. The details of the planned sequence of movements are fitted in later during the programming phase according to the circumstances of the moment (Brooks, 1986; Magill 2001; Rose 1997).

Inadequate differentiation of planning and programming results in the traditional three-level model described earlier.

The proposed theoretical framework postulates that linguistic-symbolic planning should be differentiated from phases in sensorimotor control and that sensorimotor control of speech movements comprises planning, programming, and execution phases. A clear differentiation among these processes or phases is necessary to comprehensively define the different sensorimotor speech disorders. A formulation of these four phases also provides a theoretical framework for intervention and research in the field of neurogenic speech disorders.

Speech as Sensorimotor Skill

"Sensorimotor integration is the key to motor control" (Brooks, 1986, p. 39). Most researchers today agree that sensory information or input is an integral part of movement control and coordination (Abbs & Connor, 1991; Brooks, 1986; Evarts, 1982; Gentil, 1990; Kawato & Gomi, 1992; Kent, 1990; Tatton & Bruce, 1981). Early concepts postulated that movements were controlled by peripheral reafferent sensory input. Later research determined that movements could still be performed following deafferentation. This finding suggested central programming of movements. Research aimed at determining how central nerve cells generate so-called motor programs was then initiated. Two schools of motor control originated. The one emphasizes the importance of the central program and views afferent input as relatively unimportant (open-loop control), whereas the other school takes the position that afferent input is of great significance and that movements are under continuous control by feedback (closed-loop control; Evarts, 1982). For many years experiments addressed "a null hypothesis and attempts were made to provide a general either-or solution" (Abbs & Cole, 1982, p. 160). Today a more pragmatic approach is followed, and research is geared at defining the interaction and relative role of both feedback and feedforward control.

Auditory, tactile, and proprioceptive feedback arise as consequences of speech production. Proprioception is the most important sense from inside our bodies (as opposed to "exteroceptive" senses). Proprioception is "the sense of what the muscle itself is doing" (Brooks, 1986, p. 11). This direct feedback from the muscles is faster than exteroceptive feedback (tactile and audition) and therefore presumably more involved in the control of speech movements. Sense organs (or mechanoreceptors) in the tendons signal how hard the muscles are pulling, and sense organs within the muscles, namely muscle spindles, signal how much and how fast the muscles are being stretched (Brooks, 1986). Striated muscles contract at will and muscle spindles are embedded in most striated muscles. Speech muscles are striated muscles, but not all have muscle spindles. Muscle spindles arranged in parallel with the extrafusal muscle fibers provide information about the length of the muscle and contribute to the stretch (myotatic) reflex. The stretch reflex can function as a servomechanism regulating muscle length (Gentil, 1990). Segmental and transcortical (via pyramidal tract neurons) proprioceptive reflexes exist. The major role of both is in small active movements and in active postural stability (Evarts & Fromm, 1981).

Golgi tendon organs, arranged in series with the extrafusal muscle fibers, inform the nervous system of the tension exerted by the muscle on its tendinous insertion to the bone (Gentil, 1990). Mechanoreceptors are present in the lips, the oral mucosa, the jaw muscles, the periodontium, the temporomandibular joint, the larynx, and the respiratory apparatus (Landgren & Olsson, 1982). Distribution of different receptors in different structures, however, varies. Muscle spindles have been found in the lingual and laryngeal muscles. Concerning the jaw, the deep parts of the temporal and masseter muscles contain a high number of muscle spindles. Few spindles are observed in the lateral pterygoid muscle and only occasional ones in the anterior belly of digastric. There are no muscle spindles or Golgi tendon organs in facial muscles, including the lip muscles. Tendon organs are present in the jaw system (Gentil, 1990; Persson, 1982).

McClean (1991) reported that respiratory airways are supplied with mechanoreceptors capable of signaling pressure changes. He found that changes in oral pressure produced reflex responses in lip muscles, and he concluded that mechanoreceptor responses to intraoral pressure changes are involved in sensorimotor integration for speech production. (For further reading, refer to Kent, 1990, who provides a summary of qualities, receptors, and nerve innervation of oral sensation. Also see Bowman, 1968; Bowman and Combs, 1969a,b; and Sussman, 1972.)

In addition to information fed back from the periphery, the nervous system can handle information relayed from motor to sensory areas. Reciprocal connections between sensory and motor areas of the cerebral cortex substantiate the possibility of so-called internal feedback. According to Kelso and Stelmach (1976), two sets of signals, both operating via feedforward mechanisms, are involved. One is a downward discharge to effector organs, and the other is a simultaneous central discharge from motor to sensory systems that presets the sensory area for the anticipated consequences of the motor act. The neural response in the sensory system before the arrival of response-produced feedback is referred to by Kelso and Stelmach (1976) as corollary discharge. This neural response is the result of an efference (reference) copy that tells the appropriate areas of the brain what to expect. The accuracy of the efferent command can thus be compared centrally with an internal model before the arrival of peripheral feedback. Apparently all levels of the nervous system can handle internally fed back information (Brooks, 1986; Evarts, 1971, 1982; Evarts & Fromm, 1981). Internal predictive models of the motor apparatus are developed during motor learning (Kawato & Gomi, 1992). One important function of these efference copies (re-efference) would be to detect and correct errors before movement commences.

Many studies have been conducted to determine the role of afferent feedback in speech production. The publication of the closed-loop speech production model of Fairbanks gave rise to studies on the effect of disturbed tactile feedback (Ringel, Burk, & Scott, 1968; Ringel & Ewanowski, 1965; Ringel & Steer, 1963) and proprioceptive feedback (Abbs, 1973; Goodwin & Luschei, 1974). The fact that speech was slightly impaired by such interference was interpreted as an indication of closed-loop control. Later it was found that the methods used in the tactile studies caused motor interference, too (Abbs, Folkins, & Sivarajan, 1976; Folkins & Abbs, 1977). The insubstantial effect of tactile and proprioceptive interference was also interpreted as an indication of open-loop control (Borden, 1979; Folkins & Abbs, 1975; Putnam & Ringel, 1976).

In another line of experimentation designed to evaluate sensory information on speech production, the mandible is fixed by placing a bite block between the teeth (Folkins & Zimmerman, 1981; Lindblom, Lubker, & Gay, 1979). Formant patterns typical for the speaker are obtained even at the first glottal pulse before response feedback has occurred, indicating the operation of central feedback or predictive simulation.

More recent research on the role of sensory feedback in articulatory movements has been performed by Gracco and Abbs (1986, 1988, 1989). Unanticipated perturbation of the movements of an articulator was studied. Significant magnitude compensations from the muscles and movements of the upper lip, lower lip, and jaw were observed. According to Gracco and Abbs (1987), these data suggest that sensory information is used not only to correct errors in individual movements, but also to make adjustments among the multiple movements involved in a given speech gesture.

Today it is generally accepted that sensorimotor interaction is integral to movement control and that the brain uses feedforward and feedback information in a plastic and generative manner depending on task demands or context of motor performance. Studies of the activity of single cells in cerebral motor cortex of the monkey have shown that closed-loop control of a particular neuron can rapidly change to open-loop control (Evarts, 1982).

Different modes of interaction between centrally generated motor programs and sensory feedback may exist (Tatton & Bruce, 1981). During motor learning the control mode is presumably predominantly based on feedback control, which aids in optimizing accuracy. After that, feedback may only be vital when the brain's predictive model is changed by extraordinary circumstances (Finocchio & Luschei, 1988; Grillner, 1982; Kelso & Stelmach, 1976). Sensory feedback is continually present, but the option of ignoring it seems to exist (Brooks, 1986).

During the time course of movement, progress, it seems, is assessed by an integration of peripheral sensory signals and corollary discharge. During the production of speech, auditory feedback together with tactile and proprioceptive feedback might also be utilized for this purpose. Auditory feedback can provide information about completion of speech movements and might therefore play a role in speech timing. Auditory feedback can also monitor accuracy of articulation on a long-term basis. It cannot serve to monitor ongoing skilled articulation as the information provided to the speaker arrives too late for on-line speech motor control.

In the proposed framework, the presence of different feedback circuits is indicated. Feedback and feedforward information is probably utilized at multiple levels of processing.

The exact nature of sensorimotor interface during all of these phases is not yet known, but it is evident that sensory information is an integral part of speech motor control.

Contextual Sensitivity of Speech Sensorimotor Control

The proposed framework depicts speech production as being context-sensitive. It is hypothesized that contextual factors affect the dynamics of sensorimotor control by exerting an influence on (1) the mode of coalition of neural structures involved during a particular phase; (2) the skill required from the planning, programming, and execution mechanisms; and (3) the processing and attentional resources. Certain variants of a specific contextual factor may require more complex control strategies than others. Differences in the level of activity of certain neural structures during different motor tasks (e.g., self-initiated vs. stimulus-induced) (Alexander and Crutcher, 1990a,b; Crutcher & Alexander, 1990; Jahanshahi, Jenkins, Brown, Marsden, Passingham, & Brooks, 1995; Lang, Beisteiner, Lindinger, & Deecke, 1992; Mushiake, Inase, & Tanji, 1990; Romo, Scarnati, & Schultz, 1992; Romo & Schultz, 1992; Schultz & Romo, 1992) substantiate this viewpoint. It also seems that precise fine or unfamiliar movements versus ballistic or well-learned movements require greater implementation of sensory input and thus greater involvement of sensory areas that again influence the coalition of neural areas (Evarts, 1982; Evarts & Fromm, 1977; Kelso & Stelmach, 1976). Different contextual factors may place different processing demands (McNeil, Odell, & Tseng, 1991) on the control system. These factors may operate along a continuum rendering some speech tasks easier and others more difficult to control and produce (Theron, 2003; Van der Merwe, 2002).

The contextual factors identified in the proposed framework are hypothetical and may be incomplete. A review of the literature indicates that degree of automaticity (voluntary as opposed to automatized speech) (Klein, 1976; Luria, 1966; Oberg & Divac, 1981; Van der Merwe, 2002), initiation mode (imitated as opposed to self-initiated) (Van der Merwe, 2002), sound or syllable structure (Van der Merwe, Uys, Loots, & Grimbeek, 1987, 1988), motor complexity of the utterance (Tasko & McClean, 2004), length of the utterance (Klapp, Anderson, & Berrian, 1973; Tasko & McClean, 2004), familiar versus unfamiliar utterances such as first and second language words and sentences (Kim & Corlew, 1979; Sharkey & Folkins, 1985; Theron, 2003), rate of speech (Gay, 1981; Kelso, Tuller, & Harris, 1983; MacNeilage, 1980; Shaiman, 2002), and linguistic complexity (Strand & McNeil, 1996; Tasko & McClean, 2004) may be factors that influence the process of speech sensorimotor control. Research has already indicated that variation of such factors may cause variation in the features of apraxia of speech, stuttering, and at least some types of dysarthria (Aichert & Ziegler, 2004; Kempler & Van Lancker, 2002; Kleinow & Smith, 2000; Maner, Smith, & Grayson, 2000; Strand & McNeil, 1996; Theron 2003; Van der Merwe & Grimbeek, 1990; Van der Merwe et al, 1987, 1988; Van der Merwe, Uys, Loots, Grimbeek, & Jansen, 1989). The role of contextual factors in the different phases of the speech act will have to be determined by research. Contextual factors may influence

progress in treatment and also research results. The context-sensitivity of speech features may hold the key to a better understanding of the nature of different neurogenic speech disorders as the effects of contextual changes may reveal the underlying pathogenesis.

♦ The Proposed Framework of Speech Sensorimotor Control

The proposed four-level framework of speech sensorimotor control is depicted in **Fig. 1–1**. The hypothetical processes that occur during the different phases of the transformation of the speech code together with the different neural structures that are involved during a specific phase are indicated in the model.

The different phases are identified as linguistic-symbolic planning, which is a nonmotor (or premotor) process; motor planning; motor programming; and execution. The differentiation of the three motor levels is in accord with the motor hierarchy as accepted by most neurophysiologists (Allen & Tsukahara, 1974; Brooks, 1986; Marsden, 1984; Rose 1997; Schmidt, 1978). The concept of division of the events underlying the production of speech into phases may be somewhat simplistic, but it is useful in discussing brain behavior during speech production and in localizing levels of dysfunction. The serial analytic model is implicit in many contemporary theories of motor control (Alexander & Crutcher, 1990a). It would be wrong to assume multilevel processing as strictly hierarchical and thereby implying one-way information flow. It will be noticed in the framework that information flows in both directions and in loops, indicating sensorimotor interaction.

The different neural structures involved in each phase of speech production operate by forming coalitions. They are listed in the framework, as the exact function of each structure in relation to every other structure during different movements is highly complex and not yet fully known. Research in this field is abundant and often contradictory due to differences in the criteria for inclusion of subjects, differences in experimental techniques, and the nature of the movements studied. Indication of which neural structures are involved during a specific phase, however, is as essential for the speech pathologist charged with managing neurogenic communication disorders as it is for the speech researcher. This knowledge enhances our understanding of the level and nature of the breakdown.

Intention in Verbal Communication

Intention or readiness to commence intentional behavior is regulated by frontal-limbic formations of the forebrain (Devinsky, Morrell, & Vogt, 1995; Kornhuber, 1977; Lamendella, 1977; Mogenson, Jones, & Yim, 1980; Nolte, 1999; Pribram, 1976). The most basic function of the limbic system is to govern biological drives, but it also generates emotional motivation to act. Limbic drives are transformed into motor goals or general plans through corticocortical processing in the higher association cortex. Brooks (1986)

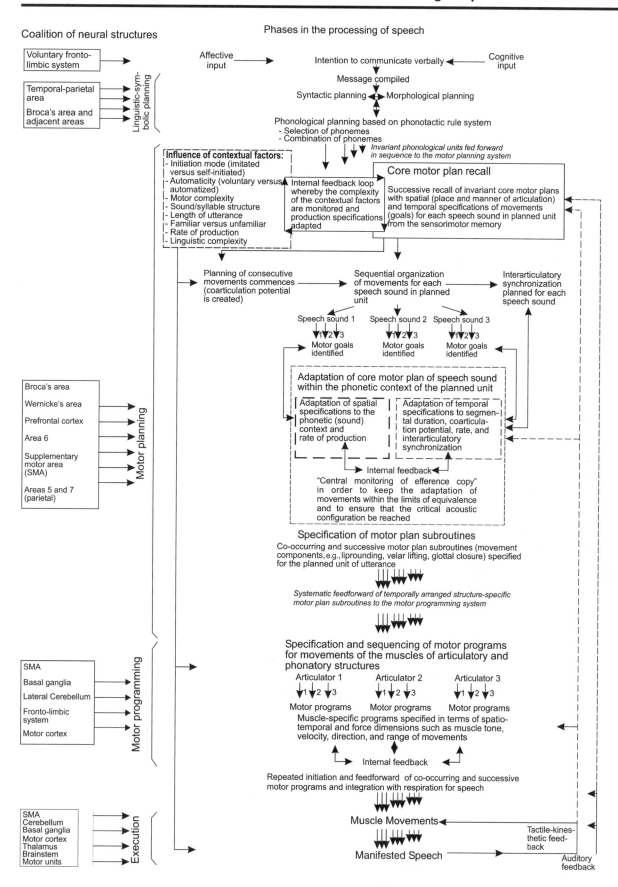

Figure 1–1 Theoretical framework of speech sensorimotor control.

further states that "motivational limbic influences are needed to enact motor plans and to assemble their programs and subprograms" (p. 33).

In a discussion of motor behavior one should differentiate between the general intention to react and the initiation of movements. There is considerable evidence that limbic forebrain structures are important in "drives" and "motivational" processes contributing to the initiation of actions, but little is known about the neural mechanisms by which limbic processes gain access to the motor system. Mogenson et al (1980) provide a tentative model for a limbic–motor interface. They consider the nucleus accumbens to be the functional link between the limbic structures and the basal ganglia. Nauta and Domesick (1984) also state that the limbic afferented striatal sector suggests itself as an interface between the motivational and the more strictly motor aspects of movement. Nolte (1999), in a discussion of basal ganglia circuits, indicate that the ventral striatum connects with the limbic system and thereby plays a role in the initiation of drive-related behavior. There are indications that the supplementary motor area (SMA), too, has a role in the initiation of movement including speech movements (Jonas, 1981; Orgogozo & Larsen, 1979). According to Ploog (1981), this area is functionally connected to the limbic cortex. Both the SMA and basal ganglia are involved in motor programming (see later discussion). It is proposed, therefore, that the frontolimbic system is involved not only in the initial intention to communicate but also in motor programming and most probably with regard to repeated initiation or feedforward of motor programs for different muscles of the speech apparatus.

In the proposed framework the initial intention to communicate verbally closely links with affective input as the needs and motivation of the speaker influence the drive to communicate. Therefore, there has to be limbic support of sensorimotor processing. Motivation of clients can be of great assistance in motor training and is a clinically important factor to keep in mind (Magill, 2001).

Linguistic-Symbolic Planning

During verbal communication, semantic, syntactic, lexical, morphological, and phonological planning have to take place. This phase in the process of verbal communication requires linguistic-symbolic planning based on knowledge of the linguistic rules of the language. The term *linguistic-symbolic planning* indicates the nonmotor nature of this level of processing.

The intention to communicate verbally originates in the internal biological or cognitive needs of the person or in the external demands exerted by the environment. A message is compiled that reflects both the internal and external sources of input. The interaction between these areas is indicated by double arrows in the framework.

Research indicates that planning of the complete utterance occurs simultaneously and not word for word (Holmes, 1984). Semantic construction of the message, recall and selection of lexical units, and syntactic, morphological, and phonological planning occur in coherence. The phonological plan is invariant, and changes therein influence the

meaning or intelligibility of the utterance. Phonological planning, which is also referred to as the covert aspect of phonology (Edwards & Shriberg, 1983), entails the selection and sequential combination of phonemes in accordance with the phonotactic rules of the language, and it is portrayed as a linguistic-symbolic function in the proposed framework.

With regard to the neural structures responsible for linguistic-symbolic planning, there are indications that the temporal-parietal area, particularly Wernicke's area, and also Broca's area are involved. Negative cerebral event-related potentials and regional cerebral blood flow indicate that activity is most prominent in the precentral and parietal regions while a person prepares to produce speech (Aschoff & Kornhuber, 1975; Fried, Ojemann, & Fetz, 1981; Grozinger, Kornhuber, & Kriebel, 1977; Lassen, Ingvar, & Skinhoj, 1978; Meyer, Sakai, Yamaguchi, Yamamoto, & Shaw, 1980). Grozinger et al (1977) find that with single-word production, the prespeech cerebral potentials are more pronounced over Broca's area than over Wernicke's area. The difference in amplitude between these two areas diminishes when full sentences are produced. In other words, Wernicke's area becomes more active with an increase in semantic content whereas Broca's area remains active during any speech act. These data might indicate that these two areas are coactive during linguistic-symbolic and motor planning, and that their relative roles change depending on the nature of the speech task and the phase of preparation of an utterance.

Motor Planning

During the planning phase of the production of articulated speech (as compared, for instance, with typewritten language), a gradual transformation of symbolic units (phonemes) to a code that can be handled by a motor system has to take place. Motor planning entails formulating the strategy of action by specifying motor goals. In the proposed framework a hypothetical description of speech motor planning is presented.

Planning is mediated by the highest level of the motor hierarchy. It is widely accepted that the so-called association areas are responsible for motor planning (Allen & Tsukahara, 1974; Brooks, 1986; Evarts, 1982; Marsden, 1984; Rose, 1997; Schmidt, 1978). The motor association area, comprising the premotor cortex (lateral area 6) and the supplementary motor area (medial area 6), and the prefrontal and parietal association areas are involved in motor planning (Brooks, 1986; Burbaud, Doegle, Gross, & Bioulac, 1991; Di Pellegrino & Wise, 1991; Knight, Singh, & Woods, 1989; Mushiake et al, 1990; Romo & Schultz, 1992; Romo et al, 1992; Sakai, Ramnani, & Passingham, 2002; Schultz & Romo, 1992). Broca's area can be considered as part of the premotor cortex. The anatomical location of inferior area 6, and in particular of F5 in the monkey, corresponds in large part to that of Broca's area in the human brain (Di Pellegrino, Fadiga, Fogassi, Gallese, & Rizzolatti, 1992). Negative cerebral event-related potentials and regional cerebral blood flow indicate that Broca's area but also other cortical motor association areas such as the premotor cortex (which includes area 6 and the supplementary motor area) and the prefrontal cortex together with the somatosensory cortex (which includes areas 5 and 7) become bilaterally active immediately prior to and during speech production (Darian-Smith, Johnson, & Goodwin, 1979; Lassen et al, 1978; Marteniuk & MacKenzie, 1980; Weinrich, Wise, & Mauritz, 1984). Brooks (1986) believes that the caudate circuit of the basal ganglia is part of the higher hierarchical level in that it enables the high-level plans to be translated into motor action.

The prefrontal area seems to operate at a hierarchically superior level compared with the frontal areas (Di Pellegrino & Wise, 1991) and is necessary for formulating integrated behavior (Brooks, 1986). The association areas project to the premotor cortex and the SMA, which organize the principal output stage of the middle level (Brooks, 1986). The premotor cortex, SMA, and certain parts of the basal ganglia are richly interconnected and probably cooperate in neuronal processing and directing planning (Burbaud et al, 1991; Nolte, 1999; Martin, Phillips, Iansek, & Bradshaw, 1994).

The SMA receives a lot of attention in research. It is somatotopically organized and is not only a motor center controlling movements, but is also implicated in the initiation of movements (Kurata, 1992; Lang, Cheyne, Kristeva, Beisteiner, Undinger, & Deecke, 1991; Luppino, Matelli, & Rizzolatti, 1990; Nolte, 1999). Lang et al (1992) have observed a *bereitschaftpotential*, which starts 2.5 seconds prior to movement onset. Prior to single movements a shorter latency, of 1.2 seconds, was observed. There are indications that the SMA is involved in both motor planning and the initiation of speech movements (Jonas, 1981; Lassen et al, 1978).

However, it is not only motor areas that become active prior to movement but also the parietal association cortex (Burbaud et al, 1991; Knight et al, 1989). The exact role of the posterior parietal areas in the planning of movement is not absolutely clear. Anatomical data point to extensive connections with the frontal cortex, the cingulate gyrus, and the different motor areas (Brooks, 1986; Darian-Smith et al, 1979; Evarts, 1982). A possible explanation is that information from the sensory memory store is implemented during planning and that these areas are involved in internal feedback.

Posterior parietal areas, together with temporal areas and in particular Wernicke's, may play a similar role in speech production. Broca's and Wernicke's areas are extensively interconnected, and both are linked to other motor areas, with Broca's area more extensively so (Darian-Smith et al, 1979; Kornhuber, 1977; Ploog, 1981). The extensive connections between cortical motor and sensory areas suggest that the planning phase requires a complex coalition between these neural structures and thus between motor and sensory information. The involvement of temporal areas might imply that linguistic or covert phonological knowledge and rules are implemented during the initial phases of motor planning of speech. The participation of both Broca's and Wernicke's areas during motor and linguistic-symbolic planning would suggest that gradual transformation of the code occurs.

In the proposed framework it is indicated that Broca's and Wernicke's areas are active during the planning phase together with the prefrontal cortex, area 6, the SMA, and the parietal association areas 5 and 7. These areas are fed with a sequence of invariant phonological units from which motor plans have to be derived.

Motor planning is goal oriented, and motor goals for speech production can be found in the spatial and temporal specifications of movements for sound production. A target-based model was first proposed by MacNeilage (1970). Underlying this approach is the assumption that the speech sound within the context of the utterance is the unit of planning.

The sounds or phonemes in every language can be described in terms of place and manner of articulation. Each sound has its own specifications, and these core features can be considered as invariant (Stevens & Blumstein, 1981). The core features determine the invariant core motor plan with spatial (place and manner of articulation) and temporal specifications for each sound. The specifications of movements constitute the motor goals. Invariance, therefore, can be found in the ultimate goals of production.

The core motor plan is attained during the development of speech, and the motor specifications and sensory model (what it feels and sounds like) are stored in the sensorimotor memory. While mastering the core motor plan, proprioceptive, tactile, and auditory feedback is implemented. This feedback loop is indicated in the model.

During the production of speech, the core motor plans of the sequence of phonological units or speech sounds are recalled from the sensorimotor memory. The context within which this motor plan has to be implemented is monitored and sometimes adapted if the complexity is found to be too high. Examples of such adaptation can be found in the phenomena of shorter chunks of utterances that are produced as units (e.g., syllabic speech), phonological changes like shortening a word, or slowed rate of speech. Such compensatory strategies are observed in sensorimotor speech disorders (Kent & Rosenbek, 1983; Van der Merwe & Grimbeek, 1990; Van der Merwe et al, 1987, 1988, 1989). The normal speaker will also decrease the rate when an unfamiliar and long word is to be produced.

Following recall of the core motor plan, planning of the consecutive movements necessary to fulfill the spatial and temporal goals commences. The different motor goals for each speech sound are to be identified, and the movements that are necessary to produce the different sounds in the planned unit are then sequentially organized. It is important to point out that motor planning is articulator-specific and not muscle-specific. Motor goals such as lip rounding, jaw depression, glottal closure, or lifting of the tongue tip need to be specified. Interarticulatory synchronization is to be planned for the production of a particular speech sound.

At this stage the potential for coarticulation is created. When the different motor goals for the sounds in the planned unit, which presumably consists of a few words in the normal speaker, are specified, a certain movement such as lip rounding can be temporally prepositioned if there is no other opposing movement prior to it.

An invariant core motor plan is recalled from the sensorimotor memory and the motor goals specified, but in the realization of speech we know that "speech violates what can be called the linearity and invariance conditions" (Wanner, Teyler, & Thompson, 1977, p. 6). On the articulatory level speech movements are variant and context-dependent, and the boundaries between discrete phonological units fade away (Kent & Minifie, 1977; MacNeilage, 1980; MacNeilage & De Clerk, 1969).

Variance manifested in the spatial and temporal aspects of speech movements originates from various sources. Adaptation of articulatory movements to the sound environment, coarticulation of more than one articulator but for different speech sounds (Borden et al, 2003; Kent & Minifie, 1977), motor equivalence of speech targets with variations in the individual components (Abbs, 1986; Hughes & Abbs, 1976; Sharkey & Folkins, 1985), phonetic and linguistic influences on segmental duration (Mitleb, 1984; Nishinuma, 1984), and changes in speech rate (Gay, 1981; Kelso et al, 1983) are all factors that contribute to variance in speech production.

The core motor plan of the speech sound therefore has to be adapted to the context of the planned unit. Adaptation of spatial specifications to the phonetic (sound) context and to the rate of production has to occur. Adaptation of temporal specifications to segmental duration, coarticulation potential, and interarticulatory synchronization also takes place. The double arrows in the framework indicate that motor goals are identified in accordance with an adapted motor plan, and a kind of parallel processing (Percheron & Filion, 1991) probably takes place. The same applies to interarticulatory synchronization. Temporal adaptation of the core plan might have implications for the synchronization of movements for a specific sound.

The adaptation of movements, however, has to be kept within certain limits of equivalence to ensure that the critical acoustic configuration is reached. The spatial and temporal differences between certain sounds are in many cases absolutely minimal, and if these boundaries or limits are violated, the sound will be perceived as being distorted or even substituted by another sound.

Adaptation of the core motor plan has to take place before articulation of a specific speech sound is initiated, as adaptation determines the innervation of specific structures at particular points in time. Adaptation cannot be guided by response feedback, as the movement has not yet taken place at the moment of planning. It is, however, conceivable that internal feedback (Evarts & Fromm, 1981; Kelso, 1982; Teuber, 1974) or predictive simulation (Lindblom et al, 1979) guides adaptation. It is therefore proposed that internal feedback of an efference copy to the sensorimotor cortex is implemented to keep adaptation of the core motor plan within the limits of equivalence. Numerous reciprocal connections between sensorimotor areas could support such a hypothesis (Burbaud et al, 1991; Brooks, 1986; Darian-Smith et al, 1979; Evarts, 1982).

Central monitoring of the efference copy implies that the speaker applies a kind of predictive simulation (Lindblom et al, 1979). Keller (1987, p. 134) refers to "learned relations between specifications for the contraction of individual muscles." During adaptation, knowledge of the results of certain movements therefore is utilized. Kawato and Gomi (1992) refer to an internal predictive model. They localize this model in the cerebellum, but there seems to be no reason why such internal models are not also present in cortical sensorimotor areas. Their concept of an inverse model,

which they define as "a neural representation of the transformation from the desired movements of the controlled object (which can be an articulator) to the motor commands required to attain these movement goals" (p. 446), seems to be an attractive theory for speech sensorimotor control. They contrast this inverse model to the forward model, which is "a neural representation of the transformation from motor commands to the resultant behavior of the controlled object" (p. 445). More sophisticated feedforward control can be achieved through an inverse model of the controlled object (Kawato & Gomi, 1992). An inverse model would require knowledge of results of movements, which seems to be present in the normal adult speaker.

It will be noticed in the proposed framework that peripheral tactile-kinesthetic feedback is available during the adaptation stage of motor planning. Under extraordinary conditions such as bite-block (Folkins & Zimmerman, 1981) or weight-perturbation (Gracco & Abbs, 1989) intervention, peripheral sensory feedback might be used to adapt movements. To a certain extent this process would be in accord with the notion of autogenic (or corrective) control proposed by Gracco and Abbs (1987).

Following the identification of motor goals in accordance with the necessary adaptations to the core plan, the different subroutines that constitute the motor plan are specified. Co-occurring and successive subroutines such as lip rounding and velar lifting are specified and temporally organized. Systematic feedforward of temporally arranged structure-specific motor plan subroutines to the motor programming system then occurs.

Motor Programming

The intricacies of the programming of movement are being researched in abundance, but a comprehensive description of what programming entails is lacking (Carpenter & Jayaraman, 1987; King, 1987; Strata, 1989). The term *motor programming* originated from the centralist view of motor control that proclaims the existence of a feedforward mechanism. In 1968, Keele defined the motor program as a "set of muscle commands that are structured before a movement sequence begins, and that follows the entire sequence to be carried out uninfluenced by peripheral feedback" (MacKay, 1980, p. 98).

Many years of debate concerning the content of the program followed (Keele, 1982; Kelso, 1982; MacKay, 1980; Schmidt, 1976). Substantial evidence related to the minimal effect of unexpected perturbations and the negative effect of deafferentation on skilled movements stressed the functional importance of sensory updating and the need for a redefinition of the motor program (Brooks, 1986; Evarts, 1982; Kelso, 1982). The suggested redefinition of Marsden (1984) seems to capture the essential elements: "The motor program is a set of muscle commands that are structured before a movement sequence begins which can be delivered without reference to external feedback" (p. 228). The implication seems to be that sensory feedback can be utilized to change or update a program should the need arise. Gracco and Abbs (1987, p. 175) state that in their view, "the motor program is an algorithm which sets up the system for a process whereby on-line sensory input and general motor command pre-specifications are 'mixed' dynamically to yield appropriate intended goals."

Both these definitions reflect the generative and plastic nature of motor control in general. According to Gracco and Abbs (1987), who studied speech motor programming in particular, the ability to modify speech movements throughout the motor act indicates that movement control is a "real-time continuous process" and is sensitive to inputs during both preexecution and movement times. Interface between preplanned motor programs and real-time updating based on sensory input, therefore, seems to be intrinsic to the motor programming of movement, including speech movements.

Another major reason for the uncertainty that generally surrounds the nature of the motor program seems to be inadequate differentiation between motor plans and motor programs. To indicate central planning, terms such as *preprogramming* (Allen & Tsukahara, 1974), *central programs* (Evarts, 1982), and *generalized motor programs* (Schmidt & Lee, 1999) are used. Some researchers, however, do draw the distinction between motor plans mediated by cortical association areas and motor programs prepared by the middle level of the motor hierarchy (Brooks, 1986; Marsden, 1984; Rose, 1997; Wing & Miller, 1984). Speech motor planning is possibly mediated primarily in the dominant hemisphere (where Broca's and Wernicke's areas are), whereas programming is probably controlled in both hemispheres.

Brooks (1986) also uses the terms *strategy* and *tactics* to explain the plan-program relationship: "Strategies prescribe the general nature of plans and tactics give them particular specifications in space and time" (p. 26). At the middle level of the motor hierarchy, strategy is converted into motor programs or tactics. Programs specify muscle tone, movement direction, velocity, force, range, as well as mechanical stiffness of the joints (Brooks, 1986; Miall, Weir, & Stein, 1987; Rose, 1997; Schultz & Romo, 1992), according to the requirements of the planned movement as it changes over time (Brooks, 1986). The timing and amount of muscle contraction in agonists, antagonists, synergists, and postural fixators need to be specified prior to movement onset (Marsden, 1984). The plan-program relationship can be explained with an example. When reaching out for an object, the plan would be to reach out the arm, to open the hand, close the hand around the object, and then to take the arm to the required position. Programming would determine the spatiotemporal and force dimensions such as the amount of muscle tension needed, the velocity, the direction, and the range. Both planning and programming requires decisions based on the circumstances. By inference, uncertainty in the planning of a movement may impact on the accuracy of motor programming.

The quest for a better understanding of the process of programming has recently primarily sought a comprehensive formulation of the role of the different neural structures involved in the middle level (or programming phase) of motor processing. The neural areas involved in motor programming are indicated in the proposed framework and comprise the basal ganglia, the lateral cerebellum, the SMA, the motor cortex, and the frontolimbic system. It is generally accepted that the basal ganglia (Evarts & Wise, 1984;

Johnson, Vernon, Almeida, Grantier, & Jog, 2003; Marsden, 1980, 1984; McGeer & McGeer, 1987) and the lateral cerebellum (Allen & Tsukahara, 1974; Eccles, 1977; Houk & Gibson, 1987; Mano, Kanazawa, & Yamamoto, 1989; Miall et al, 1987) in particular are involved in programming, and that these parts perform complementary functions (Dreher & Grafman, 2002). The exact role of each, however, is not yet fully known.

The basal ganglia consist of three subcortical forebrain systems that are connected to the sensorimotor system and the limbic system. According to Brooks (1986), there are at least three circuits through the basal ganglia: the caudate circuit is linked to the higher level of the motor hierarchy, and the putamen circuit is linked to the middle level. The loop through the higher level is thought to control the assembly of overall motor plans, while the loop through the middle level is thought to update programs. Schultz and Romo (1992), however, have found that both the caudate and putamen circuits appear to be involved in "setting and maintaining central preparatory states related to the internal generation of individual behavioral acts" (p. 363). A third circuit through the ventral basal ganglia contains the ventral striatum, which has limbic innervations. The ventral basal ganglia contribute to the conversion of need-directed intentions into specific, goal-directed motor acts (Brooks, 1986; Nolte, 1999).

According to Marsden (1984), the negative signs of Parkinson's disease give the greatest clue to the normal function of the basal ganglia. Parkinson's disease causes delayed initiation, slowed execution, abnormal sequential complex movements, and an inability to automatically execute learned motor plans. The overall form of motor programs is preserved. However, the details of the number and frequency of motor neurons activated, at least in the first agonist burst, are inaccurate. There is a problem in switching from one program to another and also in procedural motor learning (Bloxham, Mindel, & Frith, 1984; Brooks, 1986; Johnson et al, 2003; Krebs, Hogan, Hening, Adamovich, & Poizner, 2001; Marsden, 1984; Van den Bercken & Cools, 1982; Wing & Miller, 1984). Dysarthria due to Parkinson's disease also indicates that the basal ganglia may have a role to play in initiation, temporal synchronization, timing, and automized production of speech (Kim & Corlew, 1979; Leanderson, Meyerson, & Persson, 1972; Leanderson, Persson, & Ohman, 1970; Nakano, Zubick, & Tyler, 1973).

The SMA acts with the basal ganglia as part of an integrated system involved in the preparation of complex movements (Evarts & Wise, 1984; Gaymard, Pierrot-Deseilligny, & Rivaud, 1990; Martin et al, 1994; Nolte, 1999; Romo & Schultz, 1992) in relation to conscious intention (Brooks, 1986). The SMA relays information to the basal ganglia via the association areas of the cortex (Brooks, 1986; Evarts & Wise, 1984; McGeer & McGeer, 1987), and the basal ganglia (globus pallidus and putamen) also send information back to the SMA (Brooks, 1986; Evarts & Wise, 1984; Mushiake et al, 1990; Romo & Schultz, 1992; Schultz & Romo, 1992) via the thalamus (Evarts & Wise, 1984). The exact role of the SMA at this middle level of motor processing is not known. However, both basal ganglia and SMA damage appears to cause deficits in spontaneously emitted motor acts and both are therefore implicated in the programming and control of movements (Evarts & Wise, 1984).

Cerebellar contributions lie in the tactical preparation of movements and postures needed for planned motor acts by making up appropriate programs. The lateral part of the cerebellum performs this programming task (Brooks, 1986; Nolte, 1999). The cerebellum provides smoothness to the contraction of synergist and antagonist muscles (Gentil, 1990) by programming muscle length, force, and relations between them and also discharge rate (Houk & Gibson, 1987). Precise timing of movement is a function of the cerebellum (Heck & Sultan, 2002; Mano et al, 1989; Nolte, 1999; Sakai et al, 2002; Salman, 2002). The cerebellum also performs a regulatory role for the middle level of the motor hierarchy (Brooks, 1986). The cerebellum receives input from the periphery, the brainstem, and the cerebral cortex (Brooks, 1986; Gentil, 1990; Nolte, 1999; Rose, 1997). The afferent and efferent connections of these zones form side loops that can function as comparators (Brooks, 1986; Rose 1997). Recent research points toward cognitive roles for the cerebellum. According to Justus and Ivry (2001), the hypothesized cognitive roles "are at least metaphorically related to movement" (p. 276).

Reports about motor commands and their execution reach the cerebellar cortex through parallel fibers. In addition, each microzone receives a small number of climbing fibers that convey information to indicate when the motor action is not being controlled optimally. Internal loops that allow for monitoring of the corollary motor commands permit corrections to begin before movements are initiated (Brooks, 1986; Heck & Sultan, 2002; Katz 2002). The regulatory role of the cerebellum and a remarkable synaptic plasticity in the cerebellar cortex suggest that the cerebellum may play important functional roles in motor learning (Kawato & Gomi, 1992; Nolte, 1999; Sanes, Dimitrov, & Hallett, 1990). However, not only the cerebellum is involved in motor learning (Muller, Kleinhans, Pierce, Kenmotsu, & Courchesne, 2002; Krebs et al, 2001; Nolte, 1999).

Cerebellar dysfunction can result in an inability to execute aimed movements correctly (dysmetria) and the failure to perform quick alternating movements (dysdiadochokinesia) (Glees, 1988; Nolte, 1999). Cerebellar dysfunction decomposes intended movements into sequential constituents and causes errors of direction, force, velocity, and amplitude. Motor programs are thus degraded because predictive control of trajectories is lost (Brooks, 1986; Larson & Sutton, 1978). Ataxic dysarthria is the result of a cerebellar lesion. Abnormalities of range, rate, force, timing, and coordination of speech movements are characteristic of this type of dysarthria (Darley et al, 1975; Joanette & Dudley, 1980; Kent & Netsell, 1975; Kent, Netsell, & Abbs, 1979). Available data suggest that the cerebellum may be involved, though not solely in the programming of spatiotemporal and force dimensions of speech movements.

The cerebellar and basal ganglia loops are separated from each other until they finally pool their influence through indirect paths via the thalamus on output neurons of the primary motor cortex (Brooks, 1986; Iversen, 1981; Marsden, 1984; McGeer & McGeer, 1987; Nolte, 1999; Schmidt, 1978). The motor cortex, however, is not only a motor effector system (Brooks, 1986; Eccles, 1977;

Kornhuber, 1977; Nolte, 1999). It seems that sensory feedback to the motor cortex via at least two corticocortical pathways during ongoing movement provides a mechanism of sensorimotor integration (Porter, 1992). Sensory feedback continuously modulates motor cortex neuron discharge during accurate positioning and precise fine movements, whereas during ballistic movements such modulation is greatly attenuated (Evarts, 1982; Evarts & Fromm, 1977). The motor cortex, therefore, is important for the execution of learned, programmed movements (Brooks, 1986; Nolte 1999).

Motor cortex or upper motor neuron lesions cause spasticity and increased reflexes that can be considered to reflect a disorder on the lowest level of the motor hierarchy. Brooks (1986) reports that loss of corticospinal projection does not paralyze muscles but eliminates their use for skilled movements.

Extrapolating from available data, it appears that the programming of speech movements entails the specification of the muscle-specific programs in terms of spatiotemporal and force dimensions such as muscle tone, velocity, direction, and range of movements and sequencing of motor programs of the muscles of the articulators (including the vocal folds). Repeated initiation and feedforward of co-occurring and successive motor programs have to be controlled, and it is possible that the frontolimbic system, the SMA, and different sources of sensory feedback or input (even auditory feedback) might play a role in this process. Updating of programs based on sensory feedback can occur, and programming is controlled by internal feedback mediated by all the neural structures involved at this stage. This discussion is mainly geared toward movement control of the articulators and the vocal folds, but it is fully realized that the processes of articulation and phonation have to be integrated with breathing patterns for speech. Very little is known about supramedullary control (Von Euler, 1980, 1981) of breathing, but it seems logical that programming or control of inspiratory and expiratory muscles during speech would also be mediated at this level.

Execution

During the execution phase, the hierarchy of plans and programs is finally transformed into nonlearned automatic (reflex) motor adjustments. Successive specifications are relayed to the lower motor centers that control joints and muscles through the "final common path" (Sherrington's famous term). Programs are translated into activity of alpha and gamma motoneurons. Reflexes that are under descending control of the middle level are modulated to meet the circumstances within which the movement occurs. Descending paths carry tactical instructions to the lowest level, where they are coordinated and finally translated into properly timed commands for muscle movements (Brooks, 1986).

The motor cortex is the last supraspinal station for conversion of the designs for movement arising in the association cortex into programs for movement. At the same time, it is the beginning of the chain of structures responsible for the execution of movement. The motor cortex, lower motor neurons, peripheral nerves, and motor units in the muscles are the last neural structures in the hierarchical chain. However, it seems that control during movement is exerted by various structures also active during the premovement phases. Efferents from the cerebellum and basal ganglia pass primarily via the thalamus to the motor cortex, but there are also efferents passing directly to the motor centers of the brainstem, indicating control by these parts at this level (Allen & Tsukahara, 1974; Nolte, 1999; Schmidt, 1978). Movement-related neuronal activity has been observed in the SMA, motor cortex, anterior striatum, and putamen (Crutcher & Alexander, 1990; Luppino et al, 1990; Romo et al, 1992), which underscores the involvement of these areas during execution. Another implication of these observations is that multiple levels of motor processing proceed in parallel within all of these motor structures (Crutcher & Alexander, 1990). The relative role of each of the controlling centers remains unclear. Closed-loop, tactile-kinesthetic feedback as a possible means of control is also available during this phase of motor execution (Eccles, 1977) (see earlier discussion). During the manifestation of speech movements there is also an acoustic result that is fed back to the cortical areas, where it is implemented especially during speech development. This loop is indicated in the framework. The broken lines suggest that the different modes of feedback are available, though it is not necessarily constantly utilized. During speech development or in unfamiliar speech acts, a closed loop indicated by full lines may control execution.

♦ The Characterization of Pathological Speech Sensorimotor Control

The proposed framework has implications for our current understanding of neurogenic speech and language disorders. The four-level framework modifies our traditional view of aphasia, apraxia of speech, and dysarthria as being disruptions on three diverse levels of a three-level model. The level and nature of breakdown in the different neurogenic communication disorders need some reconsideration within the context of this framework.

The differentiation between levels or phases of linguistic-symbolic planning, motor planning, motor programming, and execution would suggest that a distinct disorder (or disorders) on each of these levels is conceivable. A complicating factor, however, is the involvement of some neural structures on several levels of functioning. This would make co-occurring dysfunction in more than one phase of processing possible. There is also the possibility that a disorder in one phase may impact on another. One such example could be that a motor planning disorder may result in inaccurate programming. Thus each specific disorder might exhibit deviances at more than one level of the speech production process. However, before contemplating these possibilities it is necessary to delineate the nature of disruptions on a four-level model.

A dysfunction on the level of linguistic-symbolic planning would result in an inability in semantic, lexical, syntactic, morphological, and phonological planning, which are typical symptoms and signs of aphasia. Deviant phonological planning will lead to disorders in the selection and sequential combination of phonemes, resulting in phoneme substitutions and transpositions, which are characteristic of phonological (literal) paraphasias. Within the context of this framework, errors in phoneme sequencing and true sound substitutions (not distortions perceived as substitutions) would be assigned to a disorder in covert phonological ability.

The framework further proposes the possibility of a disorder in speech motor planning, which would imply that there could be an inability to do the following:

♦ Learn or recall the invariant core motor plans for specific speech sounds

♦ Identify the different motor goals of specific speech sounds

♦ Sequentially organize the movements for each speech sound and a series of movements for a sequence of speech sounds

♦ Adapt the core motor plan to the phonetic environment

♦ Control interarticulatory synchronization

♦ Implement tactile-kinesthetic feedback from the periphery for adaptation (e.g., adaptation to varying starting positions)

♦ Centrally monitor the efference copy

♦ Keep adaptation of movements within the limits of equivalence

♦ Systematically relay the structure-specific motor plan subroutines to the motor programming system

Speech signs and symptoms resulting from disorders in motor planning would be slow, struggling speech with distortion and even apparent substitutions. These are the speech features that are ascribed to apraxia of speech. Distortion that is sometimes called the core sign of apraxia of speech (Itoh & Sasanuma, 1984) can be the result of several of the disorders mentioned above. An inability to consistently make the necessary adaptations in movements, to synchronize the movements of the different articulators, to centrally monitor the parameters of all the necessary movements, and to keep these parameters within the limits of equivalence may result in sound distortion. Motor planning difficulty may impact on motor programming and also cause sound distortion (as a secondary sign). The struggling behavior often observed in apraxic speakers may be the result of an inability to recall the core motor plan for the production of a speech sound or to identify and sequence the various motor goals of a planned unit. Motor planning difficulty may vary according to contextual demands. Utterances that increase motor planning demands may result in more or more severe speech errors. An inability to plan consecutive movements of long, unfamiliar, motorically complex utterances at normal speech rate (or an increased rate) can lead to syllabic planning and slowed temporal flow of speech.

Developmental apraxia of speech may be an inability to learn and control all the parameters of motor planning, whereas acquired apraxia of speech may be an inability to control motor planning of speech. The framework thus not only offers an explanatory premise for apraxic signs and symptoms in both developmental and acquired apraxia of speech but also suggests guidelines for principles of treatment in these cases (Van der Merwe, 2002).

The differentiation of phases as proposed in the framework not only has implications for apraxia of speech but also complicates our traditional view of dysarthria as a motor execution disorder. The role of structures such as the basal ganglia and the lateral cerebellum in both motor programming and execution suggests the possibility of dual symptomatology in certain types of dysarthria. Coexisting disorders in both motor programming and motor execution would seem to be present in parkinsonian (hypokinetic) dysarthria, hyperkinetic dysarthria, ataxic dysarthria (in which dysfunction of the lateral cerebellum occurs), and even spastic dysarthria. Dysarthria due to dysfunction of areas of the cerebellum other than the lateral cerebellum and dysarthria due to lower motor neuron disorders would be the only dysarthrias with a purely execution dysfunction. In these cases muscle tone disorders and involuntary movements hamper accurate execution of movement. The possible masking role of spasticity or low muscle tone will have to be considered when studying dysarthrias in which coexisting programming and execution disorders might be present.

Based on our current conceptualization of the programming of movement, a disorder at this level would result in an impairment of the following:

♦ The programming of muscle tone, velocity, direction, and range of movements

♦ Repeated initiation and feedforward of co-occurring and successive motor programs

Theoretically speaking, such disorders can occur in the absence of muscle tone disorders or involuntary movements, and indeed many classic signs of Parkinson's disease (see earlier discussion) in particular do illustrate the nature of a programming disorder. The important implication for the speech pathologist is that pure programming speech defects do exist. Due to the involvement of different neural structures at this level, diverse programming defects are possible.

The speech signs resulting from a disorder at the programming level would probably be sound distortion, speech rate defects, or disorders in the initiation of movement. At first glance these features seem to be similar to the features characteristic of apraxia of speech, but there might be subtle differences. It is possible that distortion due to a programming disorder will be consistently present during all movements (if the contextual factors are kept consistent). Distortion in apraxic speakers is not consistently present during repeated productions of the same utterance (Itoh & Sasanuma, 1984; Van der Merwe et al, 1989). Clients with acquired apraxia of speech may also lose the core motor plan for specific speech sounds, and they display groping behaviors that do not seem to be signs compatible with a programming disorder. An acquired foreign accent after brain damage may also be an example of a pure speech programming disorder (Schmulian, Van der Merwe, & Groenewald, 1997). The programming errors may lead to distortion that is perceived as a foreign accent. These clients usually display a normal speech rate that differentiates them from apraxic (in difficult contexts) and dysarthric speakers.

Defects in speech rate may result from programming disorders. A disruption on this level may lead either to a slowed rate of production or to an increased rate as is sometimes observed in parkinsonian speakers. The defects in speech rate may be the result of initiation and feedforward disorders. Such primary disorders in speech rate, in contrast with compensatory changes in speech rate (e.g., in reaction to changes in contextual factors), may differentiate disruptions on a planning and programming level.

When contemplating the nature of motor programming speech disorders, we should perhaps also look beyond the traditional neurogenic disorders. A three-level model cannot readily accommodate disorders other than the classic neurogenic pathologies. The four-level model, however, creates an expanded theoretical scope or field of reference. The fact that the limbic system, which is involved in volitional intent and emotional drives, gains access to the motor system via the basal ganglia at this level of the motor hierarchy (see earlier discussion), may prove to be most significant in the understanding of at least some of the speech defects not yet defined as motor programming disorders, such as stuttering, cluttering, and even spasmodic dysphonia. The primary signs of stuttering seem to fit in well with a disorder in programming of speech rate and repeated initiation. Cluttering also exhibits defects in speech rate control and accurate articulation. According to Ploog (1981), the limbic system is directly linked to the vocal folds. The limbic–vocal structures–basal ganglia interface may be central to the precipitation of spasmodic dysphonia and may also play a role in some other programming disorders.

However, these are all merely hypotheses, but they are worth exploring. The theory on motor planning and programming of movement is not yet fully developed. The challenge of future research will be to define the different defects on different levels, to determine the possibility of primary and associated (secondary) defects on each level, and to distinguish between motor planning and programming disorders and also between motor programming and execution disorders (Gericke, 2004; Von Gruenewaldt, 2003). The context-sensitivity of speech features may be a key concept in this regard.

The proposed theoretical framework not only offers explanations for neurogenic disorders but also can be implemented to clarify the nature of some other communication disorders. Articulation disorders and the speech of the hard-of-hearing can be used as examples to illustrate this point. The person with an articulation defect has a core motor plan for the production of that specific sound that differs from the core plan of the other speakers in his or her communication environment. The child born deaf, on the other hand, cannot develop motor plans for the different speech sounds because of the lack of the reinforcing role of auditory feedback in building up sensorimotor memories. The hard-of-hearing child who does learn to speak probably has to build up a sensorimotor memory of the production specifications of the core motor plan based mainly on tactile-kinesthetic feedback. Knowledge of the auditory results of productions and the ability to keep within the limits of equivalence will probably be influenced negatively by the decreased auditory feedback. It is possible to continue speculating in this way, but research should rather address the issues raised by the framework.

◆ Conclusion

We should remind ourselves that a theoretical framework or model is but a simple map to guide us in our quest for a better understanding of the nature of the phenomenon we are dealing with. The proposed framework posits a novel view on the neurogenic sensorimotor speech disorders and generates many new questions to be answered by future research. The ultimate goal, however, is to gain insights that will consequently assist in optimizing clinical assessment and intervention.

References

Abbs, J.H. (1973). The influence of gamma motor system on jaw movements during speech. *Journal of Speech and Hearing Research, 16,* 175–199

Abbs, J.H. (1986). Invariance and variability in speech production: a distinction between linguistic intent and its neuromotor implementation. In: J.S. Perkell & D.H. Klatt (Eds.), *Invariance and Variability in Speech Processes.* Hillsdale, NJ: Lawrence Erlbaum

Abbs, J.H. & Cole, K.J. (1982). Consideration of bulbar and suprabulbar afferent influences upon speech motor coordination and programming. In: S. Grillner, B. Lindblom, J. Lubker, & A. Persson (Eds.), *Speech Motor Control,* vol. 36. Oxford: Pergamon Press

Abbs, J.H. & Connor, N.P. (1991). Motorsensory mechanisms of speech motor timing and coordination. *Journal of Phonetics, 19,* 333–342

Abbs, J.H., Folkins, J.W., & Sivarajan, M. (1976). Motor impairment following blockade of the infraorbital nerve: implications for the use of anesthetization techniques in speech research. *Journal of Speech and Hearing Research, 19,* 19–35

Aichert, I. & Ziegler, W. (2004). Syllable frequency and syllable structure in apraxia of speech. *Brain and Language, 88,* 148–159

Alexander, G.E. & Crutcher, M.D. (1990a). Preparation for movement: neural representations of intended direction in three motor areas of the monkey. *Journal of Neurophysiology, 64,* 133–150

Alexander, G.E. & Crutcher, M.D. (1990b). Neural representations of the target (goal) of visually guided arm movements in three motor areas of the monkey. *Journal of Neurophysiology, 64,* 164–178

Allen, G.I. & Tsukahara, N. (1974). Cerebrocerebellar communication systems. *Physiology Review, 54,* 957–997

Aschoff, J.C. & Kornhuber, H.H. (1975). Functional interpretation of somatic afferents in cerebellum, basal ganglia and motor cortex. In: H.H. Kornhuber (Ed.), *The Somatosensory System.* Stuttgart: Georg Thieme

Ballard, K.J. (2001). Response generalization in apraxia of speech treatments: taking another look. *Journal of Communication Disorders, 34,* 3–20

Bloxham, C.A., Mindel, T.A., & Frith, C.D. (1984). Initiation and execution of predictable and unpredictable movements in Parkinson's disease. *Brain, 107,* 371–384

Borden, G.J. (1979). An interpretation of research on feedback interruption in speech. *Brain and Language, 7,* 307–319

Borden, G.J., Harris, K.S., & Raphael, L.J. (2003). *Speech Science Primer: Physiology, Acoustics and Perception of Speech,* 4th ed. Philadelphia: Lippincott Williams & Wilkins

Bowman, J.P. (1968). Muscle spindles in the intrinsic and extrinsic muscles of the rhesus monkey's *(Macaca mulatta)* tongue. *Anatomical Record, 161,* 483–488

Bowman, J.P. & Combs, C.M. (1969a). The cerebrocortical projection of hypoglossal afferents. *Experimental Neurology, 23,* 291–301

Bowman, J.P. & Combs, C.M. (1969b). Cerebellar responsiveness to stimulation of the lingual spindle afferent fibers in the hypoglossal nerve of the rhesus monkey. *Experimental Neurology, 23,* 537–543

Brooks, V.B. (1986). *The Neural Basis of Motor Control.* New York: Oxford University Press

Burbaud, P., Doegle, C., Gross, C., & Bioulac, B. (1991). A quantitative study of neuronal discharge in areas 5, 2 and 4 of the monkey during fast arm movements. *Journal of Neurophysiology, 66,* 429–443

Carpenter, M.B. & Jayaraman, A. (Eds.). (1987). *The Basal Ganglia II: Structure and Function—Current Concepts.* New York: Plenum Press

Crutcher, V.I.D. & Alexander, G.E. (1990). Movement-related neuronal activity selectively coding either direction or muscle pattern in three motor areas of the monkey. *Journal of Neurophysiology, 64,* 151–163

Darian-Smith, I., Johnson, K.O., & Goodwin, A.W. (1979). Posterior parietal cortex: relations of unit activity to sensorimotor function. *Annual Review of Physiology, 41,* 141–157

Darley, F.L., Aronson, A.E., & Brown, J.R. (1975). *Motor Speech Disorders.* Philadelphia: W.B. Saunders

Devinsky, O., Morrell, M.J., & Vogt, B.A. (1995). Contributions of anterior cingulate cortex to behaviour. *Brain, 118,* 279–306

Di Pellegrino, G., Fadiga, L., Fogassi, L., Gallese, V., & Rizzolatti, G. (1992). Understanding motor events: a neurophysiological study. *Experimental Brain Research, 91,* 176–180

Di Pellegrino, G. & Wise, S.P. (1991). A neurophysiological comparison of three distinct regions of the primate frontal lobe. *Brain, 114,* 951–978

Dreher, J. & Grafman, J. (2002). The roles of the cerebellum and basal ganglia in timing and error prediction. *European Journal of Neuroscience, 16,* 1609–1620

Eccles, J.C. (1977). *The Understanding of the Brain.* New York: McGraw-Hill

Edwards, M.L. & Shriberg, L.D. (1983). *Phonology: Applications in Communicative Disorders.* San Diego: College-Hill

Evarts, E.V. (1971). Activity of thalamic and cortical neurons in relation to learned movement in the monkey. *International Journal of Neurology, 8,* 321–326

Evarts, E.V. (1982). Analogies between central motor programs for speech and for limb movements. In: S. Grillner, B. Lindblom, J. Lubker, & A. Persson (Eds.), *Speech Motor Control,* vol. 36. Oxford: Pergamon Press

Evarts, E.V. & Fromm, C. (1977). Sensory responses in motor cortex neurons during precise motor control. *Neuroscience Letters, 5,* 267–272

Evarts, E.V. & Fromm, C. (1981). Transcortical reflexes and servo control of movement. *Canadian Journal of Physiology and Pharmacology, 59,* 757–775

Evarts, E.V. & Wise, S.P. (1984). Basal ganglia outputs and motor control. In: *Ciba Foundation Symposium 107: Functions of the Basal Ganglia.* London: Pitman

Finocchio, D.V. & Luschei, E.S. (1988). Characteristics of complex voluntary mandibular movements in the monkey before and after destruction of most jaw muscle spindle afferents. *Journal of Voice, 2,* 279–290

Folkins, J.W. & Abbs, J.H. (1975). Lip and jaw motor control during speech: responses to resistive loading of the jaw. *Journal of Speech and Hearing Research, 18,* 207–220

Folkins, J.W. & Abbs, J.H. (1977). Motor impairment during inferior alveolar nerve blockade. *Journal of Speech and Hearing Disorders, 20,* 816–817

Folkins, J.W. & Zimmerman, G.N. (1981). Jaw-muscle activity during speech with the mandible fixed. *Journal of the Acoustical Society of America, 69,* 1441–1445

Fried, I., Ojemann, G.A., & Fetz, E.E. (1981). Language-related potentials specific to human language cortex. *Science, 212,* 353–355

Gay, T. (1981). Mechanisms in the control of speech rate. *Phonetica, 38,* 148–158

Gaymard, B., Pierrot-Deseilligny, C., & Rivaud, S. (1990). Impairment of sequences of memory-guided saccades after supplementary motor area lesions. *Annals of Neurology, 28,* 622–626

Gentil, M. (1990). Organization of the articulatory system: peripheral mechanisms and central coordination. In: W.J. Hardcastle & A. Marchal (Eds.), *Speech Production and Speech Modelling,* vol. 55. Dordrecht: Kluwer Academic

Gericke, C. (2004). *Dysarthria in the Context of the Four-Level Model: An Acoustic Comparison of Two Types* (title translated). Undergraduate research report, University of Pretoria, South Africa

Glees, P. (1988). *The Human Brain.* Cambridge: Cambridge University Press

Goodwin, G.M. & Luschei, E.S. (1974). Effects of destroying spindle afferents from jaw muscles on mastication in monkeys. *Journal of Neurophysiology, 37,* 967–981

Gracco, V.L. & Abbs, J.H. (1986). Variant and invariant characteristics of speech movements. *Experimental Brain Research, 65,* 156–166

Gracco, V.L. & Abbs, J.H. (1987). Programming and execution processes of speech movement control: potential neural correlates. In: E. Keller & M. Gopnik (Eds.), *Motor and Sensory Processes of Language.* Hillsdale, NJ: Lawrence Erlbaum

Gracco, V.L. & Abbs, J.H. (1988). Central patterning of speech movements. *Experimental Brain Research, 71,* 515–526

Gracco, V.L. & Abbs, J.H. (1989). Sensorimotor characteristics of speech motor sequences. *Experimental Brain Research, 75,* 586–598

Grillner, S. (1982). Possible analogies in the control of innate motor acts and the production of sound in speech. In: S. Grillner, B. Lindblom, J. Lubker, & A. Persson (Eds.), *Speech Motor Control,* vol. 36. Oxford: Pergamon Press

Grozinger, B., Kornhuber, H.H., & Kriebel, J. (1977). Human cerebral potentials preceding speech production, phonation and movements of the mouth and tongue, with reference to respiratory and extracerebral potentials. In: J.E. Desmedt (Ed.), *Language and Hemispheric Specialization in Man: Cerebral Event-related Potentials, Progress in Clinical Neurophysiology,* vol. 3. Basel: S. Karger

Heck, D. & Sultan, F. (2002). Cerebellar structure and function: making sense of parallel fibers. *Human Movement Science, 21,* 411–421

Holmes, V.M. (1984). Sentence planning in a story continuation task. *Language & Speech, 27,* 115–133

Houk, J.C. & Gibson, A.R. (1987). Sensorimotor processing through the cerebellum. In: J.S. King (Ed.), *New Concepts in Cerebellar Neurobiology, Neurology and Neurobiology,* vol. 22. New York: Alan R. Liss

Hughes, O.M. & Abbs, J.H. (1976). Labial-mandibular coordination in the production of speech: implications for the operation of motor equivalence. *Phonetica, 33,* 199–221

Itoh, M. & Sasanuma, S. (1984). Articulatory movements in apraxia of speech. In: J.C. Rosenbek, M.R. McNeil, A.E. Aronson (Eds.), *Apraxia of Speech: Physiology, Acoustics, Linguistics, Management.* San Diego: College-Hill

Iversen, S.D. (1981). Motor control. *British Medical Bulletin, 37,* 147–152

Jahanshahi, M., Jenkins, I.H., Brown, R.G., Marsden, C.D., Passingham, R.E., & Brooks, D.J. (1995). Self-initiated versus externally triggered movements. I. An investigation using measurement of regional cerebral blood flow with PET and movement-related potentials in normal and Parkinson's disease subjects. *Brain, 18,* 913–933

Jakobson, L.S. & Goodale, M.A. (1991). Factors affecting higher-order movement planning: a kinematic analysis of human prehension. *Experimental Brain Research, 86,* 199–208

Joanette, Y. & Dudley, J.G. (1980). Dysarthria symptomatology of Friedreich's ataxia. *Brain and Language, 10,* 39–50

Jonas, J. (1981). The supplementary motor region and speech emission. *Journal of Communication Disorders, 14,* 349–373

Johnson, A.M., Vernon, P.A., Almeida, Q.J., Grantier, L.L., & Jog, M.S. (2003) The role of the basal ganglia in movement: the effect of precues on discrete bidirectional movements in Parkinson's disease. *Motor Control, 7,* 71–81

Justus, T.C. & Ivry, R.B. (2001). The cognitive neuropsychology of the cerebellum. *International Review of Psychiatry, 13,* 276–282

Katz, D.B. (2002). Psychological functions of the cerebellum. *Behavioral and Cognitive Neuroscience Reviews, 1,* 229–242

Kawato, M. & Gomi, H. (1992). The cerebellum and VOR/OKR learning models. *Trends in Neuroscience, 15,* 445–453

Keele, S.W. (1982). Learning and control of coordinated motor patterns. In: Kelso JAS, ed. *Human Motor Behavior: An Introduction.* London: Lawrence Erlbaum

Keller, E. (1987). The cortical representation of motor processes of speech. In: E. Keller, M. Gopnik (Eds.), *Motor and Sensory Processes of Language.* Hillsdale, NJ: Lawrence Erlbaum

Kelso, J.A.S. (1982). Concepts and issues in human motor behavior: coming to grips with the jargon. In: J.A.S. Kelso (Ed.), *Human Motor Behavior: An Introduction.* London: Lawrence Erlbaum

Kelso, J.A.S. & Stelmach, G.E. (1976). Central and peripheral mechanisms in motor control. In: G.E. Stelmach (Ed.), *Motor Control: Issues and Trends.* New York: Academic Press

Kelso, J.A.S., Tuller, B., & Harris, K.S. (1983). A "dynamic pattern" perspective on the control and coordination of movement. In: P.F. MacNeilage (Ed.), *The Production of Speech.* New York: Springer-Verlag

Kempler, D. & Van Lancker, D. (2002). Effect of speech task on intelligibility in dysarthria: a case study of Parkinson's Disease. *Brain and Language, 80,* 449–464

Kent, R.D. (1990). The acoustic and physiologic characteristics of neurologically impaired speech movements. In: Hardcastle & A. Marchal (Eds.), *Speech Production and Speech Modelling,* vol. 55. Dordrecht: Kluwer Academic Publishers

Kent, R.D., Duffy, J.R., Slama, A., Kent, J.F., & Clift, A. (2001). Clinicoanatomic studies in dysarthria: review, critique, and directions for research. *Journal of Speech, Language, and Hearing Research, 44,* 535–551

Kent, R.D. & McNeil, M.R. (1987). Relative timing of sentence repetition in apraxia of speech and conduction aphasia. In: J.H. Ryalls (Ed.), *Phonetic Approaches to Speech Production in Aphasia and Related Disorders.* Boston: Little, Brown

Kent, R.D. & Minifie, F.D. (1977). Coarticulation in recent speech production models. *Journal of Phonetics, 5,* 115–133

Kent, R.D. & Netsell, R. (1975). A case study of an ataxic dysarthric: cineradiographic and spectrographic observations. *Journal of Speech and Hearing Disorders, 40,* 115–134

Kent, R.D., Netsell, R., & Abbs, J.H. (1979). Acoustic characteristics of dysarthria associated with cerebellar disease. *Journal of Speech and Hearing Research, 22,* 627–648

Kent, R.D. & Rosenbek, J.C. (1983). Acoustic patterns of apraxia of speech. *Journal of Speech and Hearing Research, 26,* 231–249

Kim, B.W. & Corlew, M. (1979). Electromyographic-aerodynamic study of Parkinsonian speech. *Allied Health Behavior Science, 2,* 375–382

King, J.S. (Ed.). (1987). *New Concepts in Cerebellar Neurobiology, Neurology and Neurobiology,* vol 22. New York: Alan R. Liss

Klapp, S.T., Anderson, W.G., & Berrian, R.W. (1973). Implicit speech in reading reconsidered. *Journal of Experimental Psychology, 100,* 368–374

Klein, R.M. (1976). Attention and movement. In: G.E. Stelmach (Ed.), *Motor Control: Issues and Trends.* New York: Academic Press

Kleinow, J. & Smith, A. (2000) Influences of length and syntactic complexity on the speech motor stability of the fluent speech of adults who stutter. *Journal of Speech, Language, and Hearing Research, 43,* 548–559

Knight, R.T., Singh, J., & Woods, D.L. (1989). Pre-movement parietal lobe input to human sensorimotor cortex. *Brain Research, 498,* 190–194

Kornhuber, H.H. (1977). A reconsideration of the cortical and subcortical mechanisms involved in speech and aphasia. In: J.E. Desmedt (Ed.), *Language and Hemispheric Specialization in Man: Cerebral Event-related Potentials, Progress in Clinical Neurophysiology,* vol. 3. Basel: S. Karger

Krebs, H.I., Hogan, N., Hening, W., Adamovich, S.V., & Poizner, H. (2001). Procedural motor learning in Parkinson's disease. *Experimental Brain Research, 141,* 425–437

Kurata, K. (1992). Somatotopy in the human supplementary motor area. *Trends in Neuroscience, 15,* 159–160

Lacquaniti, F. (1989). Central representations of human limb movement as revealed by studies of drawing and handwriting. *Trends in Neuroscience, 12,* 287–291

Lamendella, J.T. (1977). The limbic system in human communication. In: H. Whitaker & H.A. Whitaker (Eds.), *Studies in Neurolinguistics,* vol. 3. New York: Academic Press

Landgren, S. & Olsson, K.A. (1982). Oral mechanoreceptors. In: S. Grillner, B. Lindblom, J. Lubker, & A. Persson (Eds.), *Speech Motor Control,* vol. 36. Oxford: Pergamon Press

Lang, W., Beisteiner, R., Lindinger, G., & Deecke, L. (1992). Changes of cortical activity when executing learned motor sequences. *Experimental Brain Research, 89,* 435–440

Lang, W., Cheyne, D., Kristeva, R., Beisteiner, R., Undinger, G., & Deecke, L. (1991). Three-dimensional localization of SMA activity preceding voluntary movement: a study of electric and magnetic fields in a patient with infarction of the right supplementary motor area. *Experimental Brain Research, 87,* 688–695

Larson, C.R. & Sutton, D. (1978). Effects of cerebellar lesions on monkey jaw-force control: implications for understanding ataxic dysarthria. *Journal of Speech and Hearing Research, 21,* 309–323

Lassen, N.A., Ingvar, D.H., & Skinhoj, E. (1978). Brain function and blood flow. *Scientific American, 239,* 50–60

Leanderson, R., Meyerson, B., & Persson, A. (1972). Lip muscle function in Parkinsonian dysarthria. *Acta Oto-Laryngologica, 74,* 350–357

Leanderson, R., Persson, A., & Ohman, S. (1970). Electromyographic studies of the function of the facial muscles in dysarthria. *Acta Oto-Laryngologica, 263,* 89–94

Lindblom, B., Lubker, J., & Gay, T. (1979). Formant frequencies of some fixed-mandible vowels and a model of speech motor programming by predictive simulation. *Journal of Phonetics, 7,* 147–161

Luppino, G., Matelli, M., & Rizzolatti, G. (1990). Cortico-cortical connections of two electro-physiologically identified arm representations in the mesial agranular frontal cortex. *Experimental Brain Research, 82,* 214–218

Luria, A.R. (1966). *Higher Cortical Functions in Man.* New York: Basic Books

MacKay, W.A. (1980). The motor program: back to the computer. *Trends in Neuroscience, 3,* 97–100

MacNeilage, P.F. (1970). Motor control of serial ordering of speech. *Physiology Review, 77,* 182–196

MacNeilage, P.F. (1980). Speech production. *Language and Speech, 23,* 3–23

MacNeilage, P.F. & De Clerk, J.L. (1969). On the motor control of coarticulation in CVC monosyllables. *Journal of the Acoustical Society of America, 45,* 1217–1233

Magill, R.A. (2001). *Motor Learning: Concepts and Applications,* 6th ed. Boston: McGraw-Hill

Maner, K.J., Smith, A., & Grayson, L. (2000). Influences of utterance length and complexity on speech motor performance in children and adults. *Journal of Speech, Language, and Hearing Research, 43,* 560–573

Mano, N., Kanazawa, I., & Yamamoto, K. (1989). Voluntary movements and complex-spike discharges of cerebellar Purkinje cells. In: P. Strata (Ed.), *The Olivo-cerebellar System in Motor Control, Experimental Brain Research,* Series 17. Berlin: Springer-Verlag

Marsden, C.D. (1980). The enigma of the basal ganglia and movement. *Trends in Neuroscience, 3,* 284–287

Marsden, C.D. (1984). Which motor disorder in Parkinson's disease indicates the true motor function of the basal ganglia? In: *Ciba Foundation Symposium 107: Functions of the Basal Ganglia.* London: Pitman

Marteniuk, R.G. & MacKenzie, C.L. (1980). Information processing in movement organization and execution. In: R.S. Nickerson (Ed.), *Attention and Performance VIII.* Hillsdale, NJ: Lawrence Erlbaum

Martin, K.E., Phillips, J.G., Iansek, R., & Bradshaw, J.L. (1994) Inaccuracy and instability of sequential movements in Parkinson's disease. *Experimental Brain Research, 102,* 131–140

McClean, M.D. (1991). Lip muscle reflex and intentional response levels in a simple speech task. *Experimental Brain Research, 87,* 662–670

McGeer, P.L. & McGeer, E.G. (1987). Integration of motor functions in the basal ganglia. In: M.B. Carpenter & A. Jayaraman (Eds.), *The Basal Ganglia II: Structure and Function—Current Concepts.* New York: Plenum Press

McNeil, M.R. & Kent, R.D. (1990). Motoric characteristics of adult aphasic and apraxic speakers. In: G.R. Hammond (Ed.), *Cerebral Control of Speech and Limb Movements.* Amsterdam: North-Holland

McNeil, M.R., Odell, K., & Tseng, C.H. (1991). Toward the integration of resource allocation into a general theory of aphasia. *Clinical Aphasiology, 20,* 21–39

Meyer, J.S., Sakai, F., Yamaguchi, F., Yamamoto, M., & Shaw, T. (1980). Regional changes in cerebral blood flow during standard behavioral activation in patients with disorders of speech and mentation compared to normal volunteers. *Brain and Language, 9,* 61–77

Miall, R.C., Weir, D.J., & Stein, J.F. (1987). Visuo-motor tracking during reversible inactivation of the cerebellum. *Experimental Brain Research, 65,* 455–464

Mitleb, F.M. (1984). Voicing effect on vowel duration is not an absolute universal. *Journal of Phonetics, 12,* 23–27

Mogeson, G.J., Jones, D.L., & Yim, C.Y. (1980). From motivation to action: functional interface between the limbic system and the motor system. *Progress in Neurobiology, 14,* 69–97

Muller, R., Kleinhans, N., Pierce, K., Kenmotsu, N., & Courchesne, E. (2002). Functional MRI of motor sequence acquisition: effects of learning stage and performance. *Cognitive Brain Research, 14,* 277–294

Mushiake, H., Inase, M., & Tanji, J. (1990). Selective coding of motor sequence in the supplementary motor area of the monkey cerebral cortex. *Experimental Brain Research, 82,* 208–210

Nakano, K.K., Zubick, H., & Tyler, H.R. (1973). Speech defects of parkinsonian patients: effects of levodopa therapy on speech intelligibility. *Neurology (Minneapolis), 23,* 865–870

Nauta, W.J.H. & Domesick, V.B. (1984). Afferent and efferent relationships of the basal ganglia. In: *Ciba Foundation Symposium 107: Functions of the Basal Ganglia.* London: Pitman

Netsell, R. (1982). Speech motor control and selected neurologic disorders. In: S. Grillner, B. Lindblom, J. Lubker, & A. Persson (Eds.), *Speech Motor Control.* Oxford: Pergamon Press

Nishinuma, Y. (1984). Prediction of phoneme duration by a distinctive feature matrix. *Journal of Phonetics, 12,* 169–173

Nolte, J. (1999). *The Human Brain: An Introduction to its Functional Anatomy,* 4th ed. St. Louis: Mosby

Oberg, R.G.B. & Divac, I. (1981). Levels of motor planning: cognition and the control of movement. *Trends in Neuroscience, 4,* 122–124

Orgogozo, J.M. & Larsen, B. (1979). Activation of the supplementary motor area during voluntary movement in man suggests it works as a supramotor area. *Science, 206,* 847–850

Percheron, G. & Filion, M. (1991). Parallel processing in the basal ganglia: up to a point. *Trends in Neuroscience, 14,* 55–56

Persson, A. (1982). Some comments on the motor control of speech. In: S. Grillner, B. Lindblom, J. Lubker, & A. Persson (Eds.), *Speech Motor Control,* vol. 36. Oxford: Pergamon Press

Ploog, D. (1981). Neurobiology of primate audio-vocal behavior. *Brain Research Review, 3,* 35–61

Porter, L.L. (1992). Patterns of projections from area 2 of the sensory cortex to area 3a and to the motor cortex in cats. *Experimental Brain Research, 91,* 85–93

Pribram, K.H. (1976). Mechanisms in transmission of signals for conscious behaviour. In: T. Desiraju (Ed.), *Executive Functions of the Frontal Lobes.* Amsterdam: Elsevier Scientific

Putnam, A.H.B. & Ringel, R.L. (1976). A cineradiographic study of articulation in two talkers with temporarily induced oral sensory deprivation. *Journal of Speech and Hearing Research, 19,* 247–266

Ringel, R.L., Burk, K.W., & Scott, C.M. (1968). Tactile perception: form discrimination in the mouth. *British Journal of Disorders of Communication, 3,* 150–155

Ringel, R.L. & Ewanowski, S.J. (1965). Oral perception: two point discrimination. *Journal of Speech and Hearing Research, 8,* 389–397

Ringel, R.L. & Steer, M.D. (1963). Some effects of tactile and auditory alterations on speech output. *Journal of Speech and Hearing Research, 6,* 369–378

Romo, R., Scarnati, E., & Schultz, W. (1992). Role of primate basal ganglia and frontal cortex in the internal generation of movements. II. Movement related activity in the anterior striatum. *Experimental Brain Research, 91,* 385–395

Romo, R. & Schultz, W. (1992). Role of primate basal ganglia and frontal cortex in the internal generation of movements. III. Neuronal activity in the supplementary motor area. *Experimental Brain Research, 91,* 396–407

Rose, D.J. (1997). *A Multilevel Approach to the Study of Motor Control and Learning.* Boston: Allyn & Bacon

Sakai, K., Ramnani, N., & Passingham, R.E. (2002). Learning of sequences of finger movements and timing: frontal lobe and action-oriented representation. *Journal of Neurophysiology, 88,* 2035–2046

Salman, M.S. (2002). The cerebellum: it's about timing! But timing is not everything—new insights into the role of the cerebellum in timing motor and cognitive tasks. *Journal of Child Neurology, 17,* 1–9

Sanes, J.N., Dimitrov, B., & Hallett, M. (1990). Motor learning in patients with cerebellar dysfunction. *Brain, 113,* 103–120

Schmidt, R.A. (1976). The schema as a solution to some persistent problems in motor learning theory. In: G.E. Stelmach (Ed.), *Motor Control: Issues and Trends.* New York: Academic Press

Schmidt, R.A. & Lee, T.D. (1999). *Motor Control and Learning: A Behavioral Emphasis.* Champaign: Human Kinetics

Schmidt, R.F. (1978). Motor systems. In: R.F. Schmidt (Ed.), *Fundamentals of Neurophysiology.* New York: Springer-Verlag

Schmullian, D., Van der Merwe, A., & Groenewald, E. (1997). An exploratory study of an undefined acquired neuromotor speech disorder within the context of the Four-Level Framework for speech sensorimotor control. *South African Journal of Communication Disorders, 44,* 87–97

Schultz, W. & Romo, R. (1992). Role of primate basal ganglia and frontal cortex in the internal generation of movements. I. Preparatory activity in the anterior striatum. *Experimental Brain Research, 91,* 363–384

Scully, C. & Guerin, B. (1991). Speech production: models, methods and data. *Journal of Phonetics, 19,* 249–250

Shaiman, S. (2002). Articulatory control of vowel length for contiguous jaw cycles: The effects of speaking rate and phonetic context. *Journal of Speech, Language, and Hearing Research, 45,* 663–675

Sharkey, S.G. & Folkins, J.W. (1985). Variability of lip and jaw movements in children and adults: implications for the development of speech motor control. *Journal of Speech and Hearing Research, 28,* 8–15

Stevens, K.N. & Blumstein, S.B. (1981). A search for invariant acoustic correlates of phonetic features. In: P.D. Eimas & J.L. Miller (Eds.), *Perspectives on the Study of Speech.* Hillsdale, NJ: Lawrence Erlbaum

Strand, E.A. & McNeil, M.R. (1996). Effects of length and linguistic complexity on temporal acoustic measures in apraxia of speech. *Journal of Speech and Hearing Research, 39,* 1018–1033

Strata, P. (Ed.). (1989). *The Olivocerebellar System in Motor Control Experimental Brain Research,* Series 17. Berlin: Springer-Verlag

Sussman, H.M. (1972). What the tongue tells the brain. *Psychological Bulletin, 77,* 262–272

Tasko, S.M. & McClean, M.D. (2004). Variations in articulatory movement with changes in speech task. *Journal of Speech, Language, and Hearing Research, 47,* 85–100

Tatton, W.G. & Bruce, J.C. (1981). Comment: a schema for the interactions between motor programs and sensory input. *Canadian Journal of Physiology and Pharmacology, 59,* 691–699

Teuber, H.L. (1974). Concluding session: panel discussion on key problems in the preprogramming of movements. *Brain Research, 71,* 533–568

Theron, K. (2003). *Temporal Aspects of Speech Production in Bilingual Speakers with Neurogenic Speech Disorders.* Doctoral thesis, University of Pretoria, South Africa

Van den Bercken, J.H.L. & Cools, A.R. (1982). Evidence for a role of the caudate nucleus in the sequential organization of behaviour. *Behavioral Brain Research, 4,* 319–337

Van der Merwe, A. (2002). *The Four-Level Framework for the characterization of pathological speech sensorimotor control: Applications to treating apraxia of speech.* Keynote Address, 32nd Clinical Aphasiology Conference, Big Cedar Lodge, Missouri

Van der Merwe, A. & Grimbeek, R.J. (1990). A comparison of the influence of certain contextual factors on the symptoms of acquired apraxia of speech and developmental apraxia of speech (title translated). *South African Journal of Communication Disorders, 37,* 27–34

Van der Merwe, A., Uys, I.C., Loots, J.M., & Grimbeek, R.J. (1987). The influence of certain contextual factors on the perceptual symptoms of apraxia of speech (title translated). *South African Journal of Communication Disorders, 34,* 10–22

Van der Merwe, A., Uys, I.C., Loots, J.M., & Grimbeeck, R.J. (1988) Perceptual symptoms of apraxia of speech: indications of the nature of the disorder (title translated). *South African Journal of Communication Disorders, 35,* 45–54

Van der Merwe, A., Uys, I.C., Loots, J.M., & Grimbeeck, R.J., & Jansen, L.P.C. (1989). The influence of certain contextual factors on voice onset time, vowel duration and utterance duration in apraxia of speech (title translated). *South African Journal of Communication Disorders, 36,* 29–41

Von Euler, C. (1980). Central pattern generation during breathing. *Trends in Neuroscience, 3,* 275–277

Von Euler, C. (1981). The contribution of sensory inputs to the pattern generation of breathing. *Canadian Journal of Physiology and Pharmacology, 59,* 700–706

Von Gruenewaldt, A.M. (2003). *Acquired Dysarthria within the Context of the Four-Level Framework of Speech Sensorimotor Control.* Master's dissertation, University of Pretoria

Wanner, E., Teyler, T.J., & Thompson, R.F. (1977). The psychobiology of speech and language—an overview. In: J.E. Desmedt (Ed.), *Language and Hemispheric Specialization in Man: Cerebral Event-Related Potentials, Progress in Clinical Neurophysiology,* vol. 3. Basel: S. Karger

Weinrich, M., Wise, S.P., & Mauritz, K.H. (1984). A neurophysiological study of the pre-motor cortex in the Rhesus monkey. *Brain, 107,* 385–414

Wing, A.M. & Miller, E.D. (1984). Basal ganglia lesions and psychological analyses of the control of voluntary movement. In: *Ciba Foundation Symposium 107: Functions of the Basal Ganglia.* London: Pitman

Chapter 2

Perceptual Sensorimotor Speech Examination for Motor Speech Disorders

Ray D. Kent

Perceptual sensorimotor examination (PSME) is a set of speech assessment procedures that are performed essentially with the examiner's eyes and ears, that is, without equipment except perhaps for a tape recorder and miscellaneous inexpensive and readily available items. The procedures assess the integrity of a client's sensory and motor functions that support speech and other behaviors such as swallowing. When a suitably definitive assessment cannot be accomplished with these observations, the information gathered may help in planning referrals or designing additional (e.g., instrument-aided) assessments. It should be emphasized that despite considerable advances in technologies for the study of speech disorders, certain aspects of speech can be assessed adequately and directly only by human observers. For example, if speech intelligibility is of interest, there is little choice but to obtain ratings by one or more human judges. Although technologies are increasingly helpful in assessing speech disorders, the data produced by these technologies are almost always validated against human judgments. Auditory-perceptual assessment remains the fundamental means by which the disability fingerprint (functional loss) of a motor speech disorder is determined. A particular advantage accruing to auditory-perceptual assessment is that such assessment can be performed at little cost in diverse environments, including telehealth programs (Theodoros, Russel, Hill, Cahill, & Clark, 2003).

It cannot be assumed that any particular examination protocol can be used invariantly with every client in every clinical setting. Inevitably, modifications may have to be made in any given protocol to account for client characteristics, purpose of examination, and time or resources available. The approach taken in this chapter is to describe a general-purpose examination, components of which can be omitted, shortened, elaborated, or otherwise modified for a given client. The intention is not to describe an inflexible, prescriptive examination but rather to present a menu from which individually tailored examinations can be developed. But this is not to deny the importance of standardized procedures for selected components of an examination. Ultimately, clinicians' competence in performing a valid and reliable clinical examination rests on their experience, adherence to specified procedures, and reliance on accepted clinical guidelines for interpreting observations and data.

♦ Value of and Difficulties in Interpreting a Perceptual Sensorimotor Examination

The perceptual examination of any motor system is challenging, but the speech motor system presents challenges that are especially difficult and probably unique. Unlike limb movements, only a few of the movements of speech are visible. Most are hidden within the body and their characteristics can only be inferred from auditory-perceptual or other information on motor function. Even with endoscopy, many speech movements are not observable. In addition, the organs of interest are not all palpable, at least not by the ordinary means available to the speech-language pathologist in a typical clinical setting. The 100 or so muscles that constitute the speech motor system are distributed in the trunk, neck, and head. The speech production system is notably sexually dimorphic, and its life-span characteristics are not sufficiently well described. Its muscles appear to possess genetic, developmental, functional properties that are unique to craniofacial muscles (as reviewed in Kent, 2004), which limits the generalization of clinical features observed in the limbs and trunk to the muscles used in speech.

Auditory-perceptual assessment of the motor speech disorders is a daunting task in that the potential dimensions of abnormality are numerous, embracing nearly all aspects of speech pathology (respiration, voice, resonance, articulation, prosody, fluency, and so on). As Duffy and Kent (2001) pointed out, there are three major challenges in auditory-perceptual assessment. First, the listener frequently has to distinguish one dimension from among several co-occurring dimensions, and attending to any one dimension can be difficult. In commenting on their results on the perceptual features of ataxic dysarthria, Sheard, Adams, and Davis (1991) observed that the ratings for various dimensions often were highly intercorrelated, and they suggested that "the actual rating values [assigned] to apparently separate dimensions may in fact reflect an overall perception of a number of concurrent, crucial/salient speech characteristics" (p. 291). Second, training and experience are often neglected, and, even more bothersome, it appears that clinical experience does not always guarantee interjudge agreement, at least not for all dimensions. In their research on the perceptual rating of voice quality disorders, Kreiman, Gerratt, and Prodoca (1990) concluded that "clinical training and experience cause listeners to differ more, not less, in how they perceive voice quality, at least in tasks that involve unstructured similarity judgments" (p. 109). Third, different scaling procedures are used in auditory-perceptual assessment, and they sometimes give different results. Although equal-appearing scaling is often used clinically, other techniques, such as direct magnitude estimation, are more suitable to many perceptual dimensions (Kent, 1996; Zraick & Liss, 2000).

Unfortunately, most of the assessments described in this chapter have not been thoroughly evaluated with respect to reliability, validity, or predictive validity. Indeed, few assessment instruments in speech-language pathology have been so evaluated (see, for example, the report by the Agency for Healthcare Research and Quality [AHRQ], Biddle, Watson, Hooper, et al, 2002).

◆ Tasks and Instruments for a Perceptual Sensorimotor Examination

A combination of tasks typically constitutes a PSME. Speech tasks may include vowel prolongation, maximum-rate syllable repetition (diadochokinesis; DDK), word production (possibly including a standardized articulation test), phrase or sentence recitation, passage reading, and conversation. Each of these has its own advantages and disadvantages, but taken together, they can offer a highly informative assessment of a client's speech production system. **Table 2–1** offers an analysis of four basic tasks with respect to the kind of information that can be obtained from each.

Tasks

Nonspeech Tasks

Opinions differ on the usefulness of various nonspeech tasks and nonsense speech tasks to obtain information relative to speech performance. To be sure, several studies cast doubt on the value of nonspeech oral movements as a correlate of speech movements or as an effective intervention for speech production disorders (Clark, 2003; Forrest, 2002; Weismer, 2005). Nonetheless, nonspeech tasks may hold value in clinical assessment, particularly if the logic and limitations of that assessment are carefully specified. A particular objective in the use of these tasks is observation of isolated muscle systems in the performance of an action that is relatively free of phonetic or other linguistic purposes. These tasks also can be used to assess the strength or endurance of a given motor system. Several tasks are considered later in this chapter, and Chapter 3 considers this topic in depth. **Table 2–2** lists the association between articulators (muscle groups) and cranial nerves. Although nonsense speech tasks may come closer to actual speech behavior than nonspeech tasks, it should be noted that nonsense speech tasks may differ from speech tasks in having larger amplitudes and velocities of movement (Tasko & McClean, 2004).

High-effort nonspeech tasks (maximum performance tasks) generally assess strength, endurance, and rate of a selected nonspeech motor performance that is outside the usual definition of speech. Examples include maximum expiratory air pressure, maximum compression force of an oral articulator, and maximum rate of tongue, lip, or jaw movements (alternating motion rate or diadochokinesis). It should be noted that speech usually taps only a small amount of physiological capacity in healthy individuals. For example, forces developed in speech are only 10 to 20% of the maximum force capability registered in nonspeech tasks, such as

Table 2–1 Relationship Between Variables of Interest in a Clinical Assessment and the Various Tasks that Can Be Used to Form an Examination Protocol

Variable	Nonspeech	Simplified Speech	Citation	Formulation
Reflexes	++	+	?	?
Tone	++	++	+	+
Range of movement	++	++	+	+
Speed	++	++	++	+
Strength or endurance	++	++	++	+
Initiation time	++	++	++	+
Stability over time	++	++	+	+
Coordination	++	++	++	++
Voice quality	0	++	++	++
Prosody	0	+	++	++
Fluency	0	+	++	++
Intelligibility	0	+	++	++
Communicative adaptability	0	+	++	++

++, highly informative; +, somewhat informative; 0, not informative; ?, uncertain.

Table 2–2 Articulatory Movements and Cranial Nerve Innervation for the Muscles Performing Those Movements

Articulatory Movements	Cranial Nerve (CN) Innervation
Jaw movements	CN V
Bilabials	CN VII
All lingual sounds (vowels and consonants)	CN XII
Phonation	CN X
Velopharyngeal function (nasal vs nonnasal)	CN V, CN IX, CN X

maximum compression (Hinton & Arokiasamy, 1997; Kent, Kent, & Rosenbek, 1987). This fact, together with the fatigue resistance of most muscle fibers used in speech (Kent, 2004), accounts for the ability of most healthy individuals to speak at length, with little evidence of fatigue (except perhaps for their listeners). However, some disorders, such as amyotrophic lateral sclerosis (ALS), may reduce physiological capacity before effects are observed in speech production (DePaul, 1989). These early reductions in capacity can be important in registering disease progression. Even though early declines in maximum physiological performance may not directly or immediately impair speech, they can alert the clinician to the need for follow-up examination, especially in the case of neurodegenerative diseases. The rate of sequential movements, as assessed by the maximum rate of syllable repetition, generally is roughly comparable for nonspeech and speech tasks, indicating that speech does place nearly maximal demands on at least one aspect of motor control.

Evaluations of maximum physiological capacity also can be informative regarding possible compensations available to the speaker. An informative assessment is directed to identify not only areas of weakness but also areas of strength. The interdependency among speech production systems can allow one system to compensate for weaknesses in another. Strength and endurance in the orofacial muscles vary with age and sex (Crow & Ship, 1996; Mortimore, Fiddes, Stephens, & Douglas, 1999), which means that a clinical examination should take these characteristics into account. A recent study of auditory-perceptual ratings of dysarthia indicates that listener judgments reach acceptable standards of agreement, giving support to the clinical value of this approach (Bunton et al, 2007).

Simplified Speech Tasks

A variety of these tasks have been used in PSME construction. Many are high-effort or maximal performance tasks that are designed to assess a client's physiological capacity in a task that has a speech-like character. Some of the most frequently used measures and tasks are the following (see Kent et al, 1987, or Kent, 1994, for tables of normative data). The maximum phonation time (MPT) is the maximum length of time that a client can phonate a vowel after a maximal inspiration. MPT is commonly used as a global assessment of phonatory capacity, but it should be underlined that this measure reflects both respiratory capacity and laryngeal efficiency. MPT can be reduced because of respiratory deficiency, laryngeal dysfunction, or both. It is also important to note that age effects can be profound. It is inappropriate to use normative data from young adults when testing children or elders. The maximum frication time (MFT) is the maximum length of time that a client can sustain a fricative such as /s/ following a maximum inspiration. MFT can be determined for both voiced and voiceless fricatives. When MFT values are obtained for voiced and voiceless cognates, then it is possible to compute a ratio, such as the /s/-/z/ ratio. The physiological voice frequency range (PVFR) is the range of fundamental frequencies that can be produced by the client. This variable is also called the fundamental frequency range (FFR) or pitch range (PR). Whatever term is used, the range in healthy speakers greatly exceeds the range of vocal fundamental frequency used in typical speaking situations. The sound pressure range (SPR) is the range of sound pressure level (SPL) from the softest to loudest production of a sound (typically vowel /a/). One caution to observe in the use of this task is that phonation at maximum effort can be taxing, especially to medically fragile clients, and can carry risks. For this reason, some clinicians prefer to determine only the minimum sound pressure level. This measure presents little risk or discomfort and may provide valuable information on phonatory function. Normal values of the minimum sound pressure level of phonation are in the range of 45 to 66 dB SPL re 20 micropascals.

Probably the most frequently used high-effort task is diadochokinesis (DDK), or syllable repetition at maximal rate. When this task involves a consonant-vowel (CV) syllable, it is also known by the term *alternating motion rate* (AMR) because the task requires alternating movements between the consonant and the vowel. The clinician can select from a large number of potential syllables, but the most commonly used syllables are /pV/, /tV/, and /kV/. (*Note:* because the vowel in CV syllables can take on somewhat different phonetic qualities in the DDK task, the abbreviation V is used here to represent the vowel segment.) Normative data for these syllables are given in **Table 2–3**. Syllables containing the voiced cognates are also frequent selections in clinical testing. The trisyllabic sequence /pVtVkV/ is used by some clinicians to test sequential labial, alveolar, and dorsal movements. However, this sequence is difficult for some

Table 2–3 Diacochokinetic Rates for Three Syllables in Syllables/s.

Age	/pV/	/tV/	/kV/
3 years	4.7	4.7	4.3
4 years	4.7	4.7	4.3
5 years	4.9	4.9	4.7
6 years	5.3	5.3	4.9
Young adults	6.0 to 7.0	6.0 to 7.0	5.2 to 6.2
Older adults	5.0 to 7.0	4.8 to 6.5	4.4 to 6.0

Mean data for different age groups are drawn from published results summarized in Kent et al (1987).

clients, especially young children. Therefore, trisyllable words such as *buttercup* and *pattycake* are used as real-word alternatives. The clinical value of DDK has been noted in several studies on individuals with motor speech disorders (Ackermann, Hertrich, & Hehr, 1995; Blumberger, Sullivan, & Clement, 1995; Samlan & Weismer, 1995; Wang, Kent, Duffy, Thomas, & Weismer, 2004).

Citation Tasks: Repetition and Routinized Speech

These tasks introduce a greater degree of phonetic or linguistic complexity than the tasks considered in the previous section. Citation tasks include monosyllabic or polysyllabic words, phrases, and sentences. Frequently, citation tasks incorporate phonetic sequences that are selected to target basic articulatory functions and interarticulatory coordination. An example is the use of a word such as *pamper* or *bumper* to target nasal-nonnasal consonant sequences as part of an examination of velopharyngeal function. Another example is selection of a set of words that vary in syllabic number or complexity. These sets are often part of the examination for apraxia of speech, which tends to become more obvious as the complexity of the phonetic sequence increases. Many clinicians also examine routine (automatic) speech, such as counting, simple greetings, days of the week, or months of the year. These expressions sometimes are preserved when propositional speech is disturbed.

Language Formulation Tasks

These tasks go beyond simple repetition of a word or phrase to involve processes of language formulation as well as speech production. The objective is to evaluate speech that is executed along with the various processes of language formulation including syntactic, semantic, and phonological processes. The specific tasks can take the form of confrontational naming, conversation, describing a picture or object, retelling a story, narrating a scene on video, or answering questions.

Information from Client History and Referral

This information is important in planning the examination and interpreting the results. Examinations often must be tailored to an individual client's sensory, motor, and cognitive-linguistic capabilities. History and referrals are a source of information in these areas. To the degree possible, client characteristics should be considered in advance, because information in this area (1) may determine restrictions on performance in certain tasks (e.g., aphasia or dementia may interfere with understanding the examiner's verbal requests), (2) helps in the selection of suitable test procedures and materials (e.g., adjusting verbal materials to the language level of the client), and (3) guides the examiner to answer specific questions that may have been raised in referral or are frequently of issue for a certain disorder (e.g., assessing vocal function in individuals with idiopathic Parkinson's disease). To take a simple example, if a client's referral information indicates diplopia, right hemiplegia, and a history of vestibular problems, the clinician should be careful to select tasks that do not rely critically on visual acuity, right-sided limb movements, or unsupported body postures or whole-body movements.

Composite Examination Instruments

Composite examination instruments refer to examination tools that are multipurpose and multidimensional. The dysarthria rating scale developed by Darley, Aronson, and Brown (1969a,b) is a well-known example of such a system. The scale consists of 38 perceptual dimensions, each of which is rated on a seven-point, equal-appearing interval scale. The dimensions pertain to pitch, loudness, voice quality, articulation, resonance, speaking rate, prosody, and other aspects of speech production. With such a scale, information can be gathered on a variety of functions. However, as noted by Duffy and Kent (2001), it is unlikely that speech-language clinicians actually rate all 38 perceptual dimensions as part of a client's assessment. Rather, they probably make note of conspicuous or salient dimensions that appear to be most important in characterizing the dysarthric patterns. The *Frenchay Dysarthria Assessment* (Enderby, 1983) is a composite examination instrument divided into 11 sections that combine nonspeech and speech assessments: reflexes, respiration, lips, jaw, palate, laryngeal, tongue, intelligibility, rate, sensation, and associated factors. Robertson (1982) and Drummond (1993) introduced other instruments designed for the description of impairments in dysarthria, and Hayden (1994) described an instrument for motor speech assessment in children. Arvedson (2000) summarizes information particularly important in the assessment of feeding and swallowing. A primary advantage of these instruments is that they permit an evaluation of several aspects of speech in a single assessment tool.

Other relevant instruments or guidelines for assessment are available for children (Hodge, 1991; Potter, 2004; Robbins and Klee, 1987; Strand and McCauley, 1999) and adults (Hodge, 1988; Mason & Simon, 1977; Ruscello, St. Louis, Barry, & Barr, 1982). Several report forms are reprinted in Kent (1994) and additional forms are cited in this chapter. These sources provide general background for assessment.

◆ A Model for Selecting Assessment Tasks and Tools for a Perceptual Motor-Sensory Examination

A system or subsystem framework helps to focus observations on functional components of speech production. This framework, given in **Table 2–4**, illustrates how specific tasks are selected to assess structure or function within a circumscribed part of the speech production system. An overall assessment entails selecting tasks suitable to the components of interest.

Note: For most of the components discussed in this chapter, both screening and deep assessments are described. Screening procedures are brief and simple assessments, designed to detect an obvious problem. Many of these can be accomplished at least in part during conversation with the client. Deep assessments are more time-consuming and detailed. An examination for an individual client may consist of a combination of screening and deep assessments, depending on the issues involved. The distinction between screening and deep testing is by no means hard and fast, but it is useful to separate those procedures that can be done quickly from those that require a greater investment of time from both the examiner and client.

Respiration

Screening Screening often can be accomplished during conversation with the client, perhaps supplemented by simple nonconversational tasks that are appropriate for the client's characteristics. A general impression of the adequacy of respiratory function can be formed while listening to the client's speech, attending especially to the length of phrases and sentences, to the location of breath pauses, and to overall prosody. To assess prosodic regulation related to speech breathing, it can be helpful to ask the client to make changes in loudness or vocal effort. Patterns of speech breathing and prosody are sensitive to various parameters of the speaking task (Lowit-Leuschel & Doherty, 2001; McFarland, 2001; Mitchell, Hoit, & Watson, 1996; Sperry & Klich, 1992). Therefore, it is often necessary to perform screening with at least two or three tasks, such as ordinary conversation, passage reading, and one or both of these repeated with loudness variation. In addition, it can be informative to see if changes in posture influence the respiratory patterns. The auditory-perceptual observations can be supplemented by a simple test of respiratory function that involves blowing bubbles into a cup of liquid (Hixon, Hawley, & Wilson, 1982).

Deep Assessment More detailed assessments of respiratory function can be made of the diaphragm, rib cage, and abdominal wall according to systematic procedures described by Hixon and Hoit (1999a,b, 2000). The various tasks used in these deep assessments are noted in **Table 2–4**; see the original articles for a worksheet that can be used to summarize the observations.

Table 2–4 Assessment Protocol Menu, Showing System Component to Be Tested, Assessment Tasks, and Selected References

System Component	Tasks	References and Comments
Respiration		
Overall function: screening	Conversation or reading passage; assess adequacy of respiration, appropriateness of breath groups	
Deep assessment: diaphragm	Resting tidal inspiration, running speech inspiration, maximum inspiration, breath hold, relaxation from total lung capacity (TLC), slow expiration from TLC, soft vowel from TLC, catch breath, gasp, sniff, pant, abdominal wall distention, abdominal wall thrust against resistance	Hixon & Hoit, 1998; examination worksheet printed on pp. 43–45
Deep assessment: rib cage	Structure at rest, resting tidal breathing, running speech production, maximum inspiration, maximum rib cage expansion, Muller maneuver, maximum expiration, maximum rib cage compression, Valsalva maneuver, breath hold within inspiratory capacity, relaxation from total lung capacity, slow expiration from total lung capacity, soft vowel from total lung capacity, breath hold with expiratory reserve volume, relaxation from residual volume, slow expiration to residual volume, forced inspiratory capacity, catch breath, gasp, cough, pant, consecutive small expirations, rib cage wall thrust against resistance	Hixon & Hoit, 2000; examination worksheet printed on pp. 190–196
Deep assessment: abdominal wall	Structure at rest, resting tidal breathing, running speech production, maximum expiration, maximum abdominal wall contraction, Valsalva maneuver, repeated abdominal wall contraction, slow expiration to residual volume, breath hold within expiratory reserve volume, relaxation from residual volume, forced vital capacity, blowing out a candle, cough, laugh, pant, trunk flexion, trunk rotation	Hixon & Hoit, 1999; examination worksheet printed on pp. 343–346
Voice Screening	Informal assessment of voice based on conversation or reading; alternatively, any of the procedures listed under "Deep assessment"	
Deep assessment	Auditory-perceptual rating scales: GRBAS Buffalo Voice Profile Vocal Profile Analysis Scheme Consensus Auditory-Perceptual Examination Quick Screen for Voice (pediatric clients)	Lee et al, 2004
Jaw Function Screening	Observe jaw movements during nonspeech and speech diadochokinesis (DDK) and during conversation, giving particular notice to stability and symmetry of jaw positioning	
Deep assessment	Elaboration of screening tasks, possibly including overarticulation and imitation of examiner's jaw movements	
Velopharyngeal function Screening	*Screening test*: examiner listens for hypernasal resonance as client counts from 60 to 80 and repeats words and sentences	Dworkin et al, 2004; scoring form printed on p. 340

Table 2–4 *(Continued)* Assessment Protocol Menu

System Component	Tasks	References and Comments
Deep assessment	Anatomic survey; observation of velar activity during vowel phonation; gag reflex; speech tasks with periodic placement of laryngeal mirror beneath most patent nostril	Dworkin et al, 2004; scoring form printed on p. 340; Fox & Johns, 1970
	Tongue-anchor technique	
Lingual function Screening	Rating of strength as client presses tip of tongue against tongue blade held by examiner; both protrusion and lateralization can be tested; also, tongue function can be examined while bite-block fixes jaw position for various tasks	Clark et al, 2003
Deep assessment	Extension of screening tasks to test for sequential movements and compensatory ability (possibly with bite block)	
Labial function Screening	Observe lip movements and shape during speech and nonspeech gestures	
Deep assessment	Client is asked to hold straw or tongue depressor firmly between the lips as examiner attempts to withdraw it. Assessment of labial movements while jaw is fixed with bite block	
Oral sensation	Light static touch, kinetic touch, simultaneous stimulation, thermal stimulation (see text for detailed descriptions)	Jacobs et al, 2002; Kent et al, 1990

Voice

Voice disorder occurs frequently in dysarthria (Darley, Aronson, & Brown, 1969a,b; Duffy, 1995; Burton et al, 2007), and therefore the assessment of voice is an important component in PSME.

Screening   Voice characteristics can be assessed during conversation with the client, with special attention to pitch and loudness variations, overall voice quality, and consistency of phonatory function. The examiner may also ask the client to modify voice by asking for more vocal effort ("pretend that you are talking to someone who is far away"). Additionally, the examiner can assess the client's sustained vowel phonation in tasks such as (1) steady phonation with at attempt to keep vocal pitch and intensity uniform throughout the vowel, (2) phonation with changes in loudness or pitch, and (3) alternating start-stop phonation for the same vowel. Some clinicians may use a brief voice rating scale (such as the GRBAS [grade, roughness, breathiness, asthenia, strain] or Quick Screen for Voice, both of which are discussed in the next subsection) as a screening instrument. A relatively quick procedure to assess vocal fold movement is the laryngeal DDK task (Renout, Leeper, Bandur, & Hudson, 1995).

Deep Assessment   Auditory-perceptual voice assessment has a long history, but one that has not produced a universally accepted rating scale. Of the many scales that have been proposed, three of the most commonly used scales for which reliability data are available are the Buffalo Voice Profile, the Vocal Profile Analysis Scheme, and the GRBAS. Bhuta, Patrick, and Garnett (2004) state, "GRBAS remains the gold standard as it serves as a formal perceptual evaluation of voice attempting to clarify and organize the perceptual features of voice quality while limiting the descriptors to five key terms" (p. 303). "GRBAS" is an acronym for the five features the evaluation assesses: grade (overall degree

of deviance in voice), roughness (irregular fluctuation of the fundamental frequency), breathiness (turbulent noise produced by air leakage), aesthenia (overall weakness of the voice), and strain (impression of tenseness or excess effort). Each item is rated on a scale of 0 to 3 where 0 is normal and 3 is severe disturbance. This simple scale has been reported to have acceptable reliability (Webb et al, 2004; Wuyts, De Bodt, & Van de Heyning, 1999). Currently, GRBAS is recommended by the Japanese Society of Logopaedics and Phoniatrics and the European Research Group (Bhuta et al, 2004).

The Consensus Auditory-Perceptual Examination V (CAPE-V) was developed by a consensus meeting sponsored by the American Speech-Language-Hearing Association's (ASHA) Division 3: Voice and Voice Disorders, and the Department of Communication Science and Disorders, University of Pittsburgh, held in Pittsburgh on June 10–11, 2002. CAPE-V is intended to be a tool for clinical auditory-perceptual assessment. Its primary purpose is to describe the severity of auditory-perceptual attributes of a voice problem in a way that can be communicated among clinicians. Its secondary purpose is to contribute to hypotheses regarding the anatomical and physiological bases of voice problems, and the need for additional testing. The report form is available at http://www.asha.org/NR/rdonlyres/79EE699E-DAEE-4E2C-A69E-C11BDE6B1D67/0/22560_1.pdf.

For children, the Quick Screen for Voice has been described by Lee, Stemple, Glaze, and Kelchner (2004). The report form includes a checklist for respiration, phonation, and resonance, along with nonverbal vocal range and flexibility.

Velopharyngeal Function

Screening and deep assessments for velopharyngeal function were described by Dworkin, Marunick, and Krouse (2004).

Screening The examiner listens for hypernasal resonance as the client counts from 60 to 80 (these numbers present frequent opportunities for pressure-consonant production) and repeats words and sentences. The examiner may also make judgments of audible nasal emission, loudness, and precision of pressure consonants (Kummer & Lee, 1996). Any part of the screening test may be repeated with the client's nares occluded versus unoccluded.

Deep Assessment Dworkin et al's deep test, which affords a more detailed examination, includes an anatomical survey, observation of velar activity during vowel phonation, gag reflex, and speech tasks accompanied by a periodic placement of laryngeal mirror beneath the more patent nostril. For details, see Dworkin et al (2004). In addition, an articulation test may be administered, with special attention to the production of pressure consonants (Yorkston et al, 2001) and the consistency (or lack thereof) in consonant production. If abnormal resonance is detected, a useful follow-up procedure is to assess the client's speech production at different speaking rates and at different levels of vocal effort. For some individuals with velopharyngeal incompetence, speaking at a slow rate or with increased vocal effort reduces the severity of the problem. Asking the client to overarticulate (produce speech with exaggerated movements) can be informative regarding the dynamics of velopharyngeal function.

The modified tongue-anchor technique, introduced by Fox and Johns (1970), may be used as well. In this method, the client is asked to fill (puff up) his/her cheeks with exhaled air. Then, the client is asked to repeat the task while protruding the tongue, which is held by the examiner. As the client undertakes this task, the examiner occludes the client's nares, as though to assist the client in performing the task. Once the client's cheeks are puffed, the examiner releases the nares' occlusion to test if any air escapes through the nose.

Jaw Function

Screening A quick screen can be performed with observation of jaw movement during conversation, DDK (e.g., syllable [pa]), and selected nonspeech tasks (e.g., maximal opening, lateral movements with the teeth held together, and rapid alternating open-close movements). Positional instability, asymmetry, or any difficulty performing movements is noteworthy.

Deep Assessment Deep testing tasks can take several forms, mostly elaborated versions of tasks used in screening. Especially for clients who exhibit minimal jaw movement in the screening assessment, the examiner can request (and model) speech production with exaggerated jaw movements (overarticulation). Another procedure is to ask the client to imitate the examiner as he/she models sequences of jaw movement (e.g., maximal opening, closure, lateral movement to right, return movement to midline, movement to left, return movement to midline, maximal opening).

Lingual Function

Screening Screening assessments are typically performed by determining the adequacy of lingual articulation for tasks such as syllable repetition (especially CV syllables containing the lingual consonants), articulation tests, word lists, reading, or conversation. In addition, tongue strength can be rated by the examiner as the client presses the tip of his/her tongue against a tongue blade held by examiner (Clark, Henson, Barber, Stierwalt, & Sherrill, 2003). In this way, both protrusion and lateralization can be tested. An alternative test for lateralization is to ask the client to press the tongue against the cheek, which is palpated by the examiner to judge the strength of the tongue. It should be noted that these tasks are not typical of lingual function in speech, but they can give an indication of an overall weakness. Some clinicians also test for lingual elevation, for example by asking the client to raise the tongue against a tongue depressor or a gloved finger held against the lingual surface. If desired, a bite block can be used to fix the jaw during this examination. (Netsell [1985] describes how to make and use a bite block for clinical assessments.) Judging from the results of Solomon and Munson (2004), the best estimate of maximum lingual strength is obtained with the jaw either free or fixed at a small incisal opening. It should be noted that repeated high-effort trials may effect speech production (Solomon, 2000), so it is wise to permit adequate rest periods between high-effort tasks and other tasks directed to assess speech articulation.

Deep Assessment Deep testing by means of auditory-perceptual methods typically involves more extended examinations that build on the screening assessments. For example, if it is suspected that the client may be compensating for impaired lingual articulation by reliance on jaw movements, a bite block can be used to fix the jaw. Greater demands on lingual articulation can be achieved by using speech samples loaded with lingual consonants, occurring either singly or in clusters.

Labial Function

Screening As in the assessment of lingual function, screening may be done while observing and listening to the client's conversational speech. Because the lips are readily visible, the examiner may be able to detect asymmetries, incomplete labial closures for bilabial stops, or other abnormalities. However, a caveat is in order: oral asymmetries during speech production are rather common in healthy subjects, especially in males (Hausmann, Behrendt-Korbitz, Kautz, Lamm, Radelt, & Gunturkun, 1998). Additional information can be gathered by observing lip shapes and movements during smiling, laughing, and other emotional expressions. Lip seal can be assessed for the tasks of chewing and swallowing.

Deep Assessment Deep testing involves challenges to the labial musculature by means of changes in speaking rate, use of a bite block to eliminate possible contribution of jaw movements to labial articulation, or testing with speech materials that are heavily loaded with labial gestures (e.g., labial and labiodental consonants produced with rounded and spread-lip vowels). A simple way to assess the strength of lip compression is to ask the client to hold an object such as a straw or tongue depressor firmly between the lips, taking care not to bite the object with the teeth. Then the examiner tries to pull the object out of the client's labial embrace. This task can be repeated at different positions to test for asymmetries in lip strength.

◆ Assessment of Orosensory Function

Examination of orosensory function is probably one of the most neglected and uncertain areas in contemporary clinical assessment. Although it is true that careful, quantitative assessment of sensory function requires special-purpose equipment, the clinician can assess sensory function with inexpensive instruments and simple tasks. Sensory examination is especially indicated in trigeminal nerve damage, localized cerebral lesions, Parkinson's disease, oral apraxia, head injury, and any severe motor involvement of the orofacial system (Kent, Martin, & Sufit, 1990).

The following procedures are discussed only briefly. More detailed information is available in several sources (Jacobs, Wu, Van Loven, Desnyder, Kolenaar, & Van Steenberghed, 2002; Kent et al, 1990).

Light Static Touch   The client is asked to respond whenever the clinician touches a monofilament to the client's skin. Commercially available monofilaments come with a range of stiffnesses. This task is static insofar as the stimulation is at one location and may be sustained (but note that different mechanoreceptors may be stimulated by short- versus long-term stimulation). Sensory innervation of the face is supplied by the three branches of cranial nerve V (trigeminal nerve): ophthalmic (V_1), maxillary (V_2), and mandibular (V_3). Static touch is especially used for testing the function of slowly adapting mechanoreceptors. An advantage of testing light static touch is that no motor response is required of the client except to report when a stimulus is felt. The examination may reveal abnormalities such as hypesthesia or asymmetrical sensitivity.

Kinetic Touch   The client is asked to indicate either verbally or with a manual gesture the direction of motion of a monofilament or rod that is drawn across the skin or mucosal surface. This procedure is easily accomplished with stimulation of the lips or tongue. Kinetic touch is relayed by rapidly adapting mechanoreceptors. A degree of control over stimulus variables can be effected as follows: (1) traverse length: move the monofilament from the midline to the lateral aspects of a structure (or vice versa); (2) touch pressure: use a monofilament that bends as the desired force is applied; and (3) movement velocity: practice using a smooth, steady motion in a specified time. The primary objective in testing kinetic sensitivity is to determine if the client can reliably detect the direction of a moving stimulus.

Double-Simultaneous Touch   The clinician touches either one part of the client's face (e.g., the cheek) or two parts (e.g., the cheek and the lip). The client is asked to report whether one or two parts were touched. This task can be used with the speech structures by selecting pairs such as lip–tongue, right lip–left lip, and so on. Some neurological disorders impair the ability to detect simultaneous stimulation, and poor performance on this task may indicate the need for a more detailed examination.

◆ Assessment of Communicative Functions

In most of the assessment considered to this point, communication per se was not of central interest. Rather, the effort was to assess the sensory and motor functions of physiological components of the speech production system. As these components are harnessed to the goals of communication, a new set of issues emerges. The concern now is with intelligibility, quality, prosody, and fluency.

Intelligibility

At its root, intelligibility means understanding. A message is intelligible if a recipient can understand it. Likewise, a speaker is intelligible if listeners can understand messages produced by that speaker. A variety of tools have been developed to measure intelligibility. They differ in choice of analysis unit (typically, word or sentence), response of the examiner (rating scale, transcription, or closed-set word choice), and even the purpose of the test (overall intelligibility, analysis of intelligibility failures). The most commonly used clinical assessment is the Assessment of Intelligibility of Dysarthric Speech (AIDS) (Yorkston, Beukelman, & Traynor, 1984), which is used to quantify single-word intelligibility, sentence intelligibility, and speaking rate of adult and adolescent individuals with dysarthria. Single-word tests have been developed primarily for research purposes (Kent, Weismer, Kent, & Rosenbek, 1989), with the particular objective of analyzing the phonetic factors underlying intelligibility failures.

The clinical rating of conversational intelligibility is motivated by the beliefs that discourse has the highest external validity (Frearson, 1985) and that discourse is perhaps the single speaking task that reflects the full demands of speech communication. Netsell (1983) stated, "The activation of the speech neural mechanisms with meaningful speech may be the only valid test of function for the speech motor system" (p. 10). The methods proposed for the assessment of conversational intelligibility include transcription (Frearson, 1985; Metz, Samar, Schiavetti, Sitler, & Whitehead, 1985), comprehensibility (Beukelman & Yorkston, 1979; Yorkston, Strand, & Kennedy, 1996), equal-appearing interval scaling (De Bodt, Hernandez-Diaz Huici, & Van De Heyning, 2002), and direct-magnitude estimates (Yunusova et al, 2005).

Several approaches have been proposed for the assessment of intelligibility in children (Gordon-Brannan &

Hodson, 2000; Kent, Miolo, & Bloedel, 1994). Some of the most promising instruments are the preschool speech intelligibility measure (Morris, Wilcox, & Schooling, 1995) and the Test of Children's Speech (TOCS) under development by Megan Hodge of the University of Alberta. The TOCS+ project now underway will move the TOCS to a computer-based platform, which will greatly expand its capabilities. The new system will be called the Test of Children's Speech and Spelling Plus (TOCS+). Alternatively, the Sentence Repetition Screening Test may be suitable as a screening instrument. This test has been shown to have acceptable sensitivity, specificity, and predictive validity for language and articulation disorders (Sturner, Funk, & Green, 1996).

Quality

Voice quality is defined as "that attribute of auditory sensation in terms of which a listener can judge that two sounds similarly presented and having the same loudness and pitch are dissimilar" (ANSI Standard S1.1.12.9, p. 45). Quality is multidimensional and includes aspects of both phonation and resonance. A number of different techniques have been proposed for the assessment of quality (Kent & Ball, 2000), but there does not appear to be a single instrument that is used widely in the assessment of speech disorders. Certainly, quality is included in composite-examination instruments such as the rating scales developed by Darley et al (1969a,b).

Prosody

Prosody is an aspect of speech that includes speaking rate, rhythm, intonation, and stress. Each of these can be difficult to assess with adequate validity and reliability. Components of prosody are included in the composite instruments of Darley et al (1969a,b) and the Frenchay Dysarthria Assessment (Enderby, 1983). Instruments specific to prosody also have been developed, but these apparently have not been adequately tested with individuals with motor speech disorders. Shriberg (1993) introduced a Prosody-Voice Profile consisting of three prosody categories (phrasing, rate, stress) along with four voice categories (loudness, pitch, laryngeal features, resonance features).

Perceptual rating of prosodic dimensions is not as straightforward as it may seem. For example, studies on perceptual rating of speaking rate show that listeners' perceptual ratings may differ in some respects from quantitative measures of rate, such as syllables/s (Nishio & Niimi, 2001; Tjaden, 2000). Impressionistic judgments of speaking rate probably are biased by factors such as adequacy of articulation and overall prosody.

Fluency

Fluency is an aspect of several neurogenic disorders. Although there is a long history of research on children and adults, there are few assessment instruments with demonstrated validity and reliability. Riley's (1994) Stuttering Severity Instrument for Children and Adults meets a validity criterion, but the reliability has not been adequately established (Biddle et al, 2002). The clinician can always analyze disfluencies according to a time-honored taxonomy (Peters & Guitar, 1991), but it should be recognized that issues of validity and reliability limit confidence in the results. Chapter 14 discusses this issue.

◆ Conclusion

The clinician's ears, eyes, and sometimes fingers are the essential tools in a PSME, which remains the central, and sometimes sole, assessment for a motor speech disorder in most clinical situations. Although serious issues have yet to be addressed concerning the validity and reliability of these assessments, there is no other means readily available to answer the broad range of questions that the PSME can address. No other method of assessment can determine the presence of problems in the critical domains of intelligibility, voice, resonance, articulation, and prosody. To be sure, instrumental assessment can add much to a perceptual examination, but the former without the latter is often hollow.

Acknowledgment This work was supported in part by research grant R01 DC00319 of the National Institute on Deafness and Other Communication Disorders/National Institutes of Health.

References

Ackermann, H., Hertrich, I., & Hehr, T. (1995). Oral diadochokinesis in neurological dysarthrias. *Folia Phoniatrica et Logopaedica, 47*, 15–23

Arvedson, J.C. (2000). Evaluation of children with feeding and swallowing problems. *Language, Speech, and Hearing Services in Schools, 31*, 28–41

Beukelman, D.R. & Yorkston, K.M. (1979). The relationship between information transfer and speech intelligibility of dysarthric speakers. *Journal of Communication Disorders, 10*, 189–196

Bhuta, T., Patrick, L., & Garnett, J.D. (2004). Perceptual evaluation of voice quality and its correlation with acoustic measurements. *Journal of Voice, 18*, 299–304

Biddle, A., Watson, L., Hooper, C., et al. (2002). Criteria for determining disability in speech-language disorders. Evidence Report/Technology Assessment No. 52 (Prepared by the University of North Carolina Evidence-based Practice Center under Contract No. 290-97-0011). AHRQ Publication NO. 02-E010. Rockville, MD: Agency for Healthcare Research and Quality

Blumberger, J., Sullivan, S.J., & Clement, N., (1995). Diadochokinetic rate in persons with traumatic brain injury. *Brain Injury, 9*, 797–804

Bunton, K. Kent, R.D., Duffy, J.R., et al. (2007). Listener agreement for auditory perceptual ratings of dysarthia. *Journal of Speech, Language, and Hearing Research, 50*, 1481–1495

Clark, H.M. (2003). Neuromuscular treatments for speech and swallowing: a tutorial. *American Journal of Speech-Language Pathology, 12,* 400–415

Clark, H.M., Henson, P.A., Barber, W.D., Stierwalt, J.A.G., & Sherrill, M. (2003). Relationships among subjective and objective measures of tongue strength and oral phase swallowing movements. *American Journal of Speech-Language Pathology, 12,* 40–50

Crow, H.C. & Ship, J.A. (1996). Tongue strength and endurance in different aged individuals. *Journal of Gerontology A: Biological Sciences and Medical Sciences, 51,* M247–M250

Darley, F.L., Aronson, A.E., & Brown, J.R. (1969a). Differential diagnostic patterns of dysarthria. *Journal of Speech and Hearing Research, 12,* 249–269

Darley, F.L., Aronson, A.E., & Brown, J.R. (1969b). Cluster of deviant speech dimensions in the dysarthrias. *Journal of Speech and Hearing Research, 12,* 462–496

De Bodt, M.S., Hernandez-Diaz Huici, M.E., & Van De Heyning, P.H. (2002). Intelligibility as linear combination of dimensions in dysarthric speech. *Journal of Communication Disorders, 35,* 283–292

DePaul, R. (1989). Orofacial muscle weakness and motor control for speech in amyotrophic lateral sclerosis. Ph.D. dissertation, University of Wisconsin-Madison

Drummond, S. (1993). *Dysarthria Examination Battery.* San Antonio: Communication Skills Builders

Duffy, J.R. (1995). *Motor Speech Disorders: Substrates, Differential Diagnosis, and Management.* St. Louis: Mosby

Duffy, J.R. & Kent, R.D. (2001). Darley's contributions to the understanding, differential diagnosis, and scientific study of the dysarthrias. *Aphasiology, 15,* 275–289

Dworkin, J.P., Marunick, M.T., & Krouse, J.H. (2004). Velopharyngeal dysfunction: speech characteristics, variable etiologies, evaluation techniques, and differential treatments. *Language, Speech, and Hearing Services in Schools, 35,* 333–352

Enderby, P.M. (1983). *Frenchay Dysarthria Assessment.* San Diego: College-Hill Press

Forrest, K. (2002). Are oral-motor exercises useful in the treatment of phonological/articulatory disorders? *Seminars in Speech and Language, 23,* 15–26

Fox, D.R. & Johns, D. (1970). Predicting velopharyngeal closure with a modified tongue-anchor technique. *Journal of Speech and Hearing Disorders, 35,* 248–255

Frearson, B. (1985). A comparison of the AIDS sentence list and spontaneous speech intelligibility scores for dysarthric speech. *Australian Journal of Human Communication Disorders, 13,* 5–21

Gordon-Brannan, M. & Hodson, B.W. (2000). Intelligibility/severity measurements of prekindergarten children's speech. *American Journal of Speech-Language Pathology, 9,* 141–150

Hausmann, M., Behrendt-Korbitz, S., Kautz, H., Lamm, C., Radelt, F., & Gunturkun, O. (1998). Sex differences in oral asymmetries during word repetition. *Neuropsychologia, 36,* 1397–1402

Hayden, D.A. (1994). Differential diagnosis of motor speech dysfunction in children. *Clinics in Communication Disorders, 4,* 119–141

Hinton, V.A. & Arokiasamy, W.M.C. (1997). Maximum interlabial pressures in normal speakers. *Journal of Speech and Hearing Research, 40,* 400–404

Hixon, T.J., Hawley, J.L., & Wilson, K.J. (1982). An around-the-house device for the clinical determination of respiratory driving pressure: a note on making the simple even simpler. *Journal of Speech and Hearing Disorders, 47,* 413

Hixon, T.J. & Hoit, J.D. (1998). Physical examination of the diaphragm by the speech-language pathologists. *American Journal of Speech-Language Pathology, 9,* 37–45

Hixon, T.J. & Hoit, J. D. (1999). Physical examination of the abdominal wall by the speech-language pathologist. *American Journal of Speech-Language Pathology, 9,* 335–346

Hixon, T.J. & Hoit, J. D. (2000). Physical examination of the rib cage wall by the speech-language pathologist. *American Journal of Speech-Language Pathology, 9,* 179–196

Hodge, M. (1988). Speech mechanism assessment. In: D. Yoder & R. Kent (Eds.), *Decision Making in Speech-Language Pathology,* 104–109. Toronto: B.C. Decker

Hodge, M.M. (1993). Assessing early speech motor function. *Clinics in Communication Disorders, 2,* 69–86

Jacobs, R., Wu, C.-H., Van Loven, K., Desnyder, M., Kolenaar, B., & Van Steenberghed, D. (2002). Methodology of oral sensory tests. *Journal of Oral Rehabilitation, 29,* 720

Kent, R.D. (1994). *Reference Manual for Communicative Disorders and Sciences.* Austin: Pro-Ed

Kent, R.D. (1996). Hearing and believing: Some limits to the auditory-perceptual assessment of speech and voice disorders. *American Journal of Speech-Language Pathology, 7,* 7–23

Kent, R.D. (2004). The uniqueness of speech among motor systems. *Clinical Linguistics & Phonetics, 18,* 495–505

Kent, R.D. (in press). Speech motor control. To appear in H.-J. Freund, M. Jeannerod, M. Hallet, & R. Leiguarda (Eds.), *Higher-Order Motor Disorders.* Oxford, England: Oxford University Press

Kent, R.D. & Ball, M.J. (2000). *Voice Quality Measurement.* San Diego: Singular Publishing

Kent, R.D., Kent, J.F., & Rosenbek, J.C. (1987). Maximum performance tests of speech production. *Journal of Speech and Hearing Disorders, 52,* 367–387

Kent, R.D., Martin, R.E., & Sufit, R.L. (1990). Oral sensation: a review and clinical prospective. In H. Winitz (Ed.), *Human Communication and Its Disorders,* vol. 3 (pp. 135–191). Norwood, NJ: Ablex

Kent, R.D., Miolo, G., & Bloedel, S. (1994). The intelligibility of children's speech: a review of evaluation procedures. *American Journal of Speech-Language Pathology, 3,* 81–93

Kent, R.D., Weismer, G., Kent, J.F., & Rosenbek, J.C. (1989). Toward phonetic intelligibility testing in dysarthria. *Journal of Speech and Hearing Disorders, 54,* 482–499

Kreiman, J., Gerratt, B.R., & Prodoca, K. (1990). Listener experience and perception of voice quality. *Journal of Speech and Hearing Research, 33,* 103–115

Kummer, A. & Lee, L. (1996). Evaluation and treatment of resonance disorders. *Language, Speech, and Hearing Services in Schools, 27,* 271–281

Lee, L., Stemple, J.C., Glaze, L., & Kelchner, L. (2004). Quick screen for voice and supplementary documents for identifying pediatric voice disorders. *Language, Speech, and Hearing Sciences in Schools, 35,* 308–319

Lowit-Leuschel, A., & Doherty, G.J. (2001). Prosodic variation across sampling tasks in normal and dysarthric speakers. *Logopedics, Phoniatry, and Vocology, 26,* 151–164

Mason, R. and Simon, C. (1977). An orofacial examination checklist. *Language, Speech and Hearing Services in Schools, 10,* 155–163

McFarland, D.H. (2001). Respiratory markers of conversational interaction. *Journal of Speech, Language, and Hearing Research, 44,* 128–143

Metz, D.E., Samar, V.J., Schiavetti, N., Sitler, R.W., & Whitehead, R.L. (1985). Acoustic dimensions of hearing-impaired speakers intelligibility. *Journal of Speech and Hearing Research, 28,* 345–355

Mitchell, H.L., Hoit, J.C., & Watson, P.J. (1996). Cognitive-linguistic demands and speech breathing. *Journal of Speech, Language, and Hearing Research, 39,* 93–104.

Morris, S.R., Wilcox, K.A., & Schooling, T.L. (1995). The preschool speech intelligibility measure. *American Journal of Speech-Language Pathology, 4,* 22–28

Mortimore, I.L., Fiddes, P., Stephens, S., & Douglas, N.J. (1999). Tongue protrusion force and fatiguability in male and female subjects. *European Respiratory Journal, 14,* 191–195

Netsell, R. (1983). Speech motor control: theoretical issues with clinical impact. In: W.M. Berry (Ed.), *Clinical Dysarthria* (pp. 1–20). San Diego. College-Hill Press

Netsell, R. (1985). Construction and use of a bite-block for the evaluation and treatment of speech disorders. *Journal of Speech and Hearing Disorders, 50*, 103–106

Nishio, M. & Niimi, S. (2001). Speaking rate and its components in dysarthric speakers. *Clinical Linguistics and Phonetics, 15*, 309–317

Peters, T.J. & Guitar, B. (1991). *Stuttering: An Integrated Approach to Its Nature and Treatment.* Baltimore: Williams & Wilkins

Potter, N.L. (2004). *Oral/Speech and Manual Motor Development in Preschool Children.* Unpublished Ph.D. dissertation, University of Wisconsin-Madison

Renout, K.A., Leeper, H.A., Bandur, D.L., & Hudson, A. J. (1995). Vocal fold diadochokinetic function of individuals with amyotrophic lateral sclerosis. *American Journal of Speech-Language Pathology, 4*, 73–80

Riley, G.D. (1994). *Stuttering Severity Instrument for Children and Adults*, 3rd ed. Austin: Pro-Ed

Robbins, J. & Klee, T. (1987). Clinical assessment of oropharyngeal motor development in young children. *Journal of Speech and Hearing Disorders, 52*, 271–277

Robertson, S.J. (1982). *Dysarthria Profile.* London: Winslow Press

Ruscello, D., St. Louis, K., Barry, P., & Barr, K. (1982). A screening method for the evaluation of the peripheral speech mechanism. *Folia Phoniatrica, 34*, 324–330

Samlan, R. & Weismer, G. (1995). The relationship of selected perceptual measures of diadochokinesis to speech intelligibility in dysarthric speakers with amyotrophic lateral sclerosis. *American Journal of Speech-Language Pathology, 4*, 9–13

Sheard, C., Adams, R.D., & Davis, P.J. (1991). Reliability and agreement of ratings of ataxic dysarthric speech with varying intelligibility. *Journal of Speech and Hearing Research, 34*, 285–293

Shriberg, L.D. (1993). Four new speech and prosody measures for genetics research and other studies in developmental phonological disorders. *Journal of Speech and Hearing Research, 36*, 105–140

Solomon, N.P. (2000). Changes in normal speech after fatiguing the tongue. *Journal of Speech, Language, and Hearing Research, 43*, 1416–1428

Solomon, N.P. & Munson, B. (2004). The effect of jaw position on measures of tongue strength and endurance. *Journal of Speech, Language, and Hearing Research, 47*, 584–594

Sperry, E.E. & Klich, R.J. (1992). Speech breathing in senescent and younger women during oral reading. *Journal of Speech, Language, and Hearing Research, 35*, 1246–1255

Strand, E.A. & McCauley, R.J. (1999). Assessment procedures for treatment planning in children with phonologic and motor speech disorders. In: A.J. Caruso & E.A. Strand (Eds.), *Clinical Management of Motor Speech Disorders in Children* (pp. 73–107). New York: Thieme

Sturner, R.A., Funk, S.G., & Green, J.A. (1996). Preschool speech and language screening: further validation of the sentence repetition screening test. *Journal of Developmental and Behavioral Pediatrics, 17*, 405–413

Tasko, S.M. & McClean, M.D. (2004). Variations in articulatory movement with changes in speech task. *Journal of Speech, Language, and Hearing Research, 47*, 85–100

Theodoros, D., Russel, T.G., Hill, A., Cahill, L., & Clark, K. (2003). Assessment of motor speech disorders online: a pilot study. *Journal of Telemedicine and Telecare, 9* (suppl 2), S66–S68

Tjaden, K. (2000). A preliminary study of factors influencing perception of articulatory rate in Parkinson disease. *Journal of Speech, Language, and Hearing Research, 43*, 997–1010

Yorkston, K., Beukelman, D.R., & Traynor, C.D. (1984). *Computerized Assessment of Intelligibility and Dysarthric Speech.* Austin: Pro-Ed

Yorkston, K.M., Spencer, K., Duffy, J., Beukelman, D., Golper, L.A., Miller, R., Strand, E., & Sullivan, M. (2001). Evidence-based practice guidelines for dysarthria: management of velopharyngeal function. *Journal of Medical Speech-Language Pathology, 4*, 257–274

Yorkston, K.M., Strand, E.A., & Kennedy, M.R.T. (1996). Comprehensibility of dysarthric speech: implications for assessment and treatment planning. *American Journal of Speech-Language Pathology, 5*, 55–66

Yunusova, Y., Weismer, G., Westbury, J.R., Kent, R.D., & Rusche, N.M. (submitted). Speech intelligibility of phrasal material in dysarthria: characteristics and underlying correlates

Wang, Y.-T., Kent, R.D., Duffy, J.R., Thomas, J.E., & Weismer, G. (2004). Syllable alternating motion rates as an index of motor speech abilities in traumatic brain injury. *Clinical Linguistics and Phonetics, 18*, 57–84

Webb, A.L., Carding, P.N., Deary, I.J., MacKenzie, K., Steen, N., & Wilson, J.A. (2004). The reliability of three perceptual evaluation scales for dysphonia. *European Archives of Otorhinolaryngology, 26*, 429–434

Weismer, G. (2005). Philosophy of research in motor speech disorders. *Clinical Linguistics and Phonetics, 20*, 315–349.

Wuyts, F.L., De Bodt, M.S., & Van de Heyning, P.H. (1999). Is the reliability of a visual analog scale higher than an ordinal scale? An experiment with the GRBAS scale for the perceptual evaluation of dysphonia. *Journal of Voice, 13*, 508–517

Yunosova, Y., Weismer, G., Kent, R.D., & Rusche, N. (2005). Breath group intelligibility in dysarthria: characteristics and underlying correlates. *Journal of Speech, Language, and Hearing Research, 48*, 1294–1310.

Zraick, R.I., & Liss, J.M. (2000). A comparison of equal-appearing interval scaling and direct magnitude estimation of nasal voice quality. *Journal of Speech, Language, and Hearing Research, 43*, 979–988

Chapter 3

Nonspeech Assessment of the Speech Production Mechanism

Kirrie J. Ballard, Nancy Pearl Solomon, Donald A. Robin, Jerald B. Moon, and John W. Folkins

The assessment of nonspeech abilities has long been a part of the clinical examination of individuals with suspected speech problems, particularly those with potential motor speech disorders. The oral mechanism examination is replete with nonspeech tasks, as are other types of tests used by speech-language pathologists. For instance, Darley, Aronson, and Brown (1975), in their description of examination for dysarthria and apraxia of speech, recommend several nonspeech observations and maneuvers. There continues to be debate over the utility of nonspeech tasks for informing studies of speech motor control as well as clinical diagnosis and treatment planning (e.g., Weismer, 2006; Weismer & Liss, 1991). Studies have reached different conclusions, seemingly based on the type of motor speech disorder studied, the severity of the disorder, the purpose of the investigation, and especially the specific measurements taken. There is also debate about the utility of using nonspeech tasks during the therapeutic management of motor speech disorders (e.g., Clark, 2003; Forrest, 2002). It is not the purpose of this chapter to challenge these positions, but rather to present an approach to the evaluation of the speech production system that incorporates the use of both nonspeech and speech tasks in the clinic.

It is our contention that nonspeech tasks can provide useful information about the functioning of the motor system that aids in differential diagnosis and in understanding a person's ability to communicate using the speech production system. The combined use of nonspeech and speech tasks is beneficial if one's goal is to determine the integrity of the speech motor system. This chapter considers two different uses of nonspeech tasks in assessment of the motor speech mechanism: isolating the specific involvement of subsystems and guiding differential diagnosis. We then present examples of nonspeech procedures available to the speech-language pathologist and examine their clinical utility.

◆ Use of Nonspeech Assessment in Examining Subsystems

Assessment of motor control in performance of nonspeech tasks potentially permits the clinician to develop hypotheses about the nature and locus of primary impairments underlying difficulties in speech. Tasks can be structured to examine movement control in a single articulator, free of the demands of coordinating multiple articulators, or in a nonverbal context, free of the demands of linguistic formulation. Tasks can then be systematically manipulated through levels of complexity to examine the change in performance as coordination and interaction of multiple structures is introduced, allowing for interpretation of motor involvement and strategies of compensation (Barlow & Netsell, 1986). That is, it may be informative for the clinician to separate motoric and linguistic contributions to the motor speech disorder to more accurately define a patient's difficulties and, thus, design targeted intervention. For example, sustaining phonation on the vowel /a/ is a task that is probably included in every speech pathologist's examination of the motor speech system. It allows one to examine the integrity of the respiratory-phonatory subsystems in a relatively simple motor task without the confounds of more complex motoric adjustments or complex pragmatic, syntactic, and semantic overlays (Duffy, 1995; Folkins et al, 1995; Kent & Kent, 2000; Kent & Kim, 2003).

On the one hand, Weismer and colleagues (e.g., Weismer, 2006; Weismer & Liss, 1991) have argued against assessment of articulatory function in isolation because articulators do not operate in isolation during speech, and so this approach may not provide information relevant to functioning during speech. McClean and Tasko (2002) demonstrated considerable neural coupling of jaw, laryngeal, and respiratory systems during speech production by healthy adults. Nonetheless, others (Darley et al, 1975; Duffy, 1995; Kent & Kent, 2000; Netsell & Rosenbek, 1985; Yorkston, Beukelman, Strand, & Bell, 1999) have promoted the consideration of differential subsystem involvement during the assessment and management of motor speech disorders. Netsell and Rosenbek (1985) noted that each of the major speech production subsystems can be affected differentially following neurological insult. Furthermore, there may be differential involvement within a given major system (e.g., upper lip versus lower lip). During speech production, the structures work together as functional units to achieve the goal of perceptually accurate speech. Thus, different combinations of movements can be used for the same speech task. Consequently, during speech, individuals with motor speech disorders often show compensations between and within the components of speech motor subsystems. As a result, the clinician does not know if the resultant movements are caused by primary motor involvement of a given structure, or if they result from compensation of a given structure for the motor impairment of a different speech structure.

Murdoch and colleagues (Horton, Murdoch, Theodorus, & Thompson, 1997; Murdoch, Johnson, & Theodoros, 1997) noted that without analysis of subsystem integrity, they would not have accurately identified the underlying impairments in their patients and may not have defined appropriate treatment goals.

Functional Ranges of a System

The maximal limit of a given structure is the envelope within which it can function. Every structure has an envelope that defines the limits of its function. Although we usually think of spatial envelopes—how far a structure can move—the concept applies to other movement parameters such as velocity or force. The operating range of the system or structure for speech then defines the range within the envelope that is habitually used. The concept of operating range is important when considering the clinical utility of nonspeech tasks. For example, Zimmermann (1980) has suggested that nonfluency results when the motor system exceeds its operating range during speech and the speaker does not have the control to compensate for these excursions.

We do not know the operating range of all of the systems of speech production. Some systems or structures may have very restricted ranges and therefore be more prone to disruption than others. The operating range of speech (at least in the laboratory) appears for many different areas to be approximately 10 to 25% of the envelope. It is important for clinicians to know if the envelope is reduced, if the operating range is reduced or expanded in relation to the envelope, or if the operating range is shifted toward one extreme. Thus, for speech produced under conditions with little stress or demand, 10 to 25% of the range may well be adequate. Normal speakers have the flexibility to handle the inherent variability that occurs when producing the same speech in various contexts. However, speakers with a reduced envelope may be prone to breakdown in situations where the demands or stresses on the system are high and there is a need to exceed the typical operating range of speech, such as high velocity movements (i.e., be more likely to produce speech errors or be restricted to unnaturally slow rates of speech) (Clark, 2003; Dworkin, Aronson, & Mulder, 1980; Luschei, 1991).

As an example, it is estimated that the amount of maximal strength of the articulators used during speech production is approximately 20% maximal strength during quiet, slow production of single words or simple phrases (Barlow & Burton, 1990; Searl, 2003). The speaker whose maximal strength is reduced by 50% due to neurological involvement may produce adequate speech during word production at a relatively slow rate, but may not be able to produce perceptually accurate speech at normal or faster speech rates due to an inability to hit articulatory targets in the appropriate time frame. Reduced strength decreases the shortening velocity of muscle fibers and therefore reduces the speed of movement. This reiterates our previous point that an examination of the motor speech system ideally involves systematically varying the level of motoric and linguistic constraints to define the impairment fully and design appropriate intervention.

Flexibility, Compensation, and Plasticity

The concepts of envelopes (i.e., ranges of maximal performance) and operating ranges are closely related to the notions of flexibility, compensation, and plasticity (Folkins, 1985). Physiological parameters of speech vary when the same speech sample is reproduced repeatedly in the same context. As long as this variability remains within the operating range of the motor system, perceptually accurate speech can occur. Flexibility is the outcome of a system that is organized around functional units. With functional units, different combinations of articulatory movements can be used for the same speech task. As an extreme example, the operating range of a structure can be reduced to zero (e.g., when we place a pencil between our teeth and continue to talk with high perceptual accuracy), and other structures (e.g., lips and tongue) will adjust to ensure perfectly intelligible speech output (Ballard, Flemmer, & Moon, 2004; Gay, Lindblom, & Lubker 1981; Kelso & Tuller, 1983). However, in some cases, the context may cause or require movement to exceed the operating range. Speakers with intact motor control are flexible enough to handle most instances of divergence and are able to produce accurate speech. This inherent flexibility is critical when the neuromotor system is damaged and one or more systems are constantly driven outside the habitual operating range (i.e., the operating range is shifted toward one extreme or there is excessive variability in performance), or the relationship between the envelope and the operating range is changed. The ability to compensate for a more permanent alteration in the system would then be called compensation.

A person's ability to compensate may be dictated by several factors. Flexibility may be reduced by the impairment or, alternatively, the impact of the impairment on the system may cause excessive changes or variability in movement parameters such that normal levels of flexibility are inadequate. In these cases, speech will not be produced accurately (Ballard et al, 2004). Solomon, Garlitz, and Milbrath (2000a) noted that dysarthria may only become apparent when the maximal envelope is reduced to a "critical level" so that there is little functional reserve to accommodate changes to, or excursions outside, the habitual operating range. Flexibility and compensation are important concepts to consider when examining a person's prognosis with therapeutic intervention. Amenability of an impairment to treatment (i.e., plasticity, Folkins, 1985) is likely related to a person's ability to manipulate operating ranges of affected and unaffected structures across a range of contextual demands, defined through nonspeech assessment tasks.

Relationships Between Performance on Nonspeech and Speech Tasks

Several studies have explored whether speech deficits such as poor intelligibility correlate with measures that reflect the operating range of articulators. Three studies have examined correlations among tongue strength, endurance, and rate of repetitive movements in nonspeech tasks in individuals with traumatic brain injury (TBI) (Goozee, Murdoch, & Theodoros, 2001), cerebrovascular accident (Thompson, Murdoch, & Stokes, 1995), and Parkinson's disease (Solomon, Robin, & Luschei, 2000b). Whereas these studies and others found differences in strength, endurance, and fatigability in subjects with dysarthria compared with healthy control groups (see Clark 2003 for a review), they reported weak or insignificant correlations between the measures of tongue function and perceptual judgments of articulation such as consonant imprecision and vowel distortions. Goozee et al contended that this does not warrant abandoning nonspeech measures, but rather these results motivate further research to explore the reasons behind strong versus weak correlations and relationships across a range of tasks. For example, they suggested that the lack of a strong correlation between nonspeech and speech tasks in their study may have been due to compensatory behaviors reducing perceived deficits or insufficient overlap in articulators involved and movement requirements for the two types of tasks studied. Further, they posited that stronger correlations may have emerged if speech tasks had focused on production of lingual consonants. Indeed, Solomon (2000) found that sentences loaded with lingual consonants sounded less precise after normal speakers fatigued their tongues through exercise. Alternately, Clark (2003) suggested that measures of power, or the speed at which a given force is produced in an articulator, might yield higher correlations with measures of speech function.

In addition to the issues raised by Goozee et al (2001) and Clark (2003), other topics need to be considered in attempting to understand the relationship between nonspeech and speech function. First, perceptual judgments of speech (such as intelligibility measures) are vital to establishing the functional status of a patient (Duffy, 1995). If speech and nonspeech performance correlated strongly, then the purpose of conducting nonspeech assessments may seem unclear. Rather, we contend that nonspeech tasks can be used to add information to the clinical picture. Nonspeech assessment is not a surrogate for measuring perceptual accuracy. If some aspect of speech performance is identified as disordered, an important role of nonspeech tasks is to help identify the subsystem impairments underlying the problem and the degree to which other structures are already compensating. This will lead to more informed treatment decisions.

Whereas nonspeech tasks may seem artificial for understanding speech production, a detailed analysis of such performance may reveal underlying deficits that are otherwise obscured. However, a typical examination will also include speaking tasks to examine the integrated functioning of the subsystems with overlying linguistic demands. Ideally, the clinician should systematically vary the level of constraint (motoric and linguistic) and determine how they interact to affect speech production. Tasko and McClean (2004) caution that movement of articulators (e.g., displacement, velocity, and duration) can vary across different speech tasks and recommend testing under a range of speech tasks and conditions to evaluate integrity of the system. The level of breakdown and pattern of performance across tasks should be related to type of motor speech disorder, severity, presence of concomitant linguistic impairment, and probably a host of other factors.

◆ Use of Nonspeech Assessment in Differential Diagnosis

In their seminal work at the Mayo Clinic, Darley et al (1975) advocated for the use of both nonspeech and speech level tasks in assessing and diagnosing motor speech disorders. In this approach, performance on each task is used to identify key perceptual characteristics and clustering of characters to converge on a diagnosis. Such an approach to diagnosis can lead to testable hypotheses regarding the locus or loci of damage in the nervous system and disease processes involved. More recently, others have extended the Mayo Clinic perceptual assessment method by incorporating a host of acoustic measurements that can be made using the same basic assessment tasks (e.g., Kent & Kim 2003; Kent, Weismer, Kent, Vorperian, & Duffy, 1999). Furthermore, we now have a greater understanding about how the various forms of motor speech disorder can differentially affect different tasks. Kent & Kent (2000) stated that "The features of a given dysarthria often vary with the speaking task, and this profile of task-dependency, which varies with the locus of damage in the nervous system, affords insights into the responsible neural lesion and its effects on the motor regulation of speech" (p. 48). This has led to research aimed at developing "task-based profiles" of motor speech disorders (e.g., Kent & Kent, 2000; Ziegler, 2002).

As an example of task-dependent motor skill, we briefly review some studies examining relationships between performance on alternating motion rate (AMR) tasks, that is, rapid repetition of a single syllable such as "pa") and connected speech. Relatively high correlations between the duration of syllables during AMR tasks and of the same syllables during sentence production have been reported in healthy adults and individuals with various types of motor speech disorder (e.g., Wang, Kent, Duffy, Thomas, & Weismer, 2004; Ziegler, 2002). However, Ziegler (2002) observed that the relationship between these two tasks is not consistent across motor speech disorders. For example, ataxic speakers produced shorter syllable durations in connected speech than in AMR tasks, replicating Kent, Kent, Rosenbek, Vorperian, and Weismer (1997), whereas apraxic speakers showed the reverse pattern. In terms of variability, healthy adults are highly consistent in syllable duration during alternating syllable repetition, and protracted durations or increased variability can be important indicators of neurological damage (Kent et al, 1997, 2000; Kent & Kim, 2003; Wang et al, 2004; Ziegler, 2002). Ziegler (2002) found that all types of motor speech disorders that he studied demonstrated greater variability of syllable duration than healthy adults.

It should be noted, however, that one must be cautious when interpreting reports of relationships, or lack thereof, between tasks. Darley et al (1975) and Duffy (1995) support using a range of tasks and a consensus approach whereby a diagnosis is proposed based on performance across many tasks. For example, Ziegler (2002) reported that ataxic dysarthria and apraxia of speech have different effects on average syllable duration for speech-like AMR tasks versus connected speech tasks. Based on these observations, Ziegler has argued that these two tasks are controlled by different mechanisms and so the AMR task is not informative in evaluations of motor speech disorders. Kent et al (1997), on the other hand, found similar results to Ziegler (2002) for their ataxic group but concluded that the AMR task revealed a basic underlying impairment in temporal regulation.

In the case of apraxia of speech, the inclusion of the AMR task may be more informative when considered alongside other tasks such as sequential motion rate (SMR; i.e., repeating a three syllable sequence such as /p/-/t/-/k/). It is commonly accepted that speakers with apraxia frequently have greater difficulty performing SMR than AMR tasks. This does not necessarily mean that repeating a single syllable and repeating a three-syllable sequence are controlled by different mechanisms. Rather, the different performance might reflect the levels of articulatory complexity of these two tasks, independent of linguistic status. If so, then including a range of tasks from AMR to SMR to more complicated speech-like tasks should provide information on the influence of articulatory complexity, separate from linguistic complexity. The use of any task should be driven by the questions one needs to answer. For any task (nonspeech or speech), we would urge clinicians to evaluate the specific rationale for its use and whether or not data are available in the literature to support their rationale.

Nonspeech measures have long been part of the speech evaluation for people with sensorimotor involvement. If one is aware of the various profiles of deficit in the different motor speech disorders and how these emerge across a range of tasks, then including nonspeech tasks in an assessment may aid in differential diagnosis (Kent & Kent, 2000). They may provide information about the absence or presence of neurological diseases as well as disease progression and treatment effects (medical or behavioral). Such measures may show change before associated changes in auditory perceptual characteristics of speech occur (i.e., subclinical signs). Below we review a sampling of nonspeech tasks that can be included in the evaluation of patients with sensorimotor impairments.

◆ Examples of Nonspeech Tasks for Assessment of Motor Speech Disorders

Respiratory System

Because the respiratory system is composed of the pulmonary system and the chest-wall system, the respiratory evaluation should address these two components separately. A speech-language pathologist with a spirometer and commercially available software can conduct a variety of tests. The most common screening test for pulmonary dysfunction involves a maximal forced exhalation. If at least 80% of the forced vital capacity (FVC) is exhaled in the first second (forced expiratory volume in 1 second [FEV_1]; calculated as FEV_1/FVC) of this maneuver, then the client passes the screening. If not, then performance may be indicative of lower airway collapse, and the patient should be referred for a thorough pulmonary examination. Using the spirometer, the speech-language pathologist can also assess vital capacity, or the maximum amount of lung volume that a person can access (the total lung capacity also includes residual volume, which is inaccessible during life). If the vital capacity is markedly reduced compared with expected values for that person's gender, age, height, and other relevant factors, then the person may have a neuromuscular limitation. **Figure 3–1** illustrates the pulmonary function screening test for a woman recently diagnosed with bulbar amyotrophic lateral sclerosis (ALS). This performance, which represents her best of three attempts, passes the screening, indicating pulmonary function within normal limits. Her vital capacity is also close to that predicted for a woman of her age and size, but this should be closely monitored as her disease progresses.

Involvement of the pulmonary or neuromuscular chest-wall system can reduce the envelope or operating range of the respiratory system, which may affect a person's ability to produce speech. Consequences can include reduced utterance length, abnormal neuromuscular control, and increased effort for speaking. Respiratory dysfunction, whether pulmonary or neuromuscular, can negatively impact speech breathing, complications from dysphagia, and overall well-being. Knowledge of the speaker's speech-breathing abilities

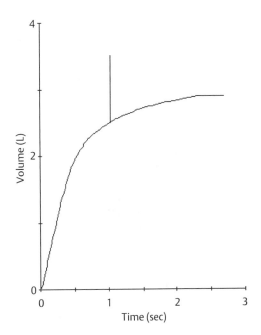

Figure 3–1 Forced vital capacity (FVC) maneuver by a 53-year-old woman recently diagnosed with bulbar amyotrophic lateral sclerosis (ALS). Maximum inspiration is plotted at 0 L volume. FVC was 2.9 L (91% of predicted) and the forced expiratory volume in 1 second (FEV_1) was 2.52 L, as indicated by the vertical line on the curve, resulting in a ratio (FEV_1/FVC) of 87%. This patient passed the screening for pulmonary dysfunction.

should assist the clinician in designing appropriate intervention strategies.

Evaluation of breathing for speech can be structured around a four-parameter approach, as taught by Hixon (1993) and described by Solomon and Charron (1998) and Hixon and Hoit (2005). The four parameters are lung pressure, lung volume, air flow, and chest-wall shape. Information regarding these parameters provides a relatively complete functional description of resting and speech breathing. The passive (recoil, rebound, gravity) and active (muscular) forces used to cause changes in these parameters are not measured directly during a typical clinical assessment, but generally can be inferred from the results. Briefly, during resting breathing, inspiration is accomplished by diaphragm contraction, and expiration occurs through passive forces until the lungs and chest wall reach a state of equilibrium. This occurs at the end-expiratory level (EEL). Relaxing the chest wall at EEL results in the resting expiratory level (REL), which serves as an important reference point for interpreting breathing events.

Much of what we know about passive and active forces for speech breathing comes from the work of Hixon (1987). During speech, a relatively constant pressure is delivered to the larynx and upper airway so that speech is adequately loud. Because passive forces vary across the lung volume, our neuromuscular systems must contend with constantly changing passive forces while we speak. This is a delicate balancing act that our brains are designed to perform with little or no awareness by us. To deliver the target net pressure, we vary contractions provided by a variety of expiratory and some inspiratory muscles at different portions of an utterance. At high lung volumes, inspiratory forces are used to hold back or brake against high recoil forces. At middle and low lung volumes, expiratory forces are needed to maintain adequate pressures and resist rebound forces. Importantly, the abdominal muscles (which provide expiratory forces) are active to varying degrees throughout speech breathing because they provide a supportive base for the other muscles to work against (Hoit, Plassman, Lansing, & Hixon, 1988).

The pressure delivered to the larynx by the lungs, necessary for phonation to occur, can be estimated by placing one end of a small tube in the mouth and connecting the other end to a pressure transducer (Rothenberg, 1973). A U-tube manometer with a leak to simulate laryngeal resistance can also be used (Netsell & Hixon, 1978). In both methods, the patient repeats a /p/+V syllable at a slow rate with the vowel sustained. A flow mask placed over the mouth and nose is used to ensure that air flow ceases during the closed phase of /p/, and the pressure peak is then used as an estimate of tracheal (subglottal) pressure during a speech-like utterance. An even simpler, more readily available, technique for measuring lung pressure was described by Hixon, Hawley, and Wilson (1982). It involves having the patient blow through a straw into a glass of water. Fix the straw so that its tip is 5 cm below the surface of the water, and have the patient blow just until bubbles come out. This indicates that the patient can generate 5 cm H_2O pressure. If she or he can sustain that pressure for 5 seconds, the pressure is considered to be adequate for speech purposes. Perceptually, tracheal pressure is reflected in vocal loudness. Thus, prolonging phonation with adequate and steady loudness indicates good generation and control of tracheal pressure. However, laryngeal interactions make this assessment somewhat difficult to interpret.

Lung volume refers to how much air is used to speak (lung volume excursion), and where within the vital capacity (VC) speech occurs. Typically, we use approximately 20% of the VC for speech, and speak in the midrange of the VC. Lung volume can be assessed with a spirometer, by integrating a flow signal obtained with a pneumotachograph, or by measuring motions of the chest wall and calibrating this to ascertain the volume measures. Lung volume excursion can be judged perceptually by the duration of speech phrases produced on one breath, assuming that air flow is within normal limits.

Air flow is a measure of the amount of lung volume expended over time, and can be assessed with a spirometer, pneumotachometer, or chest-wall kinematics. During phonation, high air flows may be perceived as breathiness. In many cases, breathy phonation may reflect laryngeal abnormalities rather than respiratory dysfunction. Assessing flow during nonspeech tasks can reveal characteristics of lower airway patency. Obstructive lung disease may lead to collapsing airways, and this can be detected during high-flow breathing tasks.

The shape and motions of the chest wall during speech can provide valuable insight regarding the muscular mechanisms used for speech. Motions of the rib cage and abdominal wall can be measured with respiratory inductive plethysmography or magnetometry. If these types of equipment are unavailable, assessment is still possible by watching or touching the patient's anterior torso during resting breathing, maximal-breathing tasks, and speech. A normal pattern of resting breathing involves outward movement of both the rib cage and abdomen during inspiration, and inward movement of both parts of the chest wall during expiration. If this pattern is abnormal, important inferences regarding the passive and active forces that affect respiration can be made (e.g., Putnam & Hixon, 1983; Solomon & Hixon, 1993). Demands for speech breathing are superimposed on these basic respiratory functions. Normal chest-wall shape for speech generally involves an inward displacement of the abdominal wall and an outward displacement of the rib cage from their resting position. Usually, but not necessarily, both parts of the chest wall move inward during the speech utterance.

The timing of breathing for speech involves a quick inspiration followed by a slow expiration. Having a patient produce this pattern of breathing without phonation can provide insight into respiratory control without the interactions of laryngeal and upper airway valving. Indeed, assessment of speech breathing aside from the rest of the speech production mechanism is possible and important for drawing conclusions regarding the respiratory system's contribution to a speech disorder and possible compensations for other disordered subsystems. In a series of articles and a textbook, Hixon and Hoit (1998, 1999, 2000, 2005) provided detailed instructions, rationales, and score sheets for evaluation of the diaphragm, abdominal wall, and rib cage by the speech-language pathologist. Included in these assessments are resting breathing, nonspeech tasks, and speech tasks.

Phonatory System

Most measures used to evaluate the function of the phonatory system require the use of speech-like tasks. Here we review measures related to vowels, prolonged sibilants, and single-syllable productions. The stimuli discussed here are operationally defined as "nonspeech" measures since they do not have linguistic or communicative intent, and are generally not as multisystem demanding as the production of words and longer units of speech. However, producing a vowel or a consonant utilizes all of the speech production system in a manner that does not allow for as clear a distinction between speech subsystems and their compensations among structures.

A voice assessment must always include visual inspection of the larynx in collaboration with a physician, usually an otolaryngologist. Although the methods used to visualize the larynx are beyond the scope of this chapter, the tasks used will be reviewed. If a rigid laryngoscope is placed in the oropharynx via the mouth, then obviously the patient cannot talk. Instead, tasks include resting breathing, prolonged vowels at various pitches and loudness, and some laryngeal maneuvers (cough, glottal stop). If flexible endonasolaryngoscopy is used, then speech is permitted. Tasks usually include vowels, pitch glides, syllable repetitions with voiceless phonemes, and sentences including voiced and voiceless phonemes. If desired, singing can be observed as well. The larynx can be examined without or with a stroboscopic light source. Straight light is best for examining the structures and gross movements; stroboscopy is helpful for appreciating the vibratory behavior of the vocal folds.

Another critical aspect of a voice evaluation is the auditory perceptual judgment of the voice by the speech-language pathologist. In 1992, a workshop sponsored by the American Speech-Language-Hearing Association (ASHA) Division 3 on Voice and Voice Disorders and the University of Pittsburgh resulted in a standard list of tasks and instructions accompanied by a rating form for the perceptual assessment of voice. Specialists in voice and perceptual analysis participated in the workshop, and developed the Consensus Auditory-Perceptual Evaluation of Voice (CAPE-V). This represents a modification and enhancement of the popular GRBAS scale (grade, roughness, breathiness, asthenia, and strain), originally introduced by Hirano (1981). The CAPE-V score sheet, shown in **Fig. 3–2**, can be downloaded from the ASHA Web site (www.asha.org). From vowels sustained 3 to 5 seconds at habitual pitch and loudness, raters judge six vocal attributes along a visual analogue scale (100-mm line). The attributes are (1) overall severity, (2) roughness, (3) breathiness, (4) strain, (5) pitch, and (6) loudness. Comments about the consistency of the attribute, resonance, and other vocal features are permitted. Judgments are repeated for speech tasks as well. This tool incorporates many aspects of a typical perceptual voice evaluation, but standardizes it so that observations can be compared across time and across clinics.

Standard assessments of phonation usually involve acoustic measures. Acoustic measures of voice should ensure meticulous recording conditions so that environmental noise or other spurious electrical events do not interfere with the analysis. A high-quality condenser microphone, preferably worn on the head to maintain a constant and close mouth-to-microphone distance is best, especially when coupled with a digital recording system. Recommendations for acoustic recordings and data analysis were developed during a meeting sponsored by the National Center for Voice and Speech and the Denver Center for the Performing Arts. A summary statement and recommendations from this workshop, written by Titze (1994a) can be found at http://www.ncvs.org/ncvs/info/rescol/sumstat/sumstat.pdf.

A maximum performance task that reveals the envelope, or operating range, of phonation is the voice range profile (VRP), also known as a "phonetogram." The VRP is a plot of voice sound pressure level (SPL) versus fundamental frequency. To obtain a VRP, patients are asked to produce the softest and loudest notes they can at several pitches across the entire frequency range. For this assessment, falsetto or loft register is included but pulse or vocal fry is not. On average, normal pitch range is approximately three octaves. Dynamic range is normally approximately 50 dB SPL, with a minimum of approximately 55 dB SPL and a maximum of approximately 105 dB SPL (see Kent, Kent, & Rosenbek, 1987 for a review). **Figure 3–3** illustrates a normal appearing VRP produced by a woman with symptoms of vocal fatigue but without dysphonia. It was obtained with the Kay Elemetrics (Pine Brook, NJ) VRP program and calibrated for SPL with a table-mounted microphone placed 15 cm from the lips. The narrowing of the dynamic range at approximately 550 Hz is associated with the passagio—the transition from modal to falsetto register. The VRP has a characteristic shape, and deviations from that shape may be indicative of phonatory difficulties (Titze, 1994b).

The ability to vary pitch without changing loudness and loudness without changing pitch can give insight to the control required to regulate phonation, although many novice voice users require practice to achieve this skill. Another task designed to assess laryngeal control, but this time at the neuromuscular level, is laryngeal AMR. Verdolini (1994) suggested that this task, involving rapid and repetitive production of glottal plosives, may serve as an index of neural integrity of the phonatory system. Clinicians should observe rate, rhythm, and accuracy of production, just as they would evaluate articulatory AMRs. The rate of production for laryngeal AMR is typically 3.6 to 5.4 per second in children and around 5.0 per second in adults. A very common maximum performance task for evaluating voice is maximum phonation duration (MPD). MPD, however, is not uniformly accepted as an index of phonatory status, because it is highly dependent on respiratory abilities and performance variables. MPD is considered to reflect adequate laryngeal valving of the airstream as well as the VC. Normative MPD values for the vowel /a/ are approximately 20 seconds for adults and 10 seconds for children (see Kent et al 1987 for review). MPD is expected to be low for abnormally decreased VC or inadequate vocal fold adduction. Generally, MPD is inversely related to the severity of the disorder (Hillel, Yorkston, & Miller, 1989; Terasawa, Hibi, & Hirano, 1987). It is assumed that the respiratory and phonatory systems work together to provide the MPD result. Solomon et al (2000a) examined the specific contributions of these two speech-production subsystems during the

Consensus Auditory-Perceptual Evaluation of Voice (CAPE-V)

Name:_____   Date:_____

The following parameters of voice quality will be rated upon completion of the following tasks:
1. Sustained vowels, /a/ and /i/ for 3-5 seconds duration each.
2. Sentence production:

    a. The blue spot is on the key again.   d. We eat eggs every Easter.
    b. How hard did he hit him?   e. My mama makes lemon muffins.
    c. We were away a year ago.   f. Peter will keep at the peak.

3. Spontaneous speech in response to: "Tell me about your voice problem." or "Tell me how your voice is functioning."

```
Legend: C = Consistent    I = Intermittent
        MI = Mildly Deviant
        MO = Moderately Deviant
        SE = Severely Deviant
```

SCORE

Overall Severity _____ C   I   ___/100
              MI   MO   SE

Roughness   _____ C   I   ___/100
              MI   MO   SE

Breathiness   _____ C   I   ___/100
              MI   MO   SE

Strain   _____ C   I   ___/100
              MI   MO   SE

Pitch   (Indicate the nature of the abnormality): _____
          _____ C   I   ___/100
              MI   MO   SE

Loudness   (Indicate the nature of the abnormality): _____
          _____ C   I   ___/100
              MI   MO   SE

_____   _____ C   I   ___/100
              MI   MO   SE

_____   _____ C   I   ___/100
              MI   MO   SE

COMMENTS ABOUT RESONANCE: NORMAL   OTHER (Provide description):_____

ADDITIONAL FEATURES (for example, diplophonia, fry, falsetto, asthenia, aphonia, pitch instability, tremor, wet/gurgly, or other relevant terms):

Clinician:_____

Figure 3–2 Consensus Auditory-Perceptual Evaluation of Voice (CAPE-V) score sheet.

MPD task in normal speakers, and found no systematic relation between MPD and VC. Furthermore, laryngeal airway resistance was correlated with MPD for only a subset of subjects. Given these and other findings, we recommend that the clinician be very careful when using and interpreting MPD data. If the goal is to assess the quality and stability of phonation, Solomon et al recommended having the patient sustain a vowel for approximately 5 seconds at a comfortable lung-volume level and with habitual vocal pitch, loudness, and quality.

Similar interpretive problems exist for the s/z ratio. This common task was developed to assist the clinician in the differentiation between respiratory and laryngeal contributions to speech production problems (Boone, 1983). The patient is asked to produce the /s/ and /z/ for as long as possible. If the respiratory and phonatory systems are functioning normally, s/z should be slightly less than 1. Normal /s/ durations are around 9 seconds in children and 16 seconds in adults (Kent et al 1987). Normal durations for /z/ are around 11 seconds in children and 19 seconds in

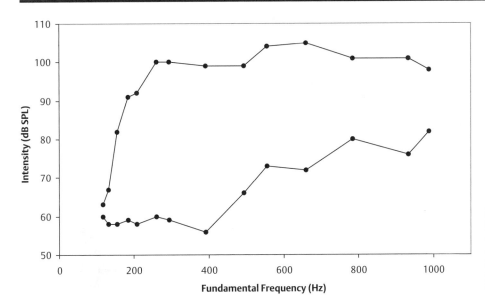

Figure 3–3 Voice range profile (VRP), also known as a "phonetogram," produced by a 44-year-old woman with symptoms of vocal fatigue. The curves represent multiple pitches (represented as voice F_0, in Hz) produced as loudly as possible (*top curve*) and as quietly as possible (*bottom curve*).

adults. The s/z ratios reported in the literature range from 0.70 to 0.99. Ratios greater than 1 are interpreted as an indication of inefficient phonation, because duration for /z/ is reduced due to air leakage at the level of the larynx. Of course, reduction in both /s/ and /z/ tends to implicate respiratory system problems. They could also be indicative of ineffective vocal tract constriction. Thus, the isolation of one subsystem from another is not easily accomplished using these measures.

Aerodynamic assessment can be an extremely helpful addition to the voice evaluation. Average airflow during a sustained vowel indicates whether the larynx is valving the air efficiently from the lungs to the upper airway. Typically, airflow is measured during the production of an /a/ or an /i/. Netsell, Lotz, and Barlow (1989) suggested examination of airflow during production of /pa/ at a rate of 1.5 per second and 3.0 per second, /pi/ as described above for /pa/, sustaining /a/ and /i/ for 3 seconds each, maximum phonation time, and possibly at different levels of pitch or loudness. Such tasks allow one to quantify airflow characteristics in a variety of contexts and gain information about the consistency of flow. Normal airflow for vowels is approximately 150 mL/s.

As discussed for the respiratory system, lung pressure can be estimated from the mouth rather than from the trachea. This finding has allowed lung pressure assessment to become common in clinical practice as well as in research. This estimate closely approximates the pressure generated by the lungs and delivered to the larynx for the production of speech, particularly vowels. This pressure, often termed *tracheal* or *subglottal pressure*, correlates strongly with the perception of vocal loudness. The task, as described by Smitheran and Hixon (1981), was designed to be easy enough for children and persons with movement disorders to perform. Data collection is straightforward, brief, and comfortable for the patient. From pressure and flow data collected during this syllable repetition task at a comfortable loudness level, laryngeal airway resistance (R_{law} or LAR) can be calculated. It is the ratio between subglottal pressure and translaryngeal airflow (measured with a face mask and pneumotachometer). R_{law} indicates the ability of the larynx to "valve" the airstream for phonation. R_{law} is quite common as a clinical and research assessment parameter, and has been used to evaluate a wide variety of disorders such as vocal tremor, vocal fatigue, spasmodic dysphonia, and unilateral vocal fold paralysis.

An additional assessment of subglottal pressure is conducted while the patient speaks as quietly as possible without using a whispered voice. The pressure peaks during /pi/ repetitions produced in this way gives a measure of phonation threshold pressure (PTP or P_{th}) (Titze, 1992). PTP is particularly sensitive to vocal function at high pitches. **Figure 3–4** illustrates two trials of the softest possible syllable productions for a woman who sustained iatrogenic recurrent laryngeal nerve (RLN) damage, resulting in unilateral vocal fold paralysis. Trials were recorded before (**Fig. 3–4A**) and after (**Fig. 3–4B**) thyroidectomy. Before surgery, PTP values were normal at this pitch (30% of her pitch range = D#3). After RLN damage, PTPs were greater at a similar pitch. This was associated with her perception of greater effort needed to produce quiet phonation. Airflow is not measured during this task, but is always included to confirm cessation of airflow during the pressure peak. If airflow is not recorded, then the pressure values cannot be considered an accurate estimate of tracheal pressure because they are likely to be underestimated. However, having the airflow record in this case also revealed higher air flows during her vowel production. This is consistent with the patient's breathy voice quality. PTP has been used in the literature to assess the effects of mass lesions of the vocal folds, vocal fatigue, hydration, and neurological diseases.

Recent studies have attempted to develop an index of overall dysphonia using logistic regression analysis with a wide variety of voice measures. Piccirillo, Painter, Fuller, Haiduk, and Fredrickson (1998) developed a vocal function index to discriminate between normal and dysphonic voices. Their index relied upon subglottal pressure, air flow, vocal efficiency, and MPD. Wuyts, DeBodt, Molenberghs, et al (2000) derived the dysphonia severity index (DSI)

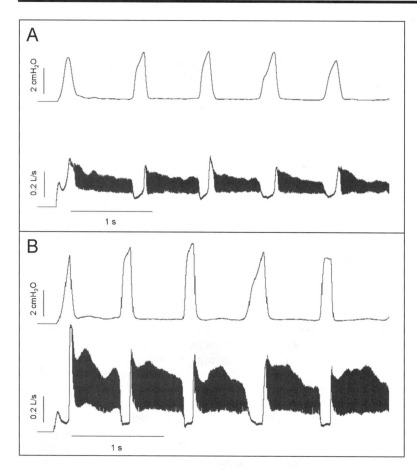

Figure 3–4 Pressure *(upper traces)* and flow *(lower traces)* signals used to determine phonation threshold pressure (PTP). The patient is a 53-year-old woman seen before **(A)** and after **(B)** unilateral vocal fold paralysis as a complication of thyroidectomy. Shown are five repetitions of /pi/ said as quietly as possible but above a whisper (indicated by high-frequency flow data during the vowels). Pressure peaks averaged 3.8 cm H_2O before and 5.7 cm H_2O after recurrent laryngeal nerve injury. Flow signals are used to confirm the lack of airflow during the pressure peaks, but also reveal higher flow during the vowels, which was associated with breathy voice quality.

based on weighted combinations of the highest voice fundamental frequency, the lowest voice intensity, jitter (cycle-to-cycle frequency variation), and MPD. A single index of dysphonia could be a valuable tool for characterizing voice disorders, and for documenting changes in pathology or with treatment. Wuyts et al (2000) recommend including the DSI along with the patient's subjective assessment, the speech-language pathologist's auditory-perceptual evaluation, and laryngeal inspection.

Velar-Pharyngeal System

Like the phonatory system, there are few tasks involving velar function used clinically that are truly nonspeech in nature. However, some tasks may allow for assessment of the envelope or maximal range. For instance, Kuehn and Moon (1995a) assessed electromyograph (EMG) activity of the soft palate during blowing versus speech in normal adult speakers. The blowing task was performed at relatively low pressures (0.5 kPa) and at maximal pressure generation. Blowing with maximal effort forced the levator veli palatini muscle to its maximal activity level. EMG activity recorded during speech production was approximately 10 to 30% of the maximal EMG activity as assessed during blowing. However, speakers with repaired palatal clefts exhibiting moderate levels of hypernasality displayed much higher EMG activation levels relative to their maximum during conversational speech attempts (Kuehn and Moon,

1995b). As a consequence, these speakers had a reduced EMG activation range and speech was considered an effortful task with respect to levator muscle activity. When forced to produce speech with added stress placed on the necessity to maintain velopharyngeal closure, these speakers experienced muscle fatigue, with concomitant loss of oral-nasal separation (Moon and Kuehn, 1998).

Similarly, patients with neurological involvement of the palate that reduces their maximal range may produce perceptually accurate speech under nonstressful conditions. However, when placed in situations of increased demand, they may not have the range to accommodate the added stress and, as a result, speech accuracy will be adversely affected. Nonspeech tasks to evaluate the velar-pharyngeal system are relatively few in number. Clinicians may ask patients to blow with the lips sealed to determine if there is leakage of the velar-pharyngeal (VP) valve. As well, one might observe the patients while they are swallowing a liquid (typically water) to determine if water leaks around the VP valve and into the nasal cavities.

Articulatory System

There are more nonspeech tasks used in the clinic to assess the function of articulatory structures (i.e., lips, tongue, jaw) than for the other speech subsystems. This is partially because these structures are more readily observed by the clinician than are the other speech production systems.

Surprisingly, however, there are few standardized tests available to guide assessment. A few published tests are available, each with its own strengths and limitations. Two of the most commonly cited tests are the Frenchay Dysarthria Assessment (Enderby, 1983) and the Dworkin-Culatta Oral-Mechanism Examination (Dworkin & Culatta, 1980). These include items addressing reflexes and nonspeech and speech tasks. The primary purpose of an oral-motor assessment is to assist with cranial nerve function testing and differential diagnosis of dysarthria. Results may also be useful for directing treatment toward a specific impairment, but efficacy data for oral-motor treatments are scarce and equivocal (Forrest, 2002).

Hall (1995) reviewed the oral mechanism examination for nonspeech and speech function. Relative to lip function, the clinician frequently asks for a pucker, retraction (unilateral and bilateral), and sequential movements of the lips. Similar activities are also used to assess tongue function. The clinician may ask the client to protrude the tongue, move it from side to side, touch the nose or chin with the tip of the tongue, or perform a series of movements in sequence. The purpose of these tasks is to assess the speed, symmetry, distance, and accuracy of movements of the tongue, lips, and jaw. As well, observations by the clinician are used to determine if there are abnormal movements associated with the structure such as tremor, hypokinesia, or groping movements.

Nonspeech AMR tasks are also used to assess nonspeech control of the speech articulators. These tasks are similar to the speech-like AMR tasks discussed previously except that these involve movements without producing speech-like sounds and that may not even resemble speech movements. For example, the patient may be asked to move the tongue tip back and forth from the right to left corner of the mouth as rapidly as possible until told to stop. The speed, rhythmicity, and accuracy of placement are noted. Performance on this task is thought to be indicative of the underlying neural integrity of the system.

The drawbacks of these tasks are that the assessments are "subjective" in nature, normative data are not well developed, and measurement reliability has not been established. This is certainly the case with measures of maximal strength (discussed below), where the typical subjective measures (see Hall, 1995; Clark, 2003) may be unreliable and insensitive to changes over time that occur as a result of treatment or disease progression (Robin, Somodi, & Luschei, 1991). Clark, Henson, Barber, Stierwalt, and Sherrill (2003) reported significant but only moderate correlations (r^2 between 0.29 and 0.32) between subjective and instrumental measures of tongue strength. Of interest, correlations were lower for more experienced clinicians compared with less experienced clinicians.

Some effort has been invested in developing more objective and reliable measures of strength, endurance, fatigability, and control of oral articulators. Some of these measures involve nonspeech movements that are closer to the control requirement during speech than movements used in traditional clinical nonspeech tasks (Clark, 2003) and often serve to define the envelope or operating range of an articulator. Tasks have included controlling static position or isometric force/pressure (e.g., Barlow & Abbs, 1986; Goozee et al, 2001; McNeil, Weismer, Adams, & Mulligan, 1990; Thompson et al 1995), dynamic ramp-and-hold force control (Barlow & Burton, 1990), and articulator visuomotor tracking (VMT; e.g., Hageman, Robin, Moon, & Folkins, 1994; McClean, Beukelman, & Yorkston, 1987; Moon, Zebrowski, Robin, & Folkins, 1993).

The basic force or position control paradigm requires the placement of a force or position transducer on the articulator of interest (e.g., upper lip). A target level of force or a position is displayed visually (e.g., on a screen). The patient's transduced signal is also present on the screen. The patient is told to reach a given target force level, or a target position, and hold it there as steadily as possible for a specific period of time (e.g., 5 seconds). One can test multiple force levels or positions. Motor control or stability is indexed by examination of the distance of the patient's force or position from the target level as well as variability of performance.

The dynamic ramp-and-hold force task is a modification of the above procedure in which subjects are asked to generate a given force level as rapidly and accurately as possible (Barlow & Burton, 1990). The duration of a trial has typically been approximately 5 seconds. The rationale for this procedure is to make the nonspeech movement more speech-like by having a dynamic, not a static, task. Measures used to index articulatory stability include the reaction time, the peak rate of force change, the peak force during the ramping maneuver, and the mean and standard deviation for the force output during the hold phase.

Results from these tasks have shown utility in the evaluation of neuromotor involvement in speech disorders. For instance, McNeil et al (1990) demonstrated that subjects with apraxia of speech or dysarthria performed abnormally on the static position and force tasks. Barlow and Abbs (1984) studied lip, jaw, and tongue force instability in subjects with spastic muscle conditions. They found that the subjects with spasticity had less stability than normal subjects. Moreover, their results showed that force instability correlated well with listener judgments of speech intelligibility ($r = 0.886$). Barlow and Burton (1990) reported data on four subjects who had sustained a TBI; they performed more poorly than normal subjects on the ramp-and-hold force task.

Another area of nonspeech research that has received attention in the literature has to do with articulatory strength and fatigability. Studies in our laboratory have used the Iowa Oral Performance Instrument (IOPI; **Fig. 3–5**) (Blaise Medical, Inc.) to assess strength and fatigue of the tongue in a variety of subject groups. The paradigm we use requires subjects to push on an air-filled bulb with the anterior portion of the tongue. The IOPI contains a digital readout of pressure as well as a series of lights that indicate how much pressure is being generated. **Figure 3–6** illustrates performance by a man with Parkinson's disease on three such tasks. The task in **Fig. 3–6A** assess maximal tongue elevation strength, **Fig. 3–6B** assesses maximum duration of tongue endurance at 50% of maximum strength, and **Fig. 3–6C** assesses constant effort beginning at 50% of maximum strength, for the purpose of assessing the exponential decline in pressure, used as an indicator of fatigue. These tasks are described briefly here, and in more detail in recent reviews

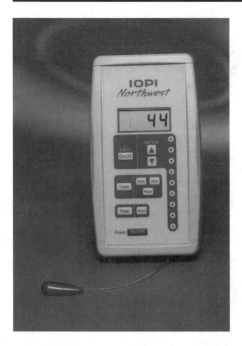

Figure 3–5 The Iowa Oral Performance Instrument (IOPI, Blaise Medical, Hendersonville, TN).

by Solomon (2004, 2006). To test maximal strength using the IOPI, patients are required to push against the bulb with their tongue as hard as possible. Patients are encouraged by verbal cheerleading (e.g., "PUSH, PUSH REALLY HARD!!"). The best of three trials is used. To test endurance, patients are asked to hold 50% of their maximal pressure for as long as possible. Here the light display is utilized, and patients are told to keep the middle light on, which is set to 50% of the maximal pressure. Along with tests of fatigue one can include a sense of effort task (Somodi, Robin, & Luschei, 1995), and a task where patients are told to hold effort constant (Solomon, Drager, & Luschei, 2002; Solomon & Robin, 2005; Solomon, Robin, Mitchinson, VanDaele, & Luschei, 1996).

Results from a variety of patient groups have been promising. Lower than normal tongue endurance has been documented in children with apraxia of speech and adults with spastic dysarthria (Robin et al, 1991) and individuals with traumatic brain injury (Stierwalt, Robin, Solomon, Weiss, & Max 1996; Theodoros et al, 1995; but see Goozee et al, 2001). Also, tongue weakness and fatigue have variably been shown in adults with Parkinson's disease (Solomon, Lorell, Robin, Rodnitzky, & Luschei, 1995; Solomon & Robin, 2005; Solomon et al, 2000b) and TBI (Goozee et al, 2001). A modest but significant correlation was identified between perceptual rating of the speech of subjects with Parkinson's disease and tongue strength (Solomon et al, 1995), but this relationship did not hold up when a larger number of subjects was evaluated (Solomon et al 2000b). Horton et al (1997) presented an interesting comparison of nonspeech and speech measures in a young boy with TBI. On a phonetic intelligibility test, the boy demonstrated reduced precision of lingual consonants. Using a pressure transducer, the authors found intact tongue strength but reduced

endurance and slow rate of repetitive tongue movements. These nonspeech findings suggest that tongue strength should not be a focus of intervention. Despite positive reports such as this one, correlations between perceptual ratings of speech (e.g., consonant imprecision) in TBI subjects and measures of strength and fatigue of the tongue have been equivocal (Goozee et al, 2001; Horton et al, 1997; Stierwalt et al, 1996). It is likely that impairment of tongue function needs be quite diminished, and perhaps affected across a range of domains (e.g., strength, endurance, and power), before speech articulation is affected functionally (Solomon, 2000).

A final task reviewed here is the VMT task, first described in the speech system by McClean et al (1987). Visuomotor tracking requires patients to follow a moving target on a screen with a given speech structure (e.g., jaw, lower lip, voice; **Fig. 3–7**). A transducer (e.g., strain gauge for the lips and jaw or a microphone for the voice) is placed on the appropriate structure(s) and the transduced signal appears as a dot on the screen. The target signal is represented on the screen by a horizontal bar that moves up and down. The patient is told to keep the dot in the bar as it moves. Targets are either predictable (sine wave motion) or unpredictable (random motion). Target speed and amplitude can be varied systematically. Dependent measures include the cross-correlation between the target signal and the signal produced by the patient, the phase relationship between the two signals, the gain ratio (an index of how closely in amplitude the two signals match), and the absolute difference between the target signal and the signal produced by the patient (e.g., in millimeters for the lips and jaw, in hertz for the voice).

Visuomotor tracking permits assessment of control of timing and amplitude parameters of movement in a single articulator without the demands of interarticulatory coordination or of language formulation. The advantages are similar to some of those for the ramp-and-hold maneuver described above. The task better reflects some of the motor demands placed on the articulators during speech production than the traditional nonspeech tasks routinely used by clinicians. In addition to utilizing dynamic movements, the predictable tracking task requires a movement with the peak velocity approximately in its center, much like speech. Moreover, one can change the complexity of the task in several different ways. For instance, increasing the speed of tracking or the predictability of the target alters task complexity. Such changes in complexity may have potential for prognosis and monitoring changes due to decline in progressive disease or to treatment.

Ballard, Robin, Woodworth, and Zimba (2001) have provided normative data across the life span on VMT performance in the lips, jaw, and voice. In addition, different profiles of performance on VMT tasks have been shown for healthy adults and those with acquired language deficits (i.e., conduction aphasia) versus individuals with motor speech disorders such as ataxic dysarthria and apraxia of speech (Hageman, Robin, Moon, & Folkins 1993, 1994). Specifically, subjects with apraxia of speech showed poorer performance than healthy or aphasic adults when tracking predictable targets (**Fig. 3–7**), but performed normally when

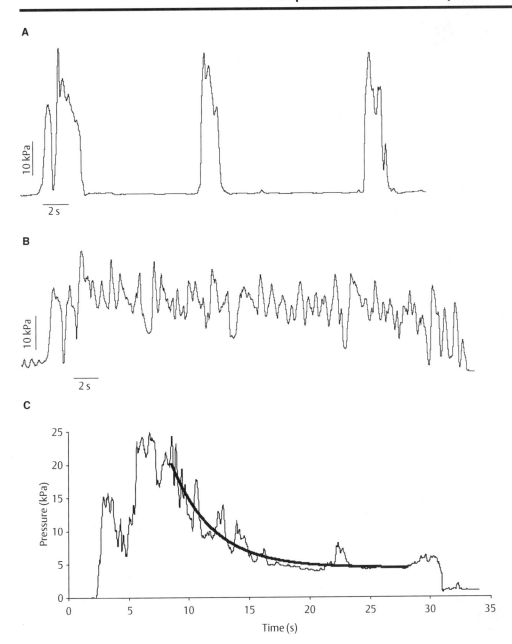

Figure 3–6 Three tongue-function tasks performed with the IOPI by a 71–year-old man with Parkinson's disease: **(A)** strength, **(B)** endurance, and **(C)** constant effort. Tongue strength (the greatest of three trials) was 42 kPa. Endurance at 50% of strength was 29 seconds; for this task, the patient uses the IOPI's light-emitting diode (LED) display for visual feedback. The constant-effort trial, performed without visual feedback, reveals the typical decreasing exponential function. The thick curve in this graph represents the curve fitting procedure, which calculated a 3.5-second time constant.

tracking unpredictable targets. Subjects with conduction aphasia tracked both predictable and unpredictable targets normally. Subjects with ataxic dysarthria had difficulty tracking predictable and unpredictable targets (Hageman et al, 1993). Data from subjects with apraxia of speech have shown strong correlations, ranging from 0.82 to 0.96, between predictable target tracking and judgments of speech (Robin, Hageman, Moon, Clark, Woodworth, & Folkins, unpublished data).

The VMT data suggest that subjects with apraxia of speech have difficulty developing or executing a model of target

motion. It has been suggested that the ability to track predictable signals is best performed based on an internal representation of target motion (Flowers, 1978). When tracking a predictable target, subjects typically are in phase or are phase advanced of the target signal. Thus, they do not follow the target, but rather anticipate the movement. We interpret this as evidence for an internal model of the target. Moreover, subjects can maintain tracking accuracy when the feedback is removed, suggesting that an internal representation of the target movement pattern drives performance. The tracking of unpredictable signals requires feedback from the

A: Healthy Adult

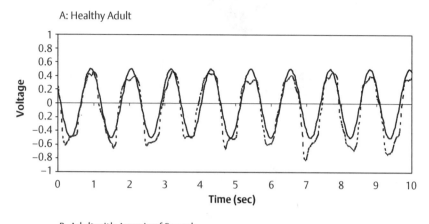

B. Adult with Apraxia of Speech

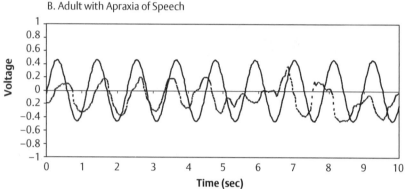

Figure 3–7 An example of performance on the visuomotor tracking task for the jaw (*dotted line*) tracking the predictable 0.9–Hz target signal (*solid line*). **(A)** Performance of an older healthy adult. **(B)** Performance of an individual with severe apraxia of speech (1 V = 10 mm).

external signal, since one cannot develop a model of random motion. In the unpredictable conditions, subjects' tracking lags behind the target. That the subjects with apraxia of speech (AOS) were able to track the unpredictable, but not the predictable target, seems reasonable. These speakers were chosen because they have difficulty with the development or execution of high-level motoric planning. By contrast, speakers with ataxia had difficulty with both predictable and unpredictable targets. This result is consistent with their disorder because ataxia affects the planning and programming of movements (see Chapter 1).

♦ Conclusion

This chapter reviewed nonspeech assessments of the speech production mechanism. Such assessment tasks are viewed in the context of a broader approach that incorporates the use of both nonspeech and speech tasks for differential diagnosis of motor speech disorders. The motor control tasks described allow the clinician to systematically vary task requirements, such as the level of force or the distance traveled by the articulator. Each of the tasks allows assessment of individual articulators, and differential involvement is often found following neurological disease. As well, each task provides insight into the motor system, without the

constraints or influences of the language system. In summary, some of the nonspeech tasks that assess strength, fatigue, or motor control of the speech production system continue to show promise as clinical assessment tools. These procedures enable the evaluation of the integrity of a given structure without the constraint of the linguistic system, but with similar motor demands as found during speech. With the development and increased availability of modern imaging methods such as electropalatography (EPG), pressure-sensing EPG (Murdoch, Goozee, Veidt, Scott, & Meyers, 2004), electromagnetic articulography (Carstens Medizinelektronik, Göttingen, Germany), and optical tracking systems (e.g., Optotrak, Northern Digital, Waterloo, Ontario, Canada), our understanding of the relationships between various nonspeech and speech tasks and their utility in diagnosis and treatment should be enhanced. Further research will determine which nonspeech tasks and measurements are most useful in differential diagnosis and treatment planning of motor speech disorders, which measures reveal relationships across nonspeech and speech maneuvers, and whether diagnosis, prognosis, or the ability to monitor disease progress is enhanced by these methods.

Acknowledgments We thank Matthew Makashay, for assistance with compiling the figures. The opinions or assertions contained herein are the private views of the authors and are not to be construed as official or as reflecting the views of the Department of the Army or the Department of Defense.

References

Ballard, K.J., Flemmer, V., & Moon, J. (2004). Effect of bite-block on oral-laryngeal timing in Apraxia of Speech. Conference on Motor Speech and Motor Speech Disorders, Albuquerque, NM

Ballard, K.J., Robin, D.A., & Folkins, J.W. (2003). An integrative model of speech motor control: a response to Ziegler. *Aphasiology, 17,* 37–48

Ballard, K.J., Robin, D.A., Woodworth, G., & Zimba, L. (2001). Age-related changes in motor control during articulator visuomotor tracking. *Journal of Speech, Language, and Hearing Research, 44,* 763–777

Barlow, S.M. & Abbs, J.H. (1984). Orofacial fine-motor control impairments in congenital spasticity: evidence against hyper-tonus related performance deficits. *Neurology, 34,* 145–150

Barlow, S.M. & Abbs, J.H. (1986). Fine force and position control of select orofacial structures in the upper motor neuron syndrome. *Experimental Neurology, 94,* 699–713

Barlow, S.M. & Burton, M.K. (1990). Ramp-and-hold force control in the upper and lower lips: developing new neuromotor assessment applications in traumatically brain injured adults. *Journal of Speech and Hearing Research, 33,* 660–675

Barlow, S.M. & Netsell, R. (1986). Differential fine force control of the upper and lower lips. *Journal of Speech and Hearing Research, 29,* 163–169

Boone, D.R. (1983). *The Voice and Voice Therapy,* 3rd ed. Englewood Cliffs, NJ: Prentice-Hall

Clark, H.M. (2003). Neuromuscular treatments for speech and swallowing: a tutorial. *American Journal of Speech and Language Pathology, 12,* 400–415

Clark, H.M., Henson, P.A., Barber, W.B., Stierwalt, J.A.G., & Sherrill, M. (2003). Relationships among subjective and objective measures of tongue strength and oral phase swallowing impairments. *American Journal of Speech and Language Pathology, 12,* 40–50

Darley, F.L., Aronson, A., & Brown, J. (1975). *Motor Speech Disorders.* Philadelphia: W.B. Saunders

Duffy, J.R. (1995). *Motor Speech Disorders: Substrates, Differential Diagnosis, and Management.* St. Louis, MO: Mosby

Dworkin, J.P., Aronson, A.E., & Mulder, D.W. (1980). Tongue force in normals and in dysarthric patients with amyotrophic lateral sclerosis. *Journal of Speech and Hearing Research, 23,* 828–837

Dworkin, J.P. & Culatta, R.A. (1980). *Dworkin-Culatta Oral Mechanism Examination.* Nicholasville, KY: Edgewood Press

Enderby, P. (1983). *Frenchay Dysarthria Assessment.* Austin: Pro-Ed

Flowers, K. (1978). Some frequency response characteristics of parkinsonism on pursuit tracking. *Brain, 101,* 19–34

Folkins, J.W. (1985). Issues in speech motor control and their relation to the speech of individuals with cleft lip and palate. *Cleft Palate Journal, 22,* 106–122

Folkins, J.W., Moon, J.B., Luschei, E.S., Robin, D.A., Tye-Murray, N., & Moll, K.L. (1995). What can nonspeech tasks tell us about speech motor disabilities? *Journal of Phonetics, 23,* 139–147

Forrest, K. (2002). Are oral-motor exercises useful in the treatment of phonological/articulatory disorders? *Seminars in Speech and Language, 23,* 15–25

Gay, T., Lindblom, B., & Lubker, J. (1981). Production of bite-block vowels: Acoustic equivalence by selective compensation. *Journal of the Acoustical Society of America, 69,* 802–810

Goozee, J.V., Murdoch, B.E., & Theodoros, D.G. (2001). Physiological assessment of tongue function in dysarthria following traumatic brain injury. *Logopedics Phoniatrics Vocology, 26,* 51–65

Hageman, C., Robin, D.A., Moon, J.B., & Folkins, J.W. (1993). Visuomotor tracking in neurogenic disorders. Paper presented to the Annual Meeting of the American Speech-Language-Hearing Association, San Antonio, November

Hageman, C., Robin, D.A., Moon, J.B., & Folkins, J.W. (1994). Visuomotor tracking abilities of speakers with apraxia. *Aphasiology, 22,* 219–229

Hall, P.K. (1995). The oral mechanism. In: J.B. Tomblin, H.L. Morris, & D.C. Spriestersbach (Eds.), *Diagnosis in Speech-Language Pathology* (pp. 67–97). San Diego: Singular Press

Hillel, A.D., Yorkston, K., & Miller, R.M. (1989). Using phonation time to estimate vital capacity in amyotrophic lateral sclerosis. *Archives of Physical Medicine and Rehabilitation, 70,* 618–620

Hirano, M. (1981). *Clinical Examination of the Voice.* New York: Springer-Verlag

Hixon, T.J. (1987). *Respiratory Function in Speech and Song.* San Diego: College-Hill Press

Hixon, T.J. (1993). Clinical evaluation of speech breathing disorders: principles and methods. Telerounds #7, National Center for Neurogenic Communication Disorders, University of Arizona

Hixon, T.J., Hawley, J.L., & Wilson, K.J. (1982). An around-the-house device for the clinical determination of respiratory driving pressure: a note on making simple even simpler. *Journal of Speech and Hearing Disorders, 47,* 413–415

Hixon, T.J. & Hoit, J.D. (1998). Physical examination of the diaphragm by the speech-language pathologist. *American Journal of Speech and Language Pathology, 7,* 37–45

Hixon, T.J. & Hoit, J.D. (1999). Physical examination of the abdominal wall by the speech-language pathologist. *American Journal of Speech and Language Pathology, 8,* 35–46

Hixon, T.J. & Hoit, J.D. (2000). Physical examination of the rib cage wall by the speech-language pathologist. *American Journal of Speech and Language Pathology, 9,* 179–196

Hixon, T.J. & Hoit, J.D. (2005). *Evaluation and Management of Speech Breathing Disorders: Principles and Methods.* San Diego: Plural Publishing

Hoit, J.D., Plassman, B.L., Lansing, R.W., & Hixon, T.J. (1988). Abdominal muscle activity during speech production. *Journal of Applied Physiology, 65,* 2656–2664

Horton, S.K., Murdoch, B.E., Theodorus, D.G., & Thompson, E.C. (1997). Motor speech impairment in a case of childhood basilar artery stroke: treatment directions derived from physiological and perceptual assessment. *Pediatric Rehabilitation, 1,* 163–177

Kelso, J.A.S. & Tuller, B. (1983). Compensatory articulation under conditions of reduced afferent information: a dynamic formulation. *Journal of Speech and Hearing Research, 26,* 217–224

Kent, R.D. & Kent, J.F. (2000). Task-based profiles of the dysarthrias. *Folia Phoniatrica et Logopedica, 52,* 48–53

Kent, R.D., Kent, J.F., Duffy, J.R., Thomas, J.E., Weismer, G., & Stuntebeck, S. (2000). Ataxic dysarthria. *Journal of Speech, Language, and Hearing Research, 43,* 1275–1289

Kent, R.D., Kent, J.F., & Rosenbek, J.C. (1987). Maximum performance tests of speech production. *Journal of Speech and Hearing Disorders, 52,* 367–387

Kent, R.D., Kent, J.F., Rosenbek, J.C., Vorperian, H.K., & Weismer, G. (1997). A speaking task analysis of the dysarthria in cerebellar disease. *Folia Phoniatrica et Logopedica, 49,* 63–82

Kent, R.D. & Kim, Y.J. (2003). Toward an acoustic typology of motor speech disorders. *Clinical and Linguistic Phonetics, 17,* 427–445

Kent, R.D., Weismer, G., Kent, J.F., Vorperian, H.K., & Duffy, J.R. (1999). Acoustic studies of dysarthric speech: methods, progress, and potential. *Journal of Communication Disorders, 32,* 141–180

Kuehn, D. & Moon, J.B. (1995a). Levator veli palatini muscle activity in relation to intraoral air pressure variation. *Journal of Speech and Hearing Research, 37,* 1260–1270

Kuehn, D. & Moon, J.B. (1995b), Levator veli palatini muscle activity in relation to intraoral air pressure variation in cleft palate subjects. *Cleft Palate-Craniofacial Journal, 32,* 376–381

Luschei, E.S. (1991). Development of objective standards of nonspeech oral strength and performance: an advocate's view. In: C.A. Moore, K.M.

Yorkston, & D.R. Beukelman (Eds.), *Dysarthria and Apraxia of Speech: Perspectives on Management* (pp. 3–14). Baltimore: Paul H. Brookes

McClean, M.D., Beukelman, D.R., & Yorkston, K.M. (1987). Speech-muscle visuomotor tracking in dysarthric and nonimpaired speakers. *Journal of Speech and Hearing Research, 30,* 276–282

McClean, M.D. & Tasko, S.M. (2002). Association of orofacial with laryngeal and respiratory motor output during speech. *Experimental Brain Research, 146,* 481–489

McNeil, M.R., Weismer, G., Adams, S., & Mulligan, M. (1990). Oral structure nonspeech motor control in normal, dysarthric, aphasic, and apraxic speakers: isometric force and static position control. *Journal of Speech and Hearing Research, 33,* 255–268

Moon, J. & Kuehn, D. (1998). Induced velopharyngeal fatigue effects in speakers with repaired palatal clefts. Paper presented at annual meeting of American Cleft Palate-Craniofacial Association, Baltimore

Moon, J.B., Zebrowski, P., Robin, D.A., & Folkins, J.W. (1993). Visuomotor tracking ability of young adult speakers. *Journal of Speech and Hearing Research, 36,* 672–682

Murdoch, B.E., Goozee, J.V., Veidt, M., Scott, D.H., & Meyers, I.A. (2004) Introducing the pressure-sensing palatograph—the next frontier in electropalatography. *Clinical Linguistics and Phonetics, 18,* 433–445

Murdoch, B.E., Johnson, SM., & Theodoros, D.G. (1997). Physiological and perceptual features of dysarthria in Moebius syndrome: directions for treatment. *Pediatric Rehabilitation, 1,* 83–97

Netsell, R. & Hixon, T.J. (1978). A noninvasive method for clinically estimating subglottal air pressure. *Journal of Speech and Hearing Disorders, 43,* 326–330

Netsell, R., Lotz, W.K., & Barlow, S.M. (1989). A speech physiology examination for individuals with dysarthria. In: K.M. Yorkston & D.R. Beukelman (Eds.), *Recent Advances in Clinical Dysarthria* (pp. 3–33). Boston: College-Hill Press

Netsell, R. & Rosenbek, J.C. (1985). Treating the dysarthrias. In: J. Darby (Ed.), *Speech and Language Evaluation in Neurology: Adult Disorders* (pp. 363–392). Orlando: Grune & Stratton

Piccirillo, J.F., Painter, C., Fuller, D., Haiduk, A., & Fredrickson, J.M. (1998). Assessment of two objective voice function indices. *Annals of Otology, Rhinology, and Laryngology, 107,* 396–400

Putnam, A.H.B. & Hixon, T.J. (1983). Respiratory kinematics in speakers with motor neuron disease. In: M. McNeil, J. Rosenbeck, & A. Aronson (Eds.), *The Dysarthrias* (pp. 37–67). San Diego: College-Hill Press

Robin, D.A., Hageman, C., Moon, J.B., Clark, H.C., Woodworth, G., & Folkins, J.W. (Unpublished.). Visuomotor tracking abilities of speakers with apraxia of speech or conduction aphasia

Robin, D.A., Somodi, L., & Luschei, E.S. (1991). Measurement of tongue strength and endurance in normal and articulation disordered subjects. In: C.A. Moore, K.M. Yorkston, & D.R. Beukelman (Eds.), *Dysarthria and Apraxia of Speech: Perspectives on Management* (pp. 173–184). Baltimore: Paul H. Brookes

Rothenberg, M. (1973). A new inverse-filtering technique for deriving the glottal air flow waveform during voicing. *Journal of the Acoustical Society of America, 53,* 1632–1645

Schmidt, R.A. (1988). *Motor Control and Learning: A Behavioral Emphasis,* 2nd ed. Champaign: Human Kinetics

Searl, J.P. (2003). Comparison of transducers and intraoral placement options for measuring lingua-palatal contact pressure during speech. *Journal of Speech, Language, and Hearing Research, 46,* 1444–1456

Smitheran, J.R. & Hixon, T.J. (1981). A clinical method for estimating laryngeal airway resistance during vowel production. *Journal of Speech and Hearing Disorders, 46,* 138–146

Solomon, N.P. (2000). Changes in normal speech after fatiguing the tongue. *Journal of Speech, Language, and Hearing Research, 43,* 1416–1428

Solomon, N.P. (2004). Assessment of weakness and fatigue of the tongue. *International Journal of Orofacial Myology, 30,* 8–19

Solomon, N.P. (2006). What is orofacial fatigue and how does it affect function for swallowing and speech? *Seminars in Speech and Language, 27,* 268–282

Solomon, N.P. & Charron, S. (1998). Speech breathing in able-bodied children and children with cerebral palsy: A review of the literature and implications for clinical intervention. *American Journal of Speech and Language Pathology, 7,* 61–78

Solomon, N.P., Drager, K.D., & Luschei, E.S. (2002). Sustaining a constant effort by the tongue and hand: effects of acute fatigue. *Journal of Speech, Language, and Hearing Research, 45,* 613–624

Solomon, N.P., Garlitz, S.J., & Milbrath, R.L. (2000a). Respiratory and laryngeal contributions to maximum phonation duration. *Journal of Voice, 14,* 331–340

Solomon, N.P. & Hixon, T.J. (1993). Speech breathing in Parkinson's disease. *Journal of Speech and Hearing Research, 36,* 294–310

Solomon, N.P., Lorell, D.M., Robin, D.A., Rodnitzky, R.L., & Luschei, E.S. (1995). Tongue strength and endurance in mild to moderate Parkinson's disease. *Journal of Medical Speech-Language Pathology, 3,* 15–26

Solomon, N.P. & Robin, D.A. (2005). Perceptions of effort during handgrip and tongue elevation in Parkinson's disease. *Parkinsonism & Related Disorders, 11,* 353–361

Solomon, N.P., Robin, D.A., & Luschei, E.S. (2000b). Strength, endurance, and stability of the tongue and hand in Parkinson disease. *Journal of Speech, Language, and Hearing Research, 43,* 256–267

Solomon, N.P., Robin, D.A., Mitchinson, S.I., VanDaele, D.J., & Luschei, E.S. (1996). Sense of effort and the effects of fatigue in the tongue and hand. *Journal of Speech and Hearing Research, 39,* 114–125

Somodi, L.B., Robin, D.A., & Luschei, E.S. (1995). A model of "sense of effort" during maximal and submaximal contractions of the tongue. *Brain and Language, 51,* 371–382

Stierwalt, J.A.G., Robin, D.A., Solomon, N.P., Weiss, A.L., & Max, J. (1996). Tongue strength and endurance: relation to the speaking ability of children and adolescents following traumatic brain injury. In: D.A. Robin, K.M. Yorkston, & D.R. Beukelman (Eds.), *Disorders of Motor Speech: Assessment, Treatment, and Clinical Characterization* (pp. 241–258). Baltimore: Paul H. Brookes

Tasko, S.M. & McClean, M.D. (2004). Variations in articulatory movement with changes in speech task. *Journal of Speech, Language, and Hearing Research, 47,* 85–100

Terasawa, R., Hibi, S.R., & Hirano, M. (1987). Mean airflow rates during phonation over a comfortable duration and maximum sustained phonation. *Folia Phoniatrics (Basel), 39,* 87–89

Theodorus, D.G., Murdoch, B.E, & Stokes, P.A. (1995). Physiological analysis of articulatory dysfunction in dysarthric speakers following severe closed-head injury. *Brain Injury, 9,* 237–254.

Thompson, E.C., Murdoch, B.E., & Stokes, P.D. (1995). Tongue function in subjects with upper motor neuron type dysarthria following cerebrovascular accident. *Journal of Medical Speech-Language Pathology, 3,* 27–40

Titze, I.R. (1992). Phonation threshold pressure: a missing link in glottal aerodynamics. *Journal of the Acoustical Society of America, 91,* 2926–2935

Titze, I.R. (1994a). Workshop on acoustic voice analysis: summary statement. NCVS (http://www.ncvs.org/ncvs/info/rescol/sumstat/sumstat.pdf)

Titze, I.R. (1994b). *Principles of Voice Production.* Englewood Cliffs, NJ: Prentice-Hall

Verdolini, K. (1994). Voice disorders. In: J.B. Tomblin, H.L. Morris, & D.C. Spriestersbach (Eds.), *Diagnosis in Speech-Language Pathology* (pp. 247–306). San Diego: Singular Press

Wang, Y.-T., Kent, R.D., Duffy, J.R., Thomas, J.E., & Weismer, G. (2004). Alternating motion rate as an index of speech motor disorder in traumatic brain injury. *Clinical Linguistics and Phonetics, 18,* 57–84

Weismer, G. (2006). Philosophy of research in motor speech disorders. *Clinical Linguistics and Phonetics, 20,* 315–349

Weismer, G. & Liss, J.M. (1991). Reductionism is a dead-end in speech research: perspectives on a new direction. In: C.A. Moore, K.M. Yorkston, & D.R. Beukelman (Eds.), *Dysarthria and Apraxia of Speech: Perspectives on Management* (pp. 15–27). Baltimore: Paul H. Brookes

Wuyts, F.L., DeBodt, M.S., Molenberghs, G., et al. (2000). The Dysphonia Severity Index: An objective measure of vocal quality based on a multiparameter approach. *Journal of Speech, Language, and Hearing Research, 43,* 796–809

Yorkston, K.M., Beukelman, D.R., Strand, E.A., & Bell, K.R. (1999). *Management of Motor Speech Disorders in Children and Adults,* 2nd ed. Austin: Pro-Ed

Ziegler, W. (2002). Task-related factors in oral motor control: Speech and oral diadochokinesis in dysarthria and apraxia of speech. *Brain and Language, 80,* 556–575

Zimmermann, G. (1980). Stuttering: a disorder of movement. *Journal of Speech and Hearing Research, 23,* 122–136

Chapter 4

Acoustic Analysis of Motor Speech Disorders

Karen Forrest and Gary Weismer

Perceptual analysis is the primary tool used by speech-language pathologists to gather information about speech production characteristics of persons with various speech disorders. Although there is much to be said about the value of perceptual analysis (e.g., relation to patients' concerns, ease of interpretation), the relation between perceptual attributes and the underlying speech pathology is complex and poorly understood. Further, our perceptual abilities are influenced by linguistic exposure such that acoustic distinctions that are not phonemic in the ambient language (e.g., prevoiced versus voiced sounds in English) are difficult to perceive (Werker & Tees, 1992). As such, the subjective nature of perceptual analyses may limit measurement reliability (Kreiman & Gerratt, 1998) and thereby obscure understanding of the variables that cause a specific speech problem. In the case of motor speech disorders, where speech production characteristics may pose a particular challenge to the fragile stability of perceptual judgments (Kent, 1996; Zyski & Weisiger, 1987), such as phonetic transcription (Shriberg & Kwiatkowski, 1982), or psychophysical scaling (Schiavetti, Metz, & Sitler, 1981), instrumental analyses may be particularly attractive.

Among the different types of instrumental analysis (e.g., aerodynamic, electromyographic) that could be used in speech disorders, acoustic analysis is highly advantageous for the following reasons. First, there is a well-developed body of literature on acoustic characteristics of normal speech production (see summaries in Baken, 1987; Kent & Read, 2002; Kent, Dembowski, & Lass, 1996; Kent, Kent, & Delaney, 2004; Klatt, 1987), and a growing body of literature concerning acoustic characteristics in various speech disorders, including those speech disorders resulting from neurological disease (see summaries in Kent & Kim, 2003; Kent, Weismer, Kent, & Rosenbek, 1989; Weismer & Martin, 1992; and Weismer, 1999). Second, the acoustic output of the vocal tract can be thought of as a bridge between speech production and perception, and so the acoustic speech signal is uniquely able to shed light on both the mechanism associated with disordered speech and the effect of those problems on speech intelligibility. Third, models of speech production hypothesize that acoustic targets serve as control variables such that neural systems specify acoustic goals to guide articulatory movements (Perkell, Guenther, Lane, et al, 2000). As such, analysis of the acoustic signal may provide insight into the disturbances introduced by neural deficits. Fourth, the acoustic output of the vocal tract contains the product of the entire speech system's effort, rather than an isolated component of that effort. To the extent that a speech disorder is defined by its anomalous communication product, acoustic analysis may prove to be valuable. Fifth, acoustic analysis is completely noninvasive. Sixth, computer-based analyses of speech acoustics have become highly sophisticated, accessible, and relatively inexpensive (e.g., CSL, TF32, and Praat). Acoustic analysis of speech, therefore, is within the reach of clinicians for diagnosis, record keeping, outcomes measures, and research purposes.

Exactly what can one expect to get from an acoustic analysis of a patient's speech? Information is available in the acoustic signal concerning such factors as speaking rate, articulatory configuration for vowels and consonants, rates of change in the overall configuration of the vocal tract, flexibility of articulatory behavior, as well as aspects of phonatory behavior. The measurements made to draw inferences about articulatory and phonatory behavior often reveal a pattern that partially explains why a speaker is unintelligible, and how speech therapy may focus on a particular aspect of speech production to improve intelligibility. As with any instrumental analysis of speech production, a certain amount of training and sophistication is required to select the appropriate analyses for a given problem, and to interpret the resulting data. This chapter provides examples of the kinds of information one can obtain from acoustic analysis of selected motor speech disorders, and discusses the variables that must be considered to make informed decisions from the analyzed data. We begin by detailing procedures for acoustic analysis for typical speakers, and then discuss the application of these acoustic measures to the study of motor speech disorders and the supplementation of perceptual data.

♦ Procedures for Acoustic Analysis

Choosing a Speech Sample for Acoustic Analysis

An ideal speech sample for acoustic analysis should represent the individual's typical communication abilities. Unfortunately, this objective must be tempered by instrumental limitations and subject performance. In some cases, such as measures of vocal perturbation (see below), only steady-state vowels may be included in the analysis because neighboring sounds may impact the cycle-to-cycle glottal variations associated with vocal fold vibration. Further, most perturbation algorithms are sensitive to noise that can be introduced by recording equipment and environment. Therefore, speaking conditions must be adapted to limit sources of extraneous variations. In other situations, wherein the dynamic aspects of speech are considered, conversational speech may be desired to better approach the individual's typical performance. Although this sample may provide a more naturalistic assessment, accurate analyses of connected speech can be quite challenging. In general, though, the type of speech material chosen depends on the questions being asked. Care should be taken to utilize the same materials across repeated analyses because different speech samples are likely to yield different values of acoustic parameters (Rosen, Kent, & Duffy, 2005), although measurements across different speech samples probably are highly correlated (Weismer, Jeng, Laures, Kent, & Kent, 2001). This is similar to the results of perceptual measures wherein different speech materials (e.g., single words, sentences) are likely to provide different, though related, estimates of a speaker's intelligibility.

Acoustic Representations of Speech

There are a variety of ways that an acoustic signal can be displayed and, when it comes to the speech signal, the format of the display affects the types of measures that can be made. In an attempt to quantify aspects of the speech signal, measures of temporal and spectral characteristics often are undertaken. Temporal characteristics reflect the duration and timing of selected events, whereas spectral characteristics show how sound energy is distributed across frequency (i.e., the pattern of resonances for a given sound). This energy distribution, in turn, can reflect the vocal tract configuration for phonetic patterns. The precise nature of these

temporal and spectral measures varies with the utterance produced. Factors that influence the choice of acoustic measures include manner of production and voicing for consonants, as well as source characteristics and nasalization. This section discusses different types of acoustic displays and the measurement procedures and techniques used in the analysis of speech. These technical issues are followed by a discussion of acoustic measures that relate to some well-known perceptual descriptions of motor speech disorders.

Segmentation and Measurement of the Speech Wave

The speech wave is a complex, time-varying signal from which temporal "pieces" must be selected for analysis. Segmentation of the speech signal carries with it many theoretical assumptions that are beyond the scope of this chapter. For example, theories of speech production propose divergent "units" wherein some models uphold the phoneme as the underlying phonological element (Guenther, Hampson, & Johnson, 1998) and other theories endorse the gesture as the basic linguistic entity (Browman & Goldstein, 1990; Byrd & Saltzman, 2003). The units to be segmented, therefore, may vary with the theoretical perspective of how speech is controlled.

The selection of these units can be made from waveform displays, which show sound energy amplitude as a function of time (**Fig. 4–1A**), and from spectrograms, which are three-dimensional displays of frequency, time, and relative amplitude (**Fig. 4–1B**). The speech waveform, such as that displayed in **Fig. 4–1**, can be segmented to identify temporal

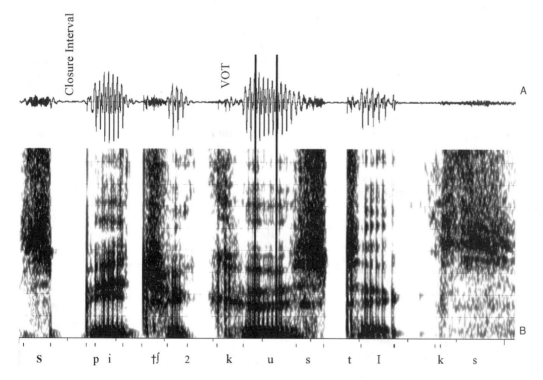

Figure 4–1 Waveform **(A)** and spectrogram **(B)** of the utterance "speech acoustics." Note the segmentation of the utterance into consonantal and vocalic elements and the correspondence between these segments on the waveform and spectrogram. Note the 30–ms window in the center of the vowel /i/ used for spectral analysis of formant frequencies.

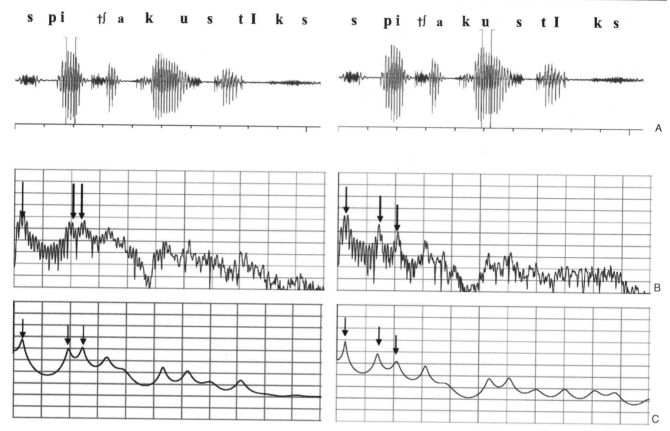

Figure 4–2 Waveform **(A)** and fast Fourier transform (FFT) displays **(B)** of the vowels /u/ (left) and /i/ (right). Each small peak in this display corresponds to a harmonic of the fundamental frequency associated with vocal fold vibration. The linear predictive coded (LPC) spectra for the vowels /u/ and /i/ **(C)** display the formant frequency peaks more clearly than can be seen in the FFT spectra, but do not provide information about the fundamental frequency.

intervals that are relevant to the structure of the utterance. Boundaries between sentences, phrases, syllables, phonemes, and so forth must be determined before temporal measurements of specific intervals can be made. Because of the interaction of speech segments due to gestural overlap or coarticulation, segment and boundary identification can be a difficult task. This is particularly true for speakers with neurological disorders wherein imprecise articulation or voicing abnormalities may blur segment boundaries. Operational definitions of the onset and offset of events must be provided and consistent application of these definitions must be maintained throughout the analysis.

The most common reasons for segmenting the speech wave are to isolate portions of the signal corresponding to durations of specific segments, such as vowels and consonants (see the segmentation in **Figs. 4–1** and **4–2**), and to select a temporal "window" for spectral analysis. Segment durations have been studied extensively because they may provide insight into principles of speech production and because they are relatively easy measures to make. Many factors influence segment durations including speaking rate, dialect, phonetic context, stress, speech materials (e.g., connected versus isolated utterances; spontaneous speech versus reading), and idiosyncratic characteristics of the speaker (e.g., vocal tract length, gender, age, neurological status). **Table 4–1** summarizes the factors that influence segment duration. In addition, variables

that are intrinsic to the phonetic element (e.g., vowel height, voicing, consonant manner) are also important determinants of segment durations. The acoustic evaluation of speech sound durations must take into account the relative nature of these measurements because the durations depend on so many interacting factors. Thus, when comparing speech segment durations from a clinical evaluation of a given patient to values found in the literature (either for neurologically

Table 4–1   Factors that Influence Segment Durations and Vowel Formant Frequencies

*†Speaking rate
*†Phonetic context
*Position-in-utterance (e.g., at end versus beginning of utterance)
*†Stress
†Inherent characteristics (e.g., vowel tongue height, advancement, lip rounding, consonant voicing)
*†Type of speech material (e.g., isolated words versus connected speech, casual versus formal speech styles)
*†Idiosyncratic speaker characteristics (e.g., dialect, age, gender, vocal tract length)

Note: Factors marked with an asterisk (*) influence segment durations, and factors marked with a dagger (†) influence formant frequencies.

normal or impaired speakers), care must be taken to ensure the equivalence of factors such as segment identity, stress, phonetic context, dialect group, and so forth. Summaries of segment duration data for normal speakers can be found in Baken and Orlikoff (2000), Crystal and House (1988a–d), and Umeda (1975, 1977). Issues concerning speaking rate characteristics in normal populations are discussed by Crystal and House (1982), Miller, Grosjean, and Lomanto (1984), Robb, MacClagan, and Chen (2004), and Tsao and Weismer (1997), among others.

Spectral measures have also been studied extensively because they can be related to vocal tract configurations, and, by inference, articulatory positions and movements. Some of the factors that affect spectral measures are noted in **Table 4–1**. In general, spectral measures that are used to describe a given sound class (e.g., vowels) are based on a rather small temporal window (30 to 50 milliseconds). Because the resonances of the vocal tract are constantly changing, as a result of constantly varying articulatory movements, a larger temporal window for spectral analysis might include too many varying acoustic features that may smear the analysis. In many cases, however, the time-varying vocal tract resonances are the critical features of interest, and analysis of formant transitions (i.e., changes in formant frequencies over time) is required. This is discussed in greater detail below.

Fant (1960), in his classic work, showed that changes in vocal tract configuration have predictable influences on the acoustic output. Although unique relations between vocal tract shape and acoustic output cannot be defined, general principles can be applied. For example, in the case of vowels (1) advancement of the tongue from a posterior to anterior location within the vocal tract results in an increase of the second formant (F2) frequency and a decrease of first formant (F1) frequency (Fant, 1960; Stevens & House, 1955, 1961); (2) lowering of the tongue from high (e.g., /i/) to low (e.g., /a/) positions within the vocal tract increases the F1 frequency; and (3) elongation of the vocal tract by lip protrusion or larynx lowering tends to result in a decrease of all formant frequencies. The relationships between articulatory configuration and spectral characteristics are somewhat more complicated for consonants, but in general it can be stated that the pattern of resonances, or formants, associated with a stop, fricative, or affricate production is related to the size of the vocal tract cavity in front of the major constriction. For example, the spectrum of the stop burst for /t/ has a higher frequency representation than the spectrum for /k/ because of the smaller front cavity in /t/ articulation.

Because of these types of relationships, information about the spectral characteristics of speech can be extremely useful in the investigation of normal and disordered production. That is, insight about the articulatory bases of perceived speech abnormalities can be obtained by analysis of the spectral characteristics of the speech signal. The types of analyses that can be made and the information that they provide are reviewed in this and following sections.

A few limitations to interpretations of speech spectra need to be emphasized. First, comparisons of spectra across subjects need to be made with care. Differences in vocal tract size as well as relative sizes of the cavities composing the vocal tract result in variations in the speech spectrum. Because information about the physical dimensions of the vocal tract is difficult, if not impossible, to obtain directly, comparison among individual speakers needs to be made cautiously. Second, as in the case of segment durations, variations in the speech material affect the spectra so that comparisons between and within speakers must be made using the same sample. Third, within-speaker variation can be quite large, so frequent repetition of the material is required to obtain a reasonable estimate of speaker characteristics.

Techniques for spectral analysis include computer-based Fourier and linear predictive analysis as well as spectrography. Fourier analysis, usually performed digitally by means of a FFT, is based on the theorem that complex periodic waveforms can be decomposed into a series of sinusoidal components of certain amplitude and phase. Each sinusoidal component derived from the analysis of a complex periodic waveform is an integer multiple of a fundamental frequency, defined as the lowest common frequency in the complex. Fourier's theorem permits the transformation of a signal with amplitude that varies in time (i.e., a waveform) into a spectrum in which the amplitude of each component frequency is represented. The importance of this theorem for speech analysis is that it provides a technique for extraction of the fundamental frequency and its associated harmonics, related to vocal fold vibration, as well as an approximation of the vocal tract resonances. As seen in **Fig. 4–2B**, the many narrow peaks in the /i/ (left) and /u/ (right) vowel spectra represent the harmonics of the fundamental frequency. However, some peaks have higher amplitude than others because they are near a vocal tract resonance that acts to further amplify those frequencies. The regions of the spectrum where a group of harmonics is of relatively great amplitude, forming a coarser-grained spectral peak, are the formants.

Formant frequencies, which represent the vocal tract resonances, can be measured more easily from linear predictive coding (LPC) of the waveform, as seen in **Fig. 4–2C**. Note that the peaks in the LPC spectra (arrows) match the peaks in the FFT spectra fairly well. LPC (Makhoul, 1975) is a procedure that derives a series of coefficients that describe the time-varying waveform. These coefficients, if properly calculated, correspond to the formant frequencies. In general, the minimum number of coefficients needed to approximate a representation of the formant frequencies is one coefficient per kilohertz (kHz) of sampling rate. Two additional coefficients are needed to allow for voice and nasalization effects (Milenkovic, 2001). By way of example, if a waveform is sampled at 22 kHz, a minimum of 24 coefficients would need to be calculated to derive the formant frequencies. TF32, (Milenkovic, 2001), the computer program used in **Fig. 4–2**, generates the LPC and Fourier spectra in fractions of a second using a few mouse clicks. A cursor can be placed on a peak in the spectrum and the value at that point, that is, the formant value, is reported on screen. Thus, the measurement of formant frequencies is simple and straightforward.

Advantages of the LPC procedure include the relative ease in estimating formant frequencies from the spectrum as

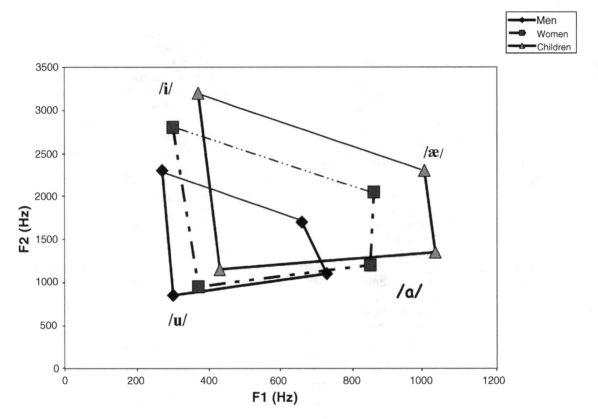

Figure 4–3 Vowel quadrilaterals for men (*diamonds*), women (*triangles*), and children (*squares*) from data reported by Peterson and Barney (1952).

well as the utility of the procedure with aperiodic signals. Because LPC can be applied to aperiodic signals, resonances associated with obstruent consonants can be derived. However, there are some limitations to the LPC procedure. Primary among these is that LPC analysis is based on the assumption that there are no side-branch resonators in the vocal tract. That is, only resonant frequencies are assumed with no provision for anti-resonances or zeroes in the signal. Anti-resonances, most commonly associated with nasal coupling in speech, interact with resonances to affect the spectral output. When anti-resonances are introduced, which may occur commonly in motorically impaired speakers who have difficulty with velopharyngeal closure, errors may be made in LPC estimates of formant frequency and bandwidth. A second limiting assumption of LPC analysis is that the vocal tract is modeled on the male speaker with a voiced source. In conventional LPC analysis, it is assumed that the source is a series of pitch pulses, each of which decays in the vocal tract prior to the next series of pitch pulses. Any deviation from this assumption results in an interaction between the source and vocal tract, which yields systematic errors of formant frequency and bandwidth. Because motor speech disorders are characterized by abnormal voice qualities (Darley, Aronson, & Brown, 1975), LPC estimates of formant frequencies may be imprecise. Although the LPC technique is powerful, easy to use, and informative, knowledge of its limitations, particularly for disordered speakers, is important.

Formant frequencies for vowels have been studied extensively (see summary in Hillenbrand and Gayvert, 1993, and Kent and Read, 2002), and many factors that affect temporal measures also impact spectral analyses (e.g., speaker characteristics, speaking rate, etc.). The same caution about comparing vowel durations from clinical settings to previously published data applies, therefore, to formant frequencies as well. Although there are numerous formants that are produced during vowel articulation, most vowels can be adequately described on the basis of their first two formants, F1 and F2. **Figure 4–3** shows an F1-F2 plot of the vowels of American English, for men, women, and children. These formant measurements were obtained in the classic way (Peterson & Barney, 1952), using a narrow temporal window centered in the middle of the vowels, as displayed on spectrograms. Note that the first and second formant frequencies for these vowels are consistent with the rules relating vocal tract configuration and vocal tract output, stated above, and help to categorize vowels on the basis of formant frequencies. For example, the low F1 and high F2 of the high front vowel /i/ follows from the rules stating that (1) moving the tongue forward raises F2 and lowers F1, and (2) raising the tongue lowers F1. The reader may want to test the logic of these rules on the other vowels plotted in **Fig. 4–3** to prove the general utility of inferring vocal tract configurations from vowel formant frequencies.

As illustrated in **Fig. 4–4**, consonant spectra are typically multipeaked with energy spread widely throughout the

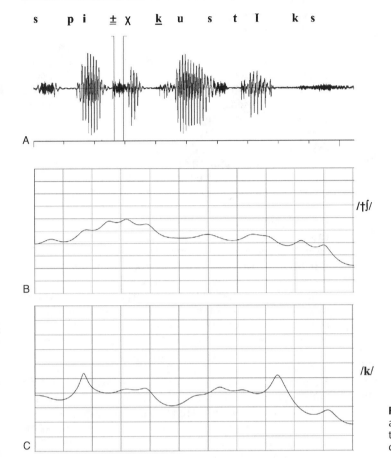

s   p i   ± χ   k   u   s   t   ɪ   k s

A

/t∫/

B

/k/

C

Figure 4–4 Waveform **(A)**, LPC spectra computed during the affricate /t∫/ **(B)** from the word *speech*, and the stop /k/ **(C)** from the word *acoustics*. Note the diffusion of peaks in the spectra for consonants.

frequency range; therefore, it is difficult to quantify the acoustic characteristics of consonants via a small group of stable formant peaks (e.g., F1-F2) as was discussed above for vowels. **Figure 4–4** shows a spectrum for a 20-ms windowed interval at the onset of the affricate /t∫/ in "speech" **(Fig. 4–4A)**, and a spectrum for the same-sized window at the onset of the first /k/ in "acoustics" **(Fig. 4–4B)**. The spectral shape of consonants depends on the overall distribution of energy across the frequency range of interest, rather than a few selected peaks. Description of acoustic characteristics of consonants, therefore, must include information about the shape of the spectrum, in addition to frequency. Quantification of spectral shape not only avoids the problem of finding stable peaks in the spectrum, but also seems to reflect the perceptual processing of consonant spectra (Jongman, Wayland, & Wong, 2000; Tomiak, 1990). As in the case of vowels, spectral analysis for consonants requires the selection of some temporal window for the analysis; the actual size of this window may vary from 20 to 100 ms, depending on the type of sound and purpose of the analysis. Additional details of spectral measurement strategies for consonants are provided below, in the discussion of the acoustic correlates of imprecise consonants. The spectral characteristics of English consonants have been reviewed by Forrest, Weismer, Milenkovic, and Dougall (1988), Kent and Read (2002), Kewley-Port (1983), Olive, Greenwood, and Coleman (1994), and Stevens (1999).

♦ Acoustic Analysis in Motor Speech Disorders

The classic departure point for understanding the speech production deficit in motor speech disorders is the Mayo classification system (Darley, Aronson, & Brown, 1969a,b, 1975). Darley et al listened to tape-recordings of the grandfather passage read by patients with a variety of known neurological diseases, and generated psychophysical scalings of 38 selected dimensions of disordered speech (see Darley et al, 1975, pp. 289–293). These perceptual dimensions were then combined in various ways to produce unique clusters of dimensions for the different dysarthria types. Here we introduce some general concepts of acoustic analysis in motor speech disorders by describing the likely acoustic correlates of some of the perceptual dimensions used in the Mayo system. We are not suggesting that the exemplar analyses described here are specific to the selected types of motor speech disorders; indeed, most of these analyses can be applied to any type of speech disorder.

Selected Perceptual Dimensions and Their Acoustic Correlates

Although the Mayo studies made use of 38 perceptual dimensions, a more limited set seemed to figure prominently

Table 4–2   Prominent Perceptual Dimensions from the Mayo Studies (Darley, et al, 1969a,b, 1975) and the Likely Acoustic Correlates of These Dimensions

Perceptual Dimension	Acoustic Correlates
Distorted vowels	Vowel durations
	Formant frequencies
	Formant transitions
Imprecise consonants	Consonant durations
	Consonant spectra
	Formant transitions
Hypernasality	Low F1 frequency
	Low-intensity formants
	Spectral zeros
Monopitch	Flat f0 contour
Monoloudness	Flat sound pressure level (SPL) contour
Harsh voice	Jitter
	Decreased signal-to-noise ratio
Stress abnormalities	Limited f0 range
	Vowel duration
	Consonant duration

in the descriptions of several different types of motor speech disorders. Some of these perceptual dimensions, along with their corresponding acoustic characteristics or measures, are listed in **Table 4–2** and discussed below.

Distorted Vowels

Although the common view of speech intelligibility is that most of the information-bearing elements of speech are to be found in the consonants, there is accumulating evidence that vowel characteristics contribute heavily to speech intelligibility deficits (Kent, Kent, Weismer, Sufit, Brooks, & Rosenbek, 1989; Turner, Tjaden, & Weismer, 1995; Ziegler & von Cramon, 1986). This contribution was probably reflected in the Mayo studies of dysarthria, where the perceptual-dimension–distorted vowels were a prominent component of several different dysarthrias (e.g., spastic, ataxic, hyperkinetic including both chorea and dystonia, and mixed dysarthria of amyotrophic lateral sclerosis [ALS]). Acoustic measures relating to perception of distorted vowels include, but are not necessarily limited to, vowel durations, vowel formant frequencies, and characteristics of formant transitions.

Vowel Durations   Measures of vowel durations are fairly straightforward, especially when the vowels are located between obstruent consonants. In **Fig. 4–1** there are four vowel segments indicated. Note that the initial and final full glottal pulses of the formant pattern are used to denote the vocalic onset and offset, respectively. A full glottal pulse is one that shows energy at least through the first two formants, indicating that the vocal tract was still open at this point in time. By contrast, glottal pulses seen during the closure intervals of voiced stops and fricatives tend to have very low amplitude in waveform displays, and show energy only along the baseline in spectrograms.

Vowel durations are quite variable during speech production, ranging anywhere from approximately 40 to 300 ms for normal speakers. The variation in vowel duration is due to factors such as stress, vowel identity, speaking rate, dialect, and phonetic context, among others (see Crystal & House, 1988a–d, for a complete review). In speakers with neurological disease, variation in vowel duration is often greater than that observed in normal speakers because slow speaking rate, which is a common feature in dysarthria, may increase the duration of vowel intervals. In addition, the contribution of abnormal vowel durations to the perception of distorted vowels may actually involve relational attributes of several vowels, rather than absolute durational characteristics of single vowels. In connected English, vowel durations are conditioned in large part by the stress patterns of the language, and therefore tend to alternate between relatively long and short intervals. When successive vowels in an utterance deviate from this pattern and have roughly equalized durations (Kent, Netsell, & Abbs, 1979), the intended short (unstressed) vowel may sound distorted in relation to the sequence in which it is embedded. The Mayo dimension "equal and excess stress" partly reflects this loss of vowel duration contrast. For example, in **Fig. 4–5** note the variability of the vowel durations for /aω/, /aI/, /æ/, and /a/ (from "...about my grandfather") produced by a normal speaker **(Fig. 4–5A)**, but the greater similarity of these vowel durations as produced by a speaker with cerebellar disease **(Fig. 4–5B;** note especially the long /æ/ in grandfather). Vowel duration measures can obviously serve as an index of the perceptual dimensions "slow rate" and "prolonged intervals," as shown in **Fig. 4–5C**, where the production of /I/ and /ɔ/ durations by a person with spastic dysarthria can be compared with the normal durations in **Fig. 4–5A**. Note that this speaker was unable to complete the first sentence of the grandfather passage within the timeframe used for the normal and ataxic speakers.

Formant Frequencies and Transitions   Vowel spectra can be used to make inferences about the vocal tract configuration. There is a rich tradition of measuring the formant frequencies of vowels as an index of vocal tract shape at a given instant in time (Peterson & Barney, 1952; and summary in Kent & Read, 2002), and a more recent focus of using formant transitions (i.e., the change in formant frequencies over time) to understand dynamic articulatory behavior (Jenkins & Strange, 1999; Kent, Kent, et al, 1990). The interpretation of the formant frequencies should follow from the rules discussed above on page 49. Other variables to consider when investigating formant frequencies of vowels include speaking rate, wherein vowel distinctiveness decreases with increased rate (Tjaden & Wilding, 2004; Turner et al, 1995); phonetic environment, in that overlapping gestures influence the spectral characteristics of vowels (Fowler, 1980; Liberman, Cooper, Shankweiler, & Studdert-Kennedy, 1967; Magen, 1997); and dialectal differences, which may cause vocalic variations (Whalen, Magen, Pouplier, Kang, & Iskarous, 2004).

The relationship between vowel identity and formant frequency may be elusive in speakers with neuromotor

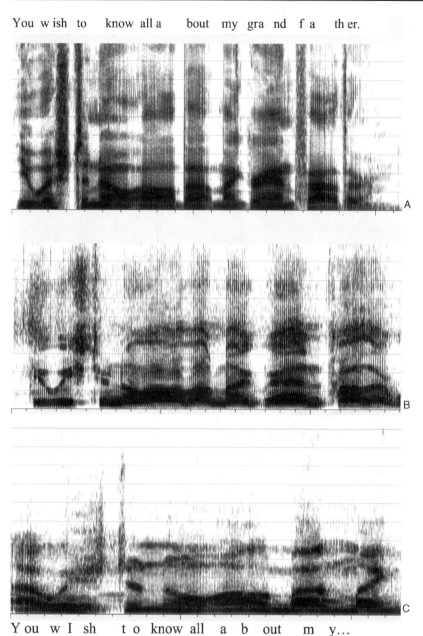

You w ish to   know all a   bout my gra nd f a   th er.

You wI sh   t o know all   a   b   out   m y...

Figure 4–5 Spectrograms of portions of the utterance "You wish to know all about my grandfather" spoken by a neurologically normal adult **(A)**, a speaker with cerebellar disease **(B)**, and a person with spastic dysarthria **(C)**. Note how these different speakers control vowel duration, with the normal speaker varying duration depending on the importance of the target word. By comparison, the speaker with cerebellar disease has similar durations for all vowels, whereas the spastic dysarthric prolongs the vocalic elements.

disorders. A primary cue to the vowel height distinction is the frequency difference between F1 and F2, with higher vowels having a greater F2-F1 distance than low vowels. This relationship ensues, in part, because of the inverse relation of F1 frequency to oral opening (Fant, 1960; Peterson & Barney, 1952). Bunton and Weismer (2001) investigated the relationship between F2-F1 and listeners' word identification from a closed-set intelligibility test (Kent et al, 1989). The prediction that speakers with neuromotor disorders, including ALS, Parkinson's disease, and cerebrovascular accident (CVA), would evidence F2-F1 reductions when their vowel height was misperceived was not supported in many cases. Rather, there was considerable overlap in the acoustic representation of correct and reduced vowels. These results support earlier assertions that speech acoustics and perception

have a complex interaction. Because there are multiple cues to any vowel distinction (e.g., vowel duration, formant frequency variation, fundamental frequency differences), it is unlikely that any single acoustic dimension accounts for the variance in listeners' judgments. In fact, acoustic cues are likely to have a "trading" relation with one another wherein different weights of cues combine to yield a perceptual distinction between phones (Repp, 1982).

Despite the potential for cue trading, some acoustic measures can lead to distinct hypotheses about articulatory control in speakers with neurological disorders. **Fig. 4–6** shows F1-F2 plots for the corner vowels (/i/, /u/, /a/, /æ/) produced by five neurologically normal speakers **(Fig. 4–6A)** and five patients with ALS **(Fig. 4–6B)**. The plotted values are means based on five repetitions for each speaker. Note

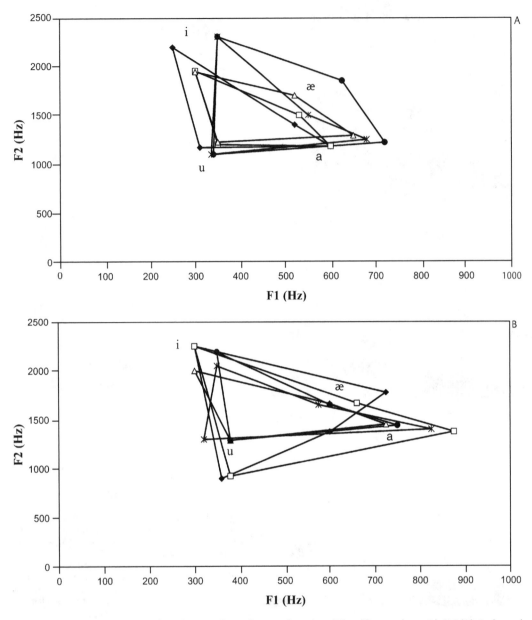

Figure 4–6 Vowel quadrilaterals from five neurologically normal speakers **(A)** and five speakers with ALS **(B)**. Each speaker within a group is represented by a different symbol. Note the compression of the F2 range for some of the ALS speakers, as evidenced by decreased spacing of F2 for /i/ and /u/.

the compression of the vowel space in the /i/ and /u/ regions for three of the speakers with ALS, and the apparent expansion of the vowel space in the /a/ region for three of the patients (compare with the plot for normal speakers). One possible articulatory interpretation of these data is that some of these patients have restricted anteroposterior movements of the tongue (hence the compressed F1-F2 plot, especially along the F2 axis) and excessive opening of the jaw for low vowels (inferred from the very high F1 values for /a/). The excessive opening of the jaw could be a compensation for the poor tongue control that appears to be a prominent feature in ALS (DePaul & Brooks, 1993). Taken together, these acoustic characteristics are likely to

explain some components of distorted vowels in these patients, and could serve as a basis for evaluation of treatment effects or of change in speech production deficits due to disease progression.

On the spectrogram shown in **Fig. 4–7**, the formant trajectories (formant frequencies as a function of time) are traced by gray lines for F1, F2, and F3 throughout the vowel nucleus. These trajectories are composed of the formant frequencies at consecutive instants in time projected throughout the duration of the vocalic elements. Formant trajectories provide information on the changing configuration of the vocal tract, rather than the single position measurement associated with a set of formant frequencies at one point in time. The trajectories

"You ...

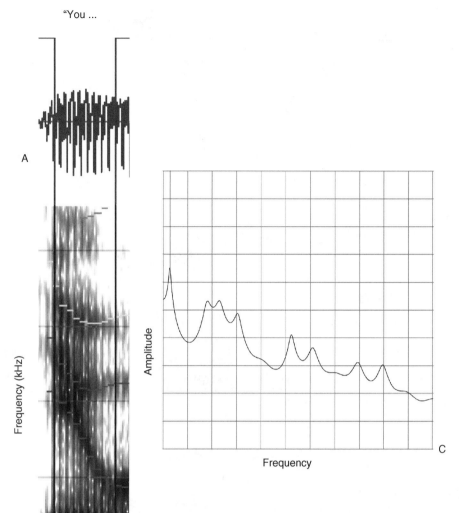

A

B   Time

C   Frequency

Figure 4–7 **(A)** Computer-generated waveform, **(B)** spectrogram, and **(C)** LPC spectrum that provide easy access to acoustic analysis. Formant trajectories, the instantaneous formant frequencies, are marked with a line through the midpoint of each formant on the spectrogram.

for different formants may change by different amounts and at different times, and parts of any one trajectory may change dramatically over some interval and then remain at the same frequency for some subsequent interval. The parts of any trajectory associated with large frequency change, reflecting relatively large changes in vocal tract configuration, are often referred to as transitions.

Figure 4–8 shows schematic F1 and F2 formant trajectories for the diphthong /aI/, together with measurements derived from the transitional segment. The transition extent (TE) is the range of frequencies covered by a transition, and reflects the amount of change in vocal tract configuration; larger TEs are associated with greater alterations in vocal tract configuration. The transition duration (TD) is the time taken to complete the transitional segment. Both TE and TD depend on an operational definition of the onset and offset of a formant transition, which is discussed in greater detail by Weismer and his colleagues (Weismer & Berry, 2003; Weismer, Kent, Hodge, & Martin, 1988; Weismer & Martin, 1992;

Weismer, Martin, Kent, & Kent, 1992). When TE and TD are known, the derived measure transition rate (TR) can be computed by dividing TE by TD. This measure is an index of the slope of the formant transition, which can be interpreted in articulatory terms as the speed of change in vocal tract configuration. Small values of TE and TR, and small or large values of TD, may all be associated with the perceptual dimension of distorted vowels. The small values of TE indicate some limitation on changing vocal tract configuration for a given articulatory gesture, perhaps reflecting a failure to reach a target configuration for a vowel or a general restriction on the range of articulatory movements. Small values of TR reflect slow articulatory gestures, a common problem in motor speech disorders (see Weismer & Martin, 1992, Table 2, p. 86). Small or large values of TD suggest abbreviated or elongated articulatory transitions, respectively, both of which are seen in various forms of motor speech disorders. Care must be taken in the interpretation of these measures, because TE, TD, and TR are not independent (Weismer et al,

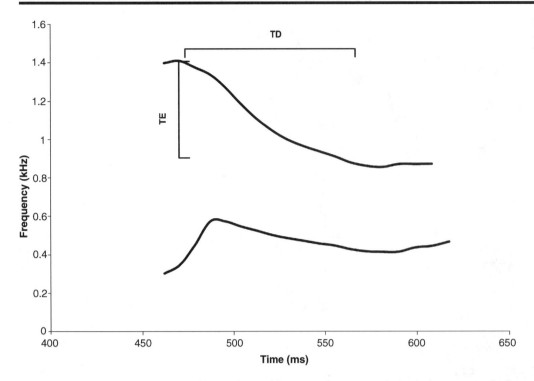

Figure 4–8 Schematic representation of first and second formants. The transition duration (TD) is the time taken to complete the part of the F2 transition associated with movement in the vocal tract. The transition extent (TE), which represents the frequency excursion of the F2 transition, is a measure that corresponds to the amount change in the vocal tract shape.

1992). Further, many aspects of the transition, such as linearity of frequency change, may vary with speaking rate and accuracy (Weismer & Berry, 2003).

Figure 4–9 shows formant trajectories for the word *sigh* for a group of neurologically healthy men and a group of men with ALS and poor speech intelligibility (Weismer et al, 1992). Note that the trajectories from the ALS speakers are relatively long as compared with those for the normal talkers. In addition, the transitional portions of the trajectories from the men with ALS are much shallower than the normal trajectories, especially for F2. These extended and slow formant transitions may be another component of the perceptual dimension of "distorted vowels." Abnormal formant transitions also may relate to the perception of imprecise consonants in that the transitions reflect changes in vocal tract configurations for varying speech segments (see later discussion).

Imprecise Consonants

The perceptual impression of imprecise consonants is common in all types of motor speech disorders, and presumably is influenced by a range of consonant production anomalies (e.g., distortions, omissions, and substitutions). As such, this perceptual dimension may not be useful to differentiate different dysarthria types, although acoustic analysis may help distinguish the articulatory variations that lead to this ubiquitous percept. We assume for this discussion that consonant distortions contribute heavily to the impression of imprecise consonants, and consider the relevant temporal and spectral measures.

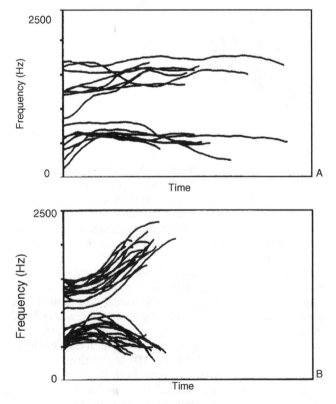

Figure 4–9 F2 trajectories for the word *sigh* in neurologically normal males **(A)** and male speakers with ALS **(B)**. Notice the difference in the slopes and durations of the trajectories for these two groups of speakers.

Consonant Durations As in the case of vowel durations, the temporal measures for consonants are quite straightforward and in most cases easily obtained from either waveform or spectrographic displays (see **Fig. 4–1**). The intervals that are measured depend on the manner of consonant production. Stop and affricate consonants include intervals of vocal tract closure, release, and voice onset time (VOT), whereas sonorant consonants are characterized by a single, prolonged interval. Typically, stop closure durations, the time during which the vocal tract is completely occluded for the buildup of intraoral air pressure, are measured from the final, full glottal pulse of the preceding vowel to the subsequent stop burst. Stop closure durations are usually on the order of 70 to 120 ms, and rarely exceed 150 ms (Stathopoulos & Weismer, 1985). The burst is the acoustic manifestation of the sudden release of the impounded air pressure and typically is extremely short. The duration of voiced and voiceless fricatives is measured from the final full glottal pulse preceding the frication energy to the first full glottal pulse following the frication.

The commonly measured interval VOT is measured from the burst to the first full glottal pulse of the following vowel and is an index of the time from the release of the vocal tract occlusion to the onset of voicing. VOTs are usually in excess of 35 ms for voiceless stops, and less than 20 ms for voiced stops. The closure interval and VOT are measured in a similar way for affricates, which have VOTs greater than those observed in stops of the same voicing status.

Consonant durations in dysarthric speech are often abnormal, and may be either too long or too short. The influence of abnormal consonant durations, in general, on the perception of imprecise consonants is unknown, and it is not clear why such abnormalities would affect a perception of precision. In fact, Chen and Stevens (2001) found that /s/ duration did not correlate with listeners' ratings of speech quality or intelligibility of eight speakers with varying types of dysarthria. Other time-varying features, particularly the amplitude variation through the fricative's duration, were more strongly predictive of the intelligibility deficits experienced by these dysarthric speakers.

Voice onset time abnormalities, especially those in a region in which the voicing characteristics of the sound are ambiguous (i.e., between approximately 20 and 40 ms), may be a component of imprecise consonants. For example, consonant errors in apraxia of speech have been shown to reflect VOT distortions rather than phoneme substitutions (Blumstein, Cooper, Goodglass, Statlender, & Gottlieb, 1980). Further, unusually long VOT durations often are seen in spastic dysarthria (Kent & Rosenbek, 1983; Weismer, 1984) in part because of the slow speaking rate, and may affect consonant precision. The very brief closure durations seen for the speaker with Parkinson's disease are likely to contribute to the impression of distorted consonants, probably because the contrasts between the consonant and adjacent vowels are blurred (Kent & Rosenbek, 1983; Weismer, 1984) by the brief closure duration. Also, reduced closure duration may reflect articulatory weakness or hypokinesia in that the oral structures cannot maintain a pressure buildup. In these cases, there may be evidence of spirantization, wherein the stop consonant is realized as a fricative (Weismer, 1984).

Consonant Spectra The spectra of stop bursts and fricative noises would seem to be a valuable source of information concerning articulatory configurations for consonants. There is a fairly well developed literature concerning the normally articulated acoustic characteristics of consonants (see reviews and data in Forrest et al, 1988; Jongman et al, 2000; Kent & Read, 2002; Olive et al, 1994; Stevens, 1999; Stevens & Blumstein, 1978), and in many cases the theory relates acoustic characteristics to articulatory configuration in a fairly straightforward way (Fant, 1960). It therefore may seem surprising to encounter so few data in the literature concerning spectral analysis of consonant production in motor speech disorders.

The lack of these data can be explained by considering the measurement issues in quantifying consonant spectra. As discussed above, consonant spectra are typically multi-peaked, with energy spread widely throughout the frequency range, and investigators have long felt that some index of the shape of consonant spectra was important (see above). Several investigators have used a categorical system to measure spectral shape, wherein spectral templates related to place of articulation are used to categorize consonant spectra (Kewley-Port, 1983; Stevens & Blumstein, 1978). Shinn and Blumstein (1983) have demonstrated the use of the Stevens and Blumstein template system in understanding stop consonant production in aphasia, but little other work has been done in this area. The application of the template system to persons with motor speech disorders is very time-consuming, requiring a human observer to generate and classify the spectra on an individual basis. This is an unlikely scenario for the clinician who wishes to use spectral analysis of consonants in a work setting.

Forrest et al (1988) developed a simple quantitative, observer-free approach to the measurement of consonant spectra. In their approach, the spectrum is treated as a statistical distribution that can be described by values for the mean, skewness, and kurtosis. The mean quantifies the central tendency of the energy in the spectrum (see also the centroid measure of Harmes, Daniloff, Hoffman, Lewis, Kramer, & Absher, 1984); the skewness, which is the degree to which the spectral energy is tilted toward the low or high frequencies; and the kurtosis, which is the degree to which the spectrum has sharp peaks or is relatively flat. More recent investigations demonstrate that the variance of the spectral distribution (i.e., the second moment) is useful in differentiating place of articulation for fricatives produced by neurologically healthy adults (Jongman et al, 2000) and children (Bunnell, Polikoff, & McNicholas, 2004; but see later discussion). These numerical indices of spectral shape can be generated very quickly with a computer program.

Figure 4–10 shows some sample spectra of stop bursts from [t] and frication noises from [z] produced by both neurologically normal and dysarthric speakers, along with the values of the mean and coefficients of skewness and kurtosis. There appears to be some relationship between "articulatory precision" obtained by perceptual ratings and the first moment coefficient, that is, the spectral mean (Tjaden & Turner, 1997). In their investigation of speakers with ALS and neurologically healthy adults, Tjaden and Turner showed that a significant amount of the variance in listeners'

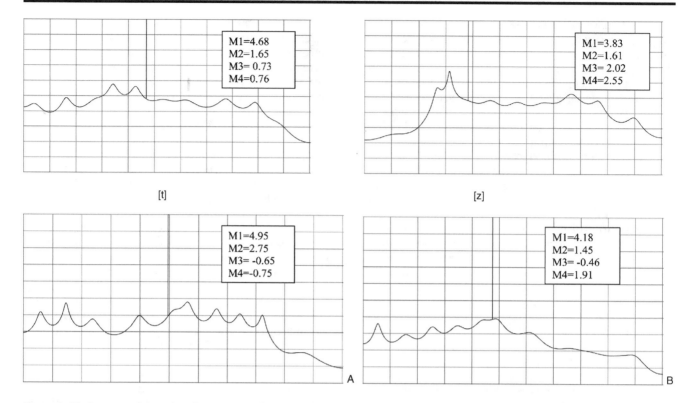

Figure 4–10 Spectra and corresponding moments for neurologically normal speaker **(A)** and a speaker with ALS **(B)**. The top panels present the waveforms and spectra for /t/ in "tile" and the bottom panels show the spectra for /z/ in "ease." M1 is the first moment, or centroid, of the spectrum; M2 is the spectral variance; M3 is the coefficient of skewness, a measure of the tilt of the spectrum; and M4 is the coefficient of kurtosis, an index that captures the "peakedness" of the spectrum.

ratings of sibilant precision was determined by the difference in spectral means of /s/ and /ʃ/. Further, McRae, Tjaden, and Schoonings (2002) used the first spectral moment (mean) to demonstrate a reduction in articulatory working space in people with Parkinson's disease compared with age-matched control subjects. More work is needed in this area to determine if spectral moments provide a useful acoustic measure to relate to listeners' judgments of consonant precision.

Hypernasality

Hypernasality is a prominent perceptual dimension in several of the disorders studied by Darley et al (1969a,b), including flaccid, spastic, and forms of mixed dysarthria, such as that seen in ALS. The underlying articulatory problem in hypernasality is a chronically open velopharyngeal port due to paralysis or paresis of the relevant musculature (i.e., the levator veli palatini and superior constrictor muscles of the pharynx) or inappropriately timed closure and opening of the port. The typical acoustic correlates of nasal articulation are (1) an intense, low-frequency F1 around 250 to 300 Hz; (2) a series of low-intensity formants roughly at 1000, 2000, 3000, and 4000 Hz; (3) regions of the spectrum showing little or no energy; and (4) a relatively low, overall intensity compared with vowel intensities. The low-frequency F1 is a resonance of the nasal cavities and the pharynx, and the low intensity of the higher formants is a result of anti-resonances and large amounts of sound energy absorption in the

nasal cavities (see Kent and Read, 2002, for an explanation of anti-resonances). These qualitative features are often fairly easy to spot in a spectrographic display, but it is difficult to quantify degrees of nasality using this type of acoustic technique. In certain patients with chronic hypernasality, as in selected cases of flaccid dysarthria, the presence of the acoustic markers of nasality described above can actually prevent meaningful analysis of any part of the signal. This is because the chronic presence of anti-resonances and absorption of sound energy in the nasal cavities obscures vocalic formant structures and consonantal landmarks, as shown in **Fig. 4–11**, where the phrase "he dresses himself" has been spoken by a neurologically healthy male **(Fig. 4–11A)** and a speaker with ALS **(Fig. 4–11B)** who evidences hypernasality. Note the very dark F1 that extends throughout the entire utterance, and the loss of the boundaries between and vowels and vowels and consonants, as compared with the spectrogram in **Fig. 4–11A**.

Several procedures have been detailed to quantify hypernasality (Chen, 1995, 1997; Kataoka, Warren, Zajac, Mayo, & Lutz, 2001; Lee, Ciocca, & Whitehill, 2003). These procedures use the relative energy in frequency bands between F1 and F2. Lee et al demonstrated increased energy in the one-third octave centered at 630, 800, and 1000 Hz as well as decreased energy in the filter band centered at 2500 Hz in speakers with hypernasal speech, including three individuals with dysarthria. Although this study had a small number of speakers with dysarthria, as well as production of only an isolated /i/ vowel, the results suggest a promising

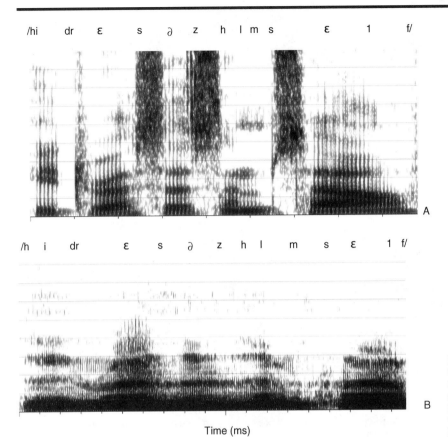

/hi dr ε s ∂ z h l m s ε 1 f/

A

/h i dr ε s ∂ z h l m s ε 1 f/

B

Time (ms)

Figure 4–11 Spectrograms of a normal production of the sequence "he dresses himself" **(A)** and the same utterance produced by a speaker with spastic dysarthria who exhibited excessive nasality **(B).** Note the ambiguity of vowel formants in the hypernasal production and the continuous low-frequency energy, typical of nasalization.

technique for quantifying hypernasality associated with dysarthric speech.

Voice Dimensions

Various voice dimensions figured prominently in Darley et al's (1975) description of the motor speech disorders. Some of these dimensions, such as harsh voice, breathy voice, and strained-strangled voice, are perceptual impressions of voice quality. **Figure 4–12** shows time and amplitude variation indicated on a waveform of a normal voice, and a waveform of a voice of someone with dystonia that is perceived to be harsh. Note that the waveform in **Fig. 4–12A**, there is minimal time and amplitude variation from cycle to cycle of this sustained /a/. In contrast, the waveform for the harsh /a/, shown in **Fig. 4–12B**, clearly contains time and amplitude variation.

To a first approximation, voice quality can be said to be determined by the shape of the glottal spectrum and the relative amount of periodic and aperiodic energy in that spectrum. Physiologically, these two acoustic components of voice quality are likely to be interdependent, and so we discuss the acoustic measures of voice quality without differentiating their relationship to different aspects of the glottal spectrum. As we will suggest, this is one of the weaknesses of acoustic measures of voice quality.

Much has been written about the influence of cycle-to-cycle variability of glottal periods on voice quality. The term *jitter* is used to describe variability occurring in time, wherein successive glottal periods differ from cycle to cycle. Variability in the amplitude of successive cycles is referred to as *shimmer*. A certain amount of jitter and shimmer give the normal voice a quality of fullness or richness, but too much variability in the period or amplitude of successive glottal cycles will typically result in the perception of a noisy voice quality. As described in detail by Baken (1987, pp. 113–119, 166–188), there are many ways to measure jitter and shimmer, and little agreement on which ways should be preferred (see also Pinto & Titze, 1990; Titze, 1991). We will not review the different approaches to making these measurements, but will note that many speech analysis programs include some form of jitter and shimmer analysis. Generally, the voice quality abnormality, as judged perceptually, will seem increasingly severe as the jitter or shimmer values become more different from normal values. In this sense, the jitter and shimmer measures may serve as useful "hardcopy" indices of perceptual events. A major limitation of these measures, however, is the lack of a straightforward relationship between the specific values and the underlying physiological behavior (see Titze, 1991). Thus jitter and shimmer values cannot help differentiate between, for example, a neurologically versus mechanically based problem in the larynx. Further, jitter and shimmer require highly refined recording procedures to be interpretable; therefore, other measures of perturbation such as signal-to-noise ratio may be more useful in clinical settings.

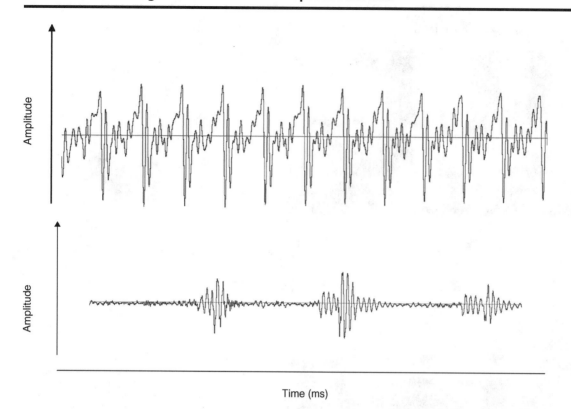

Figure 4–12 Waveform of the vowel /a/ showing the cycle-to-cycle variation found in a normal voice **(A)** and a voice that is perceived to be harsh **(B)**. Notice the temporal and amplitude variation across cycles in the harsh voice.

The signal-to-noise ratio, sometimes called the harmonic-to-inharmonic ratio or harmonic-to-noise ratio, can also be considered an acoustic counterpart of voice quality. This acoustic index is designed to capture the balance between periodic energy, generated by the cyclic vocal fold vibration, and aperiodic energy, resulting largely from turbulent flows generated in the vicinity of the glottis. High signal-to-noise ratios are typically associated with vocal fold vibration that involves good closure and symmetric action of the two folds; low signal-to-noise ratios are associated with poor closure (i.e., the kind of vocal fold vibration often resulting in the perception of a breathy or hoarse voice). Signal-to-noise values are likely to covary with jitter and shimmer values, so the measures may be somewhat redundant with respect to each other. Like jitter and shimmer values, signal-to-noise ratios may covary with perceptual judgments, but are difficult to interpret in terms of underlying mechanisms. Some predictive advantage may be gained, however, if the acoustic measures are processed through auditory filters (Shrivastav, 2001). For example, Shrivastav and Sapienza (2003) demonstrated a strong relation between perceived breathiness and partial loudness of the signal and aspiration noise when the acoustic signal was processed through the auditory model of Moore, Glasberg, and Baer (1997). Interesting hypotheses regarding the acoustic correlates of voice dysfunction in dysarthria may be tested with this procedure.

Finally, Darley et al (1975) employed several voice dimensions designed to reflect insufficient or excessive variability in the output of the larynx. Monopitch, monoloudness, and excess and equal stress are three of these dimensions, and each has acoustic counterparts. The acoustic counterpart of monopitch requires an analysis of a fundamental frequency (F0) contour of a sentence, such as the one shown in **Fig. 4–13A**, where the speech waveform and F0 contour are shown for the utterance, "A yellow lion roared." In this sentence the F0 varies by as much as 50 Hz, which is not unusual for simple declarative utterances spoken by neurologically normal individuals; this variation is shown by the up and down movement of the F0 trace in the top figure. In contrast, the relatively flat F0 contour shown in **Fig. 4–13B** is the result of an aberrant production of "A yellow lion roared." The F0 contour for this speaker would almost certainly be scaled as more severe on the monopitch scale than the F0 contour for the normal speaker, but the precise relationship between features of F0 contours and the perceptual monopitch scale is unknown. Studies have shown reduced fundamental frequency range for dysarthric speakers with Parkinson's disease (King, Ramig, Lemke, & Horii, 1993) and ALS (Ramig, Scherer, Klasner, Titze, & Horii, 1990). These reductions in F0 range certainly would contribute to the mono-perceptions discussed above. Similarly, computer programs like TF32 (Milenkovic, 2001) and the Multi-Dimensional Voice Program (Kay Pentax, Pine Brook, NJ, 1993) can display sound-pressure-level (SPL) traces for an utterance that should correspond at some level to the perceptual dimension of monoloudness. When either the F0 or SPL trace indicates flatness, one can interpret the underlying mechanism as lacking flexibility, but the reasons for this are not revealed by the acoustic analysis.

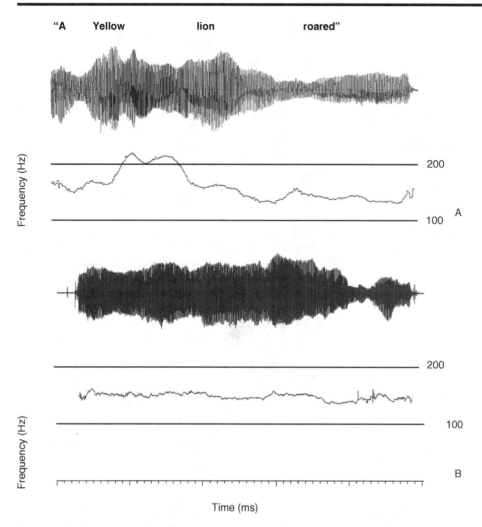

Figure 4–13 Waveforms and fundamental frequency traces for the sentence "A yellow lion roared," spoken normally **(A)** and by a female who was perceived to speak with monopitch **(B)**. The fundamental frequency traces are plotted with time on the abscissa and frequency along the ordinate.

The perceptual dimension of equal and excess stress has already been mentioned in the context of duration measures of vowels, but it is also relevant here because of the effect of F0 and SPL on stress judgments. Stress contrasts in words or at the sentence level are typically characterized by higher F0 and SPL on stressed, as compared with unstressed, syllables. A succession of syllables having roughly equivalent and extreme values of peak F0 and SPLs is likely to promote the perceptual impression of equal and excess stress. The kind of acoustic analysis of sentence-level prosodic events presented here could be used to track progress associated with a naturalness training program (see Yorkston, Beukelman, Strand, & Bell, 1999).

References

♦ Conclusion

The application of acoustic analysis as a clinical tool in motor speech disorders is a valuable application for this powerful procedure. A combination of greater understanding of acoustic characteristics of disordered speech, paired with the call for greater explanatory power in the analysis of motor speech disorders (Kent, Weismer, et al, 1989) provides motivation for the clinician to gain facility with acoustic analysis. The advent of user-friendly and relatively inexpensive computer algorithms makes it likely that acoustic analysis will find increasing acceptance in the diagnosis and management of motor speech disordered clients.

Baken, R. (1987). *Clinical Measurement of Speech and Voice.* Boston: Little, Brown

Baken, R.J. & Orlikoff, R.F. (2000). *Clinical Measurement of Speech and Voice.* San Diego: Singular

Boersma, P. & Weenink, D. (2008). Praat: doing phonetis by computer (Version 5.0. 10) [Computer program]. http://www.pratt.org/

Browman, C.P. & Goldstein, L.M. (1990). Gestural Specification using dynamically defined articulatory structures. *Journal of Phonetics, 18,* 299–320.

Blumstein S.E., Cooper W.E., Goodglass H., Statlender S., Gottlieb J., (1980). Production deficits in aphasia: a voice-onset time analysis. *Brain and Language, 9,* 153–170

Byrd, D. & Saltzman, E. (2003). The elastic phrase: Modeling the dynamics of boundary-adjacent lengthening. *Journal of Phonetics, 31,* 149–181

Bunnell, H.T., Polikoff, J.B., & McNicholas, J. (2004). Spectral moment vs. bark spectral analysis of children's word-initial voiceless stops. In: *Proceedings of the Eighth International Conference on Spoken Language Processing,* October 4–8, Jeju, Korea

Bunton, K. & Weismer, G. (2001). The relationship between perception and acoustics for a high-low vowel contrast produced by speakers with dysarthria. *Journal of Speech, Language, and Hearing, 44,* 1215–1228

Chen, M. Y. (1995). Acoustic parameters of nasalized vowels in hearing-impaired and normal-hearing speakers. *Journal of the Acoustical Society of America, 98,* 2443–2453

Chen, M.Y. (1997). Acoustic correlates of English and French nasalized vowels. *Journal of the Acoustical Society of America, 102,* 2360–2370

Chen, H. & Stevens, K.N. (2001). An acoustical study of the fricative /s/ in the speech of individuals with dysarthria. *Journal of Speech, Language, and Hearing Research, 44,* 1300–1314

Crystal, T.H. & House, A.S. (1982). Segmental durations in connected-speech signals: Preliminary results. *Journal of the Acoustical Society of America, 72,* 705–716

Crystal, T.H. & House, A.S. (1988a). Segmental durations in connected-speech signals: Current results. *Journal of the Acoustical Society of America, 83,* 1553–1573

Crystal, T.H. & House, A.S. (1988b). Segmental durations in connected-speech signals: Syllabic stress. *Journal of the Acoustical Society of America, 83,* 1574–1585

Crystal, T.H. & House, A.S. (1988c). The duration of American English stop consonants: an overview. *Journal of Phonetics, 16,* 285–294

Darley, F., Aronson, A., & Brown, J. (1969a). Differential diagnostic patterns of dysarthria. *Journal of Speech and Hearing Research, 12,* 246–269

Darley, F., Aronson, A., & Brown, J. (1969b). Clusters of deviant speech dimensions in the dysarthrias. *Journal of Speech and Hearing Research, 12,* 462–496

Darley, F., Aronson, A., & Brown, J. (1975). *Motor Speech Disorders.* Philadelphia: W.B. Saunders

DePaul, R. & Brooks, B.R. (1993). Multiple orofacial indices in amyotrophic lateral sclerosis. *Journal of Speech and Hearing Research, 36,* 1158–1167

Fant, G. (1960). *Acoustic Theory of Speech Production.* The Hague: Mouton

Forrest, K., Weismer, G., Milenkovic, P., & Dougall, R.N. (1988). Statistical analysis of word-initial voiceless obstruents: preliminary data. *Journal of the Acoustical Society of America, 84,* 115–123

Fowler, C.A. (1980). Coarticulation and theories of extrinsic timing. *Journal of Phonetics, 8,* 113–133

Guenther, F.H., Hampson, M., & Johnson, D. (1998). A theoretical investigation of reference frames for the planning of speech movements. *Psychological Review, 105,* 611–633

Harmes, S., Daniloff, R., Hoffman, P., Lewis, J., Kramer, M., & Absher, R. (1984). Temporal and articulatory control of fricative articulation by speakers with Broca's aphasia. *Journal of Phonetics, 12,* 367–385

Hillenbrand, J. & Gayvert, R.T. (1993). Vowel classification based on fundamental frequency and formant frequencies. *Journal of Speech and Hearing Research, 36,* 694–700

Jenkins, J.J. & Strange, W. (1999). Perception of dynamic information for vowels in syllable onsets and offsets. *Perception & Psychophysics, 61,* 1200–1210

Jongman, A., Wayland, R., & Wong, S. (2000). Acoustic characteristics of English fricatives. *Journal of the Acoustical Society of America, 108,* 1252–1263

Kataoka, R., Warren, D.W., Zajac, D.J., Mayo, R., & Lutz, R.W. (2001). The relationship between spectral characteristics and perceived hypernasality in children. *Journal of the Acoustical Society of America, 109,* 2181–2189

Kent, R.D. (1996). Hearing and believing: some limits to the auditory-perceptual assessment of speech and voice disorders. *American Journal of Speech-Language Pathology, 5,* 7–23

Kent, R.D., Dembowski, J., & Lass, N.J. (1996). The acoustic characteristics of American English. In N.J. Lass (Ed.) *Principles of Experimental Phonetics* (pp. 185–225). St. Louis: Mosby- Year Book

Kent, R.D., Kent, J.F., & Delaney, A.L. (2004). Technology and normative data available for clinical implementation. *Perspectives on Speech Science and Orofacial Disorders* (ASHA Special Interest Division 5), *14,* 6–10

Kent, R.D., Kent, J.F., Weismer, G., Sufit, R.L., Brooks, B.R., & Rosenbek, J.C. (1989). Relationships between speech intelligibility and the slope of second-formant transitions in dysarthric subjects. *Clinical Linguistics and Phonetics, 3,* 347–358

Kent, R.D. & Kim, Y.-J. (2003). Toward an acoustic typology of motor speech disorders. *Clinical Linguistics and Phonetics, 17,* 227–245

Kent, R.D., Netsell, R., & Abbs, J.H. (1979). Acoustic characteristics of dysarthria associated with cerebellar disease. *Journal of Speech and Hearing Research, 22,* 627–648

Kent, R.D. & Read, C. (2002). *The Acoustic Analysis of Speech.* San Diego: Singular Publishing Group

Kent, R.D. & Rosenbek, J.C. (1983). Acoustic patterns of apraxia of speech. *Journal of Speech and Hearing Research, 26,* 231–249

Kent, R.D., Weismer, G., Kent, J.F., & Rosenbek, J.C. (1989). Toward phonetic intelligibility testing in dysarthria. *Journal of Speech and Hearing Research, 54,* 482–499

Kewley-Port, D. (1983). Time-varying features as correlates of place of articulation in stop consonants. *Journal of the Acoustical Society of America, 73,* 322–335

King, J.B., Ramig, L.O., Lemke, J.H., Horii, Y. (1993). Parkinson's disease: Longitudinal changes in acoustic parameters of phonation. *NCVS Status and Progress Report, 4,* 135–149

Klatt, D.H. (1987). Review of text-to-speech conversion for English. *Journal of the Acoustical Society of America, 82,* 737–793

Kreiman, J. & Gerratt, B.R. (1998). Validity of rating scale measures of voice quality. *Journal of the Acoustical Society of America, 104,* 1598–1608

Lee, A.S-Y., Ciocca, V., & Whitehill, T.L. (2003). Acoustic correlates of hypernasality. *Clinical Linguistics and Phonetics, 17,* 259–264

Liberman, A. Cooper, F.S., Shankweiler, D., & Studdert-Kennedy, M. (1967). Perception of the speech code. *Psychological Review, 74,* 431–461

Magen, H.S. (1997). The extent of vowel-to-vowel coarticulation in English. *Journal of Phonetics, 25,* 187–205

Makhoul, J. (1975). Linear predication: a tutorial review. *Proceedings of the IEEE, 63,* 561–580

McRae, P.A., Tjaden, K., & Schoonings, B. (2002). Acoustic and perceptual consequences of articulatory rate change in Parkinson's disease. *Journal of Speech, Language, and Hearing Research, 45,* 35–50

Milenkovic, P. (2001). *TF32 User's Manual.* Madison, WI

Miller, J.L., Grosjean, F., & Lomanto, C. (1984). Articulation rate and its variability in spontaneous speech: A reanalysis and some implications. *Phonetica, 41,* 215–225

Moore, B.C.J., Glasberg, B.R., & Baer, T. (1997). A model for the prediction of thresholds, loudness, and partial loudness. *Journal of the Audio Engineering Society, 45,* 224–240

Olive, J.P., Greenwood, A., & Coleman, J.S. (1994). *Acoustics of American English Speech: A Dynamic Approach.* New York: Springer-Verlag

Perkell, J.S., Guenther, F.H., Lane, H., Matthies, M.L., Perrier, P., Vick, J., Wilhelms-Tricarico, R., & Zandipour, M. (2000). A theory of speech motor control and supporting data from speakers with normal hearing and profound hearing loss. *Journal of Phonetics, 28,* 233–272

Peterson, G.E. & Barney, H.E. (1952). Control methods used in a study of vowels. *Journal of the Acoustical Society of America, 24,* 175–184

Pinto, N. & Titze, I. (1990). Unification of perturbation measures in speech analysis. *Journal of the Acoustical Society of America, 87,* 1278–1289

Ramig, L.O., Scherer, R.C., Klasner, E.R., Titze, I.R., & Horii, Y. (1990). Acoustic analysis of voice in amyotrophic lateral sclerosis: a longitudinal case study. *Journal of Speech and Hearing Disorders, 55*, 2–14

Repp, B. (1981). Phonetic trading relations and context effect: New experimental evidence for a speech mode of perception. *Psychological Bulletin, 92*, 81–110

Robb, M.P., MacClagan, M.A., & Chen, Y. (2004). Speaking rates of American and New Zealand varieties of English. *Clinical Linguistics and Phonetics, 18*, 1–15

Rosen, K.R., Kent, R.D., & Duffy, J.R. (2005). Task-based profile of vocal intensity decline in Parkinson's disease. *Folia Phoniatrica et Logopaedica, 57*, 28–37

Schiavetti, N., Metz, D.E., & Sitler, R.W. (1981). Construct validity of direct magnitude estimation and interval scaling of speech intelligibility: evidence from a study of the hearing impaired. *Journal of Speech and Hearing Research, 24*, 441–445

Shinn, P. & Blumstein, S.E. (1983). Phonetic disintegration in aphasia: acoustic analysis of spectral characteristics for place of articulation. *Brain and Language, 20*, 90–114

Shriberg, L.D. & Kwiatkowski, J. (1982). Phonological disorders III: a procedure for assessing severity of involvement. *Journal of Speech and Hearing Disorders, 47*, 256–270

Shrivastav, R. (2001). *Perceptual structure of breathy voice quality and auditory modeling of its acoustic cues.* Unpublished Doctoral Dissertation, Indiana University, Bloomington

Shrivastav, R. & Sapienza, C. (2003). Objective measures of breathy voice quality obtained using an auditory model. *Journal of the Acoustical Society of America, 114*, 2217–2224

Stathopoulos, E.T. & Weismer, G. (1985). Oral air flow and intraoral air pressure: a comparative study of children, youths, and adults. *Folia Phoniatrica, 37*, 152–159

Stevens, K.N. (1999). *Acoustic Phonetics.* Cambridge, MA: MIT Press

Stevens, K.N. & Blumstein, S.E. (1978). Invariant cues for place of articulation in stop consonants. *Journal of the Acoustical Society of America, 64*, 1358–1368

Stevens, K.N. & House, A.S. (1955). Development of a quantitative description of vowel articulation. *Journal of the Acoustical Society of America, 27*, 484–493

Stevens, K.N. & House, A.S. (1961). An acoustical theory of vowel production and some of its implications. *Journal of Speech and Hearing Research, 4*, 303–320

Thompson, P.F., McLean, M.D., & Summers, W.V. (1992). Discriminant analysis of stop consonant spectra in dysarthria. Poster presented at the American Speech, Language, and Hearing Association Convention, San Antonio, TX

Titze, I.R. (1991). A model for neurologic sources of aperiodicity. *Journal of Speech and Hearing Research, 34*, 460–472

Tjaden, K. & Turner, G. (1997). Spectral properties of fricatives in amyotrophic lateral sclerosis. *Journal of Speech, Language, and Hearing Research, 40*, 1358–1372

Tjaden, K. & Wilding, G.E. (2004). Rate and loudness manipulations in dysarthria: acoustic and perceptual findings. *Journal of Speech, Language, and Hearing Research, 47*, 766–783

Tomiak, G. (1990). *An Acoustic and Perceptual Analysis of the Spectral Moments Invariant with Voiceless Fricative Obstruents.* Unpublished Ph.D. dissertation, State University of New York, Buffalo

Tsao, Y.C. & Weismer, G. (1997). Interspeaker variation in habitual speaking rate: evidence for a neuromuscular component. *Journal of Speech, Language, and Hearing Research, 40*, 858–866

Turner, G. S., Tjaden, K., & Weismer, G. (1995). The influence of speaking rate on vowel space and speech intelligibility for individuals with amyotrophic lateral sclerosis. *Journal of Speech and Hearing Research, 38*, 1001–1013

Umeda, N. (1975). Vowel duration in American English. *Journal of the Acoustical Society of America, 58*, 434–445

Umeda, N. (1977). Consonant duration in American English. *Journal of the Acoustical Society of America, 61*, 846–858

Weismer, G. (1984). Articulatory characteristics of Parkinsonian dysarthria: segmental and phrase-level timing, spirantization, and glottal-supraglottal coordination. In: M.R. McNeil, J.C. Rosenbek, & A.E. Aronson (Eds.), *The Dysarthrias: Physiology, Acoustics, Perception, Management* (pp. 101–130). San Diego: College Hill Press

Weismer, G. (1999). Motor speech disorders. In: W.J. Hardcastle & J. Laver (Eds.), *A Handbook of Phonetic Science* (pp. 191–219). London: Blackwell

Weismer, G. & Berry, J. (2004). Effects of speaking rate on second formant trajectories of selected vocalic nuclei. *Journal of the Acoustical Society of America, 113*, 3362–3378

Weismer, G., Jeng, J.Y., Laures, J.S., Kent, R.D., & Kent, J.F. (2001). Acoustic and intelligibility characteristics of sentence production in neurogenic speech disorders. *Folia Phoniatrica et Logopaedica, 53*, 1–18

Weismer, G., Kent, R.D., Hodge, M., & Martin, R. (1988). The acoustic signature for intelligibility test words. *Journal of the Acoustical Society of America, 84*, 1281–1291

Weismer, G. & Martin, R. (1992). Acoustic and perceptual approaches to the study of intelligibility. In: R.D. Kent (Ed.), *Intelligibility in Speech Disorders* (pp. 67–118). Philadelphia: John Benjamins

Weismer, G., Martin, R., Kent, R.D., & Kent, J.F. (1992). Formant trajectory characteristics of males with amyotrophic lateral sclerosis. *Journal of the Acoustical Society of America, 91*, 1085–1098

Werker, J.F. & Tees, J.E. (1992). Infant speech perception and phonological acquisition. In C.A. Ferguson, L. Menn, & C. Stoel-Gammon (Eds.) *Phonological Development: Models, Research, Implications* (pp. 285–312). Timonium, MD: York press

Whalen, D. H., Magen, H.S., Pouplier, M., Kang, A.M., & Iskarous, K. (2004). Vowel production and perception: hyperarticulation without a hyperspace effect. *Language & Speech, 47*, 155–174

Yorkston, K.M., Beukelman, D.R., Strand, E., & Bell, K.R. (1999). *Management of Motor Speech Disorders in Children and Adults.* Austin: Pro-Ed

Ziegler, W. & von Cramon, D. (1986). Disturbed coarticulation in apraxia of speech: acoustic evidence. *Brain and Language, 29*, 34–47

Zyski, B.J. & Weisiger, B.E. (1987). Identification of dysarthria types based on perceptual analysis. *Journal of Communication Disorders, 20*, 367–378

Chapter 5

Aerodynamic Assessment of Motor Speech Disorders

David J. Zajac, Donald W. Warren, and Virginia A. Hinton

Speech production is a complex multisystem process that is accomplished through coordination of the sensory and motor components of respiration, phonation, articulation, and resonation. If one component is damaged, it is likely that deficits will occur in other systems as well. Specifically, events that have an impact on the sensorimotor components of the central or peripheral nervous system, such as cerebral vascular accidents, progressive neurological diseases, or neoplasms, often result in deficits that adversely affect performance of the speech motor systems at many levels. For example, neurological or neuromuscular damage causing paralysis, paresis, or incoordination in the bulbar or spinal sensorimotor systems can affect the range, velocity, force, or timing of speech movements as well as the respiratory processes that support speech production. Multiple deficits in respiration, phonation, articulation, and resonation present a significant challenge to clinicians responsible for the assessment and treatment of the resulting speech disorder.

Because all speech is produced on exhalation, adequate respiratory support and coordination are essential for normal oral communication. Patients with damage to sensory or motor components of the respiratory system may have difficulty in maintaining adequate respiratory support for speech, as well as in coordinating exhalation with phonation and articulation (Hamman & Yorkston, 1994; Putnam & Hixon, 1981; Theodoros, Murdoch, & Chenery, 1994). This type of damage can be the result of progressive neuromotor disease (e.g., parkinsonism), congenital deficits (e.g., cerebral palsy), or lesions acquired through trauma or disease. Generally, any sensory or motor impairment in the respiratory system produces weakness of or dyscoordination in the respiratory muscles, thus limiting the amount of exhaled air available for maintenance of subglottal pressure (Hixon, Putnam, & Sharpe, 1983; Moon, Folkins, Smith, & Luschei, 1993; Yorkston, Beukelman, Strand, & Bell, 1999).

In addition to impaired respiratory support for speech, laryngeal dysfunction may occur in individuals with central or peripheral nervous system lesions. In some cases, impaired laryngeal control may represent the first signs of a neuromotor disease such as the bulbar form of amyotrophic lateral sclerosis (ALS) or indicate further degeneration of a previously diagnosed medical condition (Hartelius & Svensson, 1994; Roth, Glaze, Goding, & David, 1996). Inappropriate timing of vocal fold closure, inconsistencies in fundamental frequency, as well as disorders of voice quality, such as breathiness, harshness, or hoarseness, may be associated with upper or lower motor neuron lesions (Jiang, O'Mara, Chen, Stern, Vlagos, & Hanson, 1999; Yorkston et al, 1999). The presence of these perceptual characteristics may be the result of specific damage to the processes responsible for the fine motor control of the larynx (Miller, 2004). However, they may also represent inappropriate coordination between the laryngeal and respiratory systems. The ability to determine the nature of the underlying sensorimotor deficit is crucial for developing an optimal treatment plan for these patients (Yorkston, Strand, & Kennedy, 1996).

Velopharyngeal closure is another component of speech production that frequently is disrupted by deficits in sensorimotor function. Researchers and clinicians have reported the presence of velopharyngeal dysfunction in patients with a variety of nervous system disorders that may be congenital (Kent & Netsell, 1978; Yorkston et al, 1999), acquired but nonprogressive (Aten, 1988; Darley, Aronson, & Brown, 1975; McHenry, Wilson, & Minton, 1994), or degenerative (Duffy, 1995; Tandan & Bradley, 1985). Velopharyngeal dysfunction in patients with sensorimotor disorders appears related to reduced velar movement during speech, as well as inappropriate timing of the movement of the velum relative to other structures (Netsell, 1969; Yorkston, Beukelman, & Honsinger, 1989). Velopharyngeal dysfunction can range from inconsistent borderline closure to gross inadequacy, thus limiting the ability to maintain adequate intraoral pressures necessary for obstruent consonant production, as well as producing inappropriate oral-nasal resonance balance (Dalston, Warren, Morr, & Smith, 1988; Warren, Dalston, & Dalston, 1990).

In many cases, respiratory, phonatory, and velopharyngeal components of speech production are described separately when assessing the physiological deficits of patients with sensorimotor lesions (Yorkston et al, 1999). However, in reality, these systems interact constantly to produce perceptually adequate speech. For example, maintenance of intraoral air pressure during consonant production requires a constant subglottal pressure, adequate velopharyngeal closure, and sufficient bilabial or linguapalatal obstruction. Deficits in any of these areas may yield reduced intraoral pressure and serve to decrease overall speech intelligibility. Therefore, clinical assessment and treatment of patients with sensorimotor impairments should include procedures that examine the integration and coordination of these complex systems (Theodoros et al, 1994).

This chapter describes the use of aerodynamic techniques in the evaluation of patients with sensorimotor impairments. Specifically, the use of such procedures should allow clinicians to describe more accurately the nature of a patient's speech production deficits (Theodoros et al, 1994). Furthermore, these techniques and procedures may be useful in developing new treatment approaches that focus on demonstrating quantifiable changes in physiological responses rather than judgments of speech performance alone.

The assessment techniques described below are used routinely in evaluation of patients with structural deficits such as velopharyngeal impairment. The techniques measure a patient's ability to perform certain activities that are essential for the proper production of consonant and vowel sounds. These include (1) the ability to separate the nose from the mouth during velopharyngeal closure; (2) the ability to bring the tongue, alveolar ridge, and teeth into correct approximation for frication; and (3) the ability to adduct the vocal folds for voicing. In addition, temporal aspects of motor activity in terms of the ability of structures to perform tasks within periods of time can be assessed. An example would be how long it takes to effect velopharyngeal closure in certain phonetic contexts. Recent studies have shown that this variable is strongly correlated with perceptual judgments of hypernasality or audible nasal air emission in speakers with structural impairments (Dotevall, Lohmander-Agerskov, Ejnell, & Bake, 2002; Warren, Dalston, & Mayo, 1993).

We begin by describing basic instrumentation required for aerodynamic assessment of speech. The use of aerodynamic principles for the assessment of structural performance is then described with a focus on the velopharyngeal structures. This is followed by a review of temporal assessment of speech performance. Examples are provided from normal speakers and from speakers with disordered sensorimotor processes. Practical considerations when testing individuals with sensorimotor impairments are then covered. We conclude with a discussion of the assessment of sensorimotor responses of normal speakers during experiments designed to perturb the aerodynamics of the upper airways during breathing and speech production. Such experiments might shed light on the control processes of speech aerodynamics or motivate other researchers to apply the techniques.

◆ Assessing Aerodynamic Performance

During the last two decades, the development of instruments capable of measuring aerodynamic variables associated with speech has led to improved, more objective methods for assessing the performance of vocal tract structures. These tools range from simple manometric sensing devices to elaborate combinations of pressure transducers and airflow meters (Warren, 1976). Although the former are capable only of gross determinations of function, the latter provide acceptable estimates of the performance of discrete activities.

In the past, clinicians have used several devices to provide a gross indication of such variables as nasal emission of air, which reflects, to some extent, palatal function. In most instances, the measurements obtained with simple devices related more to respiratory effort than to palatal function. Also, response times were extremely slow, and errors in measurement often occurred. In addition, these measurements were usually made during nonspeech activities such as blowing.

The deficiencies associated with simple manometric instruments led to the development of more elaborate tools for objective evaluation of the structures involved in speech. The basic components of these aerodynamic measuring systems are pressure transducers, which record airway pressures within the vocal tract, and flowmeters, which record volume rates of airflow.

Air Pressure Devices

The pressure transducers currently in use are variable resistance, variable capacitance, or variable inductance gauges. Resistance wire strain gauges respond to changes in pressure with a change in resistance when the strain-sensitive wire is exposed to stretch. Compression of bellows within the chamber results in a resistance imbalance in a Wheatston bridge that is proportional to the applied pressure. The resulting output voltage from the bridge is amplified and recorded.

The electrical capacitance transducer is a condenser formed by an electrode separated from a stiff metal membrane by a carefully adjusted air gap. Movements of the membrane in relation to the electrode vary the capacitance, which can be measured by a radiofrequency circuit. Membrane displacement is extremely small, and therefore the frequency response is excellent. However, this device is more temperature sensitive than the strain-gauge manometer. The capacitance-type pressure transducer is distinguishable from other types by its exceptional accuracy, high-level outputs, and built-in signal conditioning. Typically, these transducers do not require additional signal conditioning. In most of the examples presented below, pressure-flow traces were obtained using variable capacitance transducers.

The variable inductance pressure gauge utilizes a soft iron slug placed within two coils of wire and fastened to the center of an elastic membrane. Pressure moves the iron slug, and this movement results in a change in magnetic flux. The change in inductance of the coils is then recorded through an appropriate bridge circuit. The advantage of this type of transducer is that it can be made so small that it can be placed directly on the site to be measured.

It is common practice to amplify the signal from transducers, and usually a carrier-wave amplifier is used. An oscillator supplies an alternating current, and the amplitude is continuously affected by the varying resistance. The output of the transducer enters the capacitance-coupled amplifier, which amplifies the modulated carrier wave. The signals are then rectified and the carrier wave is filtered out, leaving a direct current (DC) voltage that powers the recording instrument.

Pressure Measurements

Pressure devices have been used in a variety of ways to measure the aerodynamics of speech production. Usually,

Table 5–1 Intraoral Pressures and Standard Deviations According to Competency of Velopharyngeal Closure

	Adequate	Adequate/ Borderline	Borderline/ Inadequate	Inadequate
Area	0–4.9 mm²	5.0–9.9 mm²	10.0–19.9 mm²	>20.0 mm²
Pressure	6.4 cm H₂O ± 2.2	5.0 cm H₂O ± 1.9	4.3 cm H₂O ± 1.8	3.7 cm H₂O ± 1.9

measurements are made of oral pressures, nasal pressures, or both. Intraoral pressure can be recorded by placing a catheter in the mouth and attaching it to a pressure transducer and appropriate recording device. Pressures in the oral cavity typically vary from 3 to 8 cm H_2O for nonnasal consonants in normal conversational speech. Voiceless consonants usually are produced with pressures approximately 20% higher than their voiced cognates (Warren, 1964; Warren & Hall, 1973). This may relate to the need for greater aerodynamic energy for voiceless sounds because there is no accompanying acoustic energy from the vocal folds. Additionally, there is a difference in energy loss across the glottis between the two consonant types (Warren & Hall, 1973).

Intraoral pressures of consonants generally remain above 3.0 cm H_2O even in individuals with impaired palatal function (Dalston et al, 1988; Warren, 1986b). **Table 5–1** lists mean intraoral pressures according to the degree of velopharyngeal closure for the plosive /p/ in the word *hamper*. Several factors are involved in maintaining intraoral pressures above 3.0 cm H_2O. Perhaps the most important factor is that the nasal airway provides approximately two thirds of the total resistance of the respiratory system. Approximately 60 to 70% of intraoral pressure can be maintained by nasal airway resistance alone even in the presence of velopharyngeal impairment. Since intraoral pressures are usually maintained at levels above 3 cm H_2O, regardless of the degree of palatal dysfunction, it should be obvious that measurements of intraoral pressures alone do not provide an accurate estimate of palatal function.

Nasal pressures have also been used as an index of velopharyngeal function (Hess & McDonald, 1960). This has usually involved the placement of a nasal olive against the more patent nostril while having the subject produce nonnasal consonants within test sounds or phrases. This approach provides a gross estimate of impairment because nasal pressure should be negligible or zero for adequate closure and in the 1 to 6 cm H_2O range for inadequacy.

If only pressure measurements are to be made, a more valid approach to screening palatal function involves measuring oral and nasal pressure simultaneously. Warren (1979) described a technique that measures the pressure difference across the velopharyngeal port for rating palatal competency. Closure of the velopharyngeal orifice creates a pressure difference between the nose and mouth. When complete closure occurs, as during production of the consonant /p/, pressure in the mouth is determined by respiratory effort and will vary from approximately 3 to 8 cm H_2O (Warren, 1964, 1976; Zajac, 2000). Pressure in the nose is atmospheric or zero because no air leaks into the nasal chamber. However, if there is a velopharyngeal opening, the difference in pressure varies with the size of the opening. Because a difference in oral and nasal pressures is used, the effect of respiratory effort is canceled out when the velopharyngeal mechanism is not completely closed.

When using differential pressures as an index of velopharyngeal closure, the speech sample should include voiceless plosive consonants in such words as *papa* and *hamper*. The voiceless plosive /p/ is used because this sound provides an aerodynamic state that varies directly with the degree of velopharyngeal closure. The /p/ is produced by closing the lips and velopharyngeal orifice and stopping airflow for a period of time. If closure is complete at the lips and velopharynx, the pressure measured is equal to intraoral pressure. Indeed, if there are no other constrictions in the vocal tract, intraoral pressure is also equivalent to subglottal air pressure. Any velopharyngeal opening during /p/, however, results in airflow into the nose, which reduces the pressure difference between the nose and mouth. The result is a lower differential pressure. Also, when airflow is stopped in the oral cavity, placement of the tongue does not affect pressure within the stagnant air column. Improper tongue placement, therefore, is eliminated as a potential problem. This is not true for other sounds. For example, fricative sounds are produced with oral airflow. If tongue-palatal contacts occur, an additional pressure drop would result, which could lead to spurious values. Voiced sounds are not preferred because they often have lower, more inconsistent pressure patterns (Warren, 1979).

The nasal-plosive sequence, as in the word *hamper*, is often used because it stresses the palatal mechanism. Pressure-flow studies have demonstrated that some individuals can close the velopharyngeal port adequately for plosives in nonnasal contexts but cannot do so when the sounds are adjacent to nasal consonants (Warren, 1979). Individuals who have such difficulties tend to experience velopharyngeal inadequacy during continuous speech. Therefore, the nasal-plosive combination is used as a test of velopharyngeal closure ability during ongoing speech. Based on studies of more than 500 patients with palatal dysfunction, we have found that velopharyngeal closure is usually adequate when differential pressure is greater than 3 cm H_2O. When differential pressure is between 1 and 2.9 cm H_2O, closure is usually borderline or marginal. When differential pressure is below 1 cm H_2O, velopharyngeal closure is always inadequate for normal speech.

Airflow Devices

The most accepted airflow device is the heated pneumotachograph, which consists of a flowmeter and a differential pressure transducer (Baken & Orlikoff, 2000; Lubker, 1970). This device utilizes the principle that as air flows across a resistance, the pressure drop that results is linearly related to the volume rate of airflow. In most cases, the resistance is a wire mesh screen that is heated to prevent condensation. A pressure tap is situated on each side of the screen, and both are connected to a very sensitive differential pressure transducer. The pressure drop is converted to an electrical voltage that is amplified and recorded. Pneumotachographs are valid, reliable, and linear devices for measuring ingressive and egressive airflow rates. In addition, they are easily calibrated with a rotometer.

Airflow Measurements

Measurements of nasal airflow frequently have been used to assess velopharyngeal competency (Lubker & Moll, 1965; Machida, 1967; Subtelny, Worth, & Sakuda, 1966). Since there should be little or no nasal air emission on any English-language sounds except /m/, /n/, and /ng/ (Thompson & Hixon, 1979; Zajac, 2000), nasal airflow during the production of other sounds usually denotes velopharyngeal dysfunction. Although nasal emission of air generally increases with increased inadequacy, several factors influence the outcome enough to result in a low correlation between the two variables (Laine, Warren, Dalston, et al, 1988; Warren, 1967). Respiratory effort and nasal airway resistance are factors that influence nasal airflow during speech when tight velopharyngeal closure cannot be attained. For example, an individual with high nasal resistance to airflow generates sufficient intraoral pressure for nonnasal consonants with less respiratory effort than another individual with the same degree of inadequacy but lower nasal resistance. Thus, the former individual requires less airflow from the lungs and has less nasal emission as well.

Caution should be exercised, therefore, when using measurements of nasal airflow to estimate velopharyngeal function. That is, it is safe to consider peak nasal airflow rates above 150 mL/s during nonnasal consonant productions to be indicative of inadequate closure. However, the converse may not always be true. That is, rates of less than 150 mL/s may occur in the presence of velopharyngeal inadequacy if there is nasal obstruction or decreased respiratory effort. Zajac (2000) reported that noncleft speakers, regardless of age, exhibited complete velopharyngeal closure during production of /p/ in consonant-vowel (CV) syllables as reflected by rates of nasal airflow that did not exceed 20 mL/s. This criterion was used to account for small magnitudes of nasal airflow that might occur as artifact due to normal velar bounce (Hoit, Watson, Hixon, McMahon, & Johnson, 1994). Artifact nasal airflow due to velar bounce often can be discerned by a negative flow peak that follows a small positive peak. Based on the findings of Zajac (2000), it is further safe to consider peak nasal airflow rates greater than 20 to 30 mL/s as indicative of some degree of velopharyngeal opening.

◆ Use of Aerodynamic Principles for Assessing Structural Performance

In general, measurements of pressure and airflow alone have not provided the definitive diagnostic information required by most clinicians. These deficiencies have led to the development of more elaborate approaches for evaluating structural performance (Barlow, 1989, 1999; Warren & DuBois, 1964). The techniques involve the application of hydrokinetic principles. Upper airway structures such as the tongue, teeth, lips, and palate form numerous constrictions that influence airflow and pressure. Hydraulic equations are used to estimate the resistance or size of these constrictions.

There is a self-contained software and related hardware package (PERCI-SARS, Microtronics, Inc., Chapel Hill, NC) available for aerodynamic assessment of speech. This system is used to collect pressure-flow data along with the acoustic speech signal. The software provides analysis modes for measuring pressures, airflows, volumes, constriction areas, resistances, and timing associated with structural movements.

Area Measurements

Constrictions that form along the vocal tract produce an orifice type of airflow pattern. The pressure drop (ΔP) that results is expressed as

$$\Delta P = \frac{d(V)^2}{2k^2(A)}$$

where d is the density of air, V is airflow, and A is area of the constriction. The discharge coefficient, k, depends upon the sharpness of the edge of the orifice and on Reynolds number. The discharge coefficient has a value of 0.6 to 0.7 in the speech airflow range (Warren & DuBois, 1964; Yates, McWilliams, & Vallino, 1990).

The relationship of pressure to airflow across vocal tract constrictions has led to the application of hydrokinetic principles to estimate the size of the constrictions formed during speech. The basis for this measurement can be explained in terms of airflow through simple pipes. The size of a constriction in a pipe can be calculated by measuring the airflow through the pipe (V) and the pressure drop across the constriction (ΔP). The area (A) of the constriction is then calculated from the following equation:

$$A = k\frac{\frac{V}{\sqrt{2\Delta P}}}{d}$$

where k equals 0.65. Because nearly 80% of patients with sensorimotor deficits are unable to achieve adequate velopharyngeal closure (Netsell et al, 1979), an accurate assessment of velopharyngeal orifice size is particularly important. **Figure 5–1** illustrates catheter placement and instrumentation for estimating velopharyngeal orifice area.

Briefly, the pressure drop across the velopharyngeal orifice (oral pressure minus nasal pressure) is measured by placing one catheter in the right nostril and another in the oral cavity. The nasal catheter is secured by a foam plug, which blocks the nostril, creating a stagnant column of air. Both catheters measure static air pressures and transmit these pressures to pressure transducers. Nasal airflow is measured by a heated pneumotachograph connected by plastic tubing to the subject's other nostril. As discussed previously, voiceless bilabial plosive sounds should be used in the speech sample. Advantages of using /p/ include the following: (1) the oral catheter needs to be inserted only

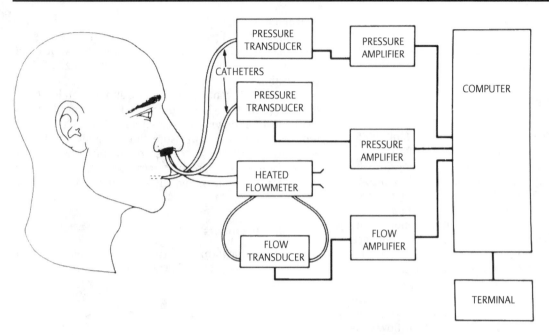

Figure 5–1 Diagrammatic representation of pressure-flow instrumentation for estimating velopharyngeal orifice size. Transducers connected to a nostril and the mouth measure the pressure drop across the velopharyngeal orifice. Airflow is measured by the flow meter and transducer connected to the other nostril. [From Warren, D.W., Dalston, R.M., & Mayo, R. (1993). Hypernasality in the presence of "adequate" velopharyngeal closure. *Cleft Palate J, 30,* 150–154 [with permission]

beyond the lips, and (2) orientation of the catheter is inconsequential given that stagnant airflow exists during the stop phase (Baken & Orlikoff, 2000). **Figure 5–2** is an audio and pressure-flow record from a normal adult producing two series of the syllable /pa/. The first series (four syllables) demonstrates complete velopharyngeal closure as indicated by (1) oral pressures above 5 cm H_2O, (2) the absence of nasal pressure, (3) the absence of nasal airflow, and (4) differential pressures that approximate oral pressures. In the second series (also four syllables), the speaker is simulating velopharyngeal inadequacy by lowering the velum. Oral pressures and nasal pressures are approximately equivalent at 2 cm H_2O, nasal airflow averages 340 mL/s, and differential pressures are well under 1 cm H_2O. The calculated velopharyngeal openings in this series exceed 90 mm², which represents a simulation of gross inadequacy.

Ratings of velopharyngeal function are based on data generated from pressure-flow studies of individuals with velopharyngeal impairment associated with cleft palate and from normal subjects (Warren, 1979). An opening greater than 20 mm² during nonnasal consonant productions is typically inadequate for normal speech. Intraoral pressure is usually low (2.5 to 3.5 cm H_2O range) in these individuals unless the nasal cavity is grossly obstructed. Similarly, nasal emission of air is excessive and usually audible, and resonance is hypernasal. **Figure 5–3** is a pressure-flow record for a patient who sustained a traumatic brain injury. The patient produced the word *hamper* three times. The velopharyngeal mechanism is grossly inadequate as indicated by a calculated area of approximately 100 mm² at peak oral pressure of the second "hamper" (dotted vertical line). Oral pressures are slightly above 3.0 cm H_2O, nasal pressures approximate

oral pressures, nasal airflow is excessive with a mean of 526 mL/s, and differential pressures (not shown in **Fig. 5–3**) are close to zero. Indeed, except for the first production of "hamper," oral and nasal pressures totally overlap indicating essentially complete oral-nasal coupling. For comparison, **Figure 5–4** is a pressure-flow record for a normal speaker producing "hamper" a single time. As illustrated, peak oral pressure is approximately 6 cm H_2O and nasal airflow is negligible, less than 30 mL/s at peak oral pressure. Typically, the rate of nasal airflow at peak pressure should be less than 30 to 60 mL/s, which results from carryover from the /m/ segment. Finally, comparison of **Fig. 5–3** and **Fig. 5–4** illustrate remarkable timing differences between the pressure and airflow pulses. These timing relationships and the airflow derivative are discussed below.

The perceptual speech characteristics of the individual in **Fig. 5–3** included excessive hypernasality, reduced loudness, and visible escape of nasal air emission. These characteristics are consistent with an estimated velopharyngeal opening that exceeds 20 mm². Except in extremely rare instances, oral-nasal resonance balance is within normal limits when the opening is less than 5 mm² during production of "hamper," and any nasal emission present is typically inaudible. Speech performance is determined by accuracy of articulation rather than palatal closure. Openings between 5 and 10 mm² are in the adequate-borderline range and are usually small enough not to interfere with an individual's ability to impound intraoral pressure. However, nasal emission will occur and, under certain circumstances, it may be audible. If the nasal airway is obstructed, turbulence produces airflow that is most audible during fricative and affricate productions because respiratory effort is increased

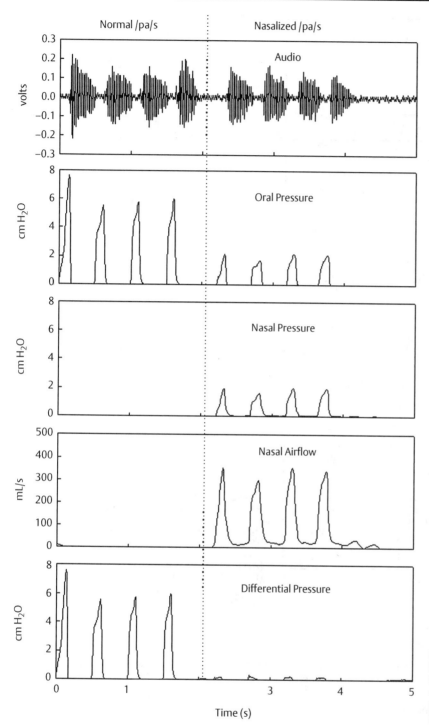

Figure 5–2 Pressure-flow traces of a neurologically intact speaker producing /pa/ normally and by lowering the velum to simulate velopharyngeal inadequacy. **(A)** Audio signal. **(B)** Oral pressure. **(C)** Nasal pressure. **(D)** Nasal airflow. **(E)** Differential oral-nasal pressure.

during production of these speech sounds. Otherwise, resonance is within normal limits or only slightly hypernasal if articulatory performance is normal. If articulatory performance is abnormal, as in the case of many individuals with dysarthrias, then even openings this small may be associated with a speech signal that is perceived by listeners as hypernasal. It must be emphasized that the indices discussed above are not based on data from individuals with sensorimotor deficits. Additional studies dealing with the effects of more generalized motor dysfunction are needed

to determine whether these criteria are valid for populations other than those with cleft palate.

The same instrumental approach can be used for measuring oral port size during fricative productions. This port represents the space between the tongue, teeth, and palate and is approximately 6 mm^2 during the production of /s/ (Smith, Allen, Warren, & Hall, 1978; Warren, Hall, & Davis, 1981). Values less than 2 mm^2 or greater than 15 mm^2 indicate an inability to achieve a proper constriction for frication. This may mean a deficiency in labial or lingual neuromotor activity.

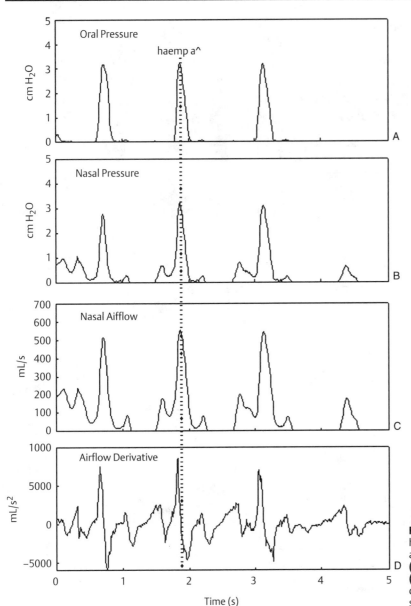

Figure 5–3 Pressure-flow traces of a speaker with a history of traumatic head injury and velopharyngeal inadequacy. The word *hamper* was produced three times. **(A)** Oral pressure. **(B)** Nasal pressure. **(C)** Nasal airflow. **(D)** Nasal airflow derivative. The dotted vertical line indicates complete overlap of oral pressure, nasal pressure, and nasal airflow during the second "hamper."

Figure 5–5 illustrates catheter placements. One catheter is placed within the oral cavity and the other within a well-fitting face mask. This measures the pressure drop across the oral port. Oral airflow is measured by a pneumotachograph attached to the oral mask.

Resistance Measurements

Resistance to airflow is opposition to air motion caused by friction (viscous drag). Friction dissipates mechanical energy in the form of heat as air moves through the vocal tract. This energy is supplied by the respiratory muscles, which require more forceful contractions as airway resistance increases. The measurement of resistance, like area, involves the simultaneous recording of the rate of airflow and the pressure drop across the structures involved. The resistance (R) to airflow is

explained by an analogy to Ohm's law for electrical currents where

$$R = \frac{\Delta P}{V}$$

where ΔP is the pressure drop across the constriction and V is the airflow. Resistance measurements can be made wherever constrictions in the vocal tract occur. Airway resistance is an important factor in maintaining stable speech pressures since the drop in pressure resulting from air moving across a structure is proportional to the reciprocal of the fourth power of the radius. Reducing the radius of an airway by one half increases the pressure drop 16-fold (Warren, Hairfield, & Seaton, 1987). Relative to velopharyngeal function, we prefer to calculate area rather than resistance given that the majority of research studies typically report areas.

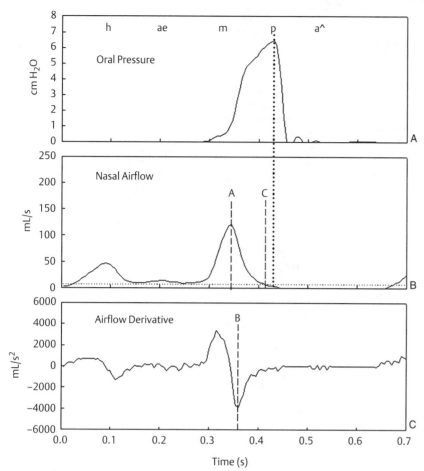

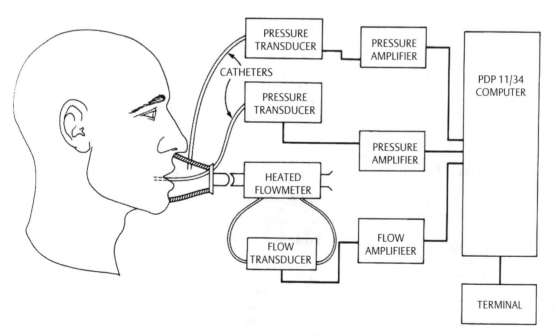

Figure 5–4 Pressure-flow traces of a neurologically intact speaker producing "hamper" a single time. **(A)** Oral pressure. **(B)** Nasal airflow. **(C)** Nasal airflow derivative. Note that nasal airflow of the /m/ segment peaks and ends before the peak of oral pressure of the /p/ segment.

Figure 5–5 Diagrammatic representation of catheter and mask placements for estimating oral port constriction area during sibilant productions. In this case, the pressure drop across the oral port is measured simultaneously with airflow through the oral port. [From Claypoole, W.H., Warren, D.W., & Bradley, D.P. (1974). The effect of cleft palate on oral port constriction during fricative productions. *Cleft Palate J, 2*, 95–104, with permission.]

Laryngeal Resistance Measurements

Laryngeal resistance during vowel production can be estimated using an approach suggested by Smitheran and Hixon (1981). Transglottal airflow and intraoral pressure is obtained during production of syllables, typically /pi/. An estimate of subglottal pressure is derived from intraoral pressure measurements. Laryngeal resistance during voicing is thus obtained. This technique and data representative of speakers with dysarthria are reviewed in Chapter 6 and thus are not discussed here. The reader should keep in mind, however, that application of this technique to obtain estimates of subglottal pressure requires closure of the velopharyngeal structures. Obviously, this condition is not always present in speakers with sensorimotor disorders.

Timing Studies

Aerodynamic assessment techniques can also be used to evaluate timing patterns associated with structural movements (Dotevall et al, 2002; Warren, Dalston, Morr, Hairfield, & Smith, 1989; Warren, Dalston, Trier, & Holder, 1985; Warren et al, 1993; Zajac & Mayo, 1996). For example, individuals with palatal dysfunction can be differentiated on the basis of specific timing parameters such as the onset, peak, and end of pressure and airflow pulses. Patients who present with differing degrees of velopharyngeal inadequacy manifest different patterns of pressure-flow pulsing over time. Pressure-flow patterns of an individual with adequate velopharyngeal function during production of the word *hamper* were previously illustrated in **Fig. 5–4.** Both peak airflow (point A) and the end of airflow (point C) for the /m/ segment occur prior to peak pressure for /p/. As illustrated in **Fig. 5–3,** however, significant timing differences are associated with palatal inadequacy. The entire airflow record shifts to the right. In fact, the peak of airflow coincides with the peak of pressure, at least for the final two productions of "hamper." In essence, this indicates that the speaker is unable to aerodynamically separate the /m/ from the /p/ segment.

Timing studies also discriminate between individuals who exhibit hypernasality associated with delayed, but adequate, velopharyngeal closure on obstruent segments. Warren et al (1993), for example, reported that the duration of the nasal airflow pulse of "hamper" was approximately 50 ms longer in speakers with repaired cleft palate who exhibited hypernasality as compared with speakers with cleft palate and normal resonance and speakers without cleft palate. Dotevall et al (2002) also reported relationships between the duration of the velopharyngeal closing phase and perceived hypernasality in Swedish-speaking children with repaired cleft palate. This phase was defined from peak nasal airflow to 5% of baseline in a nasal-plosive context (illustrated in **Fig. 5–4B**). The use of a 5% baseline avoids problems of asymptotic airflow that does not reach zero, a common occurrence in speakers with severe velopharyngeal inadequacy.

Dotevall et al (2002) also described a novel index of velopharyngeal closing dynamics based on the first derivative of nasal airflow **(Fig. 5–4C).** Called the maximum flow declination rate (MFDR), this measure indicates the fastest rate of nasal airflow change during the velopharyngeal closing phase of the nasal-plosive sequence. To control for the effects of individual variations in peak nasal airflow, Dotevall et al (2002) computed the absolute value of the quotient between the peak negative amplitude of flow declination and peak nasal airflow. They noted a strong association between this index and judgments of hypernasality among children with repaired cleft palate. Given that speakers with dysarthria typically demonstrate reduced speed and range of motion of articulators, use of the MFDR index may hold promise as a diagnostic or treatment outcome measure. For example, the value of this index for the speaker in **Fig. 5–3** is approximately 1.8 compared with a value of 28.8 for the speaker in **Fig. 5–4.**

Additional problems of pressure-flow timing are frequently observed in patients with sensorimotor deficits. **Figure 5–6** illustrates the increase in duration (196 ms) of the airflow pulse (period 1–3) in a patient with a traumatic head injury. Normally the duration would be approximately 140 ms (Warren et al, 1993). Individuals with hypernasal speech are usually in the 200-ms range. On the other hand, this subject, when producing the word *hamper,* had a normal time interval for the period that includes the beginning of airflow for /m/ at point 1 to the end of the pressure pulse at period 6. The mean duration of 190 ms compares favorably with the norm of 184 ms. This suggests that innervation of the muscles associated with velopharyngeal closure was affected (1–3), but innervation of muscles associated with labial closure was not. That is, the duration (1–6) measurement more strongly reflects labial movements while the duration (1–3) primarily reflects velopharyngeal movements.

In comparison, another patient **(Fig. 5–7),** diagnosed as being dysarthric since childhood, shows a duration of 237 ms for the period 1–6. Interestingly, this patient also has two distinct peaks: one for /m/ and the other for /p/. Usually, the two phoneme pulses blend into one when there is velopharyngeal inadequacy. In this case, there appears to be an unsuccessful attempt to separate the /m/ from the /p/. The longer (1–6) duration suggests that there is impairment of the labial musculature as well.

◆ Practical Consideration for Aerodynamic Assessment

Posture and Respiratory Effort

Individuals with speech disorders due to neurological injury or disease also may have problems with body posture control that affect their ability to participate in a speech aerodynamics evaluation. They may slump or list when seated upright, making it difficult for them to reach or stay coupled to a pressure-flow data sampling apparatus. Additional time and personnel may be required to ensure that the dysarthric subject is and remains coupled adequately to flow collecting devices and pressure sensors.

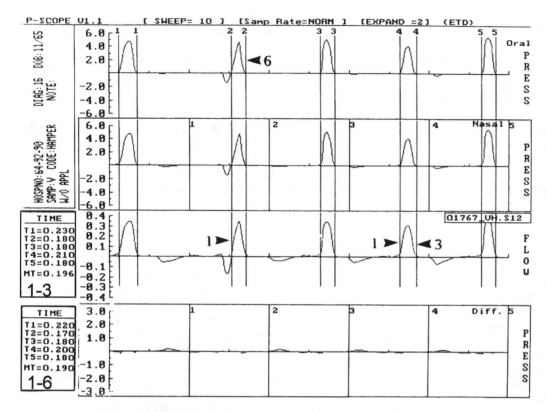

Figure 5–6 Pressure-flow traces of a patient who suffered a traumatic head injury. The word *hamper* was produced five times. **(A)** Oral pressure. **(B)** Nasal pressure. **(C)** Nasal airflow. **(D)** Differential pressure. The mean duration of the flow pulse (period 1–3) was 196 ms, which is sub-stantially longer than normal. However, the entire interval of the oral pressure pulse (period 1–6) during the /mp/ sequence was 190 ms, which compares favorably with the norm. This would occur when labial closure is not affected.

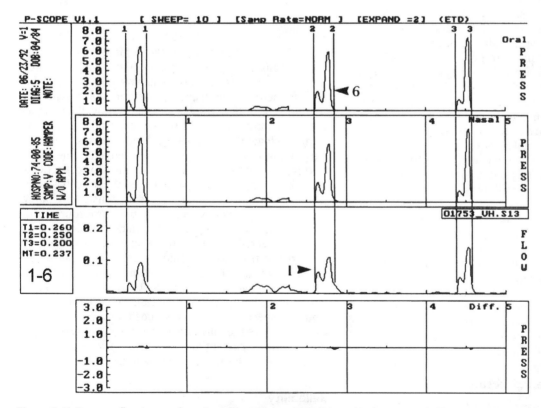

Figure 5–7 Pressure-flow traces of a patient diagnosed as dysarthric since childhood. The word *hamper* was produced three times. **(A)** Oral pressure. **(B)** Nasal pressure. **(C)** Nasal airflow. **(D)** Differential pressure. The duration of the oral pressure pulse (period 1–6) during the /mp/ sequence is 237 ms, suggesting that labial closure is affected. The oral pressure also shows a twin pulse during /mp/, which is un-usual. This suggests an unsuccessful attempt to separate the /m/ from the /p/.

The reduced trunk muscle control that compromises a subject's upright posture also may reduce or render unreliable that subject's respiratory driving pressure capabilities. When this fluctuating competence is coupled with possible velopharyngeal inadequacy, the subject may be able to generate only minimal intraoral pressures. This may be problematic if a pressure trigger is used during data sampling (an option available in PERCI-SARS). In these cases, it may be advantageous to use a continuous sampling window without a trigger threshold or lower the trigger threshold in anticipation of this phenomenon.

Limited Degrees of Freedom for Compensation, Active Participation, or Assistance

Behavioral signs suggest that subjects with injured nervous systems may be limited in their on-line compensatory abilities. The neurologically normal subject is usually able to cooperate fully with the assessor during aerodynamic testing—to swallow on command, adjust his head or trunk posture as required to approach the sampling apparatus, hold the catheter and the nasal flow-collecting tube in place, and accommodate several different catheter placements. The dysarthric subject, on the other hand, may be willing to cooperate in these ways but may be unable to perform or adjust his performance with such facility. As a general rule, examiners should allow extra time for the assessment of such patients to ensure that adequate, valid, and reliable data are obtained.

As well, some dysarthric subjects appear to be unable to accommodate the presence of the intraoral pressure catheter without adopting articulatory postures that may introduce artifacts in the pressure-flow data records. Typically, such artifacts take the form of negative-going oral pressure spikes occurring simultaneously with positive nasal airflow during production of a speech segment. One cause of these incongruent pressure-flow patterns might be a high and retropositioned tongue with velar contact such that the oral catheter is sampling pressure in an oral cul-de-sac isolated from the "real" pressure of the oropharynx during an utterance. It is not unusual to encounter artifacts of this nature during the pressure-flow assessment of individuals with moderate-severe dysarthria. Assessors, therefore, must undertake repeated samples, repositioning the intraoral pressure catheter and coaching subjects to alter their tongue positions in an attempt to find a placement that the subject can accommodate and that is legitimate for the measurement of the oropharyngeal pressure in the oral cavity. The examiner should be aware that, although the subjects may be willing to cooperate, they may be unable to make the necessary intraoral structure placement adjustments to accommodate the catheter or may tire of repeated efforts to obtain measurable data.

Bilabial Incompetence and Closure

Mandibular or labial weakness may make it difficult for some dysarthric subjects to generate valid or reliable pressure-flow records if they are unable to achieve or maintain competent bilabial closure during assessment of velopharyngeal function or laryngeal airway resistance. During the testing of velopharyngeal competence, when a subject is weak and fatigable but able to achieve bilabial closure with assistance, the assessor may choose to help the subject attain lip closure by means of a digital assist to the mandible for the bilabial plosive in the words *papa* and *hamper*. For a subject in whom aeromechanically competent bilabial closure may be impossible (for example, someone with severe expression of Möbius syndrome), the assessor may experiment with changing the sample utterance for assessment of velopharyngeal competence to "tata" or "hanter," and for laryngeal airway resistance to /ti/, and place the intraoral pressure sensor farther into the mouth to sample pressure behind the lingua-alveolar place of occlusion for /t/ or /n/.

Laryngeal airway resistance assessment may be precluded if neither labial nor lingual competence prevails, because the subject cannot produce a bilabial or lingua-alveolar stop. If only the subject's velopharyngeal closure is not competent, or competence is questionable, data for laryngeal airway resistance estimation can be collected with a mask over the oral airway only and a nose clip managing the nasal airway.

When the subject is troubled by dyscoordination such that the presence of the intraoral catheter is too disruptive altogether, an estimate of velopharyngeal adequacy can be obtained with measurement of nasal pressure and nasal flow only, preferably along with a voice signal so that interpretation of the aerodynamic data records is as unambiguous as possible.

Drooling

The presence of the intraoral catheter for aerodynamic testing normally stimulates salivation. Hence, clogging of the catheter is a pervasive operational hazard in pressure-flow measurements during speech. Dysarthric subjects who may be dysphagic or have trouble clearing and swallowing their saliva regularly or efficiently are especially at risk for catheter clogging during pressure-flow testing. Assessors must monitor the intraoral pressure signal on line and be alert for baseline shifts in the signal caused by collection of saliva in the pressure-sensing catheter. When such baseline shifts are observed (e.g., oral pressure consistently above zero during vowel segments), the procedure must be stopped, the sensor removed from the subject's mouth, the saliva cleared from the catheter, and the instruments reset to regain true baseline. Under these circumstances, it is important to clear the catheter without undue stress on the differential pressure transducer. To avoid damaging the transducer, the operator should disconnect the catheter from it, especially if suction or positive pressure is to be used to remove the saliva. Coaching subjects to swallow just prior to the placement of the catheter may help to reduce the opportunity for this problem to occur.

Reliability

Clinical and anecdotal evidence suggests that subjects who have suffered central nervous system (CNS) damage may exhibit remarkable performance variability for complex tasks such as pressure-flow measurement due to variations in medication effects, arousal levels, fatigue, and several other behavioral or physiological phenomena. Higher performance variability means poorer sample-to-sample and day-to-day sampling reliability after CNS injury. This has implications for aerodynamic data collection in the assessment of laryngeal and velopharyngeal competence. For best estimates, multiple baseline samples across several recording opportunities should be obtained to make as honest an assessment of respiratory, laryngeal, or velopharyngeal competence as possible.

♦ Assessing Sensory Sensitivity and Motor Responses

Speech is primarily a modified breathing behavior, with the respiratory system providing the energy source for sound production. Physiologists have long observed that the human body maintains a degree of constancy or "homeostasis" for its many systems. Respiration is but one example of a highly regulated system (Warren, 1986a). The essential characteristics of a regulating system include (1) regulation for the purpose of stability, and (2) control mechanisms to achieve relatively steady-state conditions (Brobeck, 1956). A system is said to be regulated if structures respond to change and, by their activity, preserve some level of constancy. That is, the purpose of a regulating system is to maintain a certain parameter at a generally steady level. For speech production, subglottal pressure appears to be maintained by providing a sufficient level of vocal tract resistance. The control process is the means by which this is accomplished. This implies that the brain receives information, processes it, and then directs control responses such as the movement of articulatory structures and respiratory muscle activity.

Because the production of speech is an overlaid function of breathing, it is not surprising that certain speech activities are similar to respiratory behaviors. Specifically, in breathing, the mechanics of respiration tend to maintain an optimal level of airway resistance in the range of 1.0 to 3.0 cm $H_2O/L/s$ (Cole, 1985; Warren, Duany, & Fischer, 1969). This level of resistance, which is maintained primarily by the nasal airway and vocal fold placement, allows sufficient time for alveolar gas exchange. Similarly, in speech, subglottal pressure is maintained at a fairly constant level by controlling airway resistance through movement of such vocal tract structures as the velum, tongue, vocal folds, lips, and respiratory muscles (Warren, 1982). The speech regulating system provides flexible, local energy sources throughout the vocal tract while maintaining a fairly constant subglottal pressure. The point to be emphasized is that, in any regulating system, there must be a relationship among sensory input, central processing, and motor output. Mechanisms to detect or identify changes in such aerodynamic variables as pressure, airflow, or resistance are necessary if responses to modify changes in the vocal tract environment are required (Warren, 1982).

Receptors that respond to pressure, airflow, volume, and resistance have been found in the trachea (Sant'Ambrogio, 1982), the larynx (Sant'Ambrogio, Matthew, Fisher, & Sant'Ambrogio, 1983), and the nasopharynx (McBride & Whitelaw, 1981). Laryngeal receptors sensing pressure, airflow, and muscle contractions have also been described (Sant'Ambrogio, 1982). Studies by England and Bartlett (1982) demonstrate that the larynx controls respiratory flow during breathing by varying the degree of glottal adduction. There is also evidence that muscles in the upper airway play a functional role in instantaneous control of airflow and compensation for changes in airway resistance (Brouillette & Thach, 1980; Cohen, 1975). Remmers and Bartlett (1977) observed a "tracking" behavior involving extrathoracic stretch receptors in which the respiratory muscles compensated for changes in upper airway resistance.

There is evidence that individuals with an intact sensorimotor system can detect imposed changes in the airway environment of approximately 20 to 40% (Elice & Warren, 1991). For example, an added resistance of less than 2.0 cm $H_2O/L/s$ during breathing is enough for most young adults to become aware of a change in the airway environment. Although the experimental conditions involved breathing in those studies, there is also evidence that individuals can detect similar changes in the aerodynamic environment during speech as well. Malecot (1966, 1970), Muller and Brown (1980), Williams, Brown, and Turner (1987), and Wyke (1981) have suggested that aerodynamic monitoring may be used to direct the movement of speech structures. They observed that pressure changes as low as 1.0 cm H_2O can be detected.

Methods of Assessment

The simplest approach to testing aerodynamic sensitivity involves using a diaphragm that has an adjustable iris. Opening or closing the aperture changes the resistance load **(Fig. 5–8)**. Data from our studies indicate that normal adults are able to detect changes in resistance that are less than 2.0 cm $H_2O/L/s$ during breathing (Elice & Warren, 1991).

The procedure is simple to perform because it merely involves breathing through a calibrated diaphragm. Determination of thresholds provides an indication of a patient's ability to detect a change in airway resistance or pressure. Such information should be useful in determining the ability of the patient to sense changes in the aerodynamic environment.

A more dynamic approach to assess vocal tract sensitivity and motor responses during speech was described by Kim, Zajac, Warren, and Mayo (1997). This approach not only provided an assessment of an individual's ability to sense pressure and resistance changes, but also revealed how fast an individual responded to such changes. The approach employed a computer-controlled "perturbator," which was considerably faster than a solenoid valve, that altered the aerodynamic environment at specified times during phonation in approximately 20 to 40 ms, depending on the magnitude of change desired. Neurologically intact speakers used a mouthpiece connected to the perturbator to produce

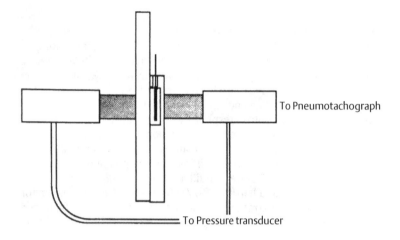

To Pneumotachograph

To Pressure transducer

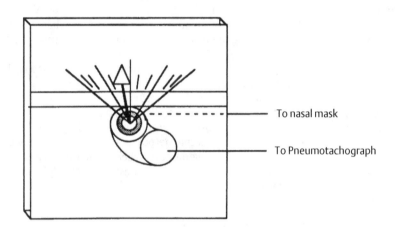

To nasal mask

To Pneumotachograph

Figure 5–8 Diagrammatic representation of the diaphragm used to create a resistance load during breathing. The calibrated diaphragm can be opened or closed to change the value of resistance.

a series of syllables consisting of /pa/. At unexpected times during pressure rise of /p/, the device created bleed openings of various magnitude. Kim et al (1997) reported that most speakers detected a loss of pressure when the bleed aperture exceeded 14 mm². In addition, there appeared to be a short-latency oral pressure recovery following the bleed that the investigators interpreted as an active response to compensate for the loss of pressure.

In a follow-up experiment, Zajac and Weissler (2004) determined the oral pressure loss to bleed openings ranging from 5 to 40 mm². They reported a systematic reduction in pressure and the slope of the rise in pressure as function of increasing bleed aperture. Of interest, even at the largest bleed opening, speakers were able to achieve oral pressures of approximately 2 to 3 cm H_2O, consistent with studies of speakers who exhibit velopharyngeal impairment. The lack of any apparent pressure stabilization across bleed openings, however, suggested that passive aeromechanical factors accounted for the oral pressure findings. Zajac and Weissler (2004) also monitored subglottal air pressure in two of the speakers during oral pressure bleeds. As illustrated in **Fig. 5–9**, while oral air pressure decreased as expected **(Fig. 5–9A)**, subglottal pressure remained relatively stable during the period of bleeds **(Fig. 5–9B).** Based on this finding, the occurrence

of respiratory reflexes to maintain subglottal pressure levels could not be ruled out.

Although the technology used to assess sensory performance is currently available, its use among patients with sensorimotor deficits is infrequent. Obviously, this special group of patients may experience a great degree of difficulty performing some of the tasks, but preliminary experience indicates that the assessment procedures are feasible, and reliable information can be obtained. We are hopeful that, by presenting our ideas on aerodynamic sensory assessments, others will become interested in pursuing these approaches, refine the techniques, and, ultimately, determine their validity.

♦ Conclusion

Aerodynamic assessment techniques can be useful for evaluating the motor and sensory abilities of patients with sensorimotor deficits. Motor assessments include measurements of velopharyngeal orifice size, oral port size, and laryngeal resistance. These techniques can also be used to assess timing behaviors associated with the movement of speech

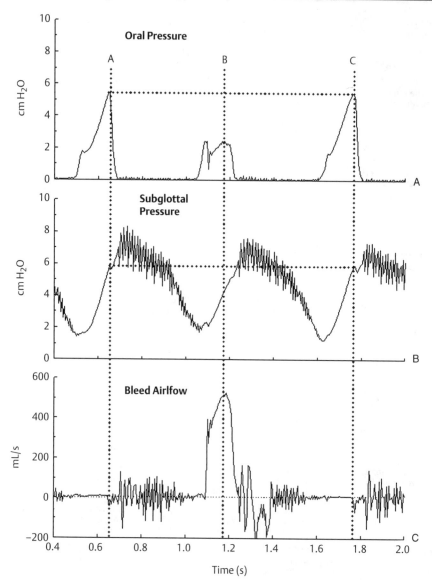

Figure 5–9 Pressure-flow traces of a neurologically intact speaker producing the syllable /pa/ three times. During the second production, oral pressure was unexpectedly bled via a mouthpiece attached to a series of valves. **(A)** Oral pressure. **(B)** Subglottal pressure. **(C)** Bleed airflow. Note that while oral pressure drops substantially during the bleed, subglottal pressure remains relatively stable.

structures such as the velopharyngeal port or the anterior oral port constriction. Such information is useful in localizing specific areas of deficiency.

Aerodynamic measurements can also be utilized in combination with apparatus that provide resistance loads to assess the sensory components of a disturbed speech system. Although sensory testing of aerodynamic performance is relatively new, data from normal subjects indicate that valuable diagnostic information can be obtained using relatively simple procedures.

Testing of patients with sensorimotor deficits is often difficult because of the limitations associated with motor problems. However, reliable measurements can be obtained on most patients when the assessor is willing to provide the time and effort necessary to obtain meaningful results.

Acknowledgment   Preparation of this chapter was supported in part by National Institute of Dental and Craniofacial Research grants DE07105, DE06957, and DE10175.

References

Aten, J.L. (1988). Spastic dysarthria: revising understanding the disorders and speech treatment procedures. *Journal of Head Trauma Rehabilitation,* 3, 63–73

Baken, R.J, & Orlikoff, R.F. (2000). *Clinical Measurement of Speech and Voice,* 2nd ed. San Diego: Singular

Barlow, S.M. (1989). A high-speed data acquisition system for clinical speech physiology. In: K.M. Yorkston, D.R. Beukelman (Eds.), *Recent Advances in Clinical Dysarthria* (pp. 39–52). Boston: College-Hill/Little, Brown

_____. (1999). *Handbook of Clinical Speech Physiology.* San Diego: Singular

Brobeck, J.R. (1956). Exchange, control and regulation. In: J.R. Brobeck & W.S. Yamamoto (Eds.), *Physiological Controls and Regulations*. Philadelphia: W.B. Saunders

Brouillette, R.T. & Thach, B.T. (1980). Control of genioglossus muscle inspiratory activity. *Journal of Applied Physiology, 49*, 801

Claypoole, W.H., Warren, D.W., & Bradley, D.P. (1974). The effect of cleft palate on oral port constriction during fricative productions. *Cleft Palate Journal, 2*, 95–104

Cohen, M.I. (1975). Phrenic and recurrent laryngeal discharge patterns and the Hering-Breuer reflex. *American Journal of Applied Physiology, 228*, 1489

Cole, P. (1985). Upper respiratory airflow. In: D.F. Proctor & I. Anderson (Eds.), *The Nose-Upper Airway Physiology and the Atmospheric Environment* (pp. 163–189). Amsterdam: Elsevier

Dalston, R.M., Warren, D.W., Morr, K.E. & Smith, L.R. (1988). Intraoral pressure and its relationship to velopharyngeal inadequacy. *Cleft Palate Journal, 25*, 210–219

Darley, E., Aronson, A., & Brown, J. (1975). *Motor Speech Disorders*. Philadelphia: W.B. Sanders

Dotevall, D.R., Lohmander-Agerskov, A., Ejnell, H., & Bake, B. (2002). Perceptual evaluation of speech and velopharyngeal function in children with and without cleft palate and the relationship to nasal airflow patterns. *Cleft Palate-Craniofacial Journal, 39*, 409–424

Duffy, J.R. (1995). *Motor Speech Disorders: Substrates, Differential Diagnosis and Management*. St. Louis: Mosby

Elice, C.E. & Warren, D.W. (1991). Perception of nasal airway resistance. *Journal of Dental Research, 70*, 341

England, S.J. & Bartlett, D., Jr. (1982). Changes in respiratory movements of human vocal cords during hypernea. *Journal of Applied Physiology, 51*, 780

Hamman, V.L. & Yorkston, K.M. (1994). Respiratory patterning and variability on dysarthric speech. *Journal of Medical Speech-Language Pathology, 2*, 253–262

Hartelius, L. & Svensson, P. (1994). Speech and swallowing symptoms associated Parkinson's disease and multiple sclerosis: a survey. *Folia Phoniatrica et Logopedica, 46*, 9–17

Hess, D.A. & McDonald, E.T. (1960). Consonantal nasal pressure in cleft palate speakers. *Journal of Speech and Hearing Research, 3*, 201–211

Hixon, T.J., Putnam, A.H., & Sharpe, J. (1983). Speech production with flaccid paralysis of the rib cage, diaphragm and abdomen. *Journal of Speech and Hearing Disorders, 19*, 297–356

Hoit, J.D., Watson, P.J., Hixon, K.E., McMahon, P., & Johnson, C.L. (1994). Age and velopharyngeal function during speech production. *Journal of Speech and Hearing Research, 37*, 295–302

Jiang, J., O'Mara, T., Chen, H.J., Stern, J.I., Vlagos, D., & Hanson, D. (1999). Aerodynamic measurements of patients with Parkinson's disease. *Journal of Voice, 13*, 583–591

Kent, R. & Netsell, R. (1978). Articulatory abnormalities in athetoid cerebral palsy. *Journal of Speech and Hearing Disorders, 43*(3):353–73

Kim, J.R., Zajac, D., Warren, D.W., & Mayo, R. (1997). The response to sudden change in vocal tract resistance during stop consonant production. *Journal of Speech, Language, and Hearing Research, 40*, 848–857

Laine, T., Warren, D.W., Dalston, R.M., et al. (1988). Screening of velopharyngeal closure based on nasal airflow rate measurements. *Cleft Palate Journal, 25*, 220–225

Lubker, J.F. (1970). Aerodynamic and ultrasonic assessment techniques in speech-dentofacial research. *American Speech and Hearing Association Reports, 5*, 203–223

Lubker, J.F. & Moll, K.L. (1965). Simultaneous oral-nasal airflow measurements and cinefluorographic observations during speech production. *Cleft Palate Journal, 2*, 257–272

Machida, J. (1967). Airflow rate and articulatory movement during speech. *Cleft Palate Journal, 4*, 240–248

Malecot, A. (1966). The effectiveness of intraoral air pressure pulse parameters in distinguishing between stop cognates. *Phonetica, 14*, 65–81

_____. (1970). The lens-fortis opposition: Its physiological parameters. *Journal of the Acoustical Society of America, 47*, 1588–1592

McBride, B. & Whitelaw, W.A. (1981). A physiological stimulus to upper airway receptors in humans. *Journal of Applied Physiology, 51*, 1179

McHenry, M.A., Wilson, R.L., & Minton, J.T. (1994). The challenge of unintelligible speech following traumatic brain injury. *Journal of Medical Speech-Language Pathology, 2*, 58–74

Miller, S. (2004). Voice therapy for vocal fold paralysis. *Otolaryngologic Clinics of North America, 37*, 105–119

Moon, J., Folkins, J.W., Smith, A.E., & Luschei, E.S. (1993). Air pressure regulation during speech production. *Journal of the Acoustical Society of America, 94*, 54–63

Muller, E.M. & Brown, W.S., Jr. (1980). Variations in the supraglottal air pressure waveform and their articulatory interpretation. In: N. Lass (Ed.), *Speech and Language: Advances in Basic Research and Practice*, vol. 4 (pp. 317–389). New York: Academic Press

Netsell, R. (1969). Evaluation of velopharyngeal dysfunction in dysarthria. *Journal of Speech and Hearing Disorders, 34*, 113–122

Netsell, R. & Daniel, B. (1979). Dysarthria in adults: physiologic approach to rehabilitation *Archives of Physical Medicine and Rehabilitation 60*(11), 502–508

Netsell, R. & Kent, R.D. (1976). Paroxysmal ataxia in dysarthria. *Journal of Speech and Hearing Disorders, 41*, 93–109

Putnam, A.H. & Hixon, T.J. (1981). Respiratory kinematics in speakers with motor neuron disease. In: M. McNeil, J. Rosenbeck, & A. Aronson (Eds.), *The Dysarthrias*. San Diego: College-Hill Press

Remmers, J.E. & Bartlett, D., Jr. (1977). Reflex control of expiratory airflow and duration. *Journal of Applied Physiology, 42*, 80

Roth, C.R., Glaze, L.E., Goding, G.S., & David, W.S. (1996). Spasmodic dysphonia symptoms as initial Presentation of amyotrophic lateral sclerosis. *Journal of Voice, 10*, 362–367

Sant'Ambrogio, G. (1982). Information arising from the tracheobronchial tree in mammals. *Physiology Review, 62*, 531

Sant'Ambrogio, G., Matthew, O.P., Fisher, J.T., & Sant'Ambrogio, F.B. (1983). Laryngeal receptors responding to transmural pressure, airflow and local muscle activity. *Respiratory Physiology, 54*, 317

Smith, Z.H., Allen, G., Warren, D.W., & Hall, D.J. (1978). The consistency of the pressure-flow technique for assessing oral port size. *Journal of the Acoustical Society of America, 64*, 1203–1206

Smitheran, R. & Hixon, T.J. (1981). A clinical method for estimating laryngeal airway resistance during vowel production. *Journal of Speech and Hearing Disorders, 46*, 138–146

Subtelny, J.D., Worth, J.H., & Sakuda, M. (1966). Intraoral pressure and rate of flow during speech. *Journal of Speech and Hearing Research, 9*, 498–518

Tandan, R. & Bradley, W.G. (1985). Amyotrophic lateral sclerosis: Part 1. Clinical features, pathology, and ethical issues in management. *Annals of Neurology, 18*, 271–280

Theodoros, D.G., Murdoch, B.E., & Chenery, H.J. (1994). Perceptual speech characteristics of dysarthric speakers following severe closed head injury. *Brain Injury, 8*, 101–124

Thompson, A.E. & Hixon, T.J. (1979). Nasal airflow during normal speech production. *Cleft Palate Journal, 16*, 412–420

Warren, D.W. (1964). Velopharyngeal orifice size and upper pharyngeal pressure-flow patterns in normal speech. *Plastic Reconstructive Surgery, 33*, 148–161

_____. (1967). Nasal emission of air and velopharyngeal function. *Cleft Palate Journal, 4*, 148–165

_____. (1976). Aerodynamics of sound production. In: N. Lass (Ed.), *Contemporary Issues in Experimental Phonetics*. Springfield, IL: Thomas

_____. (1979). Perci: a method for rating palatal efficiency. *Cleft Palate Journal, 16*, 279–285

_____. (1982). Aerodynamics of speech. In: N.J. Lass, L.V. McReynolds, J.L. Northern, & D.E. Yoder (Eds.), *Speech, Language and Hearing*. Philadelphia: Saunders

_____. (1986a). The velopharyngeal sphincter: a control factor in the speech regulating system. *American Speech-Language-Hearing Association, 28,* 103

_____. (1986b). Compensatory speech behaviors in cleft palate: a regulation/control phenomenon? *Cleft Palate Journal, 23,* 251–280

Warren, D.W., Dalston, R.M., & Dalston, E.T. (1986). Maintaining speech pressure in the presence of velopharyngeal inadequacy. *Cleft Palate Journal, 27,* 53–58

Warren, D.W., Dalston, R.M., & Mayo, R. (1993). Hypernasality in the presence of "adequate" velopharyngeal closure. *Cleft Palate Journal, 30,* 150–154

Warren, D.W., Dalston, R.M., Morr, K.E., Hairfield, W.M., & Smith, L.R. (1989). The speech regulating system: temporal and aerodynamic responses to velopharyngeal inadequacy. *Journal of Speech and Hearing Research, 32,* 566–575

Warren, D.W., Dalston, R.M., Trier, W.C., & Holder, M.B. (1985). A pressure-flow technique for quantifying temporal patterns of palatopharyngeal closure. *Cleft Palate Journal, 22,* 11–19

Warren, D.W., Duany, L.F., & Fischer, N.D. (1969). Nasal pathway resistance in normal and cleft lip and palate subjects. *Cleft Palate Journal, 6,* 134–140

Warren, D.W. & DuBois, A.B. (1964). A pressure-flow technique for measuring velopharyngeal orifice area during continuous speech. *Cleft Palate Journal, 1,* 52–71

Warren, D.W., Hairfield, W.M., & Seaton, D. (1987). The relationship between nasal airway size and nasal airway resistance. *American Journal of Orthodontics and Dentofacial Orthopedics, 92,* 390–395

Warren, D.W. & Hall, D. (1973). Glottal activity and intraoral pressures during stop consonant productions. *Folia Phoniatrica, 25,* 121–129

Warren, D.W., Hall, D.J., & Davis, J. (1981). Oral port constriction and pressure airflow relationships during sibilant productions. *Folia Phoniatrica, 33,* 380–394

Williams, W.N., Brown, W.S., & Turner, G.E. (1987). Intraoral air pressure discrimination by normal-speaking subjects. *Folia Phoniatrica, 39,* 196–203

Wyke, B. (1981). Neuromuscular control systems in voice production. In: D. Bless & J. Abbs (Eds.), *Vocal Fold Physiology: Contemporary Research and Clinical Issues* (pp. 71–76). San Diego: College-Hill Press

Yates, C.C., McWilliams, B.J., & Vallino, L. (1990). The pressure-flow method: some fundamental concepts. *Cleft Palate Journal, 27,* 193–198

Yorkston, K.M., Beukelman, D.R., & Bell, K.B. (1989). *Clinical Management of Dysarthric Speakers.* San Diego: College-Hill Press

Yorkston, K.M., Beukelman, D.R., & Honsinger, M.J. (1989). Perceived articulatory adequacy and velopharyngeal function in dysarthric speakers. *Archives of Physical Medicine and Rehabilitation, 70,* 313–331

Yorkston, K.M., Beukelman, D.R., Strand, E.A., & Bell, K.R. (1999). *Management of Motor Speech Disorders in Children and Adults.* Austin: Pro-Ed

Yorkston, K.M., Strand, E.A., & Kennedy, M.R.T. (1996). Comprehensibility of dysarthric speakers: implications for assessment and treatment planning. *American Journal of Speech-Language Pathology, 5,* 55–66

Zajac, D.J. (2000). Pressure-flow characteristics of /m/ and /p/ production in speakers without cleft palate: developmental findings. *Cleft Palate-Craniofacial Journal, 37,* 468–476

Zajac, D.J. & Mayo, R. (1996). Aerodynamic and temporal aspects of velopharyngeal function in normal speakers. *Journal of Speech and Hearing Research, 39,* 1199–1207

Zajac, D.J. & Weissler, M.C. (2004). Air pressure responses to sudden vocal tract pressure bleeds during production of stop consonants: new evidence of aeromechanical regulation. *Journal of Speech, Language, and Hearing Research, 47,* 784–801

Chapter 6

Kinematic Measurement of Speech and Early Orofacial Movements

Steven M. Barlow, Donald S. Finan, Richard D. Andreatta, and Carol Boliek

The speech motor control system, including the abdomen and ribcage, larynx, velopharynx, tongue, jaw, and lips, represents an anatomically diverse collection of connective tissue–muscle subsystems regulated by a phylogenetically elaborated and distributed neural system. An issue of special importance is the relation between orofacial motor control and speech production. Damage to select areas of the nervous system involved in the selection, sequencing, and activation of articulatory muscles will degrade speech kinematics and may reduce intelligibility (Barlow, Farley, & Andreatta, 1999; Guenther, Ghosh, & Tourville, 2006). Measurement of muscle performance variables, including kinematics, is central to advancing our understanding of the development of speech movements over the life span, and the response to neurological disease and traumatic injury.

◆ Vocal Tract Dynamics

Generating the source-excitation and shaping the anterior portion of the vocal tract to achieve a sequence of acoustic targets involves coordinated muscle actions and movements of the chest wall, larynx, velopharynx, tongue, jaw, and lips. The integrity of the underlying performance anatomy, including contractile elements, connective tissue, bone, and the neural substrate, is central to a discussion of motor proficiency during speech. In some instances, the accurate positioning of one structure (e.g., the lower lip) may be dependent on another structure (e.g., the mandible). Motor goal acquisition often involves reorganization of motor patterns for individual structures during the course of speech production. Kinematic studies of speech typically involve recording from multiple structures in an attempt to understand the trading relations between structures, patterns of organization, and reorganization during development, or following brain injury or neurological disease. Feedback and predictive or "forward looking" neural mechanisms are hypothesized to play an important role in the acquisition and maintenance of speech movements.

◆ Measures of Muscle Output

Activation of muscle yields several measurable outputs including force, displacement, heat, vibration, and electrical activity. Contractile force and displacement have been studied in the context of assessing orofacial muscle performance in normal and disordered speakers. In a limited number of experiments, select parameters of force control have been examined in relation to movement and quantitative measures of speech intelligibility in individuals with dysarthria. Force as a controlled variable is central to theories of motor control. The elaborate neural representation of sensorimotor systems subserving the static and dynamic parameters for movement and force supports this theoretical framework. Active displacement is dependent on the action(s) of the force generators (muscles) organized about joints or within soft tissues. Kinematic variables typically studied include the amplitude of displacement, velocity, acceleration, phase, and relative timing among multiple articulatory structures, spatiotemporal variability, phase relations to electromyogram (EMG) muscle patterns, and spectral properties of movement (frequency domain) (Smith, 1992).

◆ Tracking Orofacial Movements

Labial-Mandibular Strain-Gage Transduction

Strain-gage movement transducers have been used for over 30 years to capture two-dimensional (2D) movements of the upper lip, lower lip, and jaw in normal and dysarthric speakers and still represent a low-cost solution for tracking movements of accessible articulators such as the lips and mandible. Early adaptations of strain-gage movement cantilevers (Abbs & Gilbert, 1973; Müller & Abbs, 1979) were enhanced by incorporating a low-mass tubular head-frame mount (Barlow, Cole, & Abbs, 1983), which made it possible to sample speech movement disorders simultaneously in two-dimensions along with other signals such as EMGs, aerodynamics, and acoustic outputs from normal and disordered populations, including children without head restraint. The cantilevers are linear over a 30-mm range and have a stable frequency response from direct current (DC) to 18 Hz with negligible time delay.

Strain-gage systems have been used widely in studies of speech kinematics in normal adults (DeNil & Abbs, 1991; Folkins & Canty, 1986; Gracco, 1988; Moon, Zembrowski, Robin, & Folkins, 1993; Moore, 1993; Nelson, Perkell, & Westbury, 1984; Perkell & Matthies, 1992; Shaiman & Porter, 1991; Sussman & Westbury, 1981), hearing impaired speakers (Tye-Murray & Folkins, 1990), children (Sharkey & Folkins, 1985; Smith & Gartenberg, 1984; Smith & McLean-Muse, 1987a,b), geriatric adults (Forrest, Weismer, & Adams, 1990), dysfluent speakers (McClean, Kroll, & Loftus, 1990), Parkinson patients (Forrest, Weismer, & Turner, 1989), and a variety of apraxic, aphasic, and dysarthric subjects (Abbs, Hunker, & Barlow, 1983; Barlow & Abbs, 1986; Hunker, Abbs, & Barlow, 1982; McClean, Beukelman, & Yorkston, 1987; McNeil, Weismer, Adams, & Mulligan, 1990). The low cost of strain-gage movement systems maintains its appeal for certain types of kinematic studies; however, the new video-based and electromagnetic movement tracking systems offer more versatility and flexibility in data acquisition and management but at a significantly higher startup cost.

Orofacial Tracking Using X-Ray Microbeam

The x-ray microbeam is a computer-controlled system that uses a narrow beam of x-rays to localize and track the two-dimensional movements of small gold pellets attached to the various speech structures, including lips, jaw, tongue, soft palate, and eustachian tube (Abbs, Nadler, & Fujimura, 1988). Originally implemented at the University of Tokyo (Fujimura, Kiritani, & Ishida, 1973; Kiritani, Itoh, & Fujimura, 1975), the x-ray microbeam system generates an electron beam accelerated by a voltage source of up to 600 kV at a 5-mA current. The system produces a narrow beam (approximately 0.4 mm in diameter) of x-rays, which are generated by channeling the electron beam toward a tungsten target. The resulting x-rays pass through a pinhole aperture (approximately 300 mm in diameter) and are focused at the various pellets. As the x-ray beam is scanned across a pellet, a recognizable "shadow" is registered on a sodium iodide (NaI) crystal detector. The path of the x-ray beam toward a pellet is determined by predictions of the position of the pellet generated by current and previous locations. At periodic intervals, the location of each pellet (defined as the centroid of its shadow) is assigned rectangular coordinates relative to axes specified by the reference pellets. The sequence of scanning, recognition, prediction, and calculation of location for up to 10 pellets may be completed with an aggregate cycling rate of up to 700 Hz. Each pellet may be assigned its own cycle rate in the range of 40 to 180 Hz.

The x-ray microbeam system at the University of Wisconsin–Madison was designed to record the trajectories of small (2 to 3 mm in diameter) radiodense markers (gold pellets), which may be attached to various articulators (Abbs et al, 1988; Westbury, 1991). A typical application may include a total of 10 pellets that are cemented in a midsagittal plane to the tip, body, and dorsum of the tongue, the lower lip, a mandibular incisor, and in a lateral sagittal plane to a mandibular molar. The remaining two pellets are attached to the bridge of the nose and a maxillary incisor to serve as reference points that are immobile relative to the skull.

Error in the evaluated positions of pellets may arise as a result of translation (along the z-axis) or rotation of the head. Translation error relates to the proportion of the distance between the pinhole and the image plane (NaI detector) that the head moves. For example, for a pinhole to image plane distance of 500 mm, movement of the head along the z-axis ± 10 mm will generate a maximum error of $\pm 2\%$. Thus, two pellets known to be 20 mm apart may intermittently appear to be spread by 20.4 or 19.6 mm. Furthermore, head rotation of $\pm 10\%$ results in $\pm 5\%$ error. Measurements of head rotation and translation in a group of six speakers indicate high intratrial stability but somewhat variable intertrial accuracy. Also, measurement error due to head translation or rotation appeared to be within $\pm 5\%$.

The x-ray microbeam system has been used successfully in the study of speaking rate on the velocity profiles of movements of the lower lip and tongue tip during the production of stop consonants in five young normal adults (Adams, Weismer, & Kent, 1993). Fast speaking rates yielded symmetrical, single-peaked velocity functions, whereas slow speech produced asymmetrical, multipeaked velocity profiles. It was suggested that speech produced at fast rates appears to involve unitary movements that may be preprogrammed and executed with little or no dependence on sensorimotor integration, whereas articulatory gestures produced at slow speaking rates may be influenced by feedback mechanisms.

X-ray microbeam data have also been combined with cinefluorography to examine the displacement of the tongue body during opening articulatory gestures in three deaf and two hearing subjects (Tye-Murray, 1991). Speech samples consisted of consonant-vowel-consonant (CVC) syllables embedded within a carrier phrase. Displacement patterns in deaf and hearing subjects were examined for variation in vocalic contexts between subjects. As expected, the authors found that deaf speakers had less flexible tongue bodies as a result of compensatory and incorrectly learned principles for constraining tongue movement during speech.

The question of functional regionality within the tongue was studied by quantifying the strength of coupling among four different tongue locations as a function of consonantal contexts and also during swallowing in 46 participants (Green & Wang, 2003). Vertical displacements of radiodense pellets attached to the tongue were extracted from the x-ray microbeam database. Tongue-surface movement patterns were described by calculating the covariance between the vertical displacement time histories of all possible pellet pairs. Results indicated that tongue displacements for speech and swallowing clustered into distinct groups based on their coupling profiles. As suggested by these authors, the study of the coupling relations among tongue regions has the potential to elucidate modes of control for swallowing and speech, as well as advancing our understanding of the differences in the coordinative requirements for these two motor behaviors.

Orofacial Magnetometry

Alternating magnetic field devices known as magnetometers have been used extensively in a variety of settings, including industry, academics, and clinical care. The applications are diverse, ranging from magnetic measurements and theory, to biomedical research in speech production where movements of the face, jaw, tongue, soft palate, and chest wall are now tracked in real time. Part of the magnetometer's appeal in speech physiology research and clinical application is due to the fact that the kinematics of intraoral structures (tongue, velopharynx) can be observed and recorded in real time without the biohazards associated with radiological imaging methods. Historically, the study of speech kinematics has been problematic because movements within the mouth are difficult to measure and visualize.

One of the earliest versions of a magnetometer sensor for tracking tongue tip movements was described by Sonoda (1974) from Kumamoto University in Japan. A small permanent magnet was fixed on the tongue surface, and two magnetometer units sensitive to horizontal and vertical movements of the tongue were oriented at a right angle to the sagittal plane of the head. With this configuration, the position of the magnet in the mouth could be determined during speech. Sonoda concluded that this emerging technology represented a powerful method for speech physiology research due to its simplicity, safety, economy, and flexibility for signal presentation.

Hixon (1971) and van der Giet (1977) used alternating fields and various transmitter signals to track the movement trajectories of the jaw and lips, respectively. These systems did not have a provision for correcting for rotational misalignment between the magnetic field transmitters and the transducers, which could cause undetectable measurement error. By 1983 Schönle was able to register four different points within the mouth using a similar procedure.

Development of an electromagnetic articulometer was underway in 1980 at the Massachusetts Institute of Technology under the direction of Dr. Joseph Perkell. The original version used two transmitter coils and miniature biaxial sensors that were designed to enable correction for rotational misalignment. Known as the electromagnetic midsagittal articulometer (EMMA), this system offered up to 10 channels of high-resolution kinematic recordings of intraoral structures such as the tongue and velum during speech. Signals are corrected for rotational misalignment. With the EMMA system, it is possible to record movements of multiple midline points on vocal-tract structures. The EMMA system can provide the needed quantities of accurate articulatory data with minimal risk to experimental subjects. **Figure 6–1** illustrates the second-generation EMMA system that was developed at MIT (Perkell, Cohen, Svirsky, Matthies, Garabieta, & Jackson, 1992). It includes three transmitter coils, labeled *T,* which are held in a transmitter assembly, with the coil axes perpendicular to the midline plane. The transmitter assembly is positioned so its midline coincides with the subject's midsagittal plane. Each transmitter coil is excited by a sinusoidal signal at a different frequency, between 60 and 80 kHz. This generates an alternating magnetic field having a strength that decreases

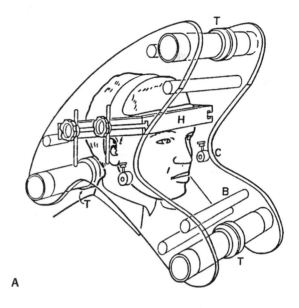

A

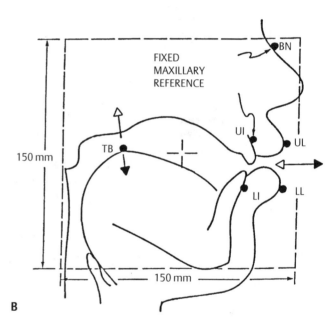

B

Figure 6–1   (A) The electromagnetic midsagittal articulometer (EMMA) system developed at the Massachusetts Institute of Technology. It includes three transmitter coils *(T),* which are held in a transmitter assembly, with the coil axes perpendicular to the midline plane. The transmitter assembly is positioned so its midline coincides with the subject's midsagittal plane. Each transmitter coil is excited by a sinusoidal signal at a different frequency, between 60 and 80 KHz. This generates an alternating magnetic field having a strength that decreases approximately in proportion to the cube of the distance from the transmitter. H = headmount, B = Spacing bars. **(B)** Small, encased transducer coils are mounted on the subject's articulators, including the tongue blade, tongue body, lower incisors, lips and possibly the velum using a special biomedical adhesive. Special care is taken to mount the transducers as close as possible to the midline, with their axes parallel to the transmitter axes BN. = bridge of nose, UL = upper lip, LL = lower lip, LI = lower incisor, UI = upper incisor, TB = tongue body. [From Perkell, J.S., Cohen, M.H., Svirsky, M.A., Matthies, M.L., Garabieta, I., & Jackson, M.T.T. (1992). Electromagnetic midsagittal articulometer systems for transducing speech articulatory movements. *Journal of the Acoustical Society of America, 92,* 3078–3096.

approximately in proportion to the cube of the distance from the transmitter.

The alternating magnetic fields from the transmitters induce alternating voltages in single-axis transducer coils, which are connected by fine wires to receiver electronics. The wires from intraoral transducers pass out of the corner of the mouth. The electronics convert the induced high-frequency signals to three slowly varying output signals from each transducer that are digitized simultaneously with the speech acoustic signal. Special signal processing software is used to convert the digitized signals to x and y coordinates in the midline plane. As the articulators move, the transducer axes can vary in their alignment, "rotational misalignment" with the transmitter axes, causing measurement error. Signal processing software includes a calculation that corrects for this rotational misalignment. The small, encased transducer coils are mounted on the subject's articulators, including the tongue blade, tongue body, lower incisors, lips, and possibly the velum using a special biomedical adhesive. As shown in the bottom panel of **Fig. 6–1**, transducers are also mounted on the bridge of the nose and upper central incisors for a maxillary frame of reference. Special care is given to mount the transducers as close as possible to the midline, with their axes parallel to the transmitter axes. The EMMA system is well suited for the study of speech production. Large quantities of kinematic and acoustic data can be safely acquired and displayed in real time to help reveal the underlying principles of speech motor control.

Motivated in part by the speech magnetometry work at the MIT laboratory, another 2D electromagnetic articulograph was developed at the medical school of the University of Göttingen, starting in 1982. By 1988, Carstens Medizinelektronik (Göttingen, Germany) developed the first commercial articulograph known as the AG100. Since 1995, Carstens Medizinelektronik, in collaboration with Professor Hans G. Tillmann (University of Munich) and with the support of Nippon Telegraph and Telephone (NTT; Tokyo, Japan), have been developing the new three-dimensional (3D) articulograph AG500. This system allows sensor placement at all positions in the oral cavity and in all orientations within a 300-mm spherical measurement area. The articulograph AG500 is currently certified for use as a laboratory apparatus. It features high timing resolution with either eight or 12 channels. Each channel is sampled at 100 kHz with 200-Hz demodulated output. A separate channel for sampling the speech acoustic signal is synchronized by the AG500 by the host microprocessor. The principal components of the AG500 include an acrylic case, known as the EMA Cube **(Fig. 6–2)**, small sensor coils that are positioned on and in the subject's mouth, and electronic signal conditioning and digital interface that are compatible with the MS Windows–compatible operating system, including 98 SE, 2000, or XP. Together with the accompanying data acquisition and analysis software, system operation includes a sensor calibration procedure to ensure accurate scaling of displacement among the sensors attached to the tongue, mouth, palate, and mandible. An extra reference sensor attached to the bridge of the nose provides for head movement correction. Each of the six transmitters fixed on the case produces an alternating magnetic field at different frequencies. The alternating magnetic field induces an alternating current in the sensors, much like in a transformer, and

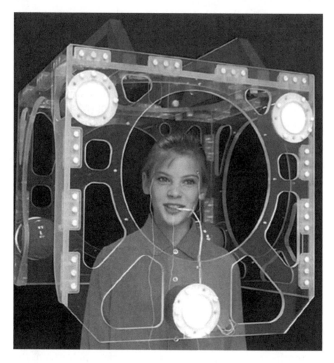

Figure 6–2 Carstens Articulograph AG500 for 3D recording of facial and intraoral movements. Transduction and subject interface is shown including the EMA Cube, and small sensor coils positioned on and in the speaker's mouth. The fixed transmitters are attached to the acrylic case. (Courtesy of Brigitta Carstens, Carstens Medizinelektronik GmbH, D37120 Lenglern, Germany.)

allows one to obtain the distances of each sensor from the six transmitters. It is then possible to calculate the x, y, and z coordinates as well as two angles, and measure, store, and display the positions of the sensors. Data analysis, however, is completed off-line.

As recognized by Sonoda (1974), the real-time data collection and kinematic monitoring rendered by orofacial magnetometry will make it applicable to speech teaching or speech correction. For example, individuals with hearing loss can observe a visual feedback analogue of their tongue movements on an oscillographic display. This approach could be applied to the rehabilitation of certain forms of dysarthria, craniofacial disorders, or second language acquisition, although such use of visual displays of articulator movements have met with limited success in the past.

◆ Optical Three-Dimensional Tracking of the Face

Developmental studies of lip and jaw coordination during speech production have benefited directly from the emergence of sophisticated multichannel video-based movement tracking systems (Green, Moore, Higashikawa, & Steeve, 2000). There are several systems available commercially that use video cameras to register marker location using either reflective markers or infrared source tracking (e.g., ViconPEAK Motion Systems, Centennial, CO; Optotrak, Northern Digital, Waterloo, Ontario, Canada; Motion Analysis, Motion Analysis Corporation, Santa Rosa, CA).

In a study of facial animation, Trotman and colleagues (Trotman & Faraway, 1998; Trotman, Faraway, Silvester, Greenlee, & Johnston, 1998; Trotman, Faraway, & Essick, 2000) used a video-based tracking system (Motion Analysis, Motion Analysis Corporation) to sample 4-mm-diameter spherical reflective markers attached to more than 30 anatomical landmarks on the face of repaired unilateral and bilateral cleft lip and palate patients and noncleft control subjects. Four analogue video cameras sampled the position of these markers at 60 frames per second. A rigid cube frame was used a priori to establish calibration in 3D space to a resolution of 0.53 mm. Using this technique, Trotman et al (2000) found that individual cleft lip patients exhibited asymmetry of facial movements and significant changes in the range of displacement during the production of facial gestures. These findings support the view that facial movements in cleft patients may be severely hampered and that assessment of facial kinematics should be considered during the course of surgical intervention.

Another approach to sampling movement patterns of the face involves attaching infrared-light–emitting diode markers to the upper lip, lower lip, jaw, and head using double-adhesive tape. Smith and Zelaznik (2004) used this technology to calculate the 3D motions of the upper lip, lower lip, and jaw markers relative to the head during the production of two sentences in 180 speakers ranging in age from 4 to 22 years. An acoustic signal sampled at 7.5 kHz was synchronized with the kinematic channels sampled at 250 Hz. Smith and Zelaznik developed an algorithm to provide an index of spatial and temporal variability in the trajectory patterns for the facial articulators over repeated productions of a particular utterance. When applied to the development of functional synergies among labial-mandibular systems, they found that the time course of development for speech motor coordination is protracted and do not reach adult-like performance until after age 14 years for both males and females, with males lagging on the spatiotemporal variability index.

An examination of spontaneous facial movements was described recently for a group of 29 normally developing infants ranging in age from 1 to 12 months (Green & Wilson, 2006). Facial movements that were not associated with vocalization, speech, or environmental stimulation were excluded from their analyses. Facial movements were tracked in 3D using a video-based movement tracking system (ViconPEAK Motion Systems). Five infrared video cameras were used to track 2-mm-diameter reflective markers placed on several facial landmarks (eyebrows, upper lip, lower lip, oral commissures, and chin) at a sampling rate of 60 frames per second. The marker locations in each two-dimensional camera image were co-registered among the five cameras to calculate its 3D location in a predefined volume. Following position tracking, movement signals were digitally low-pass filtered (LP f_c [cutoff frequency] at 10 Hz, Butterworth 8-pole) using a zero-phase shift forward and reverse algorithm. Green and Wilson found several age-related changes in labial-mandibular kinematics, including an increase in occurrence of spontaneous movements, higher movement velocities, and greater coupling among different facial regions.

♦ Orofacial Kinematics in Premature Babies and Infants

Studying the emerging speech mechanism in neonates and infants presents unique challenges to the researcher. Limited access to structures, infants' inability to perform standard tasks, distraction (or excess attentiveness to transducers and equipment), and all-important time management issues can thwart successful investigation of speech mechanism movements. In addition, calibration of some transducers used with this population may be difficult, if not impossible. However, if the transducer is characterized by a linear response, relative measures of displacement may be determined. In addition, it is often desirable to investigate temporal patterning rather than absolute displacement of structures. In such cases, calibration of the transducer's output is not necessary.

In neonates and young infants, the structures of the speech mechanism are used for biological functions such as feeding and respiration as well as for producing cry and other vocalizations. Accordingly, much of what is known about the development of neuromotor control of the speech mechanism in human neonates and infants is the result of investigations of feeding behaviors.

In human infants, the classic description of sucking behavior includes two distinct modes: nutritive suck (NS) or nonnutritive suck (NNS) (Wolff, 1968). The NS pattern is characterized by a continuous stream of suck cycles and interspersed swallows and breaths at a relatively constant frequency of approximately 1 Hz. By its nature, successful nutritive sucking behavior requires the intricate coordination of sucking, swallowing, and respiratory motor patterns, and this coordination differentiates NS from NNS patterns. The NNS mode (no milk ingestion) is characterized by bursts of approximately five to 15 suck cycles separated by pause periods. The frequency of the NNS cycles is typically approximately 2 Hz, but the rate decreases and rate variability increases throughout the sucking burst (Estep, Barlow, Fees, Stumm, Finan, Seibel, Poore, & Cannon, 2005; Finan & Barlow, 1998; Seibel, Barlow, Vantipalli, Finan, Urish, & Carlson 2005; Stumm, Barlow, Vantipalli, Finan, Estep, Seibel, Urish, & Fees, 2005). Since the spectral content of suck movements ranges from 0 to 10 Hz (Seibel et al, 2005), the transducers used should be DC-coupled and do not need an extended frequency response. Of greater importance when selecting a transducer or measurement system is a linear response, so that relative measures of structural displacement can be made.

The kinematic consequences of feeding behaviors in neonates and infants have been studied with a variety of techniques including imaging, direct observation, and transduction of jaw movements. Imaging techniques include x-ray cineradiography and ultrasound. In the 1950s and 1960s,

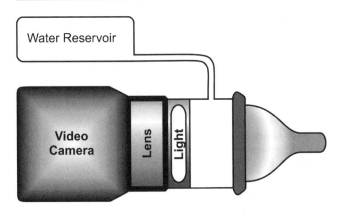

Figure 6–3 A device used in the video imaging of sucking behavior in newborn infants. [Adapted from Eishima, K. (1991). The analysis of sucking behavior in newborn infants. *Early Human Development, 27,* 163–173, with permission.]

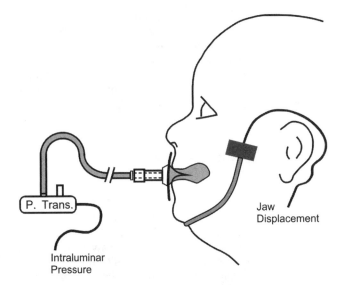

Figure 6–4 Illustration of a pressure sensor and the strain gage used to transduce kinematics of the jaw during sucking behavio. (P. Trans = pressure transducer.)

cineradiographic studies yielded the observations that NS patterns consisted of rhythmical alternating movements of the jaw and tongue (Ardran, Kemp, & Lind, 1958a,b; Bosma, 1967). Bosma also used cineradiography to describe oral and pharyngeal movements produced during infant cry. More recently, ultrasound imaging has been employed to characterize tongue and pharyngeal kinematics during NS and swallowing behaviors in neonates and infants (Bosma, Hepburn, Josell, & Baker, 1990; Mizuno & Ueda 2001; Weber, Woolridge, & Baum, 1986). Bosma and colleagues (1990) described a smooth peristaltic wave along the midline of the tongue that moved in an anterior-posterior direction, which results in expression and propulsion of milk toward the pharynx. Mizuno and Ueda (2001) observed a deficiency in the peristaltic wave during NS feeding in infants with Down syndrome.

Some investigators have used direct observation techniques to survey the motion of the tongue during NS by focusing a video camera through a transparent silicone feeding nipple (Eishima, 1991) **(Fig. 6–3).** Iwayama and Eishima (1997) reported that a bell-shaped tongue was characteristic of peristaltic movements in young infants, and this configuration began to decrease after approximately 3 months of age. Older infants did not produce peristaltic movements of the tongue involving discrete tongue movements. Tamura, Horikawa, and Yoshida (1996) used a similar method in combination with electromyographic recording of jaw opening and closing muscles, observing correlated activity between muscle activity and jaw motion.

A commonly used method of measuring the kinematics of feeding behaviors in neonates and infants involves the direct transduction of jaw movements. One technique involves the use of a strain-gage device attached to the mandible (deMonterice, Meier, Engstrom, Crichton, & Mangurten, 1992; Finan & Barlow, 1996, 1998; Hill, Kurkowski, & Garcia, 2000). In this method, a narrow Silastic silicone tube filled with mercury (and sealed at the ends) is positioned under the chin and secured at the zygomatic arches of the infant **(Fig. 6–4).** The strain gage is wired into a Wheatstone circuit and conditioned with a

bridge amplifier. Applied in this fashion, the strain gage can be used to transduce jaw displacement during NS and NNS. Unlike many techniques that may require direct line-of-sight or an appliance placed in the oral cavity, the strain gage can easily be used to measure NS behavior during breast-feeding. When properly secured to the infant's face, the frequency response of the strain gage is sufficient to measure jaw movements generated during suck behavior (including jaw tremors), and the output is suitably linear. This device cannot be calibrated easily, however, and is typically used to show relative changes in jaw displacement and to study temporal aspects of the feeding behavior.

Numerous investigators have used pressure sensors connected to feeding nipples or pacifier baglets to measure jaw kinematics during NS and NNS (Estep et al, 2005; Finan & Barlow, 1996, 1998; Gewolb, Bosma, Reynolds, & Vice, 2003; Kron, Ipsen, & Goddard, 1968; Lau, Sheena, Shulman, & Schanler, 1997; Stumm et al, 2005; Wolff, 1968) **(Fig. 6–4).** Most modern integrated circuit pressure sensors are internally temperature compensated, are easy to calibrate, have an extremely wide frequency range, and generate a highly linear response when used within operating limits. During NNS, a pressure sensor coupled to the baglet (nipple) of the pacifier transduces the jaw (and tongue) movements, realized as compression and subsequent reexpansion of the baglet. In such an arrangement, individual components cannot be parsed; thus the resulting waveform represents a composite of jaw and tongue movements. It would be very difficult to calibrate this type of measurement system for absolute jaw displacement, however, and data are typically reported as nipple pressure (expressed in centimeters of water [cm H_2O]). During NS behavior, an additional pressure sensor may be used to transduce negative pressure generation in the oral cavity, which corresponds to lowering of the tongue body during the suck cycle.

The techniques highlighted here have been used to provide a description of the kinematics and general temporal organization of neonate and infant ororhythmic behaviors. In practice, many of the above techniques are used together or in combination with methods of measuring respiratory events to overcome limitations and yield a more comprehensive representation of feeding behaviors.

◆ Tracking Tongue Movements

From the late 1940s through the mid-1970s, our understanding of tongue movements relied heavily on studies using x-ray and cineradiography (Chiba & Kajiyama, 1958; House, 1967; Kiritani, Itoh, Fujisaki, & Sawashima, 1976; Perkell, 1969; Potter, Kopp, & Green, 1947). Tongue contact patterns were studied with the popular dynamic palatometer (Fletcher, McCutcheon, & Wolf, 1975; Harley, 1972; Kuzmin, 1962; Kydd & Belt, 1964; Palmer, 1973; Shibata, 1968). Since then, technological advances have been made in optics, magnetometry, ultrasound, and x-ray microbeam for real-time tracking of the lingual surface during speech and swallowing. Some of these technologies are reviewed in the following sections.

Glossometry (Optical Tracking of the Tongue Surface)

In the late 1970s, work was underway to develop an optical distance detection system to track the superior surface of the tongue in real time for studies of speech motor control (Chuang & Wang, 1978). This system was composed of an array of four light-emitting diode (LED) and photosensor modules positioned adjacent to one another and mounted on a thin acrylic pseudoalate that was molded from a stone cast of the subjects' hard palate. LED and photosensor pairs were placed sagittally or in the coronal plane to obtain 2D or 3D representations of tongue movement. Light is reflected directly off of the tongue and received by a photosensor. The underlying principle of optical distance detection is based on the premise that a lumen (brightness) of an area illuminated by a light source is proportional to the inverse square of the distance. At distances ranging between 0 and 20 mm, the precision of distance measurement was better than 0.5 mm. The precision of distance measurement deteriorates as distance is increased beyond 20 mm. For example, error of estimation increases from 0.5 to 4 mm at a 40-mm distance. Fortunately, according to Chuang and Wang (1978), the distance between the tongue and palate usually does not exceed 25 mm in continuous speech. The effects of tongue rotation (rotation of the reflecting plane) in relation to the LED-sensor pair is another source of measurement error. The tongue surface rarely maintains a perpendicular relationship with the sagittal aspect of the hard palate during speech articulation. This leads to errors in spatial resolution of the optical track as the tongue assumes different positions relative to the pseudopalate. In summary, the optical tongue tracking system described above offers real-time signal display and temporal and submillimeter spatial resolution under optimal conditions.

Fletcher, McCutcheon, Smith, and Wilson (1989) developed an optoelectronic system, known as the glossometer, to measure tongue height, shape, and movements within the oral cavity during speech. This system consists of paired infrared LEDs and phototransistors embedded in a 0.3-mm-thick heat-pressure-molded acrylic pseudopalate. These authors claim several improvements over previous designs including a software-based linearization function, and computer-controlled activation of the LEDs for real-time sampling of tongue displacements at 100 samples per second. Each channel is calibrated in situ from zero to approximately 22 mm using intraoral spacers placed between the tongue and palate. Measurement resolution is reported to be 0.5 mm. It is important to note that discrete points on the tongue are not identified using this method, and that actions of individual muscles can only be inferred from relative changes in position.

Palatometry (Tongue and Palate Contact Patterns)

Palatometry (Fletcher, Hasegawa, McCutcheon, & Gilliom, 1980; Fletcher et al, 1975; Johnson, 1969; Michi, Suzuki, Yamashita, & Imai, 1986) is used to study and modify the place of linguapalatal contact in both consonant and vowel articulation. As described by Fletcher (1989), the palatometer employs 96 tiny (0.5 mm) bead electrodes embedded on the oral surface of an acrylic pseudopalate to sense the pattern of tongue contact during speech production. An alternating current (AC) carrier signal at 27.8 kHz is delivered to the palatal electrode array (current limited to 100 microamperes [μA]) and referenced to the wrist. The system described by Michi et al (1986) employs a palatal reference electrode and uses considerably less current, at just 8 μA. Tongue contact on any electrode in the array completes the circuit and is registered as a sensor location in a palatometric display on a videoscreen. According to Fletcher, each vowel in English is associated with a unique stationary linguapalatal contact map. For example, during the stable contact portion of /i/, the tongue is in contact with sensors extending from the cuspid-bicuspid region of the palate to the posterior border of the alveolar ridge. During the /ae/ the contact is against the most posterior-lateral sensors. Diphthongs are characterized by movements between two stable monophthong positions. The glossometer (optical tracking) and palatometer (linguapalatal contact) have been used in training or retraining vowel space and consonant production in hearing-impaired (Fletcher, 1989; Fletcher, Dagenais, & Critz-Crosby, 1991) and cleft-palate patients (Michi et al, 1986).

Ultrasonic Imaging of the Tongue

Ultrasound provides real-time images of the tongue surface in a digital video format during speech and swallowing (Gick, 2002; Peng, Jost-Brinkmann, Miethke, & Lin, 2000; Shawker, Sonies, Stone, & Baum, 1983; Stone & Lundberg, 1996; Stone, Epstein, & Iskarous, 2004; Watkin, 1999). It is now possible to combine these images with estimates of the hard palate boundary using ultrasound during the production of command swallows to establish a reference within the head space for co-registration among subjects, and calculation of select phonetic measures (Epstein & Stone, 2005).

The report by Shawker, Stone, and Sonies (1985) described the development of a method to accurately track a fixed point on the tongue surface using localized reverberation artifact from ultrasound imaging. A sector ultrasound transducer with a rotating head was used in this study. The scanner consisted of three 3-MHz transducers mounted on a central axis, with 120-degree separation between the individual transducers. Video frame rate ranged between 34 and 44 Hz, with an axial resolution of 1 mm in the coronal plane and 1.9 mm laterally. Various substances were tested to derive the best substance with the most clearly evident reverberation artifact. Lead, aluminum, copper, and stainless steel all generated sufficient artifact to be visualized on recorded ultrasonic images.

Stainless steel was chosen as the material of choice due to its inert qualities. Periodicity of the reverberation pattern was directly related to pellet size (diameter). Reverberation artifacts are produced from reflection of the sound waves from the anterior and posterior surface of the pellet. The authors suggest the possibility of using stainless steel pellets for both ultrasound and x-ray microbeam tracking, due to the pellets' high reverberation and radiopaque quality, respectively. The authors discuss several potential drawbacks to utilizing x-ray imaging techniques. These include difficulty in visualizing the tongue due to the interference of radiodense structures such as bone and teeth, the use of barium paste or liquid to highlight the image, and exposure of delicate structures to x-ray emissions. X-ray microbeam imaging presents lower doses of radiation exposure than cineradiography and is capable of tracking pellets without the need for barium pastes. However, the x-ray microbeam system is unable to visualize the surface of the tongue and is prohibitively expensive. The ability to use ultrasound and reverberation artifact for pellet tracking permits localized configuration changes in the tongue with regard to a reference point. Recent advances in ultrasound technology, such as the ability to scan and display images in real time with better resolution than older forms of x-ray imaging, may provide a cost-effective and accurate system for describing tongue kinematics in three dimensions.

Stone, Shawker, Talbot, and Rich (1988) described an ultrasound transducer holder and head restraint system for accurately imaging cross-sectional tongue movement during speech. Coarticulatory effects are also examined in light of this system. These authors outline the benefits of using real-time ultrasound data with regard to advancements in the imaging technology (i.e., motion during speech and swallowing, tracking of a single point via localized reverberation artifact, analysis of tongue shape and surface). They also discuss the drawbacks of other imaging techniques such as magnetic resonance imaging (MRI) and computed tomography (CT) scan with regard to vocal tract analysis. In general, MRI and CT scanning utilize static postures to image the shape of the vocal tract and necessitate prolonged acquisition times. Maintaining a static posture for a phoneme eliminates the possibility of any dynamic and coarticulatory

description of vocal tract structures during speech and introduces artifact into the resultant image due primarily to the subject's potential inability to reliably maintain the shape of the vocal tract over lengthy acquisition periods. Speech samples consisted of 10 English vowels embedded within two contexts, /pVp/ and /sVs/. Primary goals of the study were to assess anteroposterior (AP) coronal tongue shape, determine coarticulatory effects of /s/ on cross-sectional tongue shape of neighboring vowels, and compare cross-sectional data with models of tongue shape based on sagittal and lateral data. Subjects were seated in a dental chair with their heads stabilized by means of a Velcro strap placed over the forehead and upper skull. The strap did allow the subject a small amount of mobility. The ultrasound transducer holder consisted of several clamps and bosses equipped with solid sphere cantilever that was capable of being adjusted by means of a compression clamp. The transducer was suspended via the cantilever submentally in relation to the subject. The transducer cantilever allowed 90 degrees of rotation in the vertical plane and 180 degrees of translation in the horizontal plane and allowed only superior/inferior movement. A dual goniometer, a device used to measure joint angles, was utilized to align the ultrasound transducer with the mandible. The transducer cantilever foundation was attached to a constant force spring that acted in opposition to the load created by the transducer and the acoustic standoff. Enough superior force was applied to firmly maintain contact between the transducer and the subjects mandible. Furthermore, through this resistive spring system, the ultrasound transducer was capable of tracking all movements of the jaw during execution of the speech samples while maintaining contact submentally.

Hysteresis measures of the transducer with relation to the jaw were performed using strain gages. These data confirm that the transducer cantilever is capable of accurately tracking the movements of the mandible during speech. Two distinct scanning angles demonstrating oral and pharyngeal constriction points were performed during the protocol. Positioning of the transducer was accomplished by referencing the ramus of the mandible and utilizing the dual goniometer to localize the ultrasound beam perpendicular to the ramus. Video frames were digitized and analyzed by hand using a graphics cursor to identify surface points along the tongue dorsum. Results indicate that cross-sectional tongue shape is directly related to the position of the tongue and the lateral and sagittal shape of the tongue. In general, midsagittal grooving was evident for all vowel types, with posterior grooves being deeper than anterior grooves. In the /p/ context, posterior grooving was greater than in the /s/ context. Grooving for vowels in the /p/ context demonstrated a continuum, whereas in the anterior /s/ context two groups of vowels were identified (high group/shallower grooves, and back group with deeper grooves). In the anterior /s/ context, tongue shape for /i/ and /u/ was convex.

Ultrasound technology has been combined with x-ray microbeam data to develop a 3D model of tongue movement in one female subject (Stone, 1990). Speech materials consisted of vowel-consonant-vowel-consonant (VCVC) utterances using the consonants /s/ and /l/, and vowels /i/, /a/, and /o/. Ultrasound technology was utilized to obtain coronal views of the tongue in three locations: anteriorly, dorsally, and posteriorly. The x-ray microbeam tracked radiodense pellets that were attached to the superior surface of the tongue, midsagittally. These two distinct forms of data were combined to conclude that the tongue may be divided into a sagittal and coronal segment, with quasi-independent movements of these segments resulting in local displacements and rotation of the tongue. These two major segments were further subdivided into four functionally based sagittal sections (anterior, middle, dorsal, and posterior) and three bilateral coronal segments (medial, lateral, and most lateral). Segment boundaries were considered flexible. Movement of these segments in different combinations accounted for the total movement and rotation of the tongue during speech. Sagittal segment movements resulted in local contractions and displacements as well as AP changes. Coronal segment movements resulted in midsagittal grooving and left-right asymmetries in surface structure. A three-tiered nested organizational scheme is offered as a hypothesis for tongue movement. The first level consists of coronal segments, whose movements would result in local displacements at level two, the sagittal segments. Jaw movement is considered the third level, due to the effect jaw movement has on relative tongue positioning, which in turn affects the sagittal segments at level two.

A few laboratories have made progress on high-speed 3D reconstruction of tongue ultrasonic images (Lundberg & Stone, 1999; Stone, Epstein, & Sutton, 2003; Stone et al, 2004; Sze, Iny, Stone, & Levine, 1999; Watkin & Rubin, 1989; Yang & Stone, 2002) and tagged cineradiographic and MRI scans (Dick, Ozturk, Douglas, McVeigh, & Stone, 2000; Stone, Dick, Davis, Douglas, & Ozturk, 2000). Work using ultrasound has focused on defining predictable mathematical relations between midsagittal tongue contour shapes and five cross-sectional (coronal) contours (Stone et al, 2003). This prediction was based on earlier work that found that 3D tongue surfaces are composed of a concatenation of coronal slices, a subset of which accurately represents the 3D tongue surface (Stone & Lundberg, 1996). These relations are shown in **Fig. 6–5**. When compared among four tongue shape phonemic categories (i.e., front raising /i/, back raising /n/, continuous grooving /ae/, and two-point displacement /l/), it was found that transitional values exist that, when exceeded, predict tongue arching versus midsagittal tongue grooving. Even better predictions were noted for the three anterior coronal slices in which strong correlations exist between midline displacement and groove depth to arch height. Stone et al (2004) concluded that knowledge of both category and midsagittal displacement provides good prediction of coronal tongue shape.

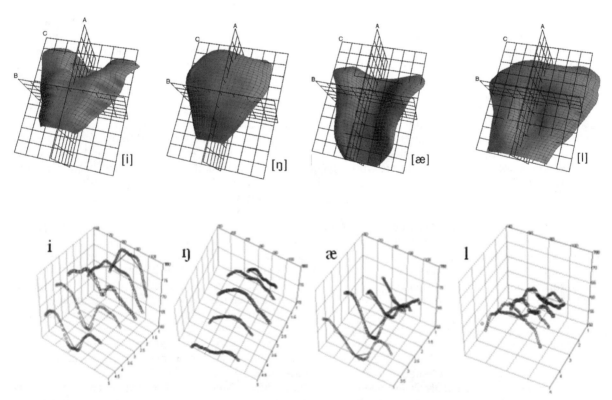

Figure 6–5   (A) Representative three-dimensional tongue surface shapes for the four shape-based categories, including front raising /i/, back raising /n/, continuous groove /ae/, and two-point displacement /l/. Tongue tip shown on the lower left. **(B)** Coronal slices and derived slopes for representation phonemes from each of the four shape-based categories, including front raising /i/, back raising /n/, continuous groove /ae/, and two-point displacement /l/. Tongue tip shown on the upper left. (Courtesy of Dr. Maureen Stone.)

◆ Tracking Velar and Laryngeal Movements

As one proceeds beyond the lips and tongue and ventures into the depths of the vocal tract, the task of recording movements generated by the "invisible valves" of speech, such as the velopharynx and larynx, becomes technologically more challenging. Acceptable sampling methods in humans usually reflects a concession between the invasiveness of the instrument and the quality of the acquired signals. The small size and inaccessibility of both the velopharynx and larynx present real problems for the bioengineer attempting to transduce these articulatory elements. Measurement error, common to all forms of transduction, becomes an even bigger concern in measures of velopharyngeal and laryngeal output. While it is acceptable to attach small sensors to the lips and jaw in the form of radiopaque pellets, reflective balls or tape, infrared diodes, cantilevers, or magnetic coils to the rib cage or abdomen, no such electromechanical device or sensor is acceptable to the delicate tissue boundary of the human vocal fold because this would disrupt the behavior and health of the organism. Instead, techniques have evolved that rely on imaging, acoustics, or fluid mechanics. These procedures are described in the following sections.

Velopharynx

The velopharynx, strategically situated to divert acoustic and aerodynamic energy through the oral and nasal cavities, constitutes a very complex anatomical region of the vocal tract. The size of the velar port determines the oral or nasal nature of speech sounds. Movements of the velum, lateral pharyngeal walls, and posterior pharyngeal wall collectively determine the size of the velar port.

Methods aimed at measuring the size and movements of select components of this port roughly fall into one of two categories: direct and indirect. Direct methods include several imaging techniques such as cineradiography (Moll, 1962; Moll & Daniloff, 1971), video nasendoscopy (Bell-Berti & Hirose, 1975), electromechanical (Christiansen & Moller, 1971; Moller, Martin, & Christiansen, 1971), optomechanical transduction (Horiguchi & Bell-Berti, 1987) of velar displacement, and others. These transducers for measuring velar activity and radiographic imaging techniques share a common limitation in that they resolve movement in only a single plane. In most radiographic studies, discrete points are tracked on a frame-by-frame basis, which is useful in resolving velocity and displacement profiles. However, because the radiographic methods are limited to one plane or slice through the velopharynx, we can never be certain if closure has occurred. It is quite possible that velar apertures may exist at locations opposite the lateral pharyngeal walls on one or both sides. It is well known that the patterns of velopharyngeal closure are highly variable both within and across speakers.

It is well known from radiography (Moll, 1962; Moll & Daniloff, 1971), nasendoscopy (Bell-Berti & Hirose, 1975), direct observation (Bloomer, 1953; Calnan, 1953), photodetection (Dalston, 1989; Keefe & Dalston, 1989;

Moon & Lagu, 1987), and acoustic analysis (House & Fairbanks, 1953) that complete velopharyngeal closure is not always obtained during vowel production. Moll's (1962) pioneering work was aimed at characterizing normal patterns of velopharyngeal closure using cinefluorographic techniques. The main results of this study indicated that high vowels exhibit greater velopharyngeal closure than low vowels, regardless of consonant context. Moll also observed that complete closure of the velopharynx was not always present during production of the low vowels. Moll also reported that velopharyngeal closure is not attained on vowels adjacent to a nasal consonant. In fact, under these conditions, the velum does not return to its rest position, but assumes what has been referred to as the "ready" position (Graber, Bzoch, & Aoba, 1959; Moll, 1962). One of the limitations of the early cinefluorographic studies was temporal resolution in that the dwell time between frames was too long to provide detailed information on the dynamics of the velopharyngeal mechanism during speech. For example, in the Moll (1962) study, lateral images of the velopharynx were sampled every 41.66 milliseconds (ms). This relatively low sampling rate would be inadequate to capture the dynamics of velopharyngeal movement during speech. Later on, the introduction of high-speed imaging has made it possible to sample lateral cinefluorographic images every 6.66 ms (Moll & Daniloff, 1971). Although this greatly improved temporal resolution, radiographic measures were still limited to 2D planar images of the port (i.e., lateral, basal, or anteroposterior). The spatial resolution was also limited in radiographic studies due to blurred or "fuzzy" boundaries, making it difficult to identify the relative positions of the velum and posterior pharyngeal wall during closure. Measurement error was reported to be 0.91 mm for velar movement toward the posterior pharyngeal wall and 0.45 mm for estimating the velopharyngeal opening. Based on area calculations of the velopharyngeal orifice, Warren and colleagues (Laine, Warren, Dalston, & Morr, 1989; Warren, 1982) have demonstrated that openings of this magnitude can yield significant airflow through the nasal cavity.

Flexible fiberoptic nasoendoscopy has the potential of becoming a powerful quantitative tool to resolve some of this uncertainty regarding the dynamics of the velopharyngeal port. The camera, fiberoptic, and recording technology has evolved to the point where very good images of the velopharynx can be acquired in real time. It should be possible to develop high-speed graphics imaging software to identify edges and features of the port in real time, including computation of portal area and edge velocity, range of displacement, and calibration schemes for determining absolute distance. Not only would data be available on the size of the port, but the added information on the kinematics would be useful for studies of motor control in patients with sensorimotor disorders affecting this important speech valve.

Indirect measures of velopharyngeal port function offer some unique perspectives on the actual behavior of this valve during speech. Compared with nasendoscopy or cineradiography, aerodynamic methods can reveal the pressure-flow dynamics of the port over a wide range of speech behaviors. Contemporary aerodynamic protocols provide reasonably accurate estimates of the aeromechanical inputs and outputs of the velopharynx during speech in fluid mechanics terms without the biohazards of cineradiography, or the invasiveness of placing a 3- or 4-mm fiberoptic bundle deep into the nasal cavity. Area functions (Warren, 1988; Warren & Dubois, 1964), resistance estimates (Smitheran & Hixon, 1981), and temporal pattern studies (Samlan & Barlow, 1999; Warren, Dalston, Trier, & Holder, 1985) have been used effectively to characterize the activity of the velopharynx during speech.

Many features of velopharyngeal and upper airway coarticulatory dynamics remain to be studied in normal speakers and explored in patients with sensorimotor speech disorders. Information gained from these experiments, involving relatively noninvasive aeromechanical measures, should prove to be of considerable value to clinicians responsible for the diagnosis and management of individuals with velopharyngeal dysfunction due to musculoskeletal abnormalities or neuromotor disease.

Numerous reports have described some of the temporal relations between pressure-flow variables during nasal-plosive blends in the hopes of stressing the velopharyngeal mechanism to reveal the coarticulatory dynamics between velopharynx and other upper airway structures in normal and cleft-palate speakers (Dalston, Warren, & Smith, 1990; Samlan & Barlow, 1999; Warren et al, 1985). For example, Dalston et al (1990) used the pressure-flow technique described in detail by Warren (1982) to study velopharyngeal aerodynamics in repaired cleft palate adults and normal controls instructed to produce five repetitions of the nasal-plosive blend /mp/ within the carrier word *hamper*. Measures of nasal air flow rate, intraoral air pressure, and timing differences between the pressure and airflow curves were obtained from the 5 /mp/ productions for each subject. Compared with control subjects, the magnitude of the average intraoral air pressure was slightly less and the average nasal airflow rate was significantly less in the repaired cleft speakers. Dalston et al (1990) also found that the nasal airflow pulse overlapped into the rising phase and peak of the pressure pulse associated with /p/ in the word *hamper*. It was suggested that a decrease in respiratory effort may have been a compensatory strategy used by patients with repaired cleft palates to achieve adequate velopharyngeal closure and minimize shunting through the velopharyngeal port. This conclusion was based on careful study of the temporal relations between the airflow and pressure curves associated with production of the nasal-plosive blend. This line of investigation is important in demonstrating the utility of indirect measurement techniques such as aerodynamics in formulating inferences about the underlying articulatory dynamics of the velopharyngeal mechanism. It is clear from this work that much remains to be learned about the factors that influence articulatory dynamics of this "invisible" speech valve.

Larynx

The larynx represents a microcosm of the entire speech mechanism in that it provides a sound source in coordination with the respiratory system, acts as a dynamic "articulator"

capable of rapid adductor and abductor adjustments, modulates pitch, and conveys emotion and personal identity (Barlow, Netsell, & Hunker, 1986).

Endoscopy

During the past 20 years, endoscopy has become a very important clinical tool in the assessment of laryngeal movement disorders affecting speech in adults (D'Antonio, Chait, & Lotz, 1986; D'Antonio, Chait, Lotz, & Netsell, 1987; D'Antonio, Netsell, & Lotz, 1988). Endoscopy is best applied in conjunction with other assessment methods and has demonstrated application in infants and children (D'Antonio et al, 1986). A detailed case history is followed by an ear, nose, and throat (ENT) exam and an auditory-perceptual evaluation of speech/voice function. Systematic application of aerodynamics is recommended to provide inferential and quantitative information concerning laryngeal and chest wall function; however, the analyses are limited to the vocal phase only and do not include a consideration of the articulatory dynamics associated with laryngeal engagement. Somewhat more invasive, fiberoptic evaluations of the nasopharynx, hypopharynx, and larynx are obtained and recorded on videotape along with an audiotape recording of the speech. Use of fiberoptic nasopharyngoscopy and laryngoscopy in conjunction with low-light cinematography allows observation of the dynamic processes of speech production. This technique allows the clinician to visualize the overall articulatory dynamics of the larynx during speech and other behaviors such as swallowing, coughing, and respiration. Information obtained during the nasoendoscopic examination has proven useful for biofeedback in the remediation of select laryngeal and velopharyngeal impairments affecting speech. To date, observation has been limited primarily to visual impressions of the video image, relative medialization of one vocal process versus another, and hyperconstriction of the ventricular folds. Videofluoroscopy offers additional information for evaluation of gross muscle activity over a large expanse of the upper airway, from the larynx to the velopharynx, pharynx, and the hypopharynx. It is most useful for evaluation of gross movement patterns and coordination of movements of the upper articulators. The combination of perceptual-physiological methods appears to have considerable value in cases where there are multiple factors involved with the speech/voice disorders, the diagnosis is elusive, or therapy has not produced adequate results.

Although endoscopy is in common clinical use today, there are significant limitations to this technique when used to assess disordered voice production. The integrity of the mucosal wave is a primary factor correlated with general impressions of clinical vocal quality. Constant-light laryngoscopy, performed via transnasal (flexible fiberoptic endoscopy) or transoral (rigid endoscopy) stroboscopic imaging, is useful in the general characterization of mucosal vibratory activity; however, the technique relies heavily on subjective interpretation by the clinical investigator (Hirano & Bless, 1993), and assumes that vocal fold vibration is periodic. Factors such as jitter and irregular vibration patterns typically demonstrated by disordered voice patients can distort the stroboscopic image, making quantification of oscillatory activity a challenge. Neither approach provides information about the vibratory behavior of the vocal folds. Stroboscopy, the application of a brief frequency-synchronized flash of light through the endoscope during phonation, provides the clinician with an apparent "slow motion" view of the vibrating vocal folds. The resulting video display is not a true cycle-by-cycle representation, however, as several phonatory cycles are "fused" into the final image. Consequently, cycle-to-cycle variations of the vibratory pattern cannot be observed via stroboscopy. In addition, pathological voicing characterized by irregular periodicity may result in the inability to synchronize the strobe light with the vibratory pattern, yielding an inaccurate display of vocal fold movements (Hirano & Bless, 1993).

Videokymography

Adjunct techniques that can provide greater objective evaluation and quantification of vibratory dynamics and cycle-by-cycle movements are thus considered important steps toward better diagnostic evaluation. One such recent adjunct technique that takes advantage of new developments in digital video recording and processing and that builds upon the exploratory work of Gall (1984) in strip kymography (the recording of wavelike motions or undulations) of the glottis, is videokymography (VKG). High-speed digital video recordings can be used, but the analysis is difficult and time-consuming, and the data storage requirements are great (švec & šram, 2002). A new technology was developed that allows for visualization of the individual cycles of phonation by analyzing only a small segment of the vibrating vocal folds. Developed in the Netherlands by Drs. Harm Schutte and Jan švec (švec & Schutte, 1996) of the University of Groningen, VKG uses a modified charge-coupled device (CCD) camera to record images of selected cross-sections of the vocal folds during motion (Verdonck-de Leeuw, Festen, & Mahieu, 2001).

The position of the horizontal measuring line is maintained throughout the analysis. VKG systems use standard videolaryngoscopic setups with a continuous light source and record images with commercial VHS videocassette recorders (Schutte, švec, & šram, 1998). Typical video frames are composed of several hundred horizontal lines. In place of recording the entire image of the vocal fold though, VKG systems allow for the collection a single line of the image (orthogonal to the longitudinal axis of the fold) at rates of 8 kHz, thus allowing for sampling rates great enough to cover the entire frequency range of fold oscillation (švec & Schutte, 1996). Successive lines are then temporally aligned and cascaded in real time on a conventional monitor, thus showing the vibratory pattern of the selected region of interest on the vocal fold for a preselected time period (Schutte et al, 1998; Sung, Kim, Koh, et al, 1999). As shown in **Fig. 6–6**, the resulting "kymogram" displays a spatiotemporal image of the vocal folds at the scanned line over time. Digital kymography, produced by analyzing high-speed digital video files of phonation, allows the clinician to select the position of the measuring line following data collection; however, line resolution and image rate are inferior to those of VKG (švec & šram, 2002). In addition to these techniques, Sung et al (1999) utilized digitized successive stroboscopic images to produce "videostrobokymographic" images. This method, while not requiring special hardware, suffers from stroboscopic limitations, and cannot reliably reveal irregular vibratory patterns (švec & šram, 2002).

The kymographic techniques of VKG and digital kymography allow for true cycle-by-cycle analysis of vocal fold vibratory patterns. Analysis of the resulting kymograms can provide clinical information on right-left vocal fold asymmetries, open and closed quotients, ventricular fold or mucous interference, mucosal wave front propagation, frequency, amplitude, speed quotient, and within-cycle perturbations (Schutte et al, 1998; švec & Schutte, 1996; švec & šram, 2002; Yumoto, 2004).

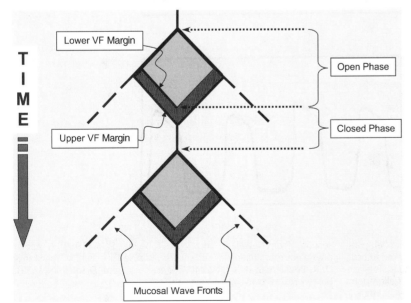

Figure 6–6 Schematic figure of normal vocal fold vibration image as obtained by videokymography.
[Redrawn from švec, J.G. & Schutte, H.K. (1996). Videokymography: high-speed line scanning of vocal fold vibration. *Journal of Voice, 10*, 201–205, with permission.]

Electroglottography

Electroglottography has been used with success to assess laryngeal activity. This instrument consists of a flexible neck collar supporting an array of electrodes and a signal conditioning unit. In electroglottography, a small DC bias current is fed through the tissues of the neck and the conditioning unit senses changes in the electrical resistance in the region of the larynx. Essentially, the electroglottogram (EGG) signal correlates with vocal fold contact area (Childers & Krishnamurthy, 1985). It is regarded as a useful assessment technique in drawing inferences about vocal fold vibration during speech.

Some of the electroglottographic measures that have been used clinically include timing measures between voiced segments and an analysis of the cycle-by-cycle dynamics of voicing (Baken, 1992; Childers & Krishnamurthy, 1985; Titze, 1990). These dynamic measures are usually obtained in combination with inverse filtered flow signals (AC flow) for the purpose of detailing the organization and timing of the open and closed phases of the glottis during voice production. Since information derived from EGGs is based on the vocal segment and subtle changes in vocal fold contact area, it would offer limited potential for drawing inferences about the aeromechanical events underlying vocal fold engagement. Furthermore, the reliability and validity of the EGG signal associated with the early phases of laryngeal engagement is questionable. The beginning phases of arytenoid rotation are associated with displacement of the vocal folds in free space. During this interval, one would not expect appreciable increases in vocal fold contact area until arytenoid advancement results in actual tissue approximation. Therefore, the EGG output during this phase of engagement may yield little or no output signal even though significant displacements of the vocal folds have occurred.

Speech Aerodynamics

The utility of laryngeal aerodynamics is underscored in neurogenic speech disorders as illustrated by the differences in pressure-flow patterns during consonant-vowel (CV) production sampled from a normal speaker and a dysarthric patient (Netsell, Lotz, & Barlow, 1989). As shown in **Fig. 6–7**, the sharp flow peaks associated with burst-release in the normal waveform are not as obvious in the dysarthric data. These peaks are presumed to correspond to the vocal fold position of maximum abduction during plosion of the /p/ consonant. The rapid decrease from peak flow in the normal subject reflects the rapid articulatory phase of vocal fold adduction toward midline for phonation. Also, the declination of flow throughout the vowel segments indicates that the folds were not abducting for the upcoming /p/ segment to the extent that they do in normal productions. Therefore, it appears that this dysarthric subject had at least two different problems with laryngeal control, including difficulties with rapid abduction/adduction of the folds as well as inefficient midline compression during vowel production.

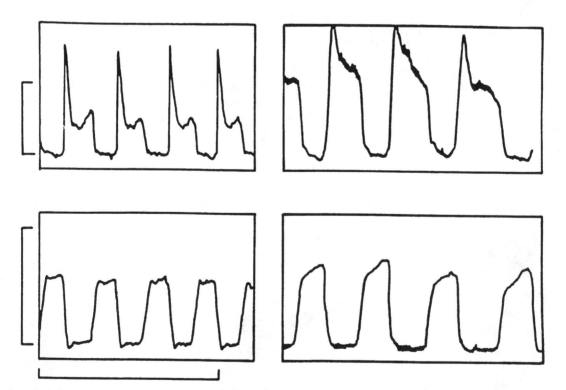

Figure 6–7 Laryngeal aerodynamic data from a normal subject (left panels) and a dysarthric subject (right panels). Subjects were asked to produce a series of [pa] syllables at a rate of four syllables per second. Total air flow (top traces) and intraoral air pressure (bottom traces). Calibration: flow = 500 cc/sec; pressure = 10 cm/sec; pressure = 10 cc H_2O; time = 1 second. [From Netsell, R., Lotz, W. K., & Barlow, S. M. (1989). A speech physiology examination for individuals with dysarthria. In K. M. Yorkston & D. R. Beukelman (Eds.), *Recent Advances in Clinical Dysarthria* (3–39). Boston: Little Brown [with permission].

Patients with sensorimotor voice disorders frequently exhibit impairments in the ability to efficiently make the transition from the plosive environment to the subsequent voiced segment (Barlow, Iacono, Paseman, Biswas, & D'Antonio, 1998; Barlow, Hammer, Pahwa, & Seibel, 2003; Ludlow & Bassich, 1984). For example, speakers with Parkinson's disease often exhibit air loss when attempting to engage (adduct) the vocal folds for voice production. In contrast, patients with adductor spasmodic dysphonia manifest exaggerated medial compression of the vocal processes of the arytenoids. This pattern of hyperadduction may include the ventricular or false folds and results in a sudden interruption of the breath stream during voicing. Therefore, it appears that a comprehensive evaluation of the vocal apparatus should include a physiological assessment of how the vocal folds/arytenoids are engaged for voicing in addition to the usual battery of tests aimed at determining glottal efficiency during phonation. Disruption of this important articulatory adjustment due to neural or biomechanical factors can dramatically influence the manner in which the vital capacity is used for speech. In cases of slow or mechanically limited engagement, it seems likely that significant portions of the lung vital capacity may be wasted by a defective laryngeal articulatory apparatus independently from the pressure-flow dynamics associated with voice production.

A new aerodynamic analysis method (Barlow, Paseman, & Philippbar, 1999; Barlow, Suing, & Andreatta, 1999; Vantipalli and Barlow, 2004) permits quantitative assessment of articulatory proficiency during laryngeal engagement. This technique, based on the simultaneous sampling of intraoral air pressure, translaryngeal air flow, and voice audio using AEROWIN RT(tm) (Neuro Logic, Inc., Rockville, MD), has been used effectively to reveal the reorganization of laryngeal function in patients with amyotrophic lateral sclerosis (ALS), idiopathic Parkinson's disease following posteroventral pallidotomy (Barlow et al, 1998), and bilateral subthalamic nucleus deep brain stimulation (Barlow, Hammer, Pahwa, & Seibel, 2003). The magnitude and time course of translaryngeal flow, described mathematically as air volume and flow rate declination functions, are presumed to reflect the underlying kinematics of vocal fold adduction toward the phonatory phase. Measures of pressure-flow dynamics and laryngeal airway resistance can also be determined for the phonatory phase of syllable production to provide for a comprehensive evaluation of the articulatory dynamics of laryngeal behavior (Holmberg, Hillman, & Perkell, 1988, 1989; Smitheran & Hixon, 1981). The net result of a hypokinetic adductory mechanism is that lung volume is wasted during translation of the arytenoids to achieve vocal fold approximation. The lung volume available for speech is depleted, and overall utterance length is decreased. Therefore, the evaluation of laryngeal function in patients with sensorimotor speech disorders benefits from an analysis of both the kinematic properties of transitory (engagement-disengagement) and phonatory (voice efficiency) phases.

Although ultrasound technology has been successfully adapted for use in the investigation of tongue kinematics (Stone et al, 2003, 2004), the application of ultrasound in other regions of the human vocal tract has been limited. For example, ultrasound use in the larynx has not historically been explored due to the limited spatial resolutions and the high-frequency movements of the vocal folds (Shau et al, 2001), yet recent advancements in signal processing may change this situation, yielding another tool for assessment and quantification of vibratory dynamics in the laryngeal system. A technique using color Doppler imaging (CDI) algorithms in conjunction with commercially available high-speed ultrasound (US) scanners has been developed and tested to noninvasively quantify parameters of mucosal wave dynamics including traveling wave and horizontal displacement velocities (Shau et al, 2001). In essence, the new system takes advantage of unique patterns of ultrasound artifact that arise from the mucosa–air interface and change systematically depending on intensity and frequency variations during vibration. By tracing the color Doppler artifacts at the tissue–air interface, the location of the vocal fold could be readily quantified using standard clinical US technology. Initial correlations between physical string models and in vivo studies with human subjects were promising and suggests that ultrasound technology may soon provide an adjunct method of investigating laryngeal kinematics that is noninvasive, has minimal interference during phonatory activities, and does not require any form of anesthesia (Shau, Wang, Hsieh, & Hsiao, 2001).

In summary, the larynx is a dynamic articulator. An individual's voice problem need not be restricted to difficulty with phonation (Netsell & Lotz, 1994, personal communication) but may include problems in abduction/adduction for consonant production and variable amounts of constriction during vowel production.

◆ Tracking Chest Wall Movements

Chest Wall Kinematics

As described by Hixon (1987), the chest wall includes, except for the lungs and airways, all parts of the respiratory apparatus including the rib cage, the diaphragm, and the abdomen and its contents. The rib cage and diaphragm constitute the thoracic cavity. The abdominal cavity is defined by the diaphragm and abdominal wall bounding an incompressible mass of liquid. According to Hixon, the chest wall is reduced to a two-structure model consisting of the rib cage and "diaphragm-abdomen." One of the central assumptions in chest wall kinematics during speech is that "the extent each of the two parts of the chest wall exhibits a fixed shape at a given volume of the part, all motions of points within a part must bear fixed relationships to the volumes that part displaces. It follows that volume displacements can be estimated from measurements of motions of a single point within the part in question, after, of course, the relationship between volume displacement and linear motion of that point is determined" (Hixon, 1987, pp. 96–97). Estimates of lung volumes derived from chest wall kinematic measurements require calibration of the chest wall. Isovolume maneuvers involve equal and opposite volume displacement by the surfaces of the abdomen and rib cage under a closed system. Movement outputs from the rib cage and abdomen can be adjusted to account for the difference in volume displacements from these two parts. Once the chest wall has been calibrated, lung volume calibrations can be achieved by measuring integrated flow at the airway opening during simultaneous chest wall kinematic measurements to establish the relationship between chest wall movement and various static inspiratory or expiratory lung volumes (Hixon, Goldman, & Mead, 1973).

Magnetometry

The transduction method preferred by Hixon and colleagues involves the use of magnetometers. Changes in the AP diameters of the rib cage and abdomen are transduced with electromagnetic devices consisting of small coils (2 cm × 0.5 cm) set up in pairs, one for signal generation and the other for sensing changes in inductance due to displacement. Typically, two generator-sensor pairs are used. The generator coils are attached midline on the anterior surface of the chest wall. The first is glued to the skin at the level of the nipples and the second coil is attached to the abdomen immediately above the umbilicus. The sensor coil mates are attached to the dorsal surface of the body on midline at the same axial level as their respective generator mate coils. All four coils are oriented with their long axes perpendicular to the sagittal plane. Subjects can be placed on a tilt table to allow for recordings of chest wall movements in the supine and prone positions, but the typical position is either seated or standing, which is the typical posture for speech. Each generator coil is driven sinusoidally at its resonant frequency: 1.53 kHz for the rib cage and 0.69 kHz for the abdomen. Signal conditioning involves coil excitation, amplification of sensor coil output, half-wave rectification, filtering, DC-coupled amplification, and output to recording or display devices. The usable frequency response for inductive systems is approximately 1/10th of the coil excitation frequency. A conservative estimate for the system used by Hixon and colleagues indicates a usable bandwidth from DC to 70 Hz. This is more than adequate to faithfully capture the relatively low-frequency displacements of the rib cage and abdomen.

Calibrating the chest wall is straightforward. A series of isovolume maneuvers are performed at several known lung volumes to reveal the functional relation between the relative motion of the abdomen and rib cage. With knowledge of the relative motion relations determined during isovolume maneuvers at constrained lung volumes, it then becomes possible to estimate the component volume contributions of the abdomen and rib cage during an unconstrained task such as speech.

Speech breathing kinematics using magnetometers has been studied in individuals with profound hearing impairments (Forner & Hixon, 1987), voice disorders (Hixon & Putnam, 1987), motor neuron disease (Putnam & Hixon, 1987), flaccid paralysis (Hixon, Putnam, & Sharp, 1987), parkinsonian dysarthria (Solomon & Hixon, 1993), spinal cord injury (Hoit, Banzett, Brown, & Loring, 1990; Watson & Hixon, 2001), and in a variety of normal subgroups where factors such as age (Hoit & Hixon, 1987; Stathopoulos & Sapienza, 1997), body type (Hoit & Hixon, 1986), and sex (Hodge & Rochet, 1989) are the dependent variables.

Strain-Gage Belt Pneumography

Another transducer system that has been used to measure chest wall kinematics is the strain-gage belt pneumograph. This setup is quite simple and involves a clip gage attached to a circumferential belt with Velcro. A bridge amplifier provides DC excitation and conditioning for each belt. Signals are typically low-pass filtered (LP at 50 Hz) and routed to a digital computer or instrumentation recorder. Murdoch and colleagues have utilized this method to study respiratory function in subjects with Parkinson's disease (Murdoch, Chenery, Bowler, & Ingram, 1989), cerebellar degeneration (Murdoch, Chenery, Stokes, & Hardcastle, 1991), pseudobulbar palsy (Murdoch, Noble, Chenery, & Ingram, 1989), closed head injury (Murdoch, Theodoros, Stokes, & Chenery, 1993), and normal subjects (Manifold & Murdoch, 1993). There is some debate concerning the exact placement of the strain-gage belt pneumographs (see Hoit, 1994; Solomon & Hixon, 1993). Much of the debate centers on the exact placement of the abdominal belt. Murdoch et al (1989) reported placement of the abdominal belt above the umbilicus in their work. According to Hixon (1987), this placement is considered appropriate for AP measurements but not for circumferential measurements because the lower ribs contribute to movement of the abdominal belt.

Variable Inductance Plethysmography

Finally, variable inductance plethysmography has been successfully used to measure chest wall kinematics in infants and very young children (Boliek, Hixon, Watson, & Morgan, 1996, 1997). A commercially available plethysmograph, Respitrace (Ambulatory Monitoring, Inc., Ardsley, NY) was used to study chest wall kinematics during breathing and vocalization in a cross section of infants and children between the ages of 5 weeks and 6 years (Boliek, Hixon, Watson, & Jones, 2004; Boliek et al, 1996, 1997; Connaghan, Moore, & Higashakawa, 2004; Moore, Caulfield, & Green, 2001). The assumptions that allow us to estimate volume displacement from measurements of motions of a single point on the thorax or abdomen of the adult chest wall do not hold true for the compliant chest wall of the infant, which has multiple degrees of freedom. Therefore, sensing movement from multiple points is essential if we want to infer lung volume events from kinematic measurements of the infant chest wall. Variable inductance plethysmography involves placing a transduction band around the rib cage just below axillae and a band around the abdomen below the costal margin (Stradling, Chadwich, Quirk, & Phillips, 1985). Each band encircles the rib cage and abdomen and senses change in size. The "average of an infinite number of cross sections through the height of the band" expresses size relative to an "ideal cylinder described by its average cross-sectional area" (Boliek et al, 1996, p. 3). Calibration of the chest wall and lung volume follow the same principles used with adults and older children. Calibration can be obtained by eliciting breath holding and measuring the attendant isovolume adjustments of the chest wall. Boliek and colleagues (1996, 1997) elicited breath holds in young infants by occluding the distal port of a face mask-pneumotachometer unit for 1 to 2 seconds. This produced a brief air struggle by the infant, resulting in an isovolume adjustment of the chest wall without the loss of lung volume. Young children can be instructed to look at their belly button or tummy, which "freezes" them, momentarily resulting in a brief breath hold and isovolume adjustment. Gently stroking their abdomens, blowing in their ears, and lightly tickling them around their neck would often elicit a similar breath hold and chest wall adjustment in these young children. Volumes can be measured at the airway opening during breathing and are used to calibrate the kinematic signals. This procedure was validated on nine infants (Boliek et al, 1996). A comparison between lung volumes derived from summing the calibrated kinematic signals of the rib cage and abdomen were compared with integration of flow at the airway opening using a face mask pneumotachometer unit. Volumes derived by the two methods were within 5% of one another across wake and sleep conditions and in upright and supine body positions.

After calibration, the infant is unencumbered by the face mask and can vocalize naturally. Baseline tidal breaths and determination of end expiratory level (EEL) are needed to assess where vocalizations are occurring relative to tidal breathing and predicted vital capacity. In addition, care must be taken to measure only kinematic signals free of extraneous limb movement and postural adjustments (Boliek et al, 1996, 1997). A total of 19 measurements of volume displacements and durations associated with vocalization and breathing can be derived from the kinematic signals. Overall, variable inductance plethysmography is capable of measuring the rapid chest wall movements of the premature infant as well as sense atypical movements associated with pediatric neurological disorders such as cerebral palsy (Boliek, Hixon, & Jones, 2008).

◆ Conclusion

Visualization and tracking movements of the vocal tract and upper airway continues to excite the interest of many in speech science and speech physiology, and those interested in movement disorders from a variety of disciplines. Technological advances abound in the area of real-time digital signal processing and improved graphical user interfaces. With most transducer systems it is possible to simultaneously acquire physiological outputs from several articulatory flesh points in combination with electromyographic, aerodynamic, acoustic, and electrical impedance measures of vocal tract function. High-speed microprocessors make it possible to reduce many channels of information, including signal processing transformations, in real time. As the technologies and scientific underpinnings of speech motor control continue to advance, so will the depth of inquiry into sensorimotor speech movement disorders. Improved instrumentation also means that the complexity of task dynamics can be increased, using more subjects and external agents to induce motor reorganization. Exciting dividends are being realized in the clinical setting as well. Many of the technologies reviewed in this chapter have been applied toward improved diagnostic methods of respiratory, laryngeal, velopharyngeal, and orofacial function in patients suffering from neurologically based speech disorders. The speed of digital signal processing and high-resolution graphics has resulted in the emergence of new biofeedback tools that await clinical trial. Increasing collaboration among the disciplines of speech science, speech pathology, physiology, neuroscience, anatomy, mechanical and bioengineering, neurology, biophysics and imaging, and computer science will undoubtedly have a dramatic impact on future studies of speech movement and neural control.

Acknowledgments   This work was supported in part by National Institutes of Health grants R01 DC03311, P30 HD02528, and P30 DC005803, the Sutherland Foundation, and Neuro Logic, LLC of Lawrence, Kansas.

References

Abbs, J.H. & Gilbert, B.W. (1973). A strain gage transducer system for lip and jaw motion in two dimensions. *Journal of Speech and Hearing Research, 16,* 248–256

Abbs, J.H., Hunker, C.J., & Barlow, S.M. (1983). Differential speech motor subsystem impairments with suprabulbar lesions: neurophysiological framework and supporting data. In: W.R. Berry (Ed.), *Clinical Dysarthria* (pp. 21–56). San Diego: College-Hill Press

Abbs, J.H., Nadler, R.D., & Fujimura, O. (1988). X-ray microbeams track the shape of speech. *SOMA, 2,* 29–34

Adams, S.G., Weismer, G., & Kent, R.D. (1993). Speaking rate and speech movement velocity profiles. *Journal of Speech and Hearing Research, 36,* 41–54

Ardran, G.M., Kemp, F.H., & Lind, J. (1958a). A cineradiographic study of bottle feeding. *British Journal of Radiology, 31,* 11–22

Ardran, G.M., Kemp, F.H., & Lind, J. (1958b). A cineradiographic study of breast feeding. *British Journal of Radiology, 31,* 156–162

Baken, R.J. (1992). Electroglottography. *Journal of Voice, 6,* 98–110

Barlow, S.M. & Abbs, J.H. (1986). Fine force and position control of select orofacial structures in the upper motor neuron syndrome. *Experimental Neurology, 94,* 699–713

Barlow, S.M., Cole, K.J., & Abbs, J.H. (1983). A new headmounted lip-jaw movement transduction system for the study of motor speech disorders. *Journal of Speech and Hearing Research, 26,* 283–288

Barlow, S.M., Farley, G.R., & Andreatta, R.D. (1999). Neural systems in speech physiology. In: S.M. Barlow & R.D. Andreatta (Eds.), *Handbook of Clinical Speech Physiology* (pp. 101–165). San Diego: Singular

Barlow, S.M., Hammer, M.J., Pahwa, R., & Seibel, L. (2003). The effects of subthalamic nucleus deep brain stimulation on vocal tract dynamics in Parkinson's disease (p. 2146). 55th Annual Meeting of the American Academy of Neurology, Hawaii

Barlow, S.M., Iacono, R.P., Paseman, L.A., Biswas, A., & D'Antonio, L.D. (1998). The effects of experimental posteroventral pallidotomy on force and speech aerodynamics in Parkinson's disease. In: M.P. Cannito, K.M. Yorkston, & D.R. Beukelman (Eds.), *Speech Motor Control* (pp. 117–156). Baltimore: Paul H. Brookes

Barlow, S.M., Netsell, R. & Hunker, C. (1986). Phonatory disorders associated with CNS lesion. In: C. Cummings, J. Fredrickson, L. Harker, C. Krause, & D. Schuller (Eds.), *Otolaryngology–Head and Neck Surgery* (pp. 2087–2093). St. Louis: Mosby

Barlow, S.M., Paseman, L.A., & Philippbar, S. (1999). The aerodynamics of laryngeal engagement in neurogenic voice disorders. In: S.M. Barlow & R.D. Andreatta (Eds.), *Handbook of Clinical Speech Physiology* (pp. 219–246). San Diego: Singular

Barlow, S.M., Suing, G., & Andreatta, R.D. (1999). Speech aerodynamics using AEROWIN. In: S.M. Barlow & R.D. Andreatta (Eds.), *Handbook of Clinical Speech Physiology* (pp. 165–190). San Diego: Singular

Bell-Berti, F. & Hirose, H. (1975). Palatal activity in voicing distinctions: a simultaneous fiberoptic and electromyographic study. *Journal of Phonetics, 3,* 69–74

Bloomer, H. (1953). Observations on palatopharyngeal movements in speech and deglutition. *Journal of Speech and Hearing Disorders, 19,* 230–246

Boliek, C.A., Hixon, T.J., Kunze N., & Jones, P. (2008). Vocalization and breathing in infants and young children with cerebral palsy. 14th Biennial Conference on Motor Speech. Monterey, CA,

Boliek, C.A., Hixon, T., Watson, P., & Jones, P. (2004). Refinement of speech breathing in normal young children. Paper presented at the bi-annual Conference on Motor Speech: Speech Motor Control, Albuquerque, NM

Boliek, C.A., Hixon, T., Watson, P., & Morgan, W. (1996). Vocalization and breathing during the first year of life. *Journal of Voice, 10,* 1–22

____. (1997). Vocalization and breathing during the second and third years of life. *Journal of Voice, 11,* 373–390

Bosma, J.F. (1967). Human infant oral function. In: J.F. Bosma (Ed.), *Symposium on Oral Sensation and Perception* (pp. 98–110). Springfield, IL: Charles C. Thomas

Bosma, J.F., Hepburn, L.G., Josell, S.D., & Baker, K. (1990). Ultrasound demonstration of tongue motions during suckle feeding. *Developmental Medicine and Child Neurology, 32,* 223–229

Calnan, J.S. (1953). Movements of the soft palate. *British Journal of Plastic Surgery, 5,* 286–296

Chiba, T. & Kajiyama, M. (1942). *The Vowel, Its Nature and Structure.* Tokyo:Tokyo-Kaiseikan Publishing Co., Ltd.

Childers, D.G. & Krishnamurthy, A.K. (1985). A critical review of electroglottography. *Critical Review of Biomedical Engineering, 12,* 131–161

Christiansen, R.L. & Moller, K. (1971). Instrumentation for recording velar movement. *American Journal of Orthodontics, 59,* 448–455

Chuang, C.K. & Wang, W.S. (1978). Use of optical distance sensing to track tongue motion. *Journal of Speech and Hearing Research, 21,* 482–496

Connaghan, K.P., Moore, C., & Higashakawa, M. (2004). Respiratory kinematics during vocalization and nonspeech respiration in children from 9 to 48 months. *Journal of Speech, Language, and Hearing Research, 47,* 70–84

Dalston, R.M. (1989). Using simultaneous photodetection and nasometry to monitor velopharyngeal behavior during speech. *Journal of Speech and Hearing Research, 32,* 195–202

Dalston, R.M., Warren, D.W., & Smith, L.R. (1990). The aerodynamic characteristics of speech produced by normal speakers and cleft palate speakers with adequate velopharyngeal function. *Cleft Palate Journal, 27,* 393–399

D'Antonio, L., Chait, D., & Lotz, W. (1986). Pediatric videonasendoscopy for speech and voice evaluation. *Otolaryngology–Head and Neck Surgery, 94,* 578–583

D'Antonio, L., Chait, D., Lotz, W., & Netsell, R. (1987). Perceptual-physiologic approach to evaluation and treatment of dysphonia. *Annals of Otology Rhinology and Laryngology, 96,* 182–190

D'Antonio, L., Netsell, R., & Lotz, W. (1988). Clinical aerodynamics for the evaluation and management of voice disorders. *Ear Nose Throat Journal, 67,* 394–399

deMonterice, D., Meier, P.P., Engstrom, J.L., Crichton, C.L., & Mangurten, H.H. (1992). Concurrent validity of a new instrument for measuring nutritive sucking in preterm infants. *Nursing Research, 41,* 342–346

DeNil, L.F. & Abbs, J.H. (1991). Influence of speaking rate on the upper lip, lower lip, and jaw peak velocity sequencing during bilabial closing movements. *Journal of the Acoustical Society of America, 89,* 845–849

Dick, D., Ozturk, C., Douglas, A., McVeigh, E., & Stone, M. (2000). Three-dimensional tracking of tongue motion using tagged MRI. 8th International Society Magnetic Resonance in Medicine

Eishima, K. (1991). The analysis of sucking behavior in newborn infants. *Early Human Development, 27,* 163–173

Epstein, M.A. & Stone, M. (2005). The tongue stops here: ultrasound imaging of the palate. *Journal of the Acoustical Society of America, 118,* 2128–2131

Estep, M., Barlow, S.M., Vantipalli, R., et al. (2008). Non-nutritive suck burst parametrics in preterm infants with RDS and oral feeding complications. *J. Neonatal Nursing, 14*(1), 28–34

Finan, D.S. & Barlow, S.M. (1996). The actifier: a device for neurophysiological studies of orofacial control in human infants. *Journal of Speech and Hearing Research, 39,* 833–838

____. (1998). Intrinsic dynamics and mechanosensory modulation of non-nutritive sucking in human infants. *Early Human Development, 52,* 181–197

Fletcher, S.G. (1989). Palatometric specification of stop, affricate, and sibilant sounds. *Journal of Speech and Hearing Research, 32,* 736–748

Fletcher, S.G., Dagenais, P.A., & Critz-Crosby, P. (1991). Teaching vowels to profoundly hearing-impaired speakers using glossometry. *Journal of Speech and Hearing Research, 34,* 943–956

Fletcher, S.G., Hasegawa, A., McCutcheon, M.J., & Gilliom, J. (1980). Use of linguapalatal contact patterns to modify articulation in a deaf adult. In: D.L. McPherson (Ed.), *Advances in Prosthetic Devices for the Deaf: A Technical Workshop.* Rochester, NY: National Technical Institute for the Deaf

Fletcher, S.G., McCutcheon, J., Smith, S.C., & Wilson, H.S. (1989). Glossometric measurements in vowel production and modification. *Clinical Linguistics and Phonetics, 3,* 359–375

Fletcher, S.G., McCutcheon, M.J., & Wolf, M.B. (1975). Dynamic palatometry. *Journal of Speech and Hearing Research, 18,* 812–819

Folkins, J.W. & Canty, J.L. (1986). Movements of the upper and lower lips during speech: interactions between lips with the jaw fixed at different positions. *Journal of Speech and Hearing Research, 29,* 348–356

Forner, L.L. & Hixon, T.J. (1987). Respiratory kinematics in profoundly hearing-impaired speakers. In: T.J. Hixon (Ed.), *Respiratory Function in Speech and Song* (pp. 199–236). Boston: Little, Brown

Forrest, K., Weismer, G., & Adams, S. (1990). Statistical comparison of movement amplitudes from groupings of normal geriatric speakers. *Journal of Speech and Hearing Research, 33,* 386–389

Forrest, K., Weismer, G., & Turner, G.S. (1989). Kinematic, acoustic, and perceptual analyses of connected speech produced by Parkinsonian and normal geriatric adults. *Journal of the Acoustical Society of America, 85,* 2608–2622

Fujimura, O., Kiritani, S., & Ishida, H. (1973). Computer controlled radiography for observation of articulatory and other human organs. *Computes in Biology and Medicine, 3,* 371–384

Gall, V. (1984). Strip kymography of the glottis. *Archives in Otorhinolaryngology, 240,* 287–293

Gewolb, I.H., Bosma, J.F., Reynolds, E.W., & Vice, F.L. (2003). Integration of suck and swallow rhythms during feeding in preterm infants with and without bronchopulmonary dysplasia. *Developmental Medicine and Child Neurology, 45,* 344–348

Gick, B. (2002). The use of ultrasound for linguistic phonetic fieldwork. *Journal of the International Phonetics Association, 32,* 113–122

Graber, T.M., Bzoch, K.R., & Aoba, T. (1959). A functional study of the palatal and pharyngeal structures. *Angle Orthodontics, 29,* 30–40

Gracco, V.L. (1988). Timing factors in the coordination of speech movements. *Journal of Neuroscience, 8,* 4628–4639

Green, J.R., Moore, C.A., Higashikawa, M., & Steeve, R.W. (2000). The physiologic development of speech motor control: lip and jaw coordination. *Journal of Speech, Language, and Hearing Research, 43,* 239–255

Green, J.R. & Wang, Y.-T. (2003). Tongue-surface movement patterns during speech and swallowing. *Journal of the Acoustical Society of America, 113,* 2820–2833

Green, J.R. & Wilson, E.M. (2006). Spontaneous facial motility in infancy: a 3D kinematic analysis. *Developmental Psychobiology, 48,* 16–28

Guenther, F.H., Ghosh, S.S., & Tourville, J.A. (2006). Neural modeling and imaging of the cortical interactions underlying syllable production. *Brain and Language, 96,* 280–301

Hammer, M.J. (2007). Laryngeal mechanosensory detection and laryngeal engagement in parkinson's disease. Doctrinal dissertation. University of Kansas, 1–94, AAT 3261055

Harley, W.T. (1972). Dynamic palatography—a study of linguapalatal contacts during the production of selected consonant sounds. *Journal of Prosthetic Dentistry, 27,* 364–376

Hill, A.S., Kurkowski, T.B., & Garcia, J. (2000). Oral support measures used in feeding the preterm infant. *Nursing Research, 49,* 2–10

Hirano, M. & Bless, D.M. (1993). *Videostroboscopic Examination of the Larynx.* San Diego: Singular

Hixon, T.J. (1971). An electromagnetic method for transducing jaw movements during speech. *Journal of the Acoustical Society of America, 49,* 603–606

____. (1987). Respiratory function in speech. In: T.J. Hixon (Ed.), *Respiratory Function in Speech and Song* (pp. 1–54). Boston: Little, Brown

Hixon, T.J., Goldman, M.D., & Mead, J. (1973). Kinematics of the chest wall during speech production: volume displacements of the rib cage, abdomen, and lung. *Journal of Speech and Hearing Research, 16,* 78–115

Hixon, T.J. & Putnam, A.H.B. (1987). Voice abnormalities in relation to respiratory kinematics. In: T.J. Hixon (Ed.), *Respiratory Function in Speech and Song* (pp. 259–280). Boston: Little, Brown

Hixon, T.J., Putnam, A.H.B., & Sharp, J.T. (1987). Speech production with flaccid paralysis of the rib cage, diaphragm, and abdomen. In: T.J. Hixon (Ed.), *Respiratory Function in Speech and Song* (pp. 311–336). Boston: Little, Brown

Hodge, M.M. & Rochet, A. (1989). Characteristics of speech breathing in young women. *Journal of Speech and Hearing Research, 32,* 466–480

Hoit, J.D., Banzett, R., Brown, R., & Loring, S. (1990). Speech breathing in individuals with cervical spinal cord injury. *Journal of Speech and Hearing Research, 33,* 798–807

Hoit, J.D. & Hixon, T.J. (1986). Body type and speech breathing. *Journal of Speech and Hearing Research, 29,* 313–324

____. (1987). Age and speech breathing. *Journal of Speech and Hearing Research, 30,* 351–366

Hoit, J.U. (1994). A critical analysis of speech breathing data from the University of Queensland (letter). *Journal of Speech and Hearing Research, 37,* 572–580

Holmberg, E.B., Hillman, R.E., & Perkell, J.S. (1988). Glottal airflow and transglottal air pressure measurements for male and female speakers in soft, normal, and loud voice. *Journal of the Acoustical Society of America, 84,* 511–529

____. (1989). Glottal airflow and transglottal air pressure measurements for male and female speakers in low, normal, and high pitch. *Journal of Voice, 3,* 294–305

Horiguchi, S. & Bell-Berti, F. (1987). The velotrace: a device for monitoring velar position. *Cleft Palate Journal, 24,* 104–111

House, A.S. & Fairbanks, G. (1953). The influence of consonant environment upon the secondary acoustical characteristics of vowels. *Journal of the Acoustical Society of America, 25,* 105–113

House, R.A. (1967). *A study of tongue body motion during selected speech sounds.* Doctoral dissertation, University of Michigan

Hunker, C.J., Abbs, J.H., & Barlow, S.M. (1982). The relationship between parkinsonian rigidity and hypokinesia in the orofacial system: a quantitative analysis. *Neurology, 32,* 755–761

Iwayama, K. & Eishima, M. (1997). Neonatal sucking behavior and its development until 14 months. *Early Human Development, 47,* 1–9

Johnson, K. (1969). Mapping the movements of the human tongue. *The Atom, 6,* 12–16

Keefe, M.J. & Dalston, R.M. (1989). An analysis of velopharyngeal timing in normal adult speakers using a microcomputer based photodetector system. *Journal of Speech and Hearing Research, 32,* 39–48

Kiritani, S., Itoh, K., & Fujimura, O. (1975). Tongue-pellet trackig by a computer-controlled x-ray microbeam system. *Journal of the Acoustical Society of America, 57,* 1516–1520

Kiritani, S., Itoh, K., Fujisaki, H., & Sawashima, M. (1976). Tongue pellet movement for the Japanese CV syllables—observations using the x-ray microbeam system. *Annual Bulletin of the Research Institute Logopaedica Phoniatrica (University of Tokyo), 10,* 19–27

Kron, R.E., Ipsen, J., & Goddard, K.E. (1968). Consistent individual differences in the nutritive sucking behavior of the human newborn. *Psychosomatic Medicine, 30,* 151–161

Kuzmin, Y.I. (1962). Mobile palatography as a tool for acoustic study of speech sounds. *Report of Fourth International Congress on Acoustics* (p. G35), Copenhagen

Kydd, W.L. & Belt, D.A. (1964). Continuous palatography. *Journal of Speech and Hearing Disorders, 29,* 489–492

Laine, T., Warren, D.W., Dalston, R.M., & Morr, K.E. (1989). Effects of velar resistance on speech aerodynamics. *European Journal of Orthodontics, 11,* 52–58

Lau, C., Sheena, H.R., Shulman, R.J., & Schanler, R.J. (1997). Oral feeding in low birth weight infants. *Journal of Pediatrics, 130,* 561–569

Ludlow, C.L. & Bassich, C.J. Relationships between perceptual ratings and acoustic measures of hypokinetic speech. In Mcneil, M.R., Rosenbek, J.C., & Aronson, A.E. (Eds.) *The Dysarthrias.* (1984). San Diego: College-Hill Press, 163–195

Lundberg, A.J. & Stone, M. (1999). Three-dimensional tongue surface reconstruction: practical considerations for ultrasound data. *Journal of the Acoustical Society of America, 106,* 2858–2867

Manifold, J.A. & Murdoch, B. (1993). Speech breathing in young adults: effect of body type. *Journal of Speech and Hearing Research, 36,* 657–671

McClean, M.D., Beukelman, D.R., & Yorkston, K.M. (1987). Speech-muscle visuomotor tracking in dysarthric and non-impaired speakers. *Journal of Speech and Hearing Research, 30,* 276–282

McClean, M.D., Kroll, R.M., & Loftus, N.S. (1990). Kinematic analysis of lip closure in stutterer's fluent speech. *Journal of Speech and Hearing Research, 33,* 755–760

McNeil, M.R., Weismer, G., Adams, S., & Mulligan, M. (1990). Oral structure non-speech motor control in normal, dysarthric, aphasic, and apraxic speakers: isometric force and static position control. *Journal of Speech and Hearing Research, 33,* 255–268

Michi, K., Suzuki, N., Yamashita, Y., & Imai, S. (1986). Visual training and correction of articulation disorders by use of dynamic palatography: serial observation in a case of cleft palate. *Journal of Speech and Hearing Disorders, 51,* 226–238

Mizuno, K. & Ueda, A. (2001). Development of sucking behavior in infants with Down's syndrome. *Acta Paediatrica, 90,* 1384–1388

Moll, K.L. (1962). Velopharyngeal closure on vowels. *Journal of Speech and Hearing Research, 5,* 30–37

Moll, K.L. & Daniloff, R.G. (1971). Investigation of the timing of velar movements during speech. *Journal of the Acoustical Society of America, 50,* 673–684

Moller, K.T., Martin, R., & Christiansen, R. (1971). A technique for recording velar movement. *Cleft Palate Journal, 8,* 263–276

Moon, J.B. & Lagu, R.K. (1987). Development of a second-generation phototransducer for the assessment of velopharyngeal activity. *Cleft Palate Journal, 24,* 240–243

Moon, J.B., Zembrowski, P., Robin, D.A., & Folkins, J.W. (1993). Visuomotor tracking ability of young adult speakers. *Journal of Speech and Hearing Research, 36,* 672–682

Moore, C.A. (1993). Symmetry of mandibular muscle activity as an index of coordinative strategy. *Journal of Speech and Hearing Research, 36,* 1145–1157

Moore, C.A., Caulfield, T.J., & Green, J.R. (2001). Relative kinematics of the rib cage and abdomen during speech and nonspeech behaviors by 15–month-old children. *Journal of Speech, Language, and Hearing Research, 44,* 80–94

Müller, E.M. & Abbs, J.H. (1979). Strain gage transduction of lip and jaw motion in the midsagittal plane: refinement of a prototype system. *Journal of the Acoustical Society of America, 65,* 481–486

Murdoch, B.E., Chenery, H., Bowler, S., & Ingram, J. (1989). Respiratory function in Parkinson's subjects exhibiting a perceptible speech deficit: a kinematic and spirometric analysis. *Journal of Speech and Hearing Disorders, 54,* 610–626

Murdoch, B.E., Chenery, H., Stokes, P., & Hardcastle, W. (1991). Respiratory kinematics in speakers with cerebellar disease. *Journal of Speech and Hearing Research, 34,* 768–780

Murdoch, B.E., Noble, J., Chenery, H., & Ingram, J. (1989). A spirometric and kinematic analysis of respiratory function in pseudobulbar palsy. *Australian Journal of Human Communication, 17,* 21–35

Murdoch, B.E., Theodoros, D., Stokes, P., & Chenery, H. (1993). Abnormal patterns of speech breathing in dysarthric speakers following severe closed head injury. *Brain Injury, 7,* 295–308

Nelson, W.L., Perkell, J.S., & Westbury, J.R. (1984). Mandible movements during increasingly rapid articulations of single syllables: preliminary observations. *Journal of the Acoustical Society of America, 75,* 945–951

Netsell, R. & Lotz, W.K. (1994). Aerodynamic abnormalities and dysphonia. Personal communication

Netsell, R., Lotz, W.K., & Barlow, S.M. (1989). A speech physiology examination for individuals with dysarthria. In: K.M. Yorkston & D.R. Beukelman (Eds.), *Recent Advances in Clinical Dysarthria* (pp. 3–39). Boston, Little, Brown

Palmer, J.M. (1973). Dynamic palatography—general implications of locus and sequencing patterns. *Phonetica, 28,* 76–85

Peng, C.L., Jost-Brinkmann, P.G., Miethke, R.R., & Lin, C.T. (2000). Ultrasonographic measurement of tongue movement during swallowing. *Journal of Ultrasound Medicine, 19,* 15–20

Perkell, J.S. (1969). *Physiology of Speech Production: Results and Implications of a Quantitative Cineradiographic Analysis.* Research Monograph No. 53. Cambridge, MA: MIT Press

Perkell, J.S., Cohen, M.H., Svirsky, M.A., Matthies, M.L., Garabieta, I., & Jackson, M.T.T. (1992). Electromagnetic midsagittal articulometer systems for transducing speech articulatory movements. *Journal of the Acoustical Society of America, 92,* 3078–3096

Perkell, J.S. & Matthies, M.L. (1992). Temporal measures of anticipatory labial coarticulation for the vowel /u/: within- and cross-subject variability. *Journal of the Acoustical Society of America, 91,* 2911–2925

Potter, R.K., Kopp, G.A., & Green, H.C. (1947). *Visible Speech.* New York: Van Nostrand

Putnam, A.H.B. & Hixon, T.J. (1987). Respiratory kinematics in speakers with motor neuron disease. In: T.J. Hixon (Ed.), *Respiratory Function in Speech and Song* (pp. 281–309). Boston: Little, Brown

Samlan, R. & Barlow, S.M. (1999). The effects of transition rate and vowel height on velopharyngeal airway resistance. In: S.M. Barlow & R.D. Andreatta (Eds.), *Handbook of Clinical Speech Physiology* (pp. 274–264). San Diego: Singular

Schutte, H.K., Svec, J.G., & Sram, F. (1998). First results of clinical application of videokymography. *Laryngoscope, 108,* 1206–1210

Seibel, L., Barlow, S.M., Vantipalli, R., Finan, D., Urish, M., & Carlson, J. (2005). Spectral dynamics of non-nutritive suck in preterm infants. *Pediatric Academy Society,* Abstract 213a, 160

Shaiman, S., Porter, R.J., Jr. (1991). Different phase-stable relationships of the upper lip and jaw for production of vowels and diphthongs. *Journal of the Acoustical Society of America, 90,* 3000–3007

Sharkey, S.G. & Folkins, J.W. (1985). Variability of lip and jaw movements in children and adults: implications for the development of speech motor control. *Journal of Speech and Hearing Research, 28,* 8–15

Shau, Y.-W., Wang, C.-L., Hsieh, F.-J., & Hsiao, T.-Y. (2001). Noninvasive assessment of vocal fold mucosal wave velocity using color Doppler imaging. *Ultrasound Medicine & Biology, 27,* 1451–1460

Shawker, T.H., Sonies, B., Stone, M., & Baum, B.J. (1983). Real-time ultrasound visualization of tongue movement during swallowing. *Journal of Clinical Ultrasound, 11,* 485–490

Shawker, T.H., Stone, M., & Sonies, B.C. (1985). Tongue pellet tracking by ultrasound: Development of a reverberation pellet. *Journal of Phonetics, 13,* 135–146

Shibata, S. (1968). A study of dynamic palatography. *Annual Bulletin of the Research Institute Logopaedica Phoniatrica (University of Tokyo), 2,* 28–36

Smith, A. (1992). The control of orofacial movements in speech. *Critical Review of Oral and Biological Medicine, 3,* 233–267

Smith, A. & Zelaznik, H.N. (2004). Development of functional synergies for speech motor coordination in childhood and adolescence. *Developmental Psychobiology, 45,* 22–33

Smith, B.L. & Gartenberg, T.E. (1984). Initial observations concerning developmental characteristics of labio-mandibular kinematics. *Journal of the Acoustical Society of America, 75,* 1599–1605

Smith, B.L. & McLean-Muse, A. (1987a). An investigation of motor equivalence in the speech of children and adults. *Journal of the Acoustical Society of America, 82,* 837–842

_____. (1987b). Effects of rate and bite block manipulations on kinematic characteristics of children's speech. *Journal of the Acoustical Society of America, 81,* 747–754

Smitheran, J.R. & Hixon, T.J. (1981). Clinical method for estimating laryngeal airway resistance during vowel production. *Journal of Speech and Hearing Disorders, 46,* 138–146

Solomon, N.P. & Hixon, T.J. (1993). Speech breathing in Parkinson's disease. *Journal of Speech and Hearing Research, 36,* 294–310

Sonoda, Y. (1974). Observation of tongue movements employing magnetometer sensor. *IEEE Transactions on Magnetics, 10,* 954–957

Stathopoulos, E.T. & Sapienza, C.M. (1997). Developmental changes in laryngeal and respiratory function with variations in sound pressure level. *Journal of Speech, Language, and Hearing Research, 40,* 595–614

Stone, M. (1990). A three dimensional model of tongue movement based on ultrasound and x-ray microbeam data. *Journal of the Acoustical Society of America, 87,* 2207–2217

Stone, M., Dick, D., Davis, E., Douglas, A., & Ozturk, C. (2000). Modeling the internal tongue using principal strains. In: *Proceedings of the 5th Speech Production Seminar* (pp. 133–136), Kloster-Seeon, Germany

Stone, M., Epstein, M.A., & Iskarous, K. (2004) Functional segments in tongue movement. *Clinical Linguistics and Phonetics, 18,* 507–522

Stone, M., Epstein, M.A., & Sutton, M.W. (2003). Predicting 3D tongue shapes from midsagittal contours. In: *Proceedings of the 6th International Seminar on Speech Production (ISSP)*

Stone, M. & Lundberg, A. (1996). Three-dimensional tongue surface shapes of English consonants and vowels. *Journal of the Acoustical Society of America, 99,* 3728–3737

Stone, M., Shawker, T.H., Talbot, T.L., & Rich, H. (1988). Cross sectional tongue shape during the production of vowels. *Journal of the Acoustical Society of America, 83,* 1586–1596

Stradling, J.R., Chadwick, G., Quirk, C., & Phillips, T. (1985). Respiratory inductance plethysmography: calibration techniques, their validation and the effects of posture. *Bulletin of the European Society of Physiopathology and Respiration, 21,* 317–324

Stumm, S. Barlow, S. M., Estep, M., et al. (2008). The relationship between respiratory distress syndrome and the fine structure of the non-intuitive suck in preterm infants. *J Neonatal Nursing, 14(1),* 9–16

Sung, M.W., Kim, H., Koh, T., Kwon, T., Mo, J., Choi, S.H., Lee, J.S., Park, K.S., Kim, E.J., & Sung, M.Y. (1999). Videostrobokymography: a new method for the quantitative analysis of vocal fold vibration. *Laryngoscope, 109,* 1859–1863

Sussman, H.M. & Westbury, J.R. (1981). The effects of antagonistic gestures on temporal and amplitude parameters of anticipatory labial co-articulation. *Journal of Speech and Hearing Research, 24,* 16–24

Svec, J.G. & Schutte, H.K. (1996). Videokymography: high-speed line scanning of vocal fold vibration. *Journal of Voice, 10,* 201–205

Švec, J.G. & Šram, F. (2002). Kymographic imaging of the vocal fold oscillations. In: J.H.L. Hansen & B. Pellom (Eds.), *Proceedings of the 7th International Conference on Spoken Language Processing*, September 16–20, Denver

Sze, C.-F., Iny, D., Stone, M., & Levine, W. (1999). Reconstructing three-dimensional tongue motion from ultrasound images. In: *Proceedings of the Conference of the International Federation for Automatic Control (IFAC)*, Beijing, China, 1, 97–102

Tamura, Y., Horikawa, Y., & Yoshida, S. (1996). Coordination of tongue movements and perioral muscle activities during nutritive sucking. *Developmental Medicine and Child Neurology, 38*, 503–510

Titze, I.R. (1990). Interpretation of the electroglottographic signal. *Journal of Voice, 4*, 1–9

Trotman, C.-A. & Faraway, J.J. (1998). Sensitivity of a method for the analysis of facial motility: II. Interlandmark separation. *Cleft Palate Craniofacial Journal, 35*, 142–153

Trotman, C.-A., Faraway, J.J., & Essick G.K. (2000). Three-dimensional nasolabial displacement during movement in repaired cleft lip and palate patients. *Plastic Reconstructive Surgery 105, 1273–1283*

Trotman, C.-A., Faraway, J.J., Silvester, K.T., Greenlee, G.M., & Johnston, L.E. (1998). Sensitivity of a method for the analysis of facial motility: I. Vector of displacement. *Cleft Palate Craniofacial Journal, 35, 132–141*

Tye-Murray, N. (1991). The establishment of open articulatory postures by deaf and hearing talkers. *Journal of Speech and Hearing Research, 34, 453–459*

Tye-Murray, N. & Folkins, J.W. (1990). Jaw and lip movements of deaf talkers producing utterances with known stress patterns. *Journal of the Acoustical Society of America, 87, 2675–2683*

van der Giet, G. (1977). Computer-controlled method for measuring articulatory activities. *Journal of the Acoustical Society of America, 61, 1072–1076*

Vantipalli, R. & Barlow, S.M. (2004). AEROWIN RT: Clinical application for motor speech disorders. 13th Bienniel National Speech Motor Control Conference, Albuquerque, New Mexico

Verdonck-de Leeuw, I.M., Festen, J.M., & Mahieu, H.F. (2001). Deviant vocal fold vibration as observed during videokymography: the effect on voice quality. *Journal of Voice, 15*, 313–322

Warren, D.W. (1982). Aerodynamics of speech. In: N.J. Lass, L.V. McReynolds, J.L. Northern, & D.E. Yoder (Eds.), *Speech, Language, and Hearing* (pp. 219–245). Philadelphia: W.B. Saunders

___. (1988). Aerodynamics of speech. In: N.J. Lass (Ed.), *Handbook of Speech-Language Pathology and Audiology*. Toronto: B.C. Decker

Warren, D.W., Dalston, R.M., Trier, W.C., & Holder, M.B. (1985). A pressure-flow technique for quantifying temporal patterns of palatopharyngeal closure. *Cleft Palate Journal, 22*, 11–19

Warren, D.W. & DuBois, A. (1964). A pressure-flow technique for measuring velopharyngeal orifice area during continuous speech. *Cleft Palate Journal, 1*, 52–71

Watkin, K.L. (1999). Ultrasound and swallowing. *Folia Phoniatrica et Logopaedica, 51*, 183–198

Watkin, K.L. & Rubin, J.M. (1989). Pseudo-three-dimensional reconstruction of ultrasonic images of the tongue. *Journal of the Acoustical Society of America, 85*, 496–499

Watson, P.J. & Hixon, T.J. (2001). Effects of abdominal trussing on breathing and speech in men with cervical spinal cord injury. *Journal of Speech, Language, and Hearing Research, 44*, 751–762

Weber, F., Woolridge, M.W., & Baum, J.D. (1986). An ultrasonographic study of the organization of sucking and swallowing by newborn infants. *Developmental Medicine and Child Neurology, 28*, 19–24

Westbury, J.R. (1991). The significance and measurement of head position during speech production experiments using the x-ray microbeam system. *Journal of the Acoustical Society of America, 89*, 1782–1791

Wolff, P.H. (1968). The serial organization of sucking in the young infant. *Pediatrics, 42*, 943–956

Yang, C.S. & Stone, M. (2002). Dynamic programming method for temporal registration of three-dimensional tongue surface motion from multiple utterances. *Speech Communication, 38*, 199–207

Yumoto, E. (2004). Aerodynamics, voice quality, and laryngeal image analysis of normal and pathologic voices. *Current Opinion in Otolaryngology & Head and Neck Surgery, 12*, 166–173

Chapter 7

Electromyographic Techniques for the Assessment of Motor Speech Disorders

Erich S. Luschei and Eileen M. Finnegan

Scientists discovered, during the mid-19th century, that very small electrical currents were generated by contracting muscles. By 1912 (Piper, 1912), instruments used for detecting these "action currents" had become sensitive enough to record voluntary muscle activity in humans. Limitations in the photographic recording devices available at that time provided records that were only 1 or 2 seconds in duration, but these records were sufficient to provide our first insights into the control of muscle by the nervous system. The signal recorded by this method was called the electromyogram (EMG) and is still known by that name today. Although the study of the EMG signal has been widely used as a research tool for studying muscle and the general principles of motor control in the body, it has also evolved into a medical procedure that is used in hospitals and clinics throughout the world.

This chapter discusses EMG procedures—where the signal comes from, the instrumentation used to record it, and how the signals may be processed and interpreted—and provides a few examples of how EMG recording is used in modern medical settings.

◆ Medical Uses of Electromyogram Recording

Diagnosis of Systemic Neurological Diseases

A patient comes to the clinic complaining of very significant weakness, which could result from diseases at several sites in the peripheral or central nervous system. One site is the neuromuscular junction, where action potentials in motor nerve fibers cause action potentials in muscle cells. Failure of the neuromuscular junction is the cause of diseases such as myasthenia gravis or the result of poisoning by toxins, for example, botulinum toxin. Another potential cause is failure of conduction in peripheral nerves (peripheral neuropathy). Another chilling possibility is amyotrophic lateral sclerosis (ALS), in which motor neurons slowly die. In considering this problem, an experienced clinician would probably have a good idea about which of these possibilities was the most likely cause of the weakness even without ordering an EMG, based on the history and the physical examination. The

prognosis and treatment of the weakness would be very different, however, for the different possible causes, so any responsible clinician would want to have as much reliable information as possible before diagnosing the patient and starting treatment. In this case, as in all others, EMG recordings yield additional information that has to be interpreted within the context of all other medical information. It is likely, in this hypothetical case of weakness, that a neurologist would order an EMG from a special diagnostic laboratory. Peripheral nerves in the forearm containing motor nerves to muscles in the hand may be percutaneously electrically stimulated while recording the EMG of the hand muscles. The synchrony of the nerve stimulation produces a large evoked EMG potential that can document the viability of the neuromuscular junction and also measure the conduction velocity of the action potentials in the peripheral nerves. The types of activity and waveforms of EMG potentials, recorded with needle electrodes inserted into the muscles, may definitively diagnose the disease of ALS.

Generally speaking, the diagnosis of motor disorders in neurological clinics is currently the main well-established clinical use of EMG recording and analysis. Texts such as that by Kimura (1989) cover the substantive issues in detail, which are not discussed here. The types of electrodes used in neurological EMG analysis are discussed later in this chapter, however, because the terminology can be a matter of significant confusion.

Evaluation of Paralyzed or Spastic Muscles

When a person cannot move a limb or articulator, it can be surprisingly difficult to know the exact cause. Damage to a particular nerve, either as the result of trauma or a surgical procedure or as a spontaneous event, can produce what appears to be paralysis. One such problem that is familiar to speech-language pathologists who work in the field of voice, and to their colleagues in the medical field of otolaryngology, is unilateral vocal fold paralysis. The condition is given this name because one of the vocal folds does not appear to move. The presumptive cause is damage to the recurrent laryngeal nerve. One of the pioneers in the use of electromyography of laryngeal muscles, Faaborg-Andersen (1957), studied EMG signals from laryngeal muscles of patients with a presumptive diagnosis of unilateral vocal fold paralysis, and observed that many of the muscles exhibited

EMG activity. Other otolaryngology studies have confirmed this observation (Blair, Berry, & Briant, 1978; Iroto, Hirano, & Tomita, 1968; Min, Finnegan, Hoffman, Luschei, & McCulloch, 1994). Failure of a limb or articulator to move, or to exhibit a normal range of motion, can have several causes: damage to motor neurons or motor nerves, mechanical changes in joints, co-contraction of antagonist muscle groups, or inappropriate reinnervation of muscles following nerve damage. Laryngeal muscle EMG recording is beginning to be used to help resolve some of these possibilities as they relate to unilateral vocal fold paralysis (Berry & Blair, 1980; Crumley, 1989; Hoffman, Brunberg, Winter, Sullivan, & Kileny, 1991), but the procedure is far less widespread and less developed than the procedures used in neurological diagnostic EMG laboratories.

Many readers may wonder at this point why voice specialists do not just send a patient with an immobile vocal fold to the neurology EMG lab. This could very well be done. The premise of this chapter, however, is that the interests of patients with dysarthrias are best served by speech-language pathologists who are directly involved in EMG procedures. An appreciation of the anatomy and physiology of the articulators, the characteristics of speech and swallowing, and certain technical aspects of doing EMG recordings from inaccessible muscles that move vigorously during function greatly improves any EMG procedures that are done. A speech-language pathologist may have more knowledge in these areas than a neurologist who has not specialized in the study of the articulators. Thus the speech-language pathologist has much to offer even if an EMG recording is conducted in a neurology EMG lab.

Many dysarthrias result from central nervous system disorders that produce abnormally high levels of activity (spasticity) in groups of muscles of the limbs and articulators. In some cases the ability of patients to walk, for instance, can be improved by surgically cutting the tendon of certain spastic muscles that are causing the most interference with the function. It may be difficult to know, ahead of time, which muscle is the culprit just using physical examination. In these cases, surgeons can use EMG recording to help make their decision about which muscle to tenotomize (Cahan, Adams, Perry, & Beeler, 1990). Although surgery of this type is not used to treat the dysarthrias, a related procedure, reversible paralysis of muscles by injection of botulinum toxin, has been widely used to treat certain dystonias (Brin et al, 1987; Cohen & Thompson, 1987; Scott, 1980; Stager & Ludlow, 1994). In this procedure, EMG recording can be used as an aid to verify the injection site (Ludlow, Naunton, Terada, & Anderson, 1991; Miller, Woodson, & Jankovic, 1987; Min, Luschei, Finnegan, McCullough, & Hoffman, 1994).

The EMG has many uses in addition to the examples given above, including the study and treatment of motor speech disorders. We recognize that technical procedures of this type are somewhat foreign to many clinical speech pathologists, not only because they appear to interfere with the person-to-person relationship, which is the heart and soul of the profession, but also because the instrumentation looks complicated. On the first point, it may be helpful to consider the fact that EMG recording is merely a way of

extending the clinician's senses to obtain information that we cannot ordinarily sense. As for the second point, it seems likely that the complexity problems will be eased a great deal in the future by new EMG instrumentation that is designed for clinical use rather than for research. In the meantime, however, most clinicians will find the instrumentation's complexity less daunting once they understand how it works.

◆ Principles of Electromyogram Recording

Source of the Electromyogram Signal

An action potential must sweep along muscle cells in order for a muscle to contract. These action potentials create, as they move along, minute electrical currents flowing outside the muscle cells (**Fig. 7–1**). These tiny currents do not really do anything. They are just there as a part of the process, like the bow and stern wave of a ship going through the water.

The nervous system activates muscles in terms of a motor unit, which is defined as a motor neuron and all the muscle cells it innervates. Because all the muscle cells in one motor unit fire (have action potentials) at the same time, the tiny extracellular currents from individual muscle cells add up to produce a current that is easily detected by recording electrodes. Because these currents are going in the same direction at the same time, the total waveform is stereotyped. Such a potential is called a single motor unit potential

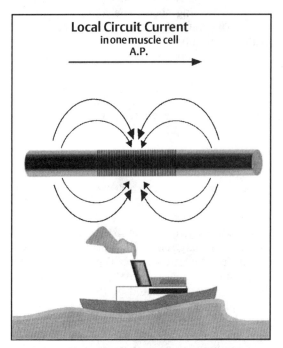

Figure 7–1 The extracellular current caused by an action potential sweeping along the muscle cell is analogous to the bow and stern wave caused by a ship going through the water.

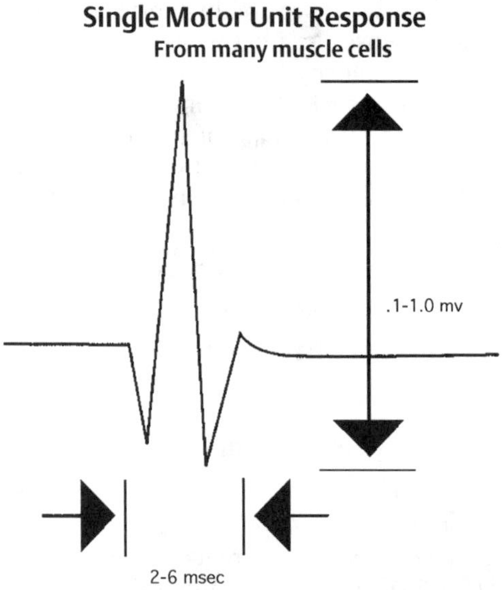

Single Motor Unit Response
From many muscle cells

.1-1.0 mv

2-6 msec

Figure 7–2 Drawing of a typical single motor unit potential caused by synchronous firing of muscle action potentials in all the muscle fibers innervated by a single motor axon.

(Fig. 7–2). This potential is equivalent to a flotilla of ships going through the water in precise synchrony; their bow waves would add up and produce quite a wave!

Because the firing of the motor neurons of a naturally activated muscle is not synchronized, the single motor unit potentials interact with one another in a complex manner and produce an interference pattern. One may imagine many flotillas of vessels sailing around a lake. Their bow waves would interact and produce a chop, which is just a hydraulic interference pattern. One may intuitively sense that the size of the chop will be related to the number of flotillas that are traveling about; the more vessels, the higher the chop. The EMG interference pattern is no different; the greater the number of motor units that are active, the higher the EMG signal. The metric to be used for describing the height of the EMG is a complicated matter, however, which will be considered later. For the moment, it can be taken as a fact that the size of the EMG signal bears a monotonic relationship to the degree to which the muscle has been activated.

Electrode Configuration in Electromyogram Recording

The EMG signal is almost always recorded with a differential amplifier, which creates an output that is proportional to (and much larger than) the *difference* in the voltage of its two inputs. How these two inputs are spaced with respect to the active muscle has a large effect on the nature of the EMG signal and on the interpretation one can apply to it. Let's go back to the hydraulic analogy. Suppose we wanted to measure the chop on the water created by the ships dashing about. The use of a differential amplifier is equivalent to measuring the height of the water between two points in the water. Suppose these two points are close together, say a foot apart. If a number of ships were steaming around miles away from our two recording points, the size of the chop would be much attenuated by the time it got to us. Also, all

the little peaky whitecaps would be gone. We would just see small slow rollers going by. Our signal, the difference in the two water heights, would be small, and it would be composed of low frequencies. However, if we had our two recording points right in the midst of all the ships, we would detect large water height differences, and many of the waves would have sharp peaks. In this case, our signal would be large and be composed of much higher frequencies than when the recording points were distant from the action.

When the electrodes are far apart, they are able to survey activity over large areas. In this case, however, the source of the activity is not known with precision. This can be a major diagnostic problem. Suppose your electrodes are far apart in a paralyzed muscle. Adjacent muscles that are active may produce a sizable EMG signal. Such distant activity would be relatively small compared with what one would expect of a normally active muscle, and it would be composed of low-frequency waveforms. Thus one would suspect (and hope) that the activity was not from the muscle under study. Close-spaced electrodes tend to reject muscle activity from distant active muscles, however, and would be preferable, therefore, in assessing a muscle suspected of being paralyzed.

Four generalizations about amplification and electrodes spacing may be offered at this points:

1. Differential amplifiers are essential.

2. Close electrode spacing is best in most cases.

3. Muscle activity close to the electrodes is represented by a signal having high frequencies, often showing characteristic single motor unit waveforms. Such signals sound crisp in the audio monitor (see later discussion).

4. Signals from distant active muscles may be picked up even by electrodes that are very close together. These signals are composed predominantly of low frequencies, however, and sound dull and muffled compared with the signals of nearby muscle fibers when they are played through an audio monitor.

For readers desiring a more rigorous treatment of this topic, an excellent article is that by DeLuca (1979). Another excellent source, covering myoelectric theory and many pragmatic issues in EMG recording, is that by Loeb and Gans (1986).

♦ Instrumentation

Overview

The scheme represented in **Fig. 7–3** identifies some of the major aspects of an overall instrumentation system. Three electrodes are attached to the patient. One of these, the reference lead, is attached to the skin with a conductive gel electrode and serves to hold the electrical reference voltage of the EMG amplifier and input stage of the isolator to the subject's body as a whole. The other two electrodes are the inputs to the differential amplifier, and their difference

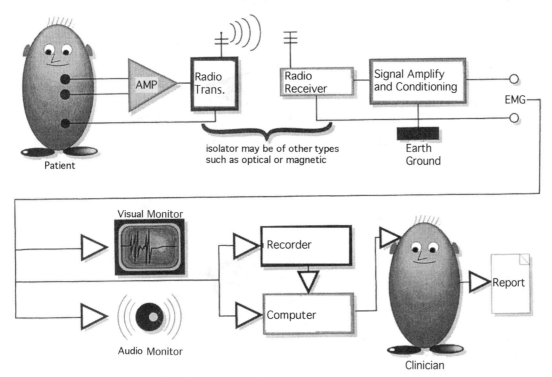

Figure 7–3 Major components of an electromyogram (EMG) instrumentation system.

in voltage is amplified by the gain of the amplifier. This amplified voltage difference is applied to the input stage of the isolator. The input stage of the isolator modulates a very low power radio transmitter as a simple linear function of the signal. The radio signal crosses an insulating gap to the output stage of the isolator, which is a radio receiver that demodulates the radio signal to recover an exact replica of the EMG signal. The signal can now be safely referenced to earth ground. (Radio transmission across a gap is only one of several ways of isolating the signal.) The rationale for use of the isolator stage is discussed in detail later.

The EMG signal may be further amplified and processed, such as being bandpass filtered, before it is presented to the eye or ear of the clinician. On-line monitors are very useful to make sure the recordings are proceeding appropriately, but documentation and objective analysis requires that the signal be permanently recorded. This can be done by tape recorders, which then may be played back off-line to a computer for analysis. Alternatively, state-of-the-art computers may now be used as the data acquisition recording device as well as serve for data analysis. The last stage of this system—perhaps the most essential one—is the experience and intelligence of the clinician in interpreting the EMG signal.

The instrumentation system just described may be usefully regarded as being like a chain, which is only as strong as its weakest link. Inappropriate electrodes or amplifiers, recorders that are noisy or lacking in fidelity, or lack of experience by the clinician in recognizing artifactual (false) signals can all defeat an otherwise adequate system. It therefore is useful to consider these various parts of the system in detail.

Electrodes

There are basically three types of electrodes that have been widely used in EMG recording: skin electrodes, intramuscular fine-wire (hooked-wire) electrodes, and intramuscular rigid needle electrodes. These types are schematically illustrated, along with their usual connections to a differential amplifier, in **Fig. 7–4.**

Skin Electrodes

Muscle activity from large muscles directly under the skin may be easily detected and quantified by simply attaching metal disk electrodes to the skin surface. This approach often seems most desirable because it is noninvasive. No one seems to like needles! However, there are major limitations on the use of skin electrodes by speech-language pathologists because most of the muscles involved in speech and oral functions such as swallowing are not directly under the skin. These muscles are also relatively small and complex in their anatomy, so records obtained with skin electrodes provide only a limited measure of how these muscle systems are operating. The lips are an exception, however. Lip EMG during speech may be easily recorded with skin electrodes (Cole, Konopacki, & Abbs, 1983; McClean, 1991; Smith, McFarland, Weber, & Moore, 1987). The surface lip EMG signal can sometimes be misleading, however, because it may reflect the activity of different muscles or functionally different motor units within what is anatomically one muscle (Blair & Smith, 1986). Surface electrodes placed over the masseter muscles can record an EMG signal related to

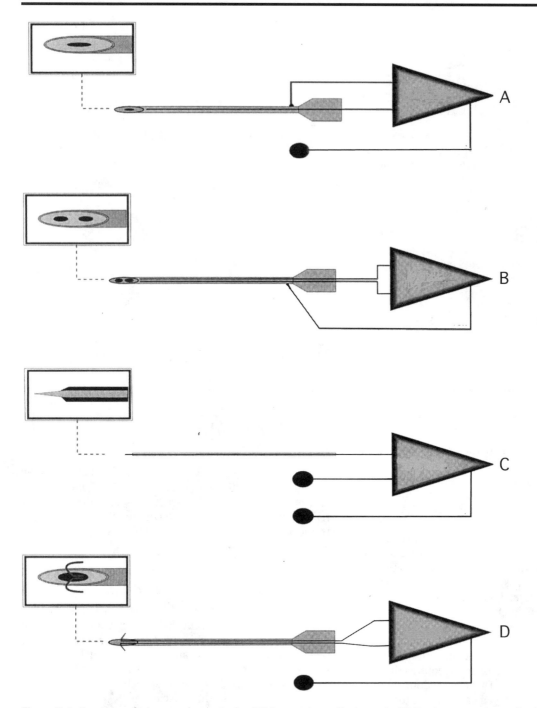

Figure 7–4 Four types of intramuscular electrodes. **(A)** Concentric needle electrode. **(B)** Bipolar concentric needle electrode. **(C)** Monopolar needle electrode. **(D)** Bipolar hooked-wire electrode.

vigorous jaw motion or relatively forcible biting. These electrodes may detect some low-level activity during speech tasks (Moore, Smith, & Ringel, 1988), but the exact source of this activity is uncertain. It could be from remote jaw muscles or from small facial muscles located under the skin close to or overlying the masseter muscle, such as the buccinator or platysma.

One skin electrode that is common to all of the recording schemes to be discussed is the electrode attached to the reference (common) input to the differential amplifier. This is a very important electrode because a stable, low-resistance contact between the skin and metal wire carrying the signal to the amplifier is critical to good noise-free recording conditions. This is facilitated by carefully cleaning the skin before the electrode is secured in place by an adhesive collar. After cleaning the skin, a conductive electrode gel is then applied to the cup of the electrode containing the metal surface, and the electrode attached to the skin.

The metal inside the electrode cup is a complicated material generally made of compressed silver powder and special ingredients known only to the manufacturer. In our experience, some commercial skin electrodes are better than others, and all of the good ones are surprisingly expensive (but well worth the cost). Large commercial disposable electrodes made for hospital recording of the electrocardiogram (ECG) are too large for placing over most muscles, but they make excellent skin electrodes for the reference electrode. They come with the gel and adhesive collar in place, and because of their large size, they provide an excellent electrical contact without excessive skin preparation.

Rigid Needle Electrodes

The needle electrode for recording the EMG is basically a long thin hypodermic needle with one or two insulated wires in the lumen. If there is one wire, the needle is usually called a concentric EMG electrode. If there are two wires, then it is called a concentric bipolar electrode. When using a concentric electrode, one input of the differential amplifier is connected to the center wire of the electrode. The other amplifier input is connected to the shaft of the hypodermic needle, which is essentially held at a neutral reference voltage by its large uninsulated area. This electrode can be quite selective in recording single motor units. The third wire, going to the reference input of the amplifier, is connected to the reference point on the patient (the skin of the forehead is often convenient when studying cranial muscles).

When using concentric bipolar electrodes, the inputs to the differential amplifier are connected to the two wires in the lumen of the needle. The uninsulated shaft of the needle is usually connected to the reference input of the amplifier. The concentric bipolar electrode is more selective than the concentric electrode, particularly if the needle can be rotated when in place. This can change the alignment of the two exposed wire tips at the lumen of the needle with respect to the direction of the muscle fibers; such alignment can have a dramatic effect on the degree to which a particular muscle action potential can be selectively isolated. From a practical standpoint, concentric bipolar electrodes are more expensive than concentric electrodes, and thus they are used mainly for research or specialized studies. They are also too selective for many EMG studies.

Monopolar EMG electrodes are insulated solid needles whose tips has been bared of the insulating material. The wire from the needle is connected to one input of the differential amplifier, and the other input of the amplifier is connected to a skin electrode placed as close as possible to the location of the needle insertion. The reference input is connected to a second skin electrode, which can be placed at a more distant location. One might suppose it would be simpler to connect the second input of the amplifier directly to the reference input, but this generally increases the response of the system to external noise. Monopolar electrodes record muscle activity just as well as the other types, but they are also more responsive to activity generated in muscles distant to the one being studied; that is, they are less selective. The monopolar arrangement is, in effect, the type of recording configuration used when one records from the tip of an insulated hypodermic needle used to inject botulinum toxin in a laryngeal muscle. This technique allows the physician to know that the electrode tip is in a laryngeal muscle when the toxin is injected.

Rigid needle electrodes are used almost exclusively in EMG diagnostic clinics, such as those found in departments of neurology. This is because the waveform and firing patterns of single motor units are of primary interest in diagnosing most neurological diseases that affect muscle activity. These electrodes can be advanced and withdrawn by the clinician to isolate particular units. When used in muscles directly under the skin during isometric contraction, in which there is relatively little actual movement of the muscle tissue, these electrodes are relatively painless to the patient and do little damage to the muscle. When used to record from small or thin muscles, particularly during functions that involve significant movements, this type of electrode has serious problems. First of all, an EMG interference pattern, as distinct from single motor unit activity, is useful for determining whether and how much a muscle can be activated. Concentric bipolar electrodes are very selective for single motor units, so one might see little, if any, evidence of activity in a normal muscle, even at fairly high levels of activation. Another serious problem is that movement of a muscle with a rigid needle in it can be quite painful. Pain from this source may have large effects on the motor neuron pool that one is attempting to study, as well as hurt the patient. If the larynx, pharynx, or other oral structure remained very still, this probably would not be a significant factor, but large, vigorous, movements occur during speaking and swallowing. Furthermore, these movements could cause the population of motor units under observation to change each time they occur. This would make it difficult to quantitatively compare a current EMG record with one taken before the movement occurred. Thus, keep in mind that rigid EMG electrodes are not the only or necessarily the best electrodes when one is attempting to study natural movements, particularly of the articulators.

The main advantage of rigid needle electrodes is that they may be advanced and withdrawn in the muscle to explore various parts of a muscle, or to explore other muscles. The potentials they record during short periods of relative immobility of muscles can provide valuable information. Such information has to do with the shape of action potentials. These potentials can confirm diagnoses of diseases such as ALS or indicate whether a muscle is being reinnervated. When these are the main diagnostic questions, the EMG recording and interpretation are obviously best done by an experienced neurologist.

Bipolar Hooked-Wire Electrodes

Hooked-wire electrodes were first used by Basmajian and Stecko (1962), who, in collaboration with several colleagues, described the activity of many muscles of the body during natural movements. These observations are summarized in a classic book, *Muscles Alive* (Basmajian & DeLuca, 1985). This type of intramuscular electrode has also been used for study and assessment of laryngeal muscles (Gartlan, Peterson,

Luschei, Hoffman, & Smith, 1993; Hirano & Ohala, 1969; Hirose, 1987; Koda & Ludlow, 1992), tongue (Hrycyshyn & Basmajian, 1972), velum (Basmajian & Dutta, 1961; Fritzell, 1969; Kuehn, Folkins, & Cutting, 1982), and pharynx (Palmer, Tanaka, & Siebens, 1989; Perlman, Luschei, & DuMond, 1989), as well as some combinations of these muscles (O' Dwyer, Neilson, Guitar, Quinn, & Andrews, 1983; Schaefer et al, 1992). They are made with two very fine, flexible, insulated wires. For recording gross EMG, approximately 1 mm of insulation is removed from each wire. These two wires are placed in the lumen of a suitable hypodermic needle so that the bared portions extend just beyond the tip, and then the ends of the wire are bent over to form a hook. When the needle is placed into the muscle and then withdrawn, the hooks catch in the muscle and the wires are left behind in the muscle. Because of the flexibility of the wires, the muscle may make large movements without causing pain. Most people find these electrodes quite comfortable. They may be left in place during repeated measures of speech and swallowing.

Although there are several good reasons for using hooked-wire electrodes, they have the major disadvantage of not permitting adjustments of the electrode position once the hypodermic needle has been withdrawn. Obviously the electrode cannot be pushed further into the muscle. One could imagine (naively) that one could gently tug on the wires and pull them along the route of the wires through the muscle. To do this, however, the hooks have to be straightened out, and once this is done, the wires do not generally remain in the muscle. For all practical purposes, we get one attempt per needle. When recording from laryngeal muscles, it is advisable to have extra electrode assemblies to try a second or third time to get the wires into the desired muscle.

Choosing the wire for these electrodes is a compromise between using wires that are too ductile and wires that are too stiff. Very ductile wires can be inserted with very fine needles and cause no sensation in the muscle. But their hooks are very weak, and they often do not hook into the muscle and get pulled out with the needle. On the other hand, their weak hooks probably do minimal damage when these wires have to be pulled out after the recording is over. Stainless steel wire with an uninsulated diameter of 50 or 75 μm (0.002 or 0.003 inch) are the most widely used types of wire. They generally hold the hook, and produce only a slight "funny feeling" in the muscle. They probably damage some muscle cells when the hook is pulled out, but there is no pain associated with this event, so the damage is quite limited (Jaffe, Solomon, Robinson, Hoffman, & Luschei, 1998). Single-strand 50- to 75-μm stainless steel wire with various types of insulation is available in small quantities from general vendors in the United States. Some companies will fabricate special configurations of fine wire (usually for a minimum order of 1000 feet). One such configuration, "bifilar," where two strands of wire are bonded together along their entire length, has two advantages over using two wires that are not bonded together. First, the bared ends of bonded wire remain in a fixed relationship, and in particular cannot "short together" in the muscle as it moves. Second, the fact that the two wires have to move together greatly reduces their tendency to produce movement artifacts and microphonics when they are mechanically disturbed. An explanation of this property is offered later in the chapter.

Once the wire is chosen, one has to select a needle size. A 25-gauge hypodermic needle is suitable for a pair of 75-μm-diameter wires. In some cases, one can choose a smaller needle that will accept the wires, but the fit is so close that the wires often get "hung up" when the needle is withdrawn, so the wires get pulled out; the wires have to have enough room in the lumen of the needle to accommodate slight bends in the wire. A single strand of insulated 75-μm wire can be inserted with a 30-gauge needle, but this requires two needle insertions for differential recording. The larger electrode spacing obtained in this case may be advantageous, however, if the goal is to sample a large area of a muscle.

When placing the electrode in a package for sterilization, it is important to use a relatively large package so that the wires may be loosely looped in a way that allows them to be straightened out without forming kinks when the package is opened. Once formed, these kinks are impossible to remove. Because the hypodermic needle cannot be pulled past a kink in the wire, such an electrode might as well be discarded before ever being inserted into the muscle.

Connecting the amplifier to fine wires can be more troublesome than one might suppose. If one uses very long pieces of fine wire, then these leads may be taken directly to the inputs to the amplifier and put under a screw-type terminal (gold-plated surfaces are a very good idea). However, these long wires have a tendency to become tangled and form kinks when removed from the sterilization packages. The wires may be kept much shorter if the amplifier has a preamplifier stage in a small box that can be placed close to the patient. Such a preamplifier stage may have screw-type terminals as well, but the small spacing usually makes it desirable to have a wire "grabber" that requires less manipulation than a screw terminal. One may use spring-loaded commercial grabbers, for example, Pamona Minigrabber 3925, but keep in mind that the very small size of the wire requires a close-tolerance fit of the jaws, and that an oxide coating on either the wires or the grabber surfaces can cause electrical noise that can interfere with recording. Grabbers with gold-plated surfaces are, for this reason, much to be preferred. We currently use gold-plated extension springs to make contact with the fine wires. The springs are bent to open a few loops, the wire inserted between them, and the spring allowed to straighten out. They seem to be a significant improvement over other methods we have used previously.

Amplifiers

To detect and study the activity of muscles requires one or more differential amplifiers that have a selection of gains between approximately 1000 and 50,000 (60 to 94 dB), with a bandpass between 30 Hz and 5 kHz. These characteristics are easily obtained with modern electronics. In a clinical situation, it is often difficult to control external sources of 60-Hz interference, so a 60-Hz notch filter in the amplifier can be quite helpful. A very important feature of the amplifier is its common mode rejection ratio (CMRR). When used with the proper electrode configuration, an amplifier with a high CMRR is the most effective way to prevent amplification of the 60-Hz electrical fields. There are companies that manufacture amplifier systems that are marketed specifically for recording EMG activity. They are expensive, but are worth the investment, because they have many if not most of the features discussed above, and are designed and built with the safety of the patient in mind.

Whatever amplifier is purchased or fabricated, it is crucial that it include an isolation stage. The function of an isolation stage is to avoid having the patient connected to earth ground. Connecting a subject to earth ground with a low-resistance electrode (the large skin electrode) is essentially like standing the patient in a bathtub. In this condition, the patient could be electrocuted by coming into contact with any equipment that is electrically "hot."

In the scheme illustrated earlier, such isolation is represented by using radio signals to transmit the output of the first stage of amplification to the earth-grounded part of the system. In this case, the patient could theoretically be on the moon! *It is nearly impossible to accidentally electrocute anyone who has no electrical connection to earth ground!* Use of the proper equipment eliminates this danger, but it is possible for a person to unwittingly defeat this safety feature by connecting the reference electrode to earth ground, or, for example, by having the patient sit on a grounded chair. It should be noted that radio transmission is certainly not the most common way of achieving isolation. It was chosen for illustration because it is intuitively easy to understand. The same effect can be achieved by using modulated light or magnetic fields to couple the signal across a gap that keeps the patient totally isolated from earth ground.

Setting the appropriate gain of an amplifier is a matter of some judgment. Usually, the gain is set so that the largest potentials observed stay within the input range of the recording instrument. If one suspects muscle paralysis, or is seeking evidence of low-level activity, one should not hesitate to try the highest gains on the amplifier, even if some other events or noise go outside the range. Some motor unit activity in a muscle is very small and can hide within the noise of the baseline if gains of 1000 to 5000 are the only ones used. Unless higher gains are used, the failure to observe activity in a muscle cannot be safely interpreted to mean that the muscle is paralyzed.

Monitors

A type of monitor that has traditionally been used with the EMG is an audio amplifier connected to a loudspeaker. This type of monitor has several advantages. It is inexpensive, it does not have to be watched, and clinicians, with some experience, can use their ears to perform an acoustic analysis that can provide critical on-line information. For example, the sound of muscle activity that is close to an intramuscular electrode sounds crisp because it has mainly high-frequency components. EMG from muscles located at greater distance has a dull sound. This is because the tissue that intervenes between the EMG source and the electrodes acts like a low-pass filter (DeLuca, 1979). Single motor unit spikes, which are produced by the near-simultaneous action potentials in

the muscle cells innervated by the same motor neuron, produce a "crack" or a "pop," which has a unitary sound. The ear can quickly detect the pattern and rate of firing of a single motor unit. In fact, subjects who can control their muscles can quickly learn to turn a unit on and off by listening to its discharges. An inexpensive receiver amplifier, which can be purchased from a commercial electronics store for a little over $100, is quite adequate for this purpose.

The limitations of an audio monitor are that it provides no permanent record and that the amplitude of the EMG cannot be determined with any precision. The audio monitor also cannot reveal the presence of some problems such as high-frequency interference (as from a nearby video monitor) and large low-frequency movement artifacts. Another problem with audio monitors is that they produce a terrible 60-Hz din when the electrode is removed or a wire becomes detached. A very good idea is to have an audio monitor with a handy volume control, or have an assistant anticipate the blast and turn the volume down before it happens.

A visual monitor such as an oscilloscope or a computer capable of providing on-line display of waveforms is very useful. It can be used to reveal the many types of artifacts that interfere with EMG recording, and by knowing the gain of the amplifier that is being used, it can be used to estimate the actual amplitude of the signals. Waveforms that cannot be discriminated by the audio monitor carry potentially important information. If an oscilloscope were to be purchased for this use, then a very basic digital oscilloscope, costing about $1000, would be quite adequate. A digital oscilloscope can "freeze" a picture on-line, and thus the EMG signal can be studied to make a decision during the procedure. Older analogue oscilloscopes are still quite useful, however, for verification of the signal's basic characteristics.

There are also computer hardware/software systems (see later discussion) that are very useful for on-line monitoring.

Data Acquisition and Storage Devices

It is very important for clinicians making decisions based on EMG recordings to be able to directly compare records from different patients. Historically, polygraph records or tape recorders have been used for permanent storage of EMG records. Both of these instruments have been historically important, but both have limitations for storing data and for its subsequent display and analysis. Another approach, made possible by the recent development of powerful but inexpensive computer systems, is direct digitization of EMG records and streaming of these data to a computer disk. Commercial software systems operating on personal computers are currently capable of continuously acquiring and storing 16-bit data at 50,000 samples per second. This would make it possible, for example, to acquire data on four channels of EMG at a sampling rate of 12,500 samples per second, quite fast enough to resolve the finest details of the waveform of a motor unit response. Some software/-hardware data acquisition systems provide a continuous display of the EMG traces, whether or not data are actually being stored to disk, so they provide a very good visual monitor of the records as well as a means of data storage. These same computer programs can also provide a method of quantitatively analyzing the EMG records. The use of one such data acquisition and analysis system, developed by DATAQ Instruments, Inc. (Akron, OH), will be illustrated later in the discussion on data analysis.

Direct digitization and storage of EMG recordings unquestionably produces very large data files. Consider, for example, the need to store 10 minutes of data at 50,000 samples per second. Remember each sample needs two bytes of storage (assuming 16-bit analogue/digital [A/D] conversion). This would produce a record of almost 60 megabytes. Although this is certainly a large file, the current state of computer disk technology is such that a 300-gigabyte disk is routinely available and relatively inexpensive. Such a disk could store 50,000 minutes of data at the rates mentioned above, enough for almost five weeks of continuous recording.

Although it is natural to look at data storage systems in terms of technical problems and costs, the most important factors, in the long run, are those related to ease of access. Simply put, stored data that are not looked at and analyzed are absolutely worthless. If data are stored in a way that requires a great deal of human time to access or analyze, they may never be used, and if they are, the labor costs for this process may easily wipe out any savings associated with a less expensive storage system or storage medium. In this respect, directly digitized and archived EMG recordings have great advantages. The fact that we do not already have well-established norms for using EMG for diagnostic purposes is probably a result of the prodigious task of analyzing EMG with the instruments that have previously been available for storing and analyzing these records. The development of digital data acquisition systems that are currently evolving will change this situation dramatically.

♦ Source and Recognition of Artifactual Signals and Noise

The 60-Cycle Beast

The electricity supplied to homes, hospitals, and laboratories by power companies in the United States comes out of the wall as a 60-Hz sine wave at a root-mean-square voltage of approximately 115 V. This power line signal often contaminates EMG records. In dealing with 60-cycle interference, there are three important steps to take:

1. Minimize the electrode impedance, including the impedance of the reference electrode.

2. Remove the sources of the interference.

3. Shield against the interference, and/or selectively filter it out of the amplification process.

Reducing Source Impedance

Other factors being the same, the size of the 60-cycle problem one encounters can be related to the source resistance of the electrodes, which in this case is the sum of the resistances from each electrode to the reference electrode. Consider the extreme: Suppose you directly connect both input electrodes to the reference electrode with a short piece of wire; you could put that electrode configuration in the middle of a generator and you would not have a problem! At the opposite extreme, suppose the electrodes are open, that is, there is nothing but air between the electrodes and the reference electrode. The source impedance is now the input impedance of the amplifier, which is extremely high. In this condition, very small 60-cycle fields are able to create comparatively large voltages (but see later discussion on blocking of amplifiers). There is really little that one can do about the resistance of the electrode contact when using needle or hooked-wire electrodes. One has a small area of bared stainless steel wire in the muscle, and that is that. The thing that one *can* do something about is the resistance between the reference electrode and skin of the patient. Good skin preparation or use of large gel electrodes, such as those for ECG recording in intensive care units, is helpful. Appreciation of the effect of having a high source impedance helps recognize a frequent problem in EMG recording: the mysterious appearance of high levels of 60-cycle noise where it was absent earlier in the recording, or where exactly the same conditions were used in a previous recording session. The best guess is that either a connection is open somewhere in the circuit (e.g., a tiny break in the wire), or there is an air bubble between the gel in the skin electrode and the metallic part of the electrode.

Eliminating the Source of the 60-Cycle Field

Interference from 60-cycle sources comes from two types of fields. The easy problem (usually) to solve is caused by inductive fields from transformers or wires carrying large AC currents that are physically close to the electrodes. The 60-cycle interference from inductive sources usually has a characteristic waveform, which does not contain "spikes" **(Fig. 7–5)**. We cannot shield against this type of field, but physically moving the source of the magnetic field away from the recording site is usually sufficient to solve the problem. Moving just a few feet sometimes helps a great deal.

The other type of 60-cycle interference comes from electrostatic influences. Any two conductors separated by an insulator form a capacitor. If a capacitor has a significant capacitance (a number that indicates how much charge can be stored at a given voltage difference between the conductors), then an AC voltage impressed upon one of the conductors can "couple" some fraction of that AC voltage to the other conductor. Large currents do not have to flow to cause this type of interference. Equipment that is plugged into the wall socket, even if it is not turned on, can cause problems. The power cord to the equipment, and the wires running internally to the power switch, can form a conductor having peak voltages of ±160 V with respect to ground. Any other conductor in the area, in particular the leads to the amplifier, can have a large AC voltage coupled to it if the resistance to ground is large (see earlier discussion of source impedance). In this case, the insulator between the plates of

Typical 60-cycle noise waveforms

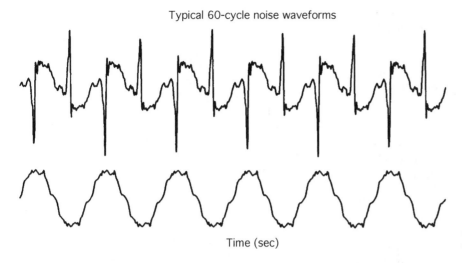

Time (sec)

Figure 7–5 Typical waveforms of 60–cycle noise from fluorescent lights **(A)** and from power cord inductive field **(B).** Traces are 0.1 second in duration, and therefore show exactly six cycles.

this capacitor is the air in the room. One strategy for finding the source of a 60-cycle interference problem is to systematically unplug any unnecessary equipment in the vicinity of the recording site. If the equipment has to be plugged in when recording, then sometimes moving the offending equipment to another location is helpful.

Fluorescent lights can be a terrible problem. They all have a ballast (a transformer) in them, which increases the voltage across the fluorescent tube to approximately 750 V. The waveform of this type of interference typically has large spikes in it **(Fig. 7–5).** The waveforms seen can vary a great deal, but they always have a period of 16.667 ms. Keep in mind that a 60-Hz notch filter does not attenuate these spikes at all, so one should check the period of regular spikes of any type having a frequency of 60 Hz, even if there is no evidence of a sinusoidal waveform. Turning off fluorescent lights close to the recording site usually gets rid of the problem, but if one has to use high amplifier gains, then one may have to turn off all the fluorescent lights. Incandescent lights, which use only 115 V, cause far less interference.

One factor that seems to greatly increase 60-cycle interference is the presence of large ungrounded metal structures of any type close to the patient or amplifier. For example, we have found it very helpful to earth-ground the metal frame holding the patient's bed so as to eliminate 60-cycle noise problems in a minor surgery room used for EMG recording. It is important to note that the patient was not in contact with this frame, so this arrangement did not ground the patient.

Shielding and Filtering

After the sources of the 60-cycle noise have been minimized, there are two additional strategies to reduce 60-cycle interference: shielding and filtering. A sound-deadened chamber can become an excellent environment for recording and is sometimes available. Its grounded metal walls absorb all electrostatic noise from outside the room. It is easy to destroy the shielding properties of a metal-shielded room, however, by bringing power cords or even an ungounded wire into the room from the outside. In particular, putting fluorescent lights inside the shielded room totally destroys its effectiveness.

Some clinicians shield the leads going from the patient to the amplifier, but this makes the leads rather stiff and much heavier than is desirable. A much more common strategy that accomplishes the same thing is to use a small input stage on the amplifier (a first-stage amplifier in a small box) that is held close to the patient. Thus the leads can be kept fairly short. If these leads are only a few feet long, then putting them in a cable with a braided shield really does not help much. Shielded input leads can also be a major source of movement artifact (discussed later), so we recommend short unshielded leads to a preamplifier located close to the patient. Although the primary attempt to control 60-cycle noise should be to get rid of the source, some environments, such as a surgical facility, make this very difficult. In this case, 60-cycle notch filters can be very helpful. They help by reducing the 60-cycle component of the noise 10-fold, compared with what it would be without the filter. They also produce corresponding amplitude and phase distortions of the biological signals in this frequency range, but that should not be a problem for diagnostic EMG recording.

Besides 60-cycle noise, one can encounter other forms of extraneous noise signals, such as high-frequency fields from televisions or computer monitors. Interference from a TV monitor is seen on the oscilloscope as a broad band of fuzz around the recorded signal. It cannot be heard on the audio monitor, because most audio amplifiers cannot reproduce it, and most older clinicians cannot hear that high a sound (about 16 kHz). Generally it is not a serious problem, but too much interference can block the input stage of the amplifier and thus affect amplification of the EMG signal. The easiest solution is to move the TV monitor as far away from the patient as possible. A few feet of movement can often totally eliminate the problem.

Movement Artifacts

Another type of artifact is related to movement of the electrode leads between the patient and the amplifier inputs. In most cases, these electrode lead movements cause large low-frequency excursions of the recording baseline. A "tap," or high-frequency vibration, of the leads may also cause artifactual signals whose frequency components are high enough to be in the pass band of the amplifier. In fact, they sound like someone tapping on the bottom of a metal can when heard over the audio monitor. An important source of movement artifact is the electrochemical system at the interface of the electrode, which is a metallic conductor in a salt solution. There is usually a significant DC junction potential at each electrode. In effect, each electrode acts like a miniature battery. The voltage from this battery charges the distributed capacitance of the electrode lead with respect to ground. Movements of the electrode leads cause changes in the distributed capacitances, and changes in these capacitors cause charging and discharging currents to flow back and forth across the electrode resistance, thus producing voltage changes. If the changes in the capacitance of both electrode leads are exactly the same, the voltage changes produced across each electrode are identical and thus are not amplified by a differential amplifier; that is, they are a "common-mode signal." This conceptual model of movement artifact would explain why the use of bi-filar wires, where both electrode leads have to move together, dramatically reduces problems with movement artifact.

Sometimes one sees a sinusoidal signal at the frequency of phonation when recording from laryngeal muscles, but one should not suppose that this is phase-locking of the EMG. This is another version of movement artifact. The wires going to the amplifier are probably vibrating at the frequency of phonation. Another type of movement artifact may be observed when using hooked-wire electrodes: rather large spikes associated with starting or stopping of voicing. They look somewhat like large single motor unit signals, except for two things. They are usually monophasic (go in only one direction from the baseline), and they typically have much longer durations than motor unit responses. Although they may occur several times in each burst, they do not exhibit a repetitive pattern at a respectable rate, such as 10 to 50 spikes per second. One possible cause of these large spikes would be intermittent contact of the two wires of the electrode within the muscle. Such contact would discharge the "standing" electrochemical junction potential (see above).

Even with bipolar hooked-wire electrodes having large tip exposures, it is fairly common to observe single motor unit activity in most muscles. One has to separate these potentials from artifacts that can produce spike-like potentials in the record. Real single motor unit potentials are distinguished by several features: (1) they are almost always biphasic; (2) they usually fire at least several times in a row at rather regular intervals; (3) they generally correlate with some aspect of motor activity; (4) they do not correspond to external events, such as a piece of electronic equipment being switched on and off; and (5) they do not fire at a steady interval of 16.667 ms (the interval of 60-cycle interference). Another thing to look for, when recording from two or more muscles, are potentials occurring simultaneously in two or more channels. Such events are very unlikely to be biological in their origin. They can result from irregular power line transients, sometimes caused by large motors in another part of the building being turned on or off. We have seen strange potentials of this variety quite often when recording in a surgical suite.

Blocking of Amplifiers

If the lead to the reference electrode or either of the input electrodes is open, that is, has an extremely high resistance, the output of many (if not most) modern EMG amplifiers will show a perplexing behavior that can be quite confusing to the novice. The amplifier output may be very quiet for extended periods of time, as if there were absolutely no muscle activity, and even noise signals will be absent. Then one may observe brief periods of high-amplitude 60-cycle noise or large movement artifacts that gradually die out, eventually leaving a quiet baseline once again.

These periods of noise recording can usually be produced at will by moving the leads to the electrodes, or by any movements of the preamplifier or the patient. This is the behavior of a blocked amplifier, and it can only be corrected by establishing a reasonable resistance from each electrode to the reference electrode and making sure the reference electrode is connected to the reference input of the amplifier. Blocking in an amplifier is caused by the very small currents that have to flow from the input transistors. In modern amplifiers these currents are in the picoampere range, and so are ordinarily of no consequence. However, if they have no path back to the reference input of the amplifier, they will create a relatively large DC differential signal at the inputs. This causes the first-stage amplifier to "saturate" its output at the plus or minus power supply voltage. Subsequent high-pass amplifier circuits, always present in an EMG amplifier system, turn this steady DC voltage into a steady zero-voltage output. Any movements of the wires or electrodes momentarily allow this input current to redistribute itself, and thereby amplify the noise signals that one ordinarily sees when the electrodes have a very high resistance. Pragmatically, the main lesson is this: if you observe a very quiet baseline, interrupted by strange episodes of recording, check to see that you have intact electrode wires and good connections to the amplifier.

◆ Analysis of Electromyogram Records

Qualitative Analysis: Using the Calibrated Eyeball

Although it is natural, from a scientific standpoint, to gravitate toward numerical comparisons when using physical measurements for diagnostic purposes, the fact remains that probably one of the most sophisticated analyzers available to us is our own senses. Therefore, it is very useful, when using EMG records to understand and diagnose dysarthrias, to be able to locate regions of interest in the record and then observe them in detail. In doing this, however, certain simple transformations of the original waveforms may improve our ability to observe relationships in the recordings. The best way to make such observations is to use a computer program specifically designed for display and analysis of physiological recordings. **Fig. 7–6** illustrates an example of how this may be done, using a program such as Windaq (DATAQ Instruments Inc.). It is the result of an

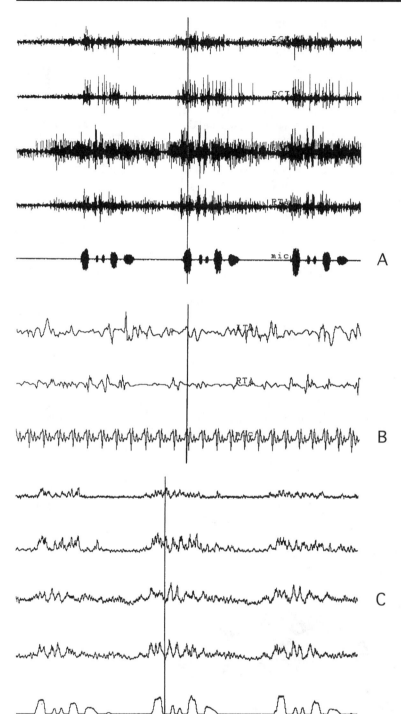

Figure 7–6 Three ways to view the same EMG record. **(A)** Compressed display. Calibration bar (upper left) represents 0.625 mV for left cricothyroid (LCT) and 1.25 mv for right cricothyroid (RCT), left thyroarytenoid (LTA), and right thyroarytenoid (RTA). **(B)** Decompressed display (bottom three traces from **A**), plotting all the data points. **(C)** Rectified and smoothed (moving average). See text for discussion.

analysis of laryngeal EMG obtained from a normal subject during three repetitions of the phrase, "Pop took his socks off." Keep in mind that this presentation is not intended as a definitive statement of how laryngeal muscles are used during speech or as a sales pitch for a particular commercial computer program. What is intended is to convey to the reader at least one approach to finding information in an EMG recording of some of the muscles involved in speech.

The recording to be presented below was obtained from a healthy and normal adult female speaker. She repeated the

phrase at normal pitch and somewhat increased loudness, using normal prosody and emphasis. Recordings were made bilaterally from the cricothyroid (CT) and thyroarytenoid (TA) muscles using bipolar hooked-wire electrodes. Amplifier gain was 2000, and the band pass of the amplifiers was 30 Hz to 5 kHz. Before being digitized on-line at a sampling rate of 5 kHz, all channels were filtered at 2.5 kHz to prevent aliasing of the signal. **Fig. 7–6A** illustrates a compressed portion of the recording. Compression of the record is accomplished by having the computer display a vertical line representing the maximum and minimum value of data in each compressed block of data (in this case, 80 data points) at each horizontal pixel of the screen. This algorithm is much preferable to other types of compression, such as just displaying every 80th data point or displaying the average of the 80 data points; it preserves the occurrence of transient responses whose duration is shorter than the duration represented by each pixel, in particular single motor unit responses. The ability to display a compressed record is very useful in locating a region in which some activity of interest is occurring. In a long record, where the subject perhaps speaks several phrases, one may determine what the subject or patient was saying by sending the data points of the microphone record to the sound-producing system of the computer being used for the analysis. It may be necessary to write or purchase special software for this task, however. It is well to keep in mind that such speech is not suitable for acoustic analysis because of the relatively low sampling rate used for recording EMG. The speech is, however, quite intelligible.

The details of the muscle activity are obscured by this degree of compression. This problem is easily solved by having the computer decrease the compression of the record corresponding to the location of the cursor. In effect, we want to magnify the record around the cursor. The decompressed record, displaying all data samples around the position of the cursor in **Fig. 7–6A,** is shown in **Fig. 7–6B.**

Even though the speaker is perfectly normal, an initial reaction to inspection of the unprocessed ("raw") EMG recordings of these laryngeal muscles is "What a bunch of junk!" There is clearly modulation of activity, but the pattern is uncertain. It might be supposed that the electrodes are not actually in the intended muscles, a possibility that always has to be considered when attempting to record from laryngeal muscles. However, certain transformation of the raw EMG

records makes it easier to recognize patterns of modulation (**Fig. 7–6C**). The raw EMG is first rectified (the sign bit of each data point is simply set to be positive). The record is then smoothed with a moving average. In this operation, the computer calculates, for each data point, the average of that data point and all the data points coming x points before and after the data point. In effect, a "window" containing $2x + 1$ samples is averaged, and the data point at the middle of this window is replaced with this average. Then the window is moved one data point to the right, and so on. In **Fig. 7–6C** the averaging window is 30 ms. The resulting record shows with more clarity the trend of EMG amplitude changes. In particular, there appears to be two peaks of activity in both TA muscles preceding the "his socks" portion of the phrase (immediately following the cursor), which correspond to two smaller peaks of activity in the CT that seem out of phase with the TA modulation. Obviously, appreciation of these features would benefit from being able to superimpose these repetitions, lining them up on some point that seems relatively invariant. This can be easily done by clipping 2.2-second portions of the record around each token, where the beginning of each of these subfiles begins exactly 1.1 second before the peak of the phrase's "his" in the microphone record. The computer program allows these subfiles to be saved in a spreadsheet format. When these files are opened in a spreadsheet program, the three tokens may be aligned in time (superimposed), and the values normalized to the highest values found in each channel. The resulting data may then be graphed, resulting in **Fig. 7–7**. In this final form, the modulation of the laryngeal muscle activity, and its repeatability, is very clear.

Even knowing that the subject studied in **Fig. 7–7** was a normal speaker, we cannot assert that this pattern of laryngeal muscle activity is normal. It could in fact be quite atypical; one would only know by applying the analysis to a

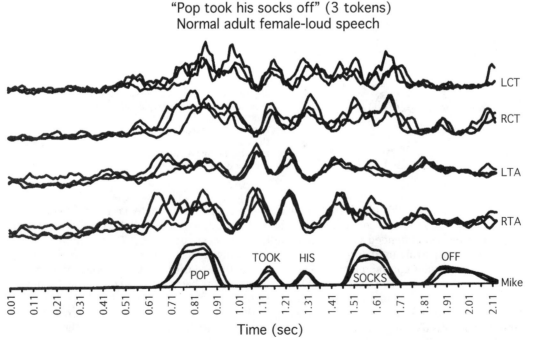

Figure 7–7 Superimposed traces of rectified and smoothed laryngeal EMG generated by a normal adult female speaker after importing the data into a spreadsheet. All trace amplitudes have been normalized to the highest value occurring in the three tokens.

large number of speakers. Had the health status of the speaker been unknown, however, the results illustrated in **Fig. 7–7** would establish important facts:

1. The nerves to the TA and CT muscle are intact bilaterally.

2. The motor neurons to these muscles are activated in a coordinated manner that seems related to speech, and thus the corticopontine neural systems controlling the laryngeal motor neurons are intact.

3. Absence of long-duration or polyphasic single motor unit waveforms would be evidence against previous nerve injury followed by reinnervation.

With additional research it eventually may be possible to make more detailed interpretations of these records. Asymmetric modulation of pairs of muscles involved in speech, or absence of modulation, may be characteristic of some diseases of the nervous system.

If one were to pursue research into the modulation of the laryngeal EMG during speech, the method described above, using Windaq and a spreadsheet, would be very laborious and time consuming. Windaq is most useful for scanning data and to make subfiles ("clippings") of interest. Matlab (The Math Works, Inc. Natick, MA) is a program that has been profitably used by many researchers, after some simple programming, to automatically perform the entire set of operations described to make **Fig. 7–6** and **Fig. 7–7**.

Quantitative Analysis of the Electromyogram

There are two basic features of the EMG signal that can be fairly easily reduced to a constrained set of numbers: its amplitude, and its temporal properties (when it starts and stops). There are some surprisingly difficult problems about making these measurements, however, and our eventual ability to say whether a measure of EMG amplitude is normal or abnormal will depend on attention to these details. Let's first consider the problem of measuring the EMG of a muscle in a patient with weakness during a static maximal response. The amplitude of this response, measured in volts, could have diagnostic value. For example, if this measure in this patient were statistically the same as in a normal subject, it would suggest that the contractile aspects of muscle, rather than muscle activation, were disordered. In arriving at this conclusion, what factors need to be considered?

Electrode Characteristics

First, the electrode type and physical configuration, such as interelectrode spacing, that is used to make the measurement has to be the same as that used to generate the normative data. For those interested in muscles of the articulators, intramuscular electrodes are usually required. Rigid needle electrodes, in which tip exposure and electrode spacing are fixed, would have advantages in this regard, but making maximal responses could be painful and thus might interfere with the patient's ability or willingness to cooperate. Hooked-wire electrodes are not painful, even for maximal responses. Historically, their tip exposure and spacing have been treated rather casually, but this could be

easily improved, particularly by the use of bi-filar wire. Let us suppose we make the measurement with hooked-wire electrodes manufactured with great attention to the uniformity of their tip characteristics. We would still have to consider that some degree of variation will occur because of differences in the geometry of the electrode in the muscle or because of its location in a particular part of the muscle. A good example of this problem is illustrated in **Fig. 7–6A.** All EMG channels were amplified at a gain of 2000. Note that the top trace (left cricothyroid [LCT]) is displayed at twice the sensitivity as the other traces (see figure legend). From this display one may see that a 2:1 difference in the general amplitude of EMGs may be expected in a normal subject when observing bilateral pairs of muscles (which we are assuming are excited to the same degree). This problem, that of difference of EMG amplitude as a function of the inherent variability of electrode placement in a muscle, could be reduced by repeated measurements in a patient. If several electrode placements in the muscle all yielded low amplitudes, then much more significance could be attached to the observations.

Measures of Electromyogram Amplitude

Periods of relatively steady EMG may be numerically summarized in two ways: (1) rectification (taking the absolute value) and then computing the mean amplitude over an established interval, or (2) computing the root-mean-square (RMS) value of the unrectified signal over an established interval. Given the same record, these two methods give somewhat different values. The squaring operation in the RMS method gives greater weight in the final value to high-amplitude portions of the record, which are usually single motor unit responses. RMS values will obviously be larger than mean rectified EMG values, but how much larger is difficult to predict from a theoretical viewpoint.

The following example presents an empirical treatment of this problem. Six 200-ms periods representing low, medium, and high levels of EMG were chosen from the "Pop took his socks off" record shown in **Fig. 7–6A**, and the ratio of the RMS value and mean rectified value was determined from each sample. For three of the muscles, the ratio was about 1.5 and did not change much as the EMG signal increased from small to large. The left thyroarytenoid (LTA) ratio, however, did decrease as the signal became larger, and the ratio for LCT was substantially smaller (1.2) than the other muscles. This is just an example, but it makes it clear that there is a complex relationship between RMS and mean rectified EMG amplitudes. The use of either measure is not right or wrong, but the use of mean rectified EMG seems much more common in current publications than the use of RMS values.

Another detail to be considered when attempting to quantify EMG amplitude is the sampling rate used to digitize the signal. Whatever rate is chosen, the signal has to be low-pass filtered at a cutoff frequency of half the sampling rate to avoid the creation of false (aliased) components. Such filters are often called anti-alias filters. Thus, all high-frequency components of the EMG signal above the cutoff frequency of the anti-alias filter will be greatly attenuated. If the EMG signal contains large high-frequency components, then the mean rectified or RMS value of this signal will obviously be spuriously low if these high frequencies are removed before they are digitized. One might avoid this problem by using a very high sampling rate, but then one would be wasting a great deal of storage space and processing time to work with the resulting large files. Spectral analysis of a typical example of EMG signal can provide this information. For example, the spectra were computed of EMG signals recorded from the wrist extensor muscles of one of the authors using skin electrodes and also an intramuscular bipolar hooked-wire electrode. Signals from both electrode pairs were anti-alias filtered at 5 kHz and digitized at 10 kHz. The skin electrodes produced an EMG signal whose high-frequency components (above 300 Hz) were attenuated by 20 dB or more. The dominant frequency component was around 100 Hz. Therefore, one can conclude that digitizing EMG from large skin electrodes at rates of around 600 Hz provides an accurate measures of EMG amplitude. The situation was very different for the intramuscular recording, however. The spectrum of this signal did not fall to an attenuation level of 20 dB until frequencies of 2 kHz were reached, and the dominant frequency was approximately 300 Hz. This little experiment illustrates why we routinely use 5-kHz sampling for our studies of intramuscular EMG.

Measuring the Temporal Characteristics of Electromyogram Activity

The duration and timing of EMG activity of muscles used in speech and swallowing have potential diagnostic value. In most respects, making these measures is merely a matter of placing the cursor at the beginning, peak, or end of periods of activity (a burst of EMG) and having the computer record the time of the cursor position. Although this sounds simple, anyone who has actually done this task has quickly come to discover that the beginning or end of EMG activity usually is somewhat difficult to establish with precision. The usual solution is to try to adopt some systematic rule, such as that the beginning is the first signal clearly larger than the baseline activity that persists and becomes larger. In making these judgments, however, it should be recognized that very different values can be obtained by honest and diligent observers if they use the EMG trace displayed at different gains. If the main body of the EMG burst is kept on the scale of the display, then very often the actual baseline activity cannot be seen with enough detail to know when it actually changes. It is perfectly acceptable to increase the gain of the display to see the baseline activity clearly, even if the larger amplitude activity in the EMG burst is clipped. In the end, people do their best, and check the reliability within and between observers. It is well to keep in mind, however, that very different measurements of EMG burst duration might result from the manner in which the signals to be measured are displayed on the computer.

Acknowledgments   We acknowledge the support of the National Center for Voice and Speech (grant No. P60 DC00976 from the National Institutes of Deafness and Other Communication Disorders).

References

Basmajian, J.V. & DeLuca, C.J. (1985). *Muscles Alive: Their Functions Revealed by Electromyography.* Baltimore: Williams & Wilkins

Basmajian, J.V. & Dutta, C.R. (1961). Electromyography of the pharyngeal constrictors and levator palati in man. *Anatomical Record, 139,* 561–563

Basmajian, J.V. & Stecko, G. (1962). A new bipolar electrode for electromyography. *Journal of Applied Physiology, 17,* 849

Berry, H. & Blair, R.L. (1980). Isolated vagus nerve palsy and vagal mononeuritis. *Archives of Otolaryngology, 106,* 333–338

Blair, C. & Smith, A. (1986). EMG recording in human lip muscles: can single muscles be isolated? *Journal of Speech and Hearing Research, 29,* 256–266

Blair, R.L., Berry, H., & Briant, T.D.R. (1978). Laryngeal electromyography: technique and application. *Otolaryngology Clinics of North America, 11,* 325–346

Brin, M.F., Fahn, S., Moskowitz, C., Friedman, A., Shale, H.M., Greene, P.E., Blitzer, A., List, T., Lange, D., Lovelace, R.E., & McMahon, D. (1987). Localized injections of botulinum toxin for the treatment of focal dystonia and hemifacial spasm. *Movement Disorders, 2,* 237–254

Cahan, L.D., Adams, J.M., Perry, J., & Beeler, L.M. (1990). Instrumented gait analysis after selective dorsal rhizotomy. *Developmental Medicine and Child Neurology, 32,* 1037–1043

Cohen, S.R. & Thompson, J.W. (1987). Use of botulinum toxin to lateralize true vocal cords: a biochemical method to relieve bilateral abductor vocal cord paralysis. *Annals of Otology, Rhinology, and Laryngology, 96,* 534–541

Cole, K., Konopacki, R., & Abbs, J. (1983). A miniature electrode for surface electromyography during speech. *Journal of the Acoustical Society of America, 74,* 1362

Crumley, R.L. (1989). Laryngeal synkinesis: its significance to the laryngologist. *Annals of Otology, Rhinology, and Laryngology, 98,* 87–92

DeLuca, C. (1979). Physiology and mathematics of myoelectric signals. *IEEE Transaction of Biomedical Engineering,* BME-26, 313–325.

Faaborg-Andersen, K. (1957). Electromyographic investigation of intrinsic laryngeal muscles in humans. *Acta Physiologica Scandinavica, 41,* 9–148

Fritzell, B. (1969). The velopharyngeal muscles in speech: an electromyographic and cineradiographic study. *Acta Oto-Laryngologica,* suppl 250, 1–81

Gartlan, M.G., Peterson, K.L., Luschei, E.S., Hoffman, H.T., & Smith, R.J. (1993). Bipolar hooked-wire electromyographic technique in the evaluation of pediatric vocal cord paralysis. *Annals of Otology, Rhinology, and Laryngology, 102,* 695–700

Hirano, M. & Ohala, J. (1969). Use of hooked-wire electrodes for electromyography of the intrinsic laryngeal muscles. *Journal of Speech and Hearing Research, 12,* 362–373

Hirose, H. (1987). Laryngeal articulatory adjustments in terms of EMG. In: M. Hirano, J. Kirchner, & D. Bless (Eds.), *Neurolaryngology: Recent Advances* (pp. 200–208). Boston: College-Hill

Hoffman, H.T., Brunberg, J.A., Winter, P., Sullivan, M.J., & Kileny, P.R. (1991). Arytenoid subluxation: diagnosis and treatment. *Annals of Otology, Rhinology, and Laryngology, 100,* 1–9

Hrycyshyn, A.W. & Basmajian, J.V. (1972). Electromyography of the oral stage of swallowing in man. *American Journal of Anatomy, 133,* 333–340

Iroto, I., Hirano, M., & Tomita, H. (1968). Electromyographic investigation of human vocal cord paralysis. *Annals of Otology, Rhinology, and Laryngology, 77,* 296–304

Jaffe, D.M., Solomon, N.P., Robinson, R.A., Hoffman, H.T., & Luschei E.S. (1998). Comparison of concentric needle versus hooked wire electrodes in the canine larynx. *Otolaryngology–Head and Neck Surgery, 118,* 655–662

Kimura, J. (1989). *Electrodiagnosis in Diseases of Nerve and Muscle: Principles and Practice,* 2nd ed. Philadelphia: F.A. Davis

Koda, J. & Ludlow, C.L. (1992). An evaluation of laryngeal muscle activation in patients with voice tremor. *Otolaryngology–Head and Neck Surgery, 107,* 684–696

Kuehn, D.P., Folkins, J.W., & Cutting, C.B. (1982). Relationships between muscle activity and velar position. *Cleft Palate Journal, 19,* 25–35

Loeb, G.E. & Gans, C. (1986). *Electromyography for Experimentalists.* Chicago: University of Chicago Press

Ludlow, C.L., Naunton, R.F., Terada, S., & Anderson, B.J. (1991). Successful treatment of selected cases of abductor spasmodic dysphonia using botulinum toxin injection. *Otolaryngology–Head and Neck Surgery, 104,* 849–855

McClean, M.D. (1991). Lip muscle EMG responses to oral pressure stimulation. *Journal of Speech and Hearing Research, 34,* 248–251

Miller, R.H., Woodson, G.E., & Jankovic, J. (1987). Botulinum toxin injection of the vocal fold for spasmodic dysphonia. A preliminary report. *Archives of Otolaryngology–Head and Neck Surgery, 113,* 603–605

Min, Y.B., Finnegan, E.M., Hoffman, H.T., Luschei, E.S., & McCulloch, T.M. (1994). A preliminary study of the prognostic role of electromyography in laryngeal paralysis. *Otolaryngology–Head and Neck Surgery, 111,* 70–75

Min, Y.B., Luschei, E.S., Finnegan, E.M., McCullough, T.M., & Hoffman, H.T. (1994). Portable telemetry system for electromyography. *Otolaryngology–Head and Neck Surgery, 111,* 849–852

Moore, C.A., Smith, A., & Ringel, R.L. (1988). Task-specific organization of jaw muscles. *Journal of Speech and Hearing Research, 31,* 670–680

O'Dwyer, N.J., Neilson, P.D., Guitar, B.E., Quinn, P.T., & Andrews, G. (1983). Control of upper airway structures during nonspeech tasks in normal and cerebral-palsied subjects: EMG findings. *Journal of Speech and Hearing Research, 26,* 162–170

Palmer, J.B., Tanaka, E., & Siebens, A.A. (1989). Electromyography of the pharyngeal musculature: technical considerations. *Archives of Physical Medicine and Rehabilitation, 70,* 283–287

Perlman, A.L., Luschei, E.S., & DuMond, C.E. (1989). Electrical activity from the superior pharyngeal constrictor during reflexive and nonreflexive tasks. *Journal of Speech and Hearing Research, 32,* 749–754

Piper, H. (1912). *Elektrophysiologie menschlicher Muskeln.* Berlin: Springer

Schaefer, S.D., Roark, R.M., Watson, B.C., Kondraske, G.V., Freeman, F.J., Butsch, R.W., & Pohl, J. (1992). Multichannel electromyographic observations in spasmodic dysphonia patients and normal control subjects. *Annals of Otology, Rhinology, and Laryngology, 101,* 67–75

Scott, A.B. (1980). Botulinum toxin injection into extraocular muscles as an alternative to strabismus surgery. *Journal of Pediatric Ophthalmology and Strabismus, 17,* 21–25

Smith, A., McFarland, D.H., Weber, C.M., & Moore, C.A. (1987). Spatial organization of human perioral reflexes. *Experimental Neurology, 98,* 233–248

Stager, S. & Ludlow, C. (1994). Responses of stutterers and vocal tremor patients to treatment with botulinum toxin. In: J. Janovic & M. Hallett (Eds.), *Therapy with Botulinum Toxin.* New York: Marcel Dekker.

Chapter 8

Flaccid Dysarthria

Carlin F. Hageman

Darley, Aronson, and Brown (1975) characterized *dysarthria* as a collective term used for a group of speech disorders that arise from disruptions in the neuromotor control of the muscular activities necessary for the production of speech. The dysarthrias arise from motor control disorders of neurological origin for respiration, articulation, resonance, and prosody. Darley et al specifically noted that dysarthria can include speech disorders arising from an isolated injury to a specific cranial nerve affecting even one speech function such as velopharyngeal competence. However, flaccid dysarthria can arise from a variety of etiologies that may affect multiple cranial nerves, and flaccid dysarthria can coexist with other types of dysarthria. This chapter discusses dysarthria that is the result of injuries to any component of the motor unit of the cranial and peripheral nerves that support speech production.

The peripheral nervous system (PNS) is either the first or final common pathway for all sensorimotor functions. For motor activities, all signals arising in the central nervous system (CNS) that will elicit muscle contractions to produce movements must pass through the final common pathway (FCP), which includes the lower motor neuron (LMN). These LMNs arise from motor nuclei in the brainstem and the spinal cord. Each LMN innervates a specific set of muscle fibers that together compose a motor unit. Yorkston, Beukelman, and Bell (1988) noted that a variety of speech problems can occur depending on the location and etiology of the injury to the motor unit. Practical questions concerning the assessment and management of flaccid dysarthria demand that we take a closer look at the components and neural excitation of the motor unit.

♦ Motor Unit

Darley et al (1975) recognized that the motor unit consists of four parts: (1) the neuron cell bodies in the cranial nerve nuclei in the brainstem and in the spinal nerve nuclei in the anterior horns of the spinal cord, (2) the axon that leaves the CNS and continues to the muscle, (3) the myoneural junction, and (4) the muscle fibers innervated by the LMN. A full discussion of the motor unit is beyond the scope of this chapter and interested readers are referred to Bear, Connors, and Paradiso (1996) or Bhatnagar (2002). However, two important points need to be made. First, a breakdown in the function of the LMN or motor unit can occur at

any of the four levels (e.g., demyelinization of the axon, disruption of neuromuscular transmitter at the synapse, or disturbance of the structural or neurochemical properties of the neuron). Second, an axon arborizes within a motor unit, innervating many muscle fibers, and individual muscle fibers from one motor unit may intermingle with fibers from another motor unit. As a result, Basmajian and DeLuca (1985) noted that a single action potential does not characterize a motor unit; rather, a motor unit is distinguished by many action potentials at several sites in the motor unit.

♦ Innervation of Muscle

A skeletal muscle can have thousands of muscle fibers but many fewer motor units. Those muscles generating large forces have a relatively larger number of muscle fibers per motor unit compared with those muscles responsible for fine, discrete movements that have relatively few muscle fibers per motor unit. The innervation ratio refers to the ratio of axons to muscle fibers (Larson, 1989). Muscles of the leg may have a few hundred fibers per motor unit (innervation ratio of 100 to 1), whereas muscles of the larynx or finger may have as few as 10 fibers per motor unit (innervation ratio of 10 to 1). A lower innervation ratio means that muscle contractions can be more finely tuned.

Contractile Properties of Muscle

Strength, power, endurance, and fatigue are four characteristics of muscle contraction (Liss, Kuehn, & Hinkle, 1994). Strength is the maximum force generated by a muscle or group of muscles, regardless of time. Power, a force measure, is time dependent (force generated over a specified time). Endurance is defined as the ability of a muscle to maintain a submaximal level of contraction for a specified time period. Finally, fatigue is exhibited by a muscle when it cannot maintain a specified level of force without increasing neural drive. Bigland-Ritchie and Woods (1984) defined the threshold for fatigue as a level of exercise that cannot be sustained indefinitely. Robin, Somodi, and Luschei (1991) noted that many variables can affect fatigue (or endurance), including motivation and central recruitment of motor units. (See Clark [2003] for systematic review of these issues for the speech-language pathologist.) Robin et al (1991) reported a technique for measuring tongue strength and fatigue (or endurance) using an instrument that became the Iowa Oral Performance Instrument (IOPI: Blaise Medical, Inc., Hendersonville, TN). Stierwalt and Robin (1996) and Youmans and Stierwalt (2006), among others, have utilized the IOPI in assessing and treating tongue strength for speaking and swallowing.

Liss et al (1994) explained the physical correlates of strength, power, and endurance, which included muscle fiber type and cross-sectional area of muscle fibers. The type of muscle fiber determines the strength, power, and endurance capabilities because the muscle fiber contractile properties specify the contraction speed, fatigability, and metabolic characteristics. Chusid (1985) noted that striated muscle can be grossly categorized as red or white. Red, or type I, muscle responds slowly (slow contracting or slow twitching) but is fatigue resistant because red muscle has an oxidative mechanism for muscle contraction. These muscles are adapted for long, slow postural control activities. White, or type II, muscle typically has fewer muscle fibers per motor unit and has short response times (fast contracting or fast twitching), but it fatigues more quickly because white muscle has an anaerobic metabolism specialized for fine skilled movements such as hand, tongue, and eye movements. Liss et al noted that muscle physiologists have further divided type II muscle into (1) type IIA, which contracts quickly but remains fatigue-resistant; (2) type IIB, which contracts quickly but is fatigue sensitive; and (3) type IIC, which is found in embryonic muscle and in degenerating and regenerating muscle and has functional contraction properties between those of type I and type II muscle fibers.

Breakdown of the Motor Unit

At the level of the motor unit, there are several possibilities for breakdown of neuromuscular function. Darley et al (1975) provided a useful model for classification of the dysarthrias based on etiology and site of lesion. One could use their model to construct **Table 8–1**, which summarizes lower motor neuron and motor unit dysarthrias without regard to speech symptoms. Specific speech problems arise depending on the cranial nerve(s) affected, the location of the lesion within the peripheral nerve pathways, and the specific muscle affected.

Table 8–1 Lower Motor Neuron and Motor Unit Dysarthria

Lesion Site	Symptoms*
Brainstem or peripheral nerve reflex	Loss of muscle contraction of affected units for and voluntary activity; flaccid muscle; reduced reflexes; hypotonia, muscle atrophy, weakness, paralysis, fasciculation
Myoneural junction	Weakness, increased fatigability over short time periods
Muscle fibers	Muscle hypertrophy or atrophy, failure to relax, failure to contract, fatty infiltration and fibrosis, hypocontraction

*Chusid (1985).

Cranial Nerves

A compendium of the cranial nerves and their general functions is available from many sources (e.g., Bhatnagar, 2002) and is not presented here. However, a summary (derived from Aronson, 1990; Bhatnager, 2002; Chusid, 1985; Darley et al, 1975; Yorkston, Beukelman, Strand, & Bell, 1999) of speech-related cranial nerves with respect to origin, distribution, etiology, and symptoms is shown in **Table 8–2**.

Cranial Nerve Syndromes

The following syndromes affect the four most inferior cranial nerves: (1) Avellis's, affecting cranial nerves IX and X; (2) Schmidt's, affecting X and XI; (3) Jackson's, affecting X, XI, and XII; (4) Tapia's, affecting X and XII; (5) Babinski-Nageotte bulbar, affecting IX, X, XI, and XII with contralateral hemiplegia; (6) Wallenberg's, similar to Babinski-Nageotte but without hemiplegia; (7) Cestan-Chenais, affecting the nuclei of V, X, and XI due to thrombosis of the vertebral artery; (8) Bonnier's, affecting VIII, IX, and X with Meniere's disease–like symptoms; (9) Vernet's, involving IX, X, and XI, often resulting from a basilar skull fracture involving the jugular foramen; and (10) Villaret's, Collet's, and Sicard's (retroparotid space injury), with ipsilateral paralysis of IX, X, XI, and XII.

Muscular Weakness and Paralysis

Weakness, paresis, and paralysis are potential outcomes from insults to the motor units. What does it mean to have a weak or paretic muscle? Sustained muscle contractions are composed of a large number of twitches (contractions) of the muscle fibers supplied by the motor units. A single twitch lasts only a few milliseconds, and it can be repeated after a delay. To produce a relatively smooth, strong contraction, there is a temporal and spatial summation of motor unit contractions. The process of developing a smooth contraction could be disrupted in several ways. First, signals could be interrupted in the peripheral nerve as it courses to the muscle (e.g., trauma or demyelinating disease). The number of axons in a nerve that are affected or unaffected will determine the number of motor units stimulating the muscle and producing a twitch. Second, if the myoneural junction is disturbed so that the action potential from the presynaptic axon does not stimulate postsynaptic receptors of the muscle, then a muscle twitch will not occur. This can occur when the neurotransmitter is depleted either from chronic stimulation (fatigue) or from a disease process that interferes with neurotransmitter uptake (e.g., myasthenia gravis). Third, if the muscle is diseased (e.g., muscular dystrophies), then it may fail to twitch properly. The result is that the greater the number of disruptions, the fewer the number of twitches that can be summed across motor units to produce a smooth, strong contraction. Muscle weakness from LMN involvement is a continuum from complete paralysis to variably reduced muscle contractions.

Titze (1994) described this process in the vocal folds in which maximum forces are generated in two muscle groups where the muscle fiber twitch amplitudes are nearly equal.

Table 8–2   Nerve, Distribution, Etiologies, and Symptoms Resulting from Lesions to Cranial Nerves

Cranial Nerve V (Trigeminal)

Sensory Distribution

Ophthalmic forehead, eyes, nose, temples, and nasal mucosa maxillary teeth, upper lip, cheeks, hard palate, nasal mucosa mandibular teeth, lower lip, buccal mucosa, tongue, auditory meatus

Motor Distribution

Motor root (pons) masseter, temporal, internal and external pterygoid

Otic ganglion tensor tympani, tensor veli palatine

Mylohyoid, anterior belly of digastric

Etiologies: neuralgias, neuritis, syphilis, tuberculosis, syringobulbia

Tumors, basilar meningitis, tic douloureux, para trigeminal

Symptoms of paralysis or weakness of muscles or mastication with mandible deviation to affected side

Cranial Nerve VII (Facial)

Nerve Distribution

Sensory

Nervous intermedius taste to anterior two thirds of the tongue

Motor: temporal frontalis, orbicularis oculi, dilator naris, nasalis

Zygomatic zygomaticus, quadratus labii superior, orbicularis oris cervicofacial risorius, mentalis, quadratus labii inferior, incisivus inferior, buccinators, posterior belly of digastric, stapedius

Etiologies: Bell's palsy, middle ear infections, chilling of the face

Tumors

Symptoms: lesion outside stylomastoid foramen-affected side of mouth droops, buccal stasis of food, no wink, decreased wrinkle of forehead on affected side

Lesion in facial canal (chorda tympani)–reduced taste and salivation

Lesion in internal auditory meatus–deafness and facial weakness

Lesion at emergence from pons–facial weakness and other cranial nerve involvement

Cranial Nerve IX (Glossopharyngeal)

Nerve Distribution

Sensory: fibers from pharynx, soft palate, taste posterior one third of tongue, fauces jugular ganglia tonsils, carotid body, and carotid sinus controlling reflexes for respiration, blood pressure, and heart rate

Motor stylopharyngeal

Parasympathetic parotid gland

Etiologies: Bonnier's syndrome, Vernet's syndrome, glossopharyngeal neuralgia (paroxysmal pain)

Symptoms: loss of gag, dysphagia, loss of taste, sensation loss in pharynx and posterior tongue, increased salivation, tachycardia

Cranial Nerve X (Vagus) *

Nerve Distribution

Sensory: auricular external auditory meatus, dura of posterior fossa, ganglion nodosum pharynx, larynx, trachea, esophageus, abdominal cavity internal superior larynx

Internal surface of larynx above vocal folds

Motor (nucleus ambiguus) pharyngeal constrictors, levator veli palatine external sup. Larynx cricothyroid recurrent laryngeal all intrinsic laryngeal muscle except cricothyroid

Etiologies: intramedullary lesions including hemorrhage, thrombosis, tumors, syphilis, syringobulbia

Peripheral lesions include primary neuritis (alcohol, diphteritic, lead, arsenic), trauma, surgery, aortic aneurysm

Symptoms: bilateral recurrent lesions-adductor/abductor paralysis of vocal folds with aphonia, dyspnea, or pseudoasthma, cardio arrhythmia and death

Unilateral recurrent lesions–unilateral vocal fold paralysis with dysphonia

Unilateral pharyngeal nerve–unilateral velar paralysis with hypernasality with deviation to strong side

Unilateral superior laryngeal nerve–anesthesia of larynx, fatigue, pitch control problems

Cranial Nerve XI (Spinal Accessory)

Nerve Distribution

Sensory: none

(Continued)

Table 8–2 *(Continued)*   Nerve, Distribution, Etiologies, and Symptoms Resulting from Lesions to Cranial Nerves

Motor

Internal medullary via X cranial nerve contributes to intrinsic laryngeal muscle

External (spinal) trapezius, sternocleidomastoid

Etiologies: meningitis, syphilis, trauma, surgery on tuberculoses nodes

Symptoms: unilateral no rotation of head to healthy side; cannot shrug shoulder on affected side, affected shoulder droops

Bilateral Difficult to rotate head or raise chin, head often drops forward

Cranial Nerve XII (Hypoglossal)

Nerve Distribution

Hypoglossal intrinsic muscle of tongue, styloglossus, genioglossus, geniohyoid, thyrohyoid, sternohyoid, sternothyroid, omohyoid

Etiologies: basal skull fractures, dislocation of upper cervical vertebrae, tuberculoses, aneurysm of circle of Willis, syphilis, and lead alcohol, arsenic, and carbon monoxide poisonings, brain abscess, syringobulbia

*See Aronson (1990) for detailed examination of cranial nerve X.

In a muscle group with a 100-motor-unit condition, the force is steady, but in a two-motor-unit condition, the force is unsteady **(Fig. 8–1)**. Thus, the strength in the two-motor-unit muscle would wax and wane, producing an unsteady movement. Because the number of functional motor units is reduced in flaccid dysarthria, the voice could be weak (poor adduction with breathiness) and unsteady. Vocal variability is actually preferred by listeners, but only to a certain extent. When the variability becomes too great, the listener perceives the voice as rough.

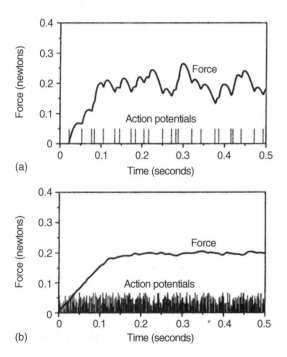

(a)

(b)

Figure 8–1 Stimulation of motor unit action potentials and corresponding muscle forces for **(A)** two motor units with equal twitch amplitudes and **(B)** 100 motor units with varying twitch amplitudes. [From Titze, I.R. (1994). *Principles of Voice Production*. Englewood Cliffs, NJ: Prentice-Hall, with permission.]

When the entire peripheral nerve is interrupted, the specialized muscle receptors receive no neural input from the CNS. In this condition, no movement is possible and muscle tone is absent. The muscle is ultimately weak or paralyzed. Fasciculation, a spontaneous twitching, may occur within individual muscle fiber bundles and muscle atrophy will be present after a time. If some of the LMN axons reach the muscle intact, then those muscle fibers are stimulated. Consequently, some degree of muscle tone is maintained, but because fewer motor units are available to contract, the muscle produces weaker and more irregular contractions. Muscle atrophy may occur because some motor units are not innervated.

When the myoneural synapse is the problem site, the effect depends on the amount of neurotransmitter available, released, and taken up postsynaptically. Because the muscle does receive some input from the CNS, atrophy and fasciculation do not occur. During the course of sustained contraction(s), neurotransmitter will be used up and motor unit dysfunction will occur, resulting in fewer motor unit twitches and muscle weakness and variability.

Neural Adaptation

After an injury to the LMN, the affected muscles often regain some amount of strength and steadiness. Neural adaptation is one mechanism leading to some recovery of strength. Within the realm of muscle strengthening, Liss et al (1994) observed that those "changes within the nervous system that correspond to muscle use and function are referred to as neural adaptation" (p. 44). Although the mechanisms of neural adaptation are not confined to LMN activities, the influence of neural adaptation on the functioning of weakened muscle due to LMN injury is potentially quite strong. Sale (1986) reported that strength and power training bring about changes in the nervous system. These changes allow the person to better organize the activation of muscle groups. Liss et al (1991) noted that muscle physiology research has shown that resistance training at any submaximal force level leads to reduced neural activity, suggesting greater efficiency. Sale (1986) reported data that suggested early or rapidly improved strength performance is likely due to neural adaptation rather than increased muscle size or metabolic capacity. Several investigators have suggested that neural adaptation occurs when one can recruit previously untapped motor units or increase the firing rate of already activated motor units (Kraemer, Deschenes, & Fleck, 1988; Liss et al, 1994; Sale, 1986; Sale, McComas, MacDougall, & Upton, 1982). With respect to dysarthria, for the most part, speech pathologists have yet to take systematic advantage of the literature in exercise physiology and apply it to muscle retraining for speech.

Muscle Training

Speech pathologists often utilize therapy time to enable the patient to strengthen weak, flaccid muscle. These strengthening trials would seem to be right on target because the hallmark of LMN disease is weakness. The success of these endeavors has been problematic and evidence of their effectiveness is improving but remains at low levels for at least two reasons. First, our attempts to strengthen weakened speech musculature have not been as successful as they could have been because we have not utilized specific muscle-training techniques. Second, systematic research has been slow to appear. Evidence-based review of specific applications of neuromuscular training has appeared (Strand & Sullivan, 2001), but much remains to be done. The literature about muscle strengthening and training suggests that neural changes resulting from muscle training are task specific (Kraemer et al, 1988). This means that neural adaptation to increase a specific pattern of motor unit recruitment occurs only when the characteristics of the target movement match those of the training movement. Kraemer et al found that type of contraction, joint angle, and velocity must be considered. Sale and MacDougall (1981) reported four kinds of training specifics: (1) movement patterns, (2) velocity, (3) contraction type, and (4) contraction force. Liss et al (1994) utilized these concepts to develop a specific training procedure for velopharyngeal musculature. They attempted to exploit the relationship between neural adaptation, which leads to more efficient muscular activity for a task, and muscle training. They believed that this could lead to more strength in a muscle that is poorly innervated due to injuries to some number of motor units innervating that muscle.

Liss et al (1994) summarized the specifics of muscle training and noted that specificity of movement means that the greatest strength increases occur when the training is done in the position(s) that the movement operates through. Thus, if we were to apply that notion to the lip, then strength training for the lip should vary according to the intended target. When the intended target is movement from an open to a closed position and then to open again, the strength training should have the lip moving against resistance from open to closed to open while fixing the mandible. If the target was tight lip closure to prevent leakage during eating, then pushing against resistance in the closed lip position while allowing the jaw to move might be more appropriate. For the tongue, it is more difficult to develop movements that operate against resistance yet mimic the movements of speech. Because the tongue is a hydrostat and does not operate around a joint, position angles and movement strategies to attain those angles (positions) during strength training may be quite different for the tongue compared with the arm. It could be argued that the first strengthening exercises should be moving the tongue through target movements as the mass of the tongue provides the resistance to the movement (Luschei, 1991). Finally, when constructing movement activities, one might want to consider compensatory postures/movements that may change the movement requirements and subsequently, change the strength training requirements. Liss and colleagues (1994) concluded that the palliative effect of strength training that is designed around these considerations resulted from neural adaptation rather than muscle change per se. If this is true, then one could expect changes in strength to occur sooner rather than later because neural adaptation seems to occur relatively quickly compared with muscle fiber change. However, the rate of change due to neural adaptation has not been systematically studied in LMN-injured patients and the dystrophies.

Muscle training should occur at similar velocities as the target movement. Again, neural adaptation is probably the mechanism responsible. Liss et al (1994) suggested that the CNS may respond differently to slow versus fast movements. This would mean that therapy to improve tongue velocity for speech using slow, protrusion movements against a tongue blade would have two strikes against it with respect to the efficiency of muscle training. The movement (or lack of it) does not approach the velocity of speech, and the position of the tongue is clearly incorrect relative to tongue positions that occur during speech. Although tongue protrusion against resistance may be a useful technique for improved Popsicle tasting, it probably does not contribute to improved tongue strength for speech, at least not in an efficient manner.

Liss et al (1994) noted that the type of contractions should match the intended movement and muscle contraction type. Three forms of contraction against resistance are possible: (1) concentric, in which muscle is shortening during the movement; (2) eccentric, in which muscle is lengthening during the movement; and (3) isometric, in which the muscle does not change length against the resistance. Many exercises used by speech pathologists are isometric (e.g., pushing against a tongue blade). Dworkin (1991) has developed some clever strategies for strengthening exercises for the speech mechanism that attempt to deal with these issues. However, it will be up to the individual speech pathologist to utilize his ideas and others to meet the muscle training guidelines noted here. For example, Kuehn (1991), Liss et al (1994), and Kuehn and Wachtel (1994) have reported the application of continuous positive airway pressure (CPAP) to utilize air pressure as a resistance for the velum to move against during muscle training exercise. Because the strength training takes place during speech, it is argued that the velum is acting against resistance at the correct angles, velocity, and distance as used in speech.

♦ Measurement, Assessment, and Management

The challenges facing the speech pathologist in treatment of the dysarthric individual are numerous and difficult. Wertz (1985) combined measurement and assessment into appraisal and suggested five objectives: (1) to measure the patient's symptoms and recognize the hierarchical relationship among them to determine the relative contribution to the speech deficit; (2) to determine the speech diagnosis (e.g., presence and type of dysarthria); (3) to determine the severity of the disorder; (4) to determine the probability for improvement (prognosis); and (5) to focus the therapy. Rosenbek and LaPointe (1985) proposed using a point-place model (Netsell, 1973) **(Table 8–3)** complemented with a process model (articulation, resonation, phonation, respiration, and prosody) to appraise speech difficulties. Yorkston et al (1999) argue for the use of consistent procedures, and proceed to elucidate guidelines and checklists for the point on the point-place mode. Yorkston et al defined consistent as a set of procedures that can be repeated and documented by the clinician and yet retain flexibility to meet the individual assessment needs of individual patients.

Models focus one's attention and should lead to more systematic appraisal. However, they may lead to a relatively inflexible mental set when the model is not revised. The mental set with which one approaches the measurement of dysarthria establishes the perceptual and cognitive filters that determine our actions and subsequently our conclusions. Arguments about whether nonspeech measures or only speech measures should be used to measure and assess dysarthria may be the result of perceptual and cognitive filters determining our direction of action. For a more in-depth discussion of these issues, see Luschei (1991), Weismer and Liss (1991), and Kent (1994). Luschei argued elegantly that just because the extent of the relationship between, for example, tongue strength and articulatory accuracy is not known with certainty, it is not sufficient reason to refrain from investigating the utility of objective nonspeech measures of tongue function. This would seem to be especially true in the case of flaccid dysarthria because it is the execution of motor commands that is disrupted and not the planning, organizing, or ideation of speech. The bottom line is that speech-language pathologists are trying to minimize the effects of dysarthria on the patient's life and to accomplish that goal in the most efficient way possible. With the present state-of-the-art measurement methods and assessment strategies, it is possible to achieve that goal in different ways, depending on the perspective and goals.

Yorkston et al (1988) noted that there are at least three perspectives from which dysarthria is addressed: neurology, speech physiology, and speech-language pathology. Yorkson et al (1999) added a fourth perspective, the speaker's point of view. To successfully manage the dysarthric patient, the speech-language pathologist must be able to change perspectives (mental set or filter) to fit the purpose at hand. One way to remain flexible, yet organized and efficient, is to utilize a model that fosters measurement and assessment from different perspectives. Because dysarthria can be viewed as a chronic disorder, models that could address dysarthria in that way (Frey, 1984; Wood, 1980; Yorkston et al, 1988, 1999) might be useful to the speech-language pathologist to create a perspective (filter set) that is adaptive. Frey's (1984) model included three levels: (1) impairment, which is "any loss or abnormality of psychological, physiological, or anatomical structure or function" (e.g., paralyzed velum); (2) disability, which is the "restriction or lack (resulting from impairment) of the ability to perform an activity in the manner or within the range considered normal for the human being" (e.g., reduced intelligibility); and (3) handicap, which is "the disadvantage for a given individual (resulting from an impairment or disability) that limits or prevents the fulfillment of a role that is normal (depending upon age, sex, social, cultural factors) for that individual" (e.g., loss of a teaching position). Other models are possible, such as that described by Yorkston et al (1999), which included five levels: (1) pathophysiology, (2) impairment, (3) functional limitation, (4) disability, and (5) societal limitations. In the discussion that follows, the management of flaccid dysarthria is addressed within the chronic disorder model. Because this chapter is devoted to flaccid dysarthria, it is assumed that the measurement and assessment procedures have been completed and that the sequelae of flaccid dysarthria have been found. Sources with more complete discussions of measurement and assessment are widely available (Duffy, 2005; Dworkin, 1991; Kent, Kent, & Rosenbek, 1987; Linebaugh, 1983; McNeil & Kennedy, 1984; Rosenbek & LaPointe, 1985; Wertz, 1985; Yorkston et al, 1999), and are found in other chapters in this text.

Management

The diagnosis of flaccid dysarthria does not mean that the therapeutic decisions regarding the treatment priorities have been determined. Dworkin (1991) proposed a hierarchical approach to management in which respiration and resonation were first-order (top-priority) subsystems, meaning that they should be addressed first to bring them to their maximum potential. He suggested that second-order (phonation) and third-order (articulation and prosody) problems should not be treated until first-order problems meet a criterion established by the clinician. In contrast,

Table 8–3 Point-Place Model

1	Muscles and structures of respiration
2	Larynx
3	Velopharyngeal port
4	Tongue blade
5	Tongue tip
6	Lips
7	Jaw

Adapted from Rosenbek, J.C. & LaPointe, L.L. (1985). The dysarthrias: description, diagnosis and treatment. In: D.F. Johns (Ed.), *Clinical Management of Communicative Disorders*, 2nd ed. (pp. 97–152). Boston: Little, Brown.

Rosenbek and LaPointe (1985) suggested that the management approach should be based on a hierarchy of symptoms. Clinicians establish the hierarchy based on their judgment about the causative relationship among symptoms and the symptoms' contribution to the intelligibility reduction of the dysarthria. Rosenbek and LaPointe's (1985) management strategy suggested eight specific treatment goals. These goals addressed each of the point-place issues in Netsell's (1973) model (e.g., modify respiration, modify phonation, etc.), targeted process-based issues (e.g., modify prosody), sought the remediation of impairments (e.g., modify abnormalities of posture, tone and strength), and finally pursued the reduction of handicap (e.g., help a person to become a productive client). Because the author of this chapter cut his therapeutic teeth following Rosenbek and LaPointe's advice, the discussion that follows borrows heavily from their ideas. However, with respect to evidenced-based practice, much work needs to be done in this area.

General Principles

Several principles of muscle training gleaned from the exercise physiology literature were discussed earlier. Briefly, the main points are that strength increases after muscle training through neural adaptation and increased contractile properties of the muscle itself. The rapid increases in strength at the early stages of training are believed to occur through neural adaptation. Liss et al (1994) observed that resistance at any submaximal force level improves neural innervation efficiency by eliciting previously untapped motor units or by increasing neural firing rates. In addition, muscle training activities are task specific for the position, velocity, and contraction type. In flaccid dysarthria, the direct management of the impairment must address the weakness caused by the loss or interruption of the LMN innervation. It should be recalled that muscle training can improve strength (maximal force), power (force over time), and endurance (sustained submaximal contraction). Strength training for flaccid muscle should attempt to increase neural activation (remaining intact pathways), and improve muscle synergist efficiency. To do this, training must be specific over four variables: (1) movement pattern, (2) velocity, (3) contraction type, and (4) contraction force.

If the LMN innervation is completely lost, then activities to strengthen muscle are a waste of time. In these cases, impairment is reduced by physical compensations (e.g., surgery), by reinnervating the muscle, or through behavioral compensations (e.g., using an artificial larynx). In the treatment suggestions offered in the following sections, an attempt is made to distinguish between therapy strategies that are muscle-strengthening activities and those that are compensatory.

Respiration

Assuming that we have flaccid respiratory muscle, the problem, then, is to decide the contribution to disability and handicap resulting from muscular impairments of the respiratory system. At least four treatment decisions need to be made: (1) Can respiratory drive itself be improved? (2) Is the maximum respiratory drive possible being utilized by the patient? (3) What compensations can be made to lessen the disability and handicap? (4) What is the prognosis for favorable outcomes at each level? In addition, it would seem prudent to note that the patient's handicap and social expectations change. The very sick (acute) patient may be concerned only with sufficient communication ability to signal for assistance, whereas the more chronic patient may be seeking more general communication goals. Thus, management of the dysarthric patient with respiratory impairments is influenced by continuous assessment and must adapt to changing ability levels as well as changing social demands.

The speech-language pathologist's first goal of intervention with a patient experiencing severe respiratory deficiencies should be to establish communication. Many patients fear their inability to speak. If the flaccid respiratory impairment is so severe that breathing for speech purposes is impossible, the immediate goal is to reduce the handicap, which at this point may be to enable the patient to signal caregivers about pain or other needs. A simple switch activating an alerting signal (e.g., a light or sound) can be used by the patient to alert caregivers. When prolonged ventilator assistance is required, the clinician should consider devices that direct airflow into the larynx, provided the patient is able to approximate the vocal folds and articulate. As it becomes apparent that the compromised respiratory support is permanent and speech breathing is impossible, then augmentative devices commensurate with the patient's cognitive abilities are recommended.

Assuming the person's immediate communication needs are met and that respiration for speech is inadequate (e.g., subglottal pressures less than 5 cm H_2O on speech-like tasks, which are unsustainable for 5 seconds; respiration does not support phonation; or respiratory support is such that a one word at a time approach is used [Yorkston, 1999]), the clinician addresses improving the respiratory support for speech (reducing impairment and disability), a first-order problem according to Dworkin (1991). For flaccid respiratory problems, there are essentially two possibilities: either improve respiratory muscle dynamic contraction, or compensate for the weakness by making maximum use of phonatory, articulatory, and postural adjustments to improve air stream management.

Strength

Strength training of the respiratory muscle is problematic for the speech-language pathologist. Shelton (1963) counseled that speech-language pathologists should leave strength training to physical therapists, an option we should consider. Certainly, efforts to improve respiration capacity beyond that needed for speech would seem to be misplaced. On the other hand, speech breathing has dynamic characteristics quite different from resting respiration for which physical therapists would have little working knowledge. Further, because muscle strength training is task specific, it would seem prudent for speech-language pathologists to explore this problem more thoroughly. Dworkin

(1991) stated that patients with flaccid respiratory muscle may need exercise to improve the strength of inspiratory and expiratory muscle. He suggests that a multidisciplinary approach is required and that any therapeutic efforts for breathing should be cleared by those professional colleagues who are specifically trained in the dynamics of respiration to support life.

Several writers have described devices or techniques believed to be useful for improving speech breathing (Dworkin, 1991; Hixon, Hawley, & Wilson, 1982; Netsell & Hixon, 1978; Rosenbek & LaPointe, 1985; Yorkston et al, 1999). The applications include practicing expiratory breath control using a glass of water 12 cm or higher with a straw inserted to 10 cm (Hixon et al, 1982), using a water manometer with a "leak" tube to mirror glottal resistance during speech (Putnam & Hixon, 1984), using a Sea-scape device (Pro-Ed, Austin, TX; Dworkin, 1991), and utilizing pressure matching tasks using an oscilloscope (Rosenbek & LaPointe, 1985). Readers are referred to those sources for specific strategies. Of concern here is whether these exercise strategies improve dynamic strength (i.e., throughout a full range of motion with appropriate velocities). When these exercises employ a "bleed tube," an analogue to laryngeal resistance, expiratory movements are completed throughout the range of motion and at nearly the same velocity as during speech (albeit not a dynamic). The goal of these strategies is usually to establish a level of pressure (5 cm H_2O) for a specific length of time (5 seconds), which is considered the minimum pressure necessary to support phonation.

These exercises used to strengthen respiratory support are problematic. First, only expiratory activity is targeted. Second, lung volumes at which these exercises occur determine which muscles are forced to work. At high lung volumes, inspiratory muscles perform a checking action, so to obtain higher expiratory breath pressures, the inspiratory muscles would relax rather than contract. At middle to low lung volumes, the expiratory muscles work to increase pressure and to maintain a constant pressure against a column of water, whereas overcoming resistance of the "leak" tube would require extra effort from the expiratory muscle. Consequently, practicing constant air pressures against leaks probably works more on control than strength per se, especially for expiratory muscle. This is not to say that exercises are not helpful; rather, it would seem that they are helpful for one aspect of respiratory support for speech, and when they fail, inspiration or control of inspiratory muscles during exhalation could be the source of the problem.

Putnam and Hixon (1984) noted that problems of inhalation are frequently found in flaccid dysarthria. The literature is sparse with respect to strengthening inspiratory muscle. Dworkin (1991) described a clever application of the Sea Scape for inspiratory muscle strengthening. His step-by-step approach has several levels of practice designed to increase lung volume and faster breathing movements. Because he approaches the exercises utilizing both prolonged and rapid inspirations, these exercises would appear to approach two of the components of muscle strengthening exercise: movement through the entire range of motion, and at a velocity similar to the task requirement (speech breathing). For most of these exercises, inspiratory resistance to the movement is provided by the natural resistance of the chest wall and viscera. Dworkin (1991) developed at least one exercise that provided external resistance in which clinicians applied light pressure with their hands to resist the patient's abdominal distention during inspiration. This may be appropriate if the target of muscle strengthening was the diaphragm. However, if the diaphragm was not active during inspiration due to paralysis, and the chest wall muscles were carrying the load, then resistance to chest wall expansion would be necessary to increase chest muscle strength.

Compensation

Learning to modify a rather automatic behavior such as speech breathing and articulation is difficult. At first, the new movements have to be highly controlled, requiring attention to be directed to the speech act. If the movements are practiced too slowly, then a closed-loop mode of control that is attention demanding and not conducive to learning an open-loop control mode is required (Schmidt & Wrisberg, 2004). If the compensations are not learned as an automatic process but remain at a slow, closed-loop level, then continuous high cognitive direction is needed. This is useful only if the compensations are used in short bursts of effort in specific situations. To be successful in the larger sense, the compensations must become automatic, and for movements to be executed automatically, they must be programmed (controlled in an open-loop manner). Feedback and time to internally process the movements are required. Schmidt and Wrisberg (2004) described two forms of feedback: knowledge of results (KR) (e.g., successful or not successful performance) and knowledge of performance (KP) (e.g., how the movements were made). Feedback that duplicates the learners' intrinsic knowledge of the outcome or their performance is neutral at best or detrimental to learning at worst (Schmidt & Wrisberg, 2004). However, many of the pathologies (not all) that affect the lower motor neuron can affect the afferent pathways as well. Thus, just as the muscle may not be completely innervated by efferent signals, neither may the sensory pathways from a muscle be completely functional. In order for the speaker with interrupted sensory pathways to know what the muscles are doing, it may be necessary for the clinician to supply KP. However, that may not be sufficient for the person to learn new movements to automaticity because the learner must be able to compare intended performance with actual performance and results to develop motor programs for new movements or to modify old ones (Schmidt & Wrisberg, 2004).

Compensations that can be learned utilizing more intact pathways would seem to make the most sense due to the possibility of utilizing intrinsic feedback about the movement. Compensation implies that more intact mechanisms can and will take over (or supplement) muscle activity in the impaired system. For respiration, the compensations can take the form of extra respiratory drive or better management of the respiratory support available. For example, Hixon, Putnam, and Sharpe (1983) described a patient with flaccid paralysis of the respiratory muscles who learned to use neck movements to store recoil energy to inspire and used glossopharyngeal pumping to extend breath groups. These strategies represented compensations for respiratory drive. Hixon et al recommended that patients with progressive LMN disorders begin to learn these compensatory movements as soon as chest wall paresis is showing moderate levels of dysfunction. Glossopharyngeal pumping to support speech can be taught (Dail, Zumwalt, & Adkins, 1983) but there are medical issues to consider. For example, Hixon et al noted that glossopharyngeal pumping may be hazardous to individuals without normal vasomotor reflexes. Again, the implementation of glossopharyngeal pumping highlights the necessity for clinicians to consult with expert pulmonary physicians and receive medical clearance before implementing respiratory training.

The report by Hixon et al (1983) points the way for downstream compensations for the respiratory difficulties of flaccid dysarthria. Their patient became efficient using his air supply that relied on only 5% of his predicted vital capacity during speech. He accomplished this by using a tighter laryngeal closure, leading to a mild strained quality and by modifying his articulation to become more efficient. He shortened fricatives, used stops instead of fricatives, and interrupted airflow with intrusive glottal stops. Even though this patient learned these compensations without specific training, his success does show that potential compensations utilizing upstream valving modifications can be learned. The challenge for the speech clinician is to provide the environment where instruction and feedback (KR or KP) are utilized by the learner to develop compensatory motor speech programs.

Postural adjustments to improve respiratory drive are valuable for some patients. Patients with predominately inspiratory difficulties may do better in a sitting position because gravity will assist in the lowering of the diaphragm during inspiration (Putnam & Hixon 1984), with the added advantage that an additional motor learning task is not necessary. On the other hand, patients with expiratory problems may do better in a supine position. Binders and corsets have been reported to improve expiratory air pressure especially in patients with good diaphragm function but weak expiratory muscles (Duffy, 1995; Rosenbek & LaPointe, 1985; Yorkston et al, 1988) and in patients with phrenic nerve pacers (Hoit, Banzett, & Brown, 2002). The necessity for medical approval is paramount due to the potential pulmonary complications from binding. Rosenbek and LaPointe (1985) pointed out that leaning into a flat surface during exhalation can assist respiratory drive, reducing the complications of binding. However, poor trunk support, poor balance, or general weakness can make this compensation difficult to implement and to time (Yorkston et al, 1988).

Phonation

Flaccid dysphonia has been widely addressed in texts devoted to voice disorders. The voice that results from LMN interruption depends on which branches of the vagus nerve has been damaged. Flaccid paralysis of the vocal folds can be unilateral or bilateral. When the external branch of the superior laryngeal nerve is affected, the pitch-changing cricothyroid muscle is affected. When the recurrent branch

is affected, all of the intrinsic laryngeal muscles, except for the cricothyroid, are weakened with impairment of laryngeal adduction, abduction, and active tensing (shortening).

Strengthening

Two medical approaches to manage flaccid laryngeal muscles address muscle strengthening directly. Pharmacological management of myasthenia gravis directly affects the ability of muscle to contract by improving neuromuscular synaptic function. Flaccid dysarthria caused by myasthenia gravis can be treated with the anticholinesterase drug pyridostigmine (Mestinon). Dworkin (1991) noted that the long-term effects of pyridostigmine on dysarthria are uncertain, but that it is most likely to assist voice return in those patients in the initial stages of the disease. Surgical interventions have been developed to reestablish neural innervation to the intrinsic laryngeal muscles. Crumley (1992) stated that the ansa cervicalis/recurrent laryngeal nerve anastomosis usually results in near-normal voice, and attributed the good results to the reinnervation of the four ipsilateral intrinsic muscles innervated by the recurrent nerve. Olson, Goding, and Michael (1998) reported in a retrospective study using a variety of acoustic and perceptual measures that laryngeal reinnervation by ansa cervicalis transfer could restore near normal or normal voice in patients with isolated unilateral vocal fold paralysis. Paniello (2000) reported reinnervation of the intrinsic laryngeal muscle using cranial nerve XII and recurrent laryngeal nerve (RLN) anastomosis, with reasonable return of voice quality.

Leddy and Canfield (1991) and Dworkin (1991) have proposed therapeutic exercise to directly strengthen the laryngeal muscle. Leddy and Canfield's contribution is a computerized home program that utilizes vowel prolongation at different pitches and pitch ranges to improve vocal function. Dworkin's programs are more complex and target improved strength (or improved vocal closure) through a hierarchical exercise program including exercises at the contextual speech level. These exercises are designed to increase the force with which the vocal folds close during phonation. The exercises make use of nonspeech or vegetative valving and hard glottal attack. Whether any of these exercises can or actually strengthen the muscles rather than improve the utilization of existing strength is not apparent. However, Dworkin provided a valuable, though complex, method to document patient change through each level and provides valuable admonitions to establish objective baselines and criteria for treatment continuation or termination.

Compensation

Compensation for laryngeal paralysis includes behavioral changes and surgical interventions. Most behavioral strategies attempt to improve vocal fold adduction, taking advantage of the closure capabilities that occur while protecting the airway (e.g., during swallowing) or when providing constriction to increase thoracic pressure during lifting, pushing, and pulling. Surgical interventions improve closure by moving the paralyzed vocal fold closer to midline or by increasing the mass of the paralyzed vocal fold.

Effort closure techniques have been reported to induce phonation while pushing, pulling, or lifting a resistance, or producing a controlled cough to improve adduction and subsequent voice (Aronson, 1990; Duffy, 2005; Rosenbek & LaPointe [1985]; Yorkston et al, 1999). Boone and McFarlane (1994) preferred to use other techniques such as the "half-boom" swallow or a change of head position to facilitate better voice. They claimed that these techniques resulted in a clearer voice than other effort closure techniques and with less hyperfunction. Rosenbek and LaPointe (1985) pointed out that the techniques that create postures that are cosmetically undesirable should be reserved for specific situations. Careful attention to the integration of closure attempts with good respiratory support without inducing hyperfunctional behavior is a must.

A variety of sources are available for specific step-by-step guidance to implement facilitating techniques. Boone and McFarlane (1994) provided detailed descriptions of 25 techniques for improving voice, of which at least six are directly applicable to flaccid weakness of the larynx. These facilitation techniques do not address muscle strengthening; rather, they are designed to elicit the most muscle contraction possible with the existing LMN innervation. Dworkin's (1991) systematic approach of charting baselines and progress could easily be combined with any facilitation approach.

Laryngeal framework surgery or phonosurgery is often completed to improve vocal fold closure. Medialization laryngoplasty improves laryngeal closure by introducing a mass between the vocal fold and the thyroid cartilage on the affected side (Koufman, 1986), which moves the paralyzed vocal fold closer to midline. Gray et al (1992) have noted that even though improvement in pitch and loudness usually results, breathiness, vocal harshness, and fatigue may continue. Because this procedure is reversible, the mass can be removed if reinnervation occurs. Ford (1999) noted that laryngeal framework surgery has seen the development of Silastic, hydroxylapatite, expanded polytetrafluoroethylene, and titanium shims as materials for medialization of the vocal folds. Ford's (1999) review of advances in phonosurgery noted that vocal fold augmentation by injection has evolved to include new applications of the rigid telescope and intraoperative videostroboscopy and anatomical studies focusing on the infrafold region combined with rheological investigations are leading to injectable materials, which more closely match the viscoelastic properties to those of vocal folds. Ford noted that alloplastic materials such as Teflon have been largely supplanted by newer bioimplantables such as fat, collagen, and fascia.

Arytenoid adduction surgery repositions the paralyzed vocal fold without lateral compression. Ford (1999) also observed that more detailed and accurate anatomical studies have been completed, which have led to improved operative precision and safety and to new variations in arytenoid repositioning, improving closure of the posterior subunit. One advantage of arytenoid repositioning is that it can place the vocal process into a position more consistent with the vocal fold position during phonation. However, medialization of the membranous portion of the vocal fold may not occur. In that case, type I thyroplasty or injection thyroplasty

may be necessary (Bauer, Valentino, & Hoffman, 1994). Zeitels (2000) reported a new procedure for paralytic vocal folds in which adduction arytenopexy, Gore-Tex medialization laryngoplasty, and cricothyroid subluxation were used simultaneously, with good results in that the patient's phonations times were within normal limits and they obtained more than two octaves of pitch range with minimal perturbation.

Bauer et al (1995) reported the successful use of autogenous fat to augment vocal fold mass persisting for at least 5 months. They noted that questions remain concerning the long-term survival of the graft and the amount of overcorrection needed. A clear advantage to the use of autogenous fat is the increased tolerance of the vocal folds to the graft. In their opinion, this would lead to a more naturally moving vocal fold during phonation.

Injectable collagen has also been used for augmenting the vocal fold bulk (Ford & Bless, 1986; Ford, Staskowski, & Bless, 1995; Remacle, Marbaiz, Hamoir, Bertrand, & Van den Eeckhout, 1990). Ford and colleagues observed that Food and Drug Administration (FDA) concerns about the potential immunological response to bovine source material, which is used in the airway, has slowed the approval for the use of collagen. They went on to describe the use of autologous collagen vocal fold injection that produced vocal fold function results comparable to those of bovine collagen. The large advantage is that the likelihood of a hypersensitivity response is negligible. Other advances accrue during the preparation of the material and should contribute to increased tolerability with longer duration of effectiveness.

Although considerable progress has been made in surgical compensation for vocal fold paralysis, McFarlane, Holt-Romeo, Laworato, and Warner (1991) concluded that a conservative approach to unilateral vocal fold paralysis (without significant dysphagia), which utilizes behavioral therapy, is the most cost-efficient and risk-free approach to restoring the voice. Voice therapy should be considered as a primary treatment to maximize voice production in cases of unilateral vocal fold paralysis because it resulted in superior voice compared with Teflon injection. An average of 9 hours of voice therapy was required for older and more severely impaired voice patients to be rated as successful as the surgery group and more successful than the Teflon group. McFarlane and colleagues (1991) suggested that most laryngologists agree that a waiting period of at least 9 months is recommended before proceeding with surgical interventions but that they may not consider voice therapy during this time. They concluded that voice therapy, utilizing facilitation techniques, can provide a cost-effective treatment during that initial waiting period without the risks of surgery. Further, Tsunoda, Kikkawa, Kumada, Higo, and Tavama (2003) reported a case with idiopathic right vocal fold paralysis that resolved completely after 18 months. They recommended waiting 18 months, even for implementing surgeries that can be reversed.

New approaches to decision making regarding management of laryngeal paralysis are on the horizon. Min, Finnegan, Hoffman, Luschei, and McCulloch (1994) have described electromyographic measures that predict innervation recovery, leading to better decisions regarding the type and timing of surgical intervention for laryngeal paralysis. Electromyography (EMG) completed prior to 6 months but preferably with 6 weeks of onset was successful in predicting recovery outcome at 89%. A positive prognosis for laryngeal recovery was present when the following EMG features were present: (1) normal motor unit waveform morphology, (2) overall EMG activity at a root-mean-square (RMS) value greater than 40 μV in any one task, and (3) no electrical silence during voluntary tasks. These data suggest that it will be possible to predict innervation outcome and assist speech pathologists and laryngologists in the management of voice disorder secondary to laryngeal paralysis. Magnetic resonance imaging (MRI) has led to better application of vocal fold imaging techniques (Ford, Unger, Zundel, & Bless, 1994). Placement and durability of the medialization medium can be precisely defined by MRI and should lead to better decisions regarding the repair of suboptimal results.

Finally, prosthetic management of voice disorders is possible. Speech amplifiers, such as the Chattervox (Copyright (c) 2003 by Asyst Communications Co., Vernon Hills, IL), can be used to amplify a weak voice. However, good articulation abilities are necessary for the best result. An audiologist may prove invaluable in providing classroom amplification when one must consider the acoustic characteristics of the room to obtain the best results. Patients with bilateral vocal fold paralysis without voice, but with good articulation, could make use of an artificial larynx.

Resonance

Even though the term *resonance* is applied to the functional outcome of the velopharyngeal port, other parameters of speech are affected by velopharyngeal function. Because speakers with velopharyngeal incompetence (VPI) are unable to impound air for intraoral pressure consonants, nasal emission or articulatory substitutions (e.g., glottal stop or pharyngeal fricative) are likely. In addition, the open velopharyngeal port allows acoustic energy to be diverted into the nasal passages, damping the acoustic signal and reducing overall loudness. To complicate matters further, respiratory air wastage makes intelligible speech even more difficult for those speakers with compromised respiratory, phonatory, or articulatory systems. VPI due to flaccid velar musculature can range from mild hypernasality to unintelligible speech. When VPI is severe, management of VPI becomes a necessity so that more intelligible speech can be produced. As with other levels of the point-place model, the handicap brought about by VPI is determined by the communication requirements of the individual patient. The management of the impairment of VPI caused by flaccid muscle can take three forms: behavioral, prosthetic, and surgical.

Behavioral

Several exercises have been put forward as ways to improve velopharyngeal closing including blowing and sucking (Johns, 1985). Johns also noted facilitation techniques such as pressure, icing, brushing, stroking, and electrical stimulation have been advocated to improve VPI due to flaccid

muscle. Johns was pessimistic because "these exercises are disappointing and generally ineffective" (p. 158). Duffy (1995) concluded that further controlled investigations of the effectiveness of palatal stimulation and strengthening may be warranted. Indeed, it could be argued that none of the previous attempts at muscle strengthening have addressed any of the known principles of muscle training. Certainly, blowing and sucking exercises require the velum to assume a static position, and although sucking can create a negative intraoral pressure that may act as a resistance (load) to the closing action of the levator palatini muscle, blowing would not. Consequently, exercises through representative velocities, ranges of movement, or types of muscle contraction would not be possible; hence, neural adaptation as a means to increase velar function would be unlikely.

Kuehn and Wachtel (1994) and Liss et al (1994) utilized CPAP to provide an exercise to strengthen the velum. CPAP, used in the treatment of sleep apnea, provides a continuous positive pressure within the nasopharyngeal and pharyngeal spaces. They took advantage of the positive pressure within the nasopharynx to provide a resistance against which the velum could operate through a full range of motion, at speech-related velocities, with the correct muscle contraction type. Liss et al (1994) developed a standard protocol to use with CPAP. The results are encouraging, but variables that continue to require investigation include exercise quantity, intensity, and frequency, as well as the role of feedback.

Dworkin (1991) described behavioral techniques that he has used with VPI. He suggested that 10 hours of concentrated (undefined) behavioral therapy be completed before alternative methods of repairing the VPI are tried. Dworkin delineated a series of exercises (and charting techniques) to reduce VPI. His techniques call for systematically increasing oral pressure capability into activities that progressively approximate conversational speech. The activities have been designed to use Sea scape and recordings to provide feedback to the patient. These exercises would not appear to address strength (power, force, or endurance) directly except in the sense that the patient is taught to make better use of existing strength. Consequently, the 10-hour limit is probably a good one because it provides a window of opportunity for the patient to demonstrate learning but does not provide an unrealistic expectation of strength change.

Prosthetic

A palatal lift prosthesis lifts the velum to approximate the posterior pharyngeal wall. Yorkston et al (1999) reported that this technique has been the most successful strategy to improve VPI in patients with dysarthria. Detailed explanations of the utilization and fitting of palatal lifts have been provided (Aten, McDonald, Simpson, & Gutierrez, 1984; Dworkin, 1991; Johns, 1985; Yorkston et al, 1999). Duffy (1995) observed that the best candidates for palatal lift management are those with minimal deficits throughout the speech production system, static rather than progressive conditions, adequate dentition, and a hypoactive gag reflex. Because the gag reflex is usually diminished or absent in flaccid dysarthria, the palatal lift is well suited for the task of improving VPI in the face of isolated flaccid paralysis of the velum. However, Shaughnessy, Netsell, and Farrage (1983) cautioned that clients may need to be taught to use the palatal lift. The amount of rehabilitation is determined by the degree of successful use of oral pressure during speech.

Surgical

Two general approaches have been tried: pharyngeal flap and injection. Noll (1982) remarked that any form of surgical management of VPI due to neuromotor problems is not as successful compared with surgical approaches with structural deficits. Johns (1985) furnished a detailed report delineating approaches to surgical management and their usefulness. He concluded that pharyngeal flap surgery is effective for some patients. Witt et al (1997), using an autogenous posterior pharyngeal wall augmentation procedure, concluded that it did not result in speech improvement in their patients. Kotz, Howard, Hengerer, and Slupchynski (2001) describe a successful autologous lipoinjection within the soft palate to treat stress VPI in musicians without recurrence of the VPI for up 18 months. Further study and documentation of the effectiveness of these procedures with patients demonstrating flaccid dysarthria remains to be completed.

Articulation

Successful articulation of speech requires the integration of all the points and places represented on Netsell's point-place model. This section deals with the anterior and posterior tongue, lips, and mandible. Because these elements are innervated by different cranial nerves, the deficits vary widely. The movement relationships among respiration, phonation, and articulatory mechanisms necessary to produce linguistic contrasts, such as the voice and voiceless distinction, are complex across space and time. Further, the systems involved are quite disparate in terms of their architecture. For example, the tongue operates as a hydrostat, whereas the muscles of the jaw operate around a joint. The effect of flaccid weakness, especially bilateral, is to slow articulatory movements and reduce the range of motion so that articulatory targets are not reached in either space or time. Management of impairment of articulation due to flaccid weakness can be behavioral, surgical, and pharmacological.

Behavioral

At first glance, strengthening of flaccid articulatory muscle would seem to be the correct target of remediation. Many authors (DePaul & Brooks, 1993; Dworkin, 1991; Duffy, 1995; Rosenbek & LaPointe, 1985; Yorkston et al, 1999) have discussed strengthening the articulatory musculature, but there is no consensus regarding the necessity of doing so. For example, it has been reported that only 10 to 30% (for the jaw, only 2%) of maximum forces are utilized during speech and that up to one third of the motor nerve fibers can be lost before functional impairments are apparent (Duffy, 1995). Indeed, I have observed dysarthric patients

for whom unilateral weakness of the tongue posed no difficulty whatsoever. On the other hand, Dworkin, Aronson, and Mulder (1980) and Robin, Goel, Somodi, and Luschei (1992) have discussed positive relationships between measures of tongue strength and amount of articulatory deficit. For the purposes of this chapter on flaccid dysarthria, strength is considered an important treatment variable. It is likely that much of the difference in opinion regarding lingual, lip, and jaw strength as targets of remediation stems from dissimilar definitions and methods of increasing and measuring strength.

To improve muscle strength of the articulators, the challenge is to design exercises that provide movement against resistance at the appropriate velocity, with the right movement pattern, and with sufficient contraction to engender neural adaptation, which is the quickest way to increased strength. Duffy (1995) noted that the "jaw can be opened, closed, or lateralized; the lips can be rounded, spread, puffed, closed isometrically with our without clinician provided resistance; the tongue can be protruded and lateralized against resistance or pushed against the alveolus, cheeks or a tongue blade and so on" (p. 398). However, we must carefully consider whether these movements of the tongue or lips capture the elements of dynamic strengthening activity necessary to generate neural adaptation for speech movements. For the most part, it would appear that they do not. For example, pushing against the alveolus with the tongue certainly approximates an appropriate target position, but utilizing that as a strengthening technique does not elicit the dynamic aspect of tongue activity for speech. To create neural adaptation, the patient should move the articulator against a resistance through a variety of movement velocities, which mimic speech movements (or are speech movements). Of course, that is easier said than done, especially for the tongue.

In my clinic, we saw an 8-year-old boy (C.T.) with congenital flaccid dysarthria. We adapted Dworkin's (1991) use of tongue blades to provide resistance against which the tongue could work. Since C.T. could attain two positions with the posterior aspect of his tongue (high and low), we had him initiate anterior tongue movements toward and from the alveolus with the posterior tongue in elevated and depressed positions. He was asked also to move the tongue quickly and slowly. The results were encouraging in that we proceeded from zero tongue tip articulations to producing a /d/ consistently in single words.

Because this patient also had flaccid lips, we attempted to strengthen lip movements. Traditional lip strengthening activities would usually have the lips press together or purse. However, these activities represent only one aspect of strength necessary for successful lip movement during speech. It especially ignores lip retraction, which is an important aspect of anterior oral shaping. Early trials with C.T. attempted to increase lip strength by having him resist the pulling of a button placed behind the lips. This exercise may have led to increased lip closure during chewing because C.T.'s parents reported less drooling and loss of food during meals. However, there was no change in his ability to produce lip closure for bilabial consonants or anterior oral shaping for vowels. Exercise was then directed toward eliciting a retraction movement from a closed position with light resistance provided by the clinician followed immediately by a closing gesture against resistance. However, we were unable to complete the clinical trial with C.T., as his family unexpectedly moved out of the area.

We have found that Dworkin's (1991) ideas about exercise provide useful starting points from which to devise other exercises. His ideas are particularly appealing to the practicing clinician because he has made creative use of routine clinical materials such as tongue blades, buttons, and string. These exercises provide a starting point to devise other exercises that more closely resemble speech movements.

On the other hand, successful tongue strengthening regimes have been described to address swallowing issues. Robbins et al (2005) utilized an 8-week progressive lingual resistance exercise program on swallowing in older individuals. Their subjects participated in an 8-week lingual resistance exercise program. The exercises consisted of compressing an air-filled bulb between the tongue and the hard palate. They reported that all of their subjects significantly improved their isometric and swallowing pressures. MRI measures showed that lingual volume increased by an average of 5.1%. Robbins and colleagues concluded that resistance exercise for patients with lingual weakness has the potential to be an effective treatment strategy for patients with lingual weakness and swallowing disability due to frailty and other age-related problems. Although they were encouraged by these results for the improvement of swallowing, it remains to be seen whether a favorable effect for speech would be seen.

Before we jump onto the exercise bandwagon completely, several admonitions can be found in the literature. Kent et al (1987) have observed that maximal strength may not be a useful measure to predict speech motor capability. Duffy (1995) advised determining that weakness is clearly related to the speech impairment and subsequent disability. To do this we need improved methods of measuring lingual and labial strength. Typical clinical measures of tongue strength, such as pushing anteriorly against a tongue blade or laterally against the cheek are inadequate. Not only do these measures fail to approximate any of the natural targets or vectors of speech movement, but they are dependent on subjective estimates of strength by the clinician.

Techniques are emerging that will allow the creation of standardized measures of tongue, lip, and jaw strength or movement. Barlow, Finan, Andreatta, and Paseman (1997) detailed the use of force transducers to quantify labial, lingual, and mandibular function in dysarthria. Robin, Solomon, Moon, and Folkins (1997) provided an extensive discussion of the relationship between nonspeech measures such as the IOPI and physiological parameters (e.g., strength or endurance). Solomon, Robin, and Luschei (2000) utilized the IOPI to examine tongue strength and endurance in persons with Parkinson's disease and demonstrated that while strength was not poorer than the controls, endurance was significantly poorer. Although they were not examining flaccid dysarthria, their study clearly demonstrated that the relationship between strength and speech is not straightforward. In another investigation of tongue strength, Clark,

Henson, Barber, Stierwalt, and Sherrill (2003) found that tongue strength measured objectively and subjectively by experienced clinicians could be used to predict oral phase swallowing impairments. Inexperienced raters of tongue strength did not reach as high a level of correlation with oral function as did the objective measures or the experienced clinicians. These data suggest that it is even more important for inexperienced clinicians to use objective measures of tongue strength (e.g., the IOPI).

Interestingly, the supranormal speakers of Robin et al (1992), who demonstrated greater than average strength and endurance of the tongue, had not "lifted weights" with their tongues, but they had practiced speaking in certain ways (i.e., speaking very rapidly while maintaining good intelligibility in the case of debaters). Luschei (1991) argued that the architecture of the tongue requires sufficient strength to overcome its intrinsic viscous load. Consequently, exercise that elicits rapid tongue movement may provide sufficient resistance to improve tongue strength. In other words, strength gains may be made by practicing speech with greater effort. Further, Robin et al suggested that the minimum strength (e.g., 20% of normal) to support sufficient movement for speech is not known. Duffy (1995) also observed that only 20 to 30% of maximum forces may be required for speech. However, to conclude that some level of strength above these levels is unnecessary may be premature. Robin et al (1992) have pointed out that "sense of effort" plays an important role in task compliance and that speakers who are weak may articulate adequately for short periods of time but not for longer times or in conditions that demand more of the speech mechanism. These notions might be particularly important in trying to reduce the handicap of an individual who articulates well enough in therapy but has trouble at work. For example, DePaul and Brooks (1993) concluded that weakness is not directly related to intelligibility, and suggested that the orofacial system can compensate for lingual weakness. Intelligibility measures in their report were obtained under optimal speaking conditions for relatively short periods of time (2 minutes). Although that might be good enough for someone who is homebound, for another person who wants to return to work in a more challenging environment (with a handicap), it might not be. Without a doubt, the influence of strength upon articulatory performance remains far from understood, especially with respect to critical levels of strength and endurance. Finally, the relationship of strength and endurance to articulatory performance in children may be different from that in adults. It is likely that the usefulness of compensatory strategies is affected by weakness and would likely be related to the competency of articulatory performance obtained before the onset of weakness. Clearly, much clinical investigation remains to be done.

Clark (2003) provided an excellent tutorial regarding neuromuscular treatments for speech. She provided in-depth discussions of neuromuscular impairments, common assessment procedures, and treatment strategies. Her discussion of exercise and the principles of strength training are particularly useful for developing research paradigms to study neuromuscular treatments and evaluate research that purports to address neuromuscular treatments for speech disorders.

Surgical

Myasthenia gravis is often managed surgically. A thymectomy is often used to change the neurochemistry at the myoneural junction (Aronson, 1990). Two surgical approaches to recovery of nerve function associated with Bell's palsy are occasionally used. Although controversial, decompression of the facial nerve has been advocated for some forms of cranial nerve VII involvement. Fisch (1981) found increased recovery with decompression surgery compared with no surgery when the surgery was performed within 24 hours of onset of the facial palsy. However, Holland and Weiner (2004) noted that middle fossa craniotomy for decompression of the facial nerve presents risks such as seizures, deafness, leakage of cerebrospinal fluid, and direct injuries to the facial nerve. They observed that for these reasons decompression surgery for Bell's palsy is not routinely utilized for Bell's palsy in the United Kingdom. Neural anastomosis has also been used to restore facial nerve innervation, typically a branch of cranial nerve XII (Mingrino & Zuccarello, 1981). These authors pointed out that hypoglossal-facial anastomosis can result in facial synkinesis during speech, which could be cosmetically unappealing and affect speech articulation. Yorkston et al (1988) stated that patients should have intact lingual function to minimize the chance of impaired tongue function after the anastomosis.

Pharmacological

Holland and Weiner (2004) have observed that systematic review of pharmacological management of Bell's palsy has shown that it can be effectively treated with corticosteroids within the first 7 days, providing an additional 17% of patients with a good outcome over the 80% that spontaneously improve. In addition, they noted that antiviral treatment is evolving to provide relief when there is an involvement of herpes viruses. Acyclovir has been used with some success, but its poor bioavailability (15 to 20%) has led to investigation of newer drugs such as valacidovir, famcidovir, and sorivudine. In addition, other methylcobalamin, an active form of vitamin B_{12} has shown some promise, as has hyperbaric oxygen in some patients with degeneration.

In myasthenia gravis, pyridostigmine bromide has been prescribed, and speech pathologists have encouraged conservation of effort to reduce fatigue. Recently, the long-term treatment of generalized myasthenia gravis with FK506 (tacrolimus) has been reported (Konishi, Yoshiyama, Takamori, & Saida, 2005). They reported that 67% of their patients showed improvement in their myasthenia gravis score or in their activities of daily living score, and that the prednisolone dosage was reduced in 58% of the patients. However, they only studied 12 patients, and more investigation is needed.

Finally, there are continued efforts to develop a vaccine against myasthenia gravis. Cohen-Kaminsky and Jambou (2005) noted that there is optimism that a vaccine can be developed for autoimmune disorders such as myasthenia gravis. Specifically, they noted that a T-cell receptor (TCR) may be boosted by a TCR vaccine because of the development of spontaneous anti-TCR antibodies directed against the pathogenic T-cells.

◆ Conclusion

We are beginning to utilize the principles of muscle training and apply them to the unique demands of the speaking mechanism. There are remarkable advances in the pharmacological treatments of some disorders and advances in the application of surgical techniques to flaccid dysarthria. Many of the clinicians cited in this chapter are striving to develop new strategies to cope with flaccid dysarthria and have reported many of them. However, we are in great need of systematic controlled studies to further raise the level of evidence that we have for intervening in flaccid dysarthria.

References

Aronson, A.E. (1990). *Clinical Voice Disorders: An Interdisciplinary Approach,* 3rd ed. New York: Thieme

Aten, J., McDonald, A., Simpson, M., & Gutierrez, B. (1984). Efficacy of modified palatal lifts for improved resonance. In: M. McNeil, J. Rosenbek, & A. Aronson (Eds.), *The Dysarthrias: Physiology, Acoustics, Perception, Management* (pp. 231–242). San Diego: College-Hill Press

Barlow, S.M., Finan, D.S., Andreatta, R.D., & Paseman, L.A. (1997) Kinematic measurement of the human vocal tract. In: M.R. McNeil (Ed.), *Clinical Management of Sensorimotor Speech Disorders.* New York: Thieme

Basmajian, J.V. & DeLuca, C.J. (1985). *Muscles Alive: Their Functions Revealed by Electromyography,* 5th ed. Baltimore: Williams & Wilkins

Bauer, C.A., Valentino, J., & Hoffman, H.T. (1995). Long-term result of vocal cord augmentation with autogenous fat. *Annals of Otology, Rhinology, and Laryngology, 104,* 871–874

Bear, M.F., Connors, B.W., & Paradiso, M.A. (1996). *Neuroscience: Exploring the Brain.* Baltimore: Williams & Wilkins

Bhatnagar, S.C. (2002). *Neuroscience for the Study of Communicative Disorders,* 2nd ed. Philadelphia: Lippincott, Williams & Wilkins

Bigland-Ritchie, B. & Woods, J.J. (1984). Changes in muscle contractile properties and neural control during human muscular fatigue. *Muscle & Nerve, 7,* 691–699

Boone, D.R. & McFarlane, S.C. (1994). *The Voice and Voice Therapy,* 5th ed. Englewood Cliffs, NJ: Prentice Hall

Chusid, J.G. (1985). *Correlative Neuroanatomy and Functional Neurology.* Los Altos, CA: LANGE Medical

Clark, H.M. (2003). Neuromuscular treatments for speech and swallowing: a tutorial. *American Journal of Speech-Language Pathology, 12,* 400–415

Clark, H.M., Henson, P.A., Barber, W.D., Stierwalt, J.A.G., & Sherrill, M. (2003). Relationships among subjective and objective measures of tongue strength and oral phase swallowing impairments. *American Journal of Speech-Language Pathology, 12,* 40–50

Cohen-Kaminsky, S. & Jambou, F. (2005). Prospects for a T-cell receptor vaccination against myasthenia gravis. *Expert Review of Vaccines, 4*, 473–492

Crumley, R.L. (1992). Response to McFarlane & co-authors. *American Journal of Speech-Language Pathology, 1*, 65–67

Dail, C., Zumwalt, M., & Adkins, H. (1983). *A Manual of Instruction for Glossopharyngeal Breathing.* New York: National Foundation for Infantile Paralysis

Darley, F.L., Aronson, A.E., & Brown, J.R. (1975). *Motor Speech Disorders.* Philadelphia: W.B. Saunders

DePaul, R. & Brooks, B.R. (1993). Multiple orofacial indices in amyotrophic lateral sclerosis. *Journal of Speech and Hearing Research, 23*, 828–837

Duffy, J.R. (1995). *Motor speech disorders: substrates, differential diagnosis and management.* St. Louis: Mosby-Year Book, Inc

Duffy, J.R. (2005). *Motor Speech Disorders: Substrates, Differential Diagnosis and Management.* St. Louis: Elsevier Mosby

Dworkin, J.P., Aronson, A., Mulder, D. (1980). Tongue force in normals and dysarthric patients with amyotrophic lateral sclerosis. *J. Speech and Hearing Research, 23*, 828–837

Dworkin, J.P. (1991). *Motor Speech Disorders: A Treatment Guide.* St. Louis: Mosby-Year Book.

Fisch, U. (1981). Surgery for Bell's palsy. *Archives of Otolaryngology, 107*, 1–11

Ford, C.N. (1999). Advances and refinements in phonosurgery: Triological Society Papers. *Laryngoscope, 109*, 1891–1900

Ford, C.N. & Bless, D.M. (1986). A preliminary study of inectable collagen in human vocal fold augmentation. *Otolaryngology–Head and Neck Surgery, 94*, 104

Ford, C.N., Staskowski, P.A., & Bless, D.M. (1995). Autologous collagen vocal fold injection: a preliminary clinical study. *Laryngoscope, 8*, 75–80

Ford, C.N., Unger, J.M., Zundel, R.S., & Bless, D.M. (1994). Magnetic resonance imaging (MRI) assessment of vocal fold medialization surgery. *Laryngoscope, 7*, 23–27

Frey, W.D. (1984). Functional assessment in the '80s: a conceptual enigma, a technical challenge. In: A.S. Halpern & M.J. Fuhrer (Eds.), *Functional Assessment in Rehabilitation.* Baltimore: Paul H. Brookes

Gray, S.D., Barkmeier, J., Druker, D., Shive, C., Van Denmark, D., Jones, D., & Alder, S. (1992). Vocal evaluation of thyroplasty surgery in treatment of unilateral vocal cord paralysis. *Laryngoscope 102*, 415–421

Hixon, T.J., Hawley, J., & Wilson, J. (1982). An around-the-house device for the clinical determination of respiratory driving pressure: a note on making the simple even simpler. *Journal of Speech and Hearing Disorders, 47*, 413

Hixon, T.J., Putnam, A.H., & Sharpe, J.T. (1983). Speech production with flaccid paralysis of the rib cage, diaphragm, and abdomen. *Journal of Speech and Hearing Disorders, 48*, 315–327

Hoit, J.D., Banzett, R.B., & Brown, R. (2002). Binding the abdomen can improve speech in men with phrenic nerve pacers. *American Journal of Speech-Language Pathology, 11*, 71–76

Holland, N.J. & Weiner, G.M. (2004) Recent developments in Bell's palsy. *British Medical Journal, 329*, 553–557

Johns, D.F. (1985). Surgical and prosthetic management of neurogenic velopharyngeal incompetency in dysarthria. In: Johns DF, (Ed.), *Clinical Management of Communicative Disorders*, 2nd ed. (pp. 153–178). Boston: Little, Brown

Kent, R.D. (1994). The clinical science of motor speech disorders: a personal assessment. In: J.A. Till, K.M. Yorkston, & D.R. Beukelman (Eds.), *Motor Speech Disorders: Advances in Assessment and Treatment* (pp. 3–18). Baltimore: Paul H. Brookes

Kent, R.D., Kent, J.F., & Rosenbek, J.C. (1987). Maximum performance tests of speech production. *Journal of Speech and Hearing Disorders, 52*, 367–387

Klotz, D.A., Howard, J., Hengerer, A.S., & Slupchynski, O. (2001). Lipoinjection Augmentation of the Soft Palate for Velopharyngeal Stress Incompetence. *Laryngoscope, 111*, 2157–2161

Konishi, T., Yoshiyama, Y., Takamori, M., & Saida, T. (2005). Long-term treatment of generalised myasthenia gravis with FK506 (tacrolimus). *Journal of Neurology Neurosurgery and Psychiatry, 76*, 448–450

Koufman, J.A. (1986). Laryngoplasty for vocal cord medialization: an alternative to Teflon. *Laryngoscope, 96*, 726–731

Kraemer, W.J., Deschenes, M.R., & Fleck, S.J. (1988). Physiological adaptations to resistance exercise: implications for athletic conditioning. *Sports Medicine, 6*, 246–256

Kuehn, D.P. (1991). New therapy for treating hypernasal speech using continuous positive airway pressure (CPAP). *Plastic Reconstructive Surgery, 88*, 959–966

Kuehn, D.P. (1997). The Development of a New Technique for Treating Hypernasality: CPAP. *American Journal of Speech-Language Pathology, 6*, 5–8

Kuehn, D.P., Imrey, P.B., Tomes, L., Jones, D.L., O'Gara, M.M., Seaver, E.J., Smith, B.E., Van Demark, D.R., & Wachtel, J.M. (2002). Efficacy of continuous positive airway pressure for treatment of hypernasality. *Cleft Palate-Craniofacial Journal, 39*, 267–276

Kuehn, D.P. & Wachtel, J.M. (1994). CPAP therapy for treating hypernasality following closed head injury. In: J.A. Till, K.M. Yorkston, & D.R. Beukelman (Eds.), *Motor Speech Disorders: Advances in Assessment and Treatment* (pp. 207–212). Baltimore: Paul H. Brookes

Larson, C. (1989). Basic neurophysiology. In: D.P. Kuehn, M.L. Lemme, & J.M. Baumgartner (Eds.), *Neural Basis of Speech, Hearing and Language.* Boston: College-Hill; Little, Brown

Leddy, M. & Canfield, M.R. (1992). Laryngeal muscle strengthening exercises: A computerized home study program. Paper presented at the Annual Convention of the American Speech-Language and Hearing Association, San Antonio, TX

Linebaugh, C. (1983). Treatment of flaccid dysarthria. In: W. Perkins (Ed.), *Dysarthria and Apraxia.* New York: Thieme Stratton

Liss, J.M., Kuehn, D.P., & Hinkle, K.P. (1994). Direct training of velopharyngeal musculature. *Journal of Medical Speech Language Pathology, 2*, 243–248

Luschei, E.S. (1991). Development of objective standards of nonspeech oral strength and performance: an advocate's perspective. In: C.A. Moore, K.M. Yorkston, D.R. Beukelman (Eds.), *Dysarthria and Apraxia of Speech: Perspectives on Management* (pp. 3–14). Baltimore: Paul H. Brookes

McFarlane, S.C., Holt-Romeo, T.L., Laworato, A.S., & Warner, L. (1991). Unilateral vocal fold paralysis: perceived vocal quality following three methods of treatment. *American Journal of Speech-Language Pathology, 1*, 45–48

McNeil, M.R. & Kennedy, J.G. (1984). Measuring the effects of treatment for dysarthria: knowing when to change or terminate. *Seminars in Speech and Language, 4*, 337–358

Min, Y.B., Finnegan, E.M., Hoffman, H.T., Luschei, E.S., & McCulloch, T.M. (1994). A preliminary study of the prognostic role of electromyography in laryngeal paralysis. *Otolaryngology–Head and Neck Surgery, 6*, 67–72

Mingrino, S. & Zuccarello, M. (1981). Anastomosis of the facial nerve with accessory or hypoglossal nerves. In: M. Samii, P.J. Jannetta (Eds.), *The Cranial Nerves.* New York: Springer-Verlag

Netsell, R. (1973). Speech physiology. In: F.D. Minifie, T.J. Hixon, & F. Williams (Eds.), *Normal Aspects of Speech, Hearing, and Language* (pp. 211–234). Englewood Cliffs, NJ: Prentice-Hall

Netsell, R. & Hixon, T.J. (1978). A noninvasive method for clinically estimating subglottal air pressure. *Journal of Speech and Hearing Disorders, 43*, 326–330

Noll, J.D. (1982). Remediation of impaired resonance among patients with neuropathologies of speech. In: N. Lass, L. McReynolds, J. Northern, & D. Yoder (Eds.), *Speech, Language and Hearing.* Vol. III: *Pathologies of Speech and Language.* Philadelphia: W.B. Saunders

Olson, D.E.L., Goding, G.S., & Michael, D.D. (1998). Acoustic and Perceptual Evaluation of Laryngeal Reinnervation by Ansa Cervicalis Transfer. *Laryngoscope, 108*, 1767–1772

Paniello, R.C. (2000). Laryngeal reinnervation with the hypoglossal nerve: II. Clinical evaluation and early patient experience. *Laryngoscope, 110*, 739–748

Putnam, A., Hixon, T.J. (1984). Respiratory kinematics in speakers with motor neuron disease. In: M. McNeil, J. Rosenbek, & A. Aronson (Eds.), *The Dysarthrias: Physiology, Acoustics, Perception, Management* (pp. 37–67). San Diego: College-Hill Press

Remacle, M., Marbiaz, E., Hamoir, M., Bertrand, B., & Van den Eeckhaut, J. (1990). Correction of glottic insufficiency of collagen injection. *Annals of Otology, Rhinology, and Laryngology, 99*, 438–444

Robbins J., Gangnon R.E., Theis S.M., Kays, S.A., Hewitt, A.L., & Hind J.A. (2005). Effects of lingual exercise on swallowing in older adults. *Journal of the American Geriatrics Society, 53*, 1483–1489

Robin, D.A., Goel, A., Somodi, L.B., & Luschei, E.S. (1992). Tongue strength and endurance: relation to highly skilled movements. *Journal of Speech and Hearing Research, 35*, 1239–1245

Robin, D.A., Solomon, N.P., Moon, J.B., & Folkins, J.W. (1997) Nonspeech assessment of the speech production mechanism. In: M.R. McNeil (Ed.), *Clinical Management of Sensorimotor Speech Disorders.* New York: Thieme

Robin, D.A., Somodi, L.B., & Luschei, E.S. (1991). Measurement of tongue strength and endurance in normal and articulation disordered subjects. In: C.A. Moore, K.M. Yorkston, D.R. Beukelman (Eds.), *Dysarthria and Apraxia of Speech: Perspectives on Management* (pp. 3–14). Baltimore: Paul H. Brookes

Rosenbek, J.C. & LaPointe, L.L. (1985). The dysarthrias: Description, diagnosis and treatment. In: D.F. Johns (Ed.), *Clinical Management of Communicative Disorders,* 2nd ed. (pp. 97–152). Boston: Little, Brown

Sale, D. & MacDougall, D. (1981). Specificity in strength training: a review for the coach and athlete. *Canadian Journal of Applied Sports Science, 6,* 87–92

Sale, D.B. (1986). Neural adaptation in strength and power training. In: N.L. Jones, N. McCartney, & A.J. Mccomas (Eds.), *Human Muscle Power* (pp. 281–305). Champaign, IL: Human Kinetics

Sale, D.G., McComas, A.J., MacDougall, J.D., & Upton, A.R.M. (1982). Neuromuscular adaptation in human thenar muscles following strength training and immobilization. *Journal of Applied Physiology, 53,* 419–424

Schmidt, R.A. & Wrisberg, C.A. (2004). *Motor Learning and Performance,* 3rd ed. Champaign: Human Kinetics

Shaughnessy, A.L., Netsell, R., & Farrage, J. (1983). Treatment of a four-year-old with a palatal lift prosthesis. In: W.R. Berry (Ed.), *Clinical Dysarthria.* San Diego: College-Hill Press

Shelton, R.L. (1963). Therapeutic exercise and speech pathology. *American Speech-Language-Hearing Association, 5,* 855

Solomon, N.P., Robin, D.A., & Luschei, E.S. (2000). Strength, endurance, and stability of the tongue and hand in Parkinson disease. *Journal of Speech, Language, and Hearing Research, 43,* 256–267

Stierwalt, J.A. & Robin, D.A. (1996). Tongue strengthening in the treatment of severe flaccid dysarthria: a single subject study. Presented at the 2006 Annual Motor Speech Conference. Amelia, VA

Strand, E. & Sullivan, M. (2001). Evidence-based practice guidelines for dysarthria: management of velopharyngeal function. *Journal of Medical Speech-Language Pathology, 9,* 257–274

Titze, I.R. (1994). *Principles of Voice Production.* Englewood Cliffs, NJ: Prentice-Hall

Tsunoda, K., Kikkawa, Y.S., Kumada, M., Higo, R., & Tavama, N. (2003). Hoarseness caused by unilateral vocal fold paralysis: how long should one delay phonosurgery? *Acta Otolaryngologica, 123,* 555–556

Weismer, G. & Liss, J. (1991). Reductionism is a deadend in speech research: perspectives on new direction. In: C.A. Moore, K.M. Yorkston, D.R. Beukelman (Eds.), *Dysarthria and Apraxia of Speech: Perspectives on Management* (pp. 3–14). Baltimore: Paul H. Brookes

Wertz, R.T. (1985). Neuropathologies of speech and language: an introduction to patient management. In: D.F. Johns (Ed.), *Clinical Management of Communicative Disorders,* 2nd ed. (pp. 1–96). Boston: Little, Brown

Witt, P.D., O'Daniel, T.G., Marsh, J.L., Grames, L.M., Muntz, H.R., & Pilgram, T.K. (1997). Surgical management of velopharyngeal dysfunction: outcome analysis of autogenous posterior pharyngeal wall augmentation. *Plastic and Reconstructive Surgery, 99,* 1287–1296.

Wood, P.H.N. (1980). Appreciating the consequences of disease: the classification of impairment, disability and handicap. *World Health Organization Chronicle, 43,* 376–380

Youmans, S.R. & Stierwalt, J.A.G. (2005). An acoustic profile of normal swallowing. *Dysphagia, 20,* 195–209

Youmans, S.R. & Stierwalt, J.A.G. (2006). Measures of tongue function related to normal swallowing. *Dysphagia, 21,* 102–111

Yorkston, K.M., Beukelman, D.R., & Bell, K.R. (1988). *Clinical Management of Dysarthric Speakers.* Boston: College-Hill; Little, Brown

Yorkston, K.M., Beukelman, D.R., Strand, E.A., & Bell, K.R. (1999) *Management of Motor Speech Disorders in Children and Adults.* Austin: Pro-Ed

Zeitels, S.M. (2000). New procedures for paralytic dysphonia: adduction arytenopexy, Goretex medialization laryngoplasty, and cricothyroid subluxation. *Otolaryngological Clinics of North America, 33,* 841–854

Chapter 9

Ataxic Dysarthria

Michael P. Cannito and Thomas P. Marquardt

Ataxic dysarthria (AD) is a disorder of sensorimotor control for speech production that results from damage to the cerebellum or to its input and output pathways. The dragging and blurred quality of AD speech has sometimes been likened to "drunken speech" (Netsell, 1986), which results from the particular vulnerability of the cerebellum to the immediate effects of alcohol ingestion. Patients with AD suffer not from inebriation, however, but from a dramatic disintegration of fundamental motor processes, termed "ataxia," due to disturbance of the essential role played by the cerebellum in the regulation of movement. The cerebellum, or "little brain," is a highly complex structure that, like the cerebrum that overlays it, consists of a convoluted outer cortex replete with gyri and sulci, two hemispheres subdivided into various lobes, subcortical white matter projections and paired deep nuclei, as well as diverse efferent and afferent projections via the cerebellar peduncles, which interconnect with other central nervous system structures. Due to its distinct complexity of structure and connectivity, the cerebellum cannot be viewed as subserving any single function. Its duties are manifold and have been described as follows: the regulation of muscle spindle activity for postural maintenance (Granit, 1977), the ongoing comparison and correction of intended with achieved postural goals (Thach, 1980), signaling the sensory discrepancy between predicted and actual sensory consequences of movement (Blakemore, Frith, & Wolpert, 2001), the rapid timing generation and ballistic motor programming (Kornhuber, 1975), sensorimotor learning (Eccles, 1977), auditory and visual information processing (Mortimer, 1975), and even cognitive linguistic behavior (Leiner, Leiner, & Dow, 1991), including temporal aspects of speech perception (Ackermann, Graber, Hertrich, & Daum, 1999).

This chapter emphasizes those aspects of sensorimotor function that are most relevant to the assessment and treatment of the speech deficits associated with AD. For a more comprehensive discussion of cerebellar structure and function, see Ito (1984). This chapter reviews the pathophysiology of ataxia and its nonspeech symptomatology; discusses existing research findings on the physiological, acoustic, and perceptual characteristics of AD speech; and provides a systematic framework for treatment, supported with efficacy data where available.

◆ Pathophysiology of Ataxia

Cerebellar Structure and Function

Gilman (1986) suggested that it is clinically useful to conceptualize the cerebellar cortex in terms of three sagittal subdivisions or zones: *a medial zone,* which includes the cerebellar vermis, a "worm-shaped" band of midline cortex that lies between the hemispheres; *a paravermal zone,* which includes the more medial aspects of each cerebellar hemisphere adjacent to the vermis; and a *lateral zone,* which includes the more lateral portions of the hemispheres. Each cortical zone projects axonal fibers to the subcortical nuclei, bilaterally paired neuronal masses, deep within the cerebellum. The medial zone comprises only approximately 5% of the human cerebellum and projects to the fastigial nuclei; the paravermal zone comprises approximately 7% of the cerebellum and projects to the globose and emboliform nuclei; and the lateral zone, comprising approximately 88% of the human cerebellum, projects to the dentate nuclei (Eccles, 1977). Major inputs to the medial (vermal) zone include spinal cord and the vestibular, reticular, and trigeminal nuclei of the brainstem, whereas major outputs (via the fastigial nuclei) include vestibulospinal and reticulospinal projections. The paravermal zone of the cerebellar hemispheres receives input from the cerebral motor cortex, brainstem, and spinal cord, and projects output (via the globose and emboliform nuclei) back to these areas. The lateral zone of the cerebellar hemispheres receives major cerebral input relayed via pontine and reticular nuclei of the brainstem, and projects its output (via the dentate nuclei) to brainstem and thalamic structures, which in turn relay information to both spinal and cerebral levels.

According to Gilman (1986), the medial zone contributes primarily to locomotion and posture; clinical symptoms associated with damage to this region include abnormalities of stance and gait, truncal titubation, rotated postures of the head, and disturbances of extraocular movement. Gilman suggests that at our present state of knowledge the functions of the paravermal zone are not well understood, and for clinical purposes it may be grouped with the lateral zone. Symptoms associated with damage of the cerebellar hemispheres relate primarily to voluntary movement and include hypotonia, dysmetria, dysdiadochokinesis, excessive rebound, impaired check, tremors, decomposition of movement, eye movement disorders, and dysarthria (Gilman, 1986).

It is clear that the cerebellum serves as a component in several control loops for sensory motor systems (e.g., cortical–pontine–cerebellar–thalamic–cortical), which appear to be involved in movement initiation and specification of muscular activation patterns necessary for coordinated movements (Alexander & Delong, 1986). The cerebral premotor cortex (which includes Broca's and supplemental motor areas in humans) and the primary motor cortex project via brainstem nuclei onto the lateral cerebellum and receive back cerebellar projections, via the ventrolateral thalamus (Leiner et al, 1991; Sasaki, 1984; Schell & Strict, 1984). Studies by Thach (1975, 1978) of neuroelectrical activity in awake monkeys during wrist flexion and extension have demonstrated that neuronal activity in the dentate nucleus precedes activity in the motor cortex, which in turn precedes the appearance of electromyograph (EMG) activity in the extremity. In contrast, the interpositus nucleus (analogous to the human globose and emboliform nuclei) is active during movement, or in response to perturbations of static holding positions. These and other similar studies collectively suggest that contributions of the cerebellum to voluntary movement control include initiation, continuation, and termination of movements, regulation of slow ramp, ballistic, and compound movements, maintenance of static postures, and compound postural adjustments (Brooks & Thach, 1981). Although few physiological data of this type are available on the role of the cerebellum in normal speech production, owing to the lack of viable animal models, cerebellar activation during speech production has been demonstrated via positron emission tomography (Petersen, Fox, Posner, Mintun, & Raichle, 1988). It is reasonable to assume that cerebellar participation in speech motor function is similar to that reported in voluntary arm movement. This assumption is reinforced by the striking speech deficits, analogous to ataxic limb impairments, observed in patients with AD in association with cerebellar lesions (Brown, Darley, & Aronson, 1970).

The neural substrate for ataxic dysarthria was originally thought to be in the cerebellar vermis region (Holmes, 1917; Mills, & Weisenburg, 1914); however, dysarthria with lesions restricted to the cerebellar hemispheres has also been reported (Holmes, 1917). Lechtenberg and Gilman (1978) examined surgical, autopsy, and radiographic data on 122 patients with focal, nondegenerative cerebellar disease, of which 32 had exhibited AD. Twenty-one of these patients had left cerebellar hemisphere damage, seven had right hemisphere damage, and two had vermal lesions. Three additional cerebellar patients who had normal speech following an initial lesion developed AD subsequent to surgical resection of the left cerebellar hemisphere. The authors interpret these findings as strong evidence of a left hemispheric lateralization of speech function in the cerebellum. The area identified by Lechtenberg and Gilman (1978) in association with AD corresponds well on the left side to cerebellar areas reported for bilateral afferent representation of the tongue and larynx (Bowman, 1971; Lam & Ogura, 1952). Although the left cerebellar hemisphere may house an important subcortical center for speech

production, Gilman, Bloedel, and Lechtenberg (1981) have recognized that the left hemisphere localization probably does not account for all manifestations of AD occurring with cerebellar disease. Orofacial structures have somatotopic input and output representation in the right cerebellar hemisphere as well as the left, and are also represented in the anterior portion of the vermis (Thach, 1980); thus is it not surprising that some cases of AD have been observed following lesions in these areas. In addition, AD is frequently associated with damage to the input and output pathways of the cerebellum in such disorders as Friedreich's ataxia and olivopontocerebellar atrophy (Gilman & Kluin, 1984).

♦ Ataxiogenic Disorders

The term *ataxia* is used with various connotations in specific circumstances. Sometimes it refers to difficulties with stance and gait, or it is a generic heading for collective symptoms of cerebellar disease (e.g., "ataxic dysarthria"); more properly it refers to a loss of motor synergy or the ability to integrate movement subcomponents in the appropriate time and space (Gilman, 1986). Etiologies of disorders that cause ataxia and related symptoms include degenerative, traumatic, vascular, infectious, metabolic, and neoplastic conditions, as well as congenital anomalies. All types of ataxiogenic disorders may be associated with AD; however, AD incidence varies greatly in different disease states. For example, AD occurs in approximately 25% of focal cerebellar lesions (Lechtenberg & Gilman, 1978) but is considered an essential criterion for diagnosis of Friedreich disease (Ackermann & Hertrich, 1993). Gilman et al (1981) provide an extensive discussion of cerebellar disorders, from which much of the following overview (unless otherwise indicated) has been condensed.

Degenerative Ataxias

These ataxias frequently result from inherited conditions which, depending on the specific disorder, may be autosomal recessive or autosomal dominant; may have their onset at any time from birth to adulthood; may be associated with hyperreflexia or hyporeflexia; and characteristically include extracerebellar loci of pathology such as the cerebrum, brainstem nuclei, dorsal columns, or peripheral nerves. Friedreich disease is an example of autosomal recessive disorder that usually has its onset between 6 and 16 years of age; involves the cerebellum, dorsal columns, and the corticospinal tracts; and exhibits hyporeflexia of the deep tendons. It presents initially as gait ataxia, then weakness and fatigability, followed by a marked dysarthria. Autosomal-dominant diseases in which dysarthria is a prominent feature include olivopontocerebellar degenerations of the Menzel and Schute-Haymaker types. Gilman and Kluin (1984) have suggested that, whereas AD of both Friedreich disease and olivopontocerebellar degeneration share perceptual symptoms of slowness, dysrhythmia, excess and equalized stress, and prolonged phonemes and intervals, they can be differentiated on the basis of strained-strangled harshness and low monopitch. These features were attributed to a spastic component related to brainstem degeneration that occurs in olivopontocerebellar degeneration but not in Freidreich disease. The hypothesis of differentiated neural substrata for spastic and ataxic components within the same dysarthric patients appears to be supported by studies of oxygen hypometabolism via positron emission tomography (Gilman & Kluin, 1992). Another degenerative disease that incorporates ataxic and spastic components is multiple sclerosis, which, although not fully understood, is thought to result from an interaction of environmental influence with genetic predisposition (Hogancamp, Rodriguez, & Weinshenker, 1997). The condition is characterized by sclerotic plaques scattered primarily in the white matter throughout the nervous system. Although this disorder is more typically associated with mixed dysarthria, it may sometimes present as AD, depending on the specific locus of demyelinization.

◆ Cerebellar Anomalies

Congenital malformations of the cerebellum and related structures include such factors as agenesis or dysgenesis of the vermis or of one hemisphere, hypoplasia of a particular fiber pathway (e.g., pontocerebellar projections), growth of posterior fossa cysts, or atresia of the foramina of the fourth ventricle, which results in hydrocephalus. Several of these factors combine in the developmental anomalad known as Dandy-Walker malformation. The various Chiari malformations include both brainstem and cerebellar pathology.

◆ Metabolic Disorders

A variety of metabolic conditions are known to affect the cerebellum; however, these typically affect other regions as well. Cerebellar Purkinje cells are among the most sensitive neurons in the nervous system to loss of oxygen associated with hypoxia, ischemia, or severe hyperthermia. Toxins that may affect the cerebellum include heavy metals (e.g., lead and thallium), drugs (e.g., certain barbiturates and anticonvulsants), and alcohol. All of these toxins may have chronic, irreversible effects. Other metabolic etiologies include vitamin and trace metal deficiencies, amino acid deficiencies, and endocrine disorders. Dysarthria is typical of ataxia secondary to hypoxia, myxedema, and Dilantin toxicity, and is variably present in alcoholic cerebellar degeneration (Victor & Ferrendelli, 1970).

◆ Focal Pathologies

Focal cerebellar lesions frequently result from vascular pathology of the posterior inferior, anterior inferior, and superior cerebellar arteries. This may take the form of transient ischemic attacks, infarction, or hemorrhage. Thrombosis is more common than embolism, but hemorrhage is more common than infarction and may result from hypertension, aneurysm and arteriovenous malformations, anticoagulant therapy, or bleeding tumors. Traumatic damage such as gunshot wounds are a frequent cause of focal cerebellar pathology (Holmes, 1917), whereas rotational forces associated with closed head injury are more likely to affect the cerebellar peduncles (Brooke, Uomoto, McLean, & Fraser, 1991). Focal lesions may also result from abscess due to bacterial or viral infections. However, meningitis and encephalitis may cause diffuse cerebellar damage, and the slow virus *kuru* causes extensive cerebellar degeneration. Cerebellar tumors are quite common, with astrocytomas and medulloblastomas occurring more frequently in children, but metastatic tumors occurring more often after middle age (French, Chou, Long, & Seljeskog, 1970). Although the mechanisms are not well understood, neoplasms elsewhere in the body (in which the cancer has not spread to the cerebellum) may also cause cerebellar degeneration and associated AD (Victor & Ferrendelli, 1970).

◆ Nonspeech Concomitants of Ataxic Dysarthria

Generalized Movement Dysfunction

Hypotonia, Hyporeflexia, and Asthenia

Reduced postural muscle tone is believed to be associated with the cerebellum's role in the proprioceptive control of posture, via both cortical and spinal pathways, and may be seen in degenerative illness or most prominently following acute injury (Gilman et al, 1981). With chronic cerebellar disease, the significant postural abnormalities, including abnormal postures of the head, may become entrenched. Diminished limb resistance to passive movement can be demonstrated by grasping the patient's forearm and shaking the relaxed hand at the wrist. Hyporeflexia takes the form of "pendular reflexes," as in clinical elicitation of the patellar reflex wherein the leg swings back and forth at least three times (Gilman et al, 1981). Asthenia and muscle fatigue are also major symptoms of cerebellar disease (Eccles, 1977); affected limbs tire easily on repetitive tasks, and strength has been demonstrated by dynomometry to be as much as 50% below normal function (Holmes, 1939). Weakness is greater in proximal than in distal musculature, and facial weakness is not uncommon. Dworkin and Aronson (1986) studied tongue strength in five AD subjects as part of a broader study of dysarthria wherein anterior and lateral lingual pushing forces were transduced electronically over time and integrated under a force line curve. Inspection of the individual subject data revealed that tongue strength in the AD subgroup ranged from 37 to 96% of average normal function based on gender-matched controls, with three subjects generating less than 50% of expected normal values. Marked instability of force maintenance over time has also been reported for the finger, tongue, lips, and jaw in ataxic subjects (McNeil, Weismer, Adams, & Mulligan, 1990). One mechanism that has been hypothesized to account for voluntary motor weakness in cerebellar disease is that decreased activation of cortical upper motor neurons by the cerebellum results in similarly diminished cortical output via the pyramidal pathway to the lower motor neurons (Eccles, 1977).

Tremor, Titubation, and Myoclonus

Both static and kinetic limb tremors are common in cerebellar disease, and are greater in proximal musculature (Dichgans & Diener, 1984). Both types of tremor manifest at frequencies of 3 to 5 Hz (Jankovic & Fahn, 1980). Static or postural tremor may be demonstrated by extending the patient's arms parallel to the floor; after a few seconds, an oscillation will develop. The kinetic or "intention" tremor may be elicited by having the patient perform the "finger-nose" or "heel-shin" tests, wherein the amplitude of the oscillation typically increases as the extremity approaches its target.

Titubation is a rhythmic rocking of the trunk or head, several times per second, in the forward-to-back, side-to-side, or rotational dimensions (Gilman, 1986). Palatal myoclonus characterized by rhythmic movements of 2 to 3 Hz is associated with dentate nucleus or dentato-olivary tract lesions, and may involve the pharynx, larynx, floor of the mouth, and lower face (Dichgans & Diener, 1984), or co-occur with muscular contractions at the base of the upper limbs (Rondot, Jedynak, & Ferrey, 1978). Marked degrees of positional unsteadiness have been quantitatively demonstrated in ataxic subjects, using a visual cursor matching task, for both cranially and spinally innervated structures (McNeil et al, 1990). Gilman et al (1981) reported that in their series of 162 cerebellar lesioned patients, kinetic tremors were present in 56%, with hemispheric lesions affecting chiefly the ipsilateral limb and vermal lesions usually resulting in bilateral disturbance. Titubation was present in only approximately 9% of their patients and had little localizing significance.

Timing of Movements

Ataxic patients present an impression of pervasive slowness. Hallett, Shahani, and Young (1975) demonstrated that on a fast elbow flexion task, the average reaction time of ataxic patients was 270 ms in comparison to a normal average of 200 ms. This slowness has also been demonstrated after acute poisoning of the cerebellum by alcohol ingestion, when mean thumb flexion reaction time increased to 218 ms over a pre-alcohol mean of 146 ms (Marsden, Merton, Morton, Hallett, Adams, & Rushton, 1977). Marsden et al suggest that motor slowness results in disruption of agonist-antagonist muscle activity during ballistic movements, which interferes with the generation of accelerative and decelerative forces. Termination or breaking of movement is also impaired (Vilis & Hore, 1981). Prolonged delay times for the attainment of peak force generation have also been observed in ataxic patients for lingual pushing activities (Dworkin & Aronson, 1986).

Most authors agree that the motor slowness should not be attributed solely to underlying hypotonia, but rather interpreted as part of a central timing and programming deficit (Eccles, 1977; Hallett et al, 1975; Marsden et al, 1977). Timing abnormalities contribute to the decomposition of movements; however, ataxic patients do not merely move through life in slow motion. Hallet et al (1975) reported that at times on their fast elbow flexion task the patient's arm would move in the opposite direction from that intended and that movement would occur inappropriately at the shoulder joint in inappropriately active muscles that should have fixed the limb. Similar reciprocity abnormalities have also been reported during slow ramp visuomotor elbow tracking (Beppu, Suda, & Tanaka, 1983).

Dysmetria, Check, and Rebound

Dysmetria refers to inappropriate trajectory toward a target during a goal-directed movement. Hypometria, or "undershoot," falls short of the intended target, whereas hypermetria, or "overshoot," surpasses the target (Hallett et al, 1975). A patient with cerebellar ataxia may on repeated occasions hit the target normally and then overshoot or undershoot the same target. Upper limb dysmetrias can be assessed using the "finger-nose" test in which the forefinger of the patient's outstretched arm touches the nose. In hypometria the finger does not reach the nose; in hypermetria the finger points past the nose, perhaps poking the patient in the eye. A dysmetric movement may be erratic throughout, but tends to culminate with a crescendo of tremor-like corrective movements around the target. Gilman et al (1981) reported dysmetria in 74% of their cerebellum-damaged patients in association with left hemisphere, right hemisphere, and vermal lesions.

Check and rebound abnormalities are conceptually similar to dysmetria. Normally, when a limb is flexed strongly against resistance and the resistance is released, the resulting movement is quickly checked. Impaired check is the inability to counteract that resulting forceful movement opposite the direction of the resistance. One clinical test (Gilman, 1986) requires the patient to extend the arms forward in space with hands pronated while keeping the eyes closed. The examiner taps the wrists (strongly enough to displace the arms). A normal individual exhibits a small displacement but rapidly returns to the original position. Impaired check appears as a wide excursion away from the displacement, with *rebound* occurring as a significant overshoot of the original position on the return swing. Dichgans and Diener (1984) speculate that a similar mechanism may underlay dysmetria and impaired check/rebound phenomena due to "a pronounced delay in or absence of the agonist pause and antagonist burst resulting in inappropriate deceleratory forces" (p. 129).

Diadochokinetic Impairments

Decomposition of movement in cerebellar ataxia includes errors in movement direction, off-course deviations during movement, discontinuous movement, dysmetria, and tremor (Dichgans & Diener, 1984). These phenomena can be strikingly demonstrated on tasks involving alternating rapid movements at a single joint or repetitive fine movement sequences. Dysdiadochokinesis appears as slowness and incompleteness of sequence on tasks such as rapid pronation supination of the hand or apposition of each finger against its thumb in rapid succession (Gilman et al, 1981). Irregularity of the rhythm of repetitive movements is also quite characteristic of ataxic patients. Slow and irregular diadochokinesis of the speech musculature has been demonstrated quantitatively using computer-automated analysis of rapidly repeated monosyllables (Portnoy & Aronson, 1982). It should be noted that diadochokinetic abnormalities are common in various neuromotor disorders and therefore are not differentially diagnostic in and of themselves. They do, however, afford a useful mechanism for highlighting the disintegration of complex motor processes in ataxia during clinical evaluation.

Other Associated Deficits

Abnormalities of Stance and Gait

Difficulties with walking and standing are among the most prominent signs of cerebellar disease, occurring frequently as isolated symptoms of vermal damage or in association with other disturbances following damage to the cerebellar hemispheres (Gilman, 1986). Postural instability manifests when standing as excessive swaying (i.e., anterior-posterior, lateral, or multidirectional), which is exacerbated by closing the eyes (Dichgans & Diener, 1984). These patients adopt a wide-based stance, which tends to be maintained when walking, to compensate for truncal instability; nevertheless, falling is common (Gilman et al, 1981). Gilman (1986) described the ataxic gait pattern as "a series of steps irregularly placed, some too far forward, some not sufficiently far forward, and some too far to the left or right" (p. 415). Clinical maneuvers for assessing gait disturbance include walking a straight line; heel-to-toe placement, or "tandem walking"; walking on heels or toes only; or walking backward (Dichgans & Diener, 1984; Gilman et al, 1981).

Oculomotor Dysfunction

Abnormal eye movements associated with cerebellar disease are many and varied. Among the most prominent are gaze-evoked nystagmus, rebound nystagmus, ocular dysmetria, and abnormal optokinetic nystagmus. Gaze-evoked nystagmus manifests as a series of jerking, to-and-fro eye movements when attempting conjugate gaze that deviates from the midline position; the eyes drift slowly back to midline, but there is a rapid corrective movement toward the intended direction of gaze (Gilman et al, 1981). Rebound nystagmus occurs following a prolonged attempt at holding an eccentric gaze (e.g., extreme lateral deviation), during which the gaze-evoked nystagmus gradually disappears, then returning the gaze to midline, whereupon a nystagmus occurs in the opposite direction from the previous gaze-evoked nystagmus (Dichgans & Diener, 1984). Similar to nystagmus is ocular dysmetria, wherein small, rapid oscillating eye movements emerge as the gaze approaches a target and the

patient attempts to correct for overshoot and undershoot of the fixation point (Gilman et al, 1981). Optokinetic nystagmus occurs normally when one observes the telephone poles on the roadside from a moving vehicle and clinically when attempting to count the stripes on a moving strip of cloth; the eyes follow the leading stripe and then jerk back to the next. According to Gilman et al (1981), patients with chronic cerebellar disease may exhibit enhanced amplitude of optokinetic nystagmus, but patients with acute cerebellar lesions may have inconsistent or diminished optokinetic nystagmus. Smooth visual pursuit of a moving target is also frequently impaired in cerebellar ataxia patients (Dichgans & Diener, 1984).

Nondysarthric Communication Disorders

Other nonspeech factors affecting communication in patients with AD include disorders of writing, cognition, and hearing. In their patient series, Gilman et al (1981) observed dysgraphia in 33% (not surprisingly given the extent of limb impairments), and more than 10% had overt psychotic symptoms including visual hallucinations, paranoid ideation, and confabulation, all of which may result in language of confusion. Dementia sometimes occurs in degenerative diseases that affect the cerebellum, but is generally attributed to damage to other structures. Although not a direct consequence of cerebellar damage itself, hearing loss commonly co-occurs with a variety of cerebellar diseases including tumors and vascular occlusions (Gilman et al, 1981).

Implications for Speech Production

The striking varieties of motoric abnormalities that are associated with cerebellar disorders affect not only the movement capabilities of the limbs and torso, but also the functions of the cranially innervated structures involved in speaking. Thus, the neurophysiological bases of AD have been postulated to be of essentially the same character as motor abnormalities found elsewhere in the body and during nonspeech functions (Brown, Darley, & Aronson, 1970). Netsell and Kent (1976) proposed three hypotheses concerning the cerebellum's role in the execution of skilled movements, including speech, all of which may be operative to different degrees in different types of cerebellar lesions.

First, the cerebellum affects sensorimotor integration by biasing muscle spindles that provide continuous feedback concerning states of muscular contraction. Depression of spindle activity deprives the motor system of proprioceptive feedback about evolving movements, and reduces expected background level of muscular activation that would normally facilitate α motor neuron discharge. This could inhibit the strength, speed, and accuracy of movement, leading to compensatory slowing. Second, the cerebellum is important to the interpretation of afferent proprioceptive information for ongoing motor control by translating the "language of tensions" into the "language of movements." Impairment of this interpretative function could result in deautomaticity of movement, leading to errors of direction, timing, and range. Third, cerebellar-cerebral interaction involves the regulation and facilitation of cortical motor commands on an ongoing basis by the cerebellum. This could lead to the phenomenon of the presence of motor gestures that are preserved in some form but lacking in precision. It is clear that much of the underlying sensorimotor symptomatology of cerebellar disease observable during nonspeech functions is also distinctively manifested during speech activities.

◆ Speech Characteristics of Ataxic Dysarthria

Studies of ataxia have utilized single subjects with well-documented lesions limited to the cerebellum/peduncle apparatus (e.g., Kent and Netsell, 1975), groups heterogeneous in etiology and severity (Kent, Netsell, & Abbs, 1979; Kent, Kent, Duffy, Thomas, Weismer, & Stuntebeck, 2000), and small-scale studies of relatively homogeneous subjects with cerebellar atrophy (Ackermann, Hertrich, & Scharf, 1995; Hertich & Ackermann, 1999). The problem with case studies is that it is difficult to determine the idiosynchronicity of the observed deficits and whether the findings are generalizable to a broader group of subjects. Group studies that have focused on subjects with diverse etiologies (e.g., Darley, Aronson, & Brown, 1969a) or degenerative lesions such as Friedreich's ataxia (Ackermann & Hertrich, 1993) or multiple sclerosis (Darley, Brown, & Goldstein, 1972; Farmakides & Boone, 1960) show damage outside the cerebellum and make it difficult to isolate deficits attributable to the cerebellum alone. Moreover, as noted by Kent, Netsell, and Abbs (1979), it is difficult to separate speech behaviors due to the lesion from motor control compensations that are a response to the impairment. These qualifications withstanding, we will present speech characteristics of ataxic dysarthria.

Early descriptions of ataxic dysarthria are rooted in the context of the clinical neurological examination. Charcot (1877) described slow, scanning speech; Holmes (1917) noted the monotonous vocal characteristics and indistinct production of consonants and vowels. Brown et al (1970), in a review of medical textbooks of neurology, used the adjectives "slow, slurred, irregular, labored, intermittent, jerky, explosive, staccato, singsong, and scanning" (p. 302) to describe the disorder. Speech deficits in ataxia are due to errors in the timing, force, range, and direction of movements that would be expected to affect respiratory, laryngeal, and articulatory structures. The first large-scale perceptual study of ataxic dysarthria with lesions specific to the cerebellum was included in a series of reports from the Mayo Clinic (Darley, Aronson, & Brown, 1969a, 1969a,b; Brown et al, 1970) that provided a comprehensive description of the primary characteristics of the disorder. Darley et al (1969a,b) studied 212 patients divided into seven groups, one group being subjects with cerebellar damage from a wide range of etiologies (stroke, progressive degeneration, and trauma). Ratings on 38 dimensions were completed from speech and reading samples. Prominent dimensions for ataxic dysarthria included imprecise consonants, irregular articulatory breakdown with

errors that were inconsistent, and sudden "telescoping" of a syllable or syllables. Also prominent were excess and equal stress ("scanning speech"), prolonged phonemes and intervals, and slow rate interactively encompassing prosodic abnormalities tied to the equalization and increase in stress. Based on the perceptual ratings, Darley et al (1969b) divided the 10 most deviant dimensions into three clusters: articulatory inaccuracy (irregular articulatory breakdown, imprecise consonants, distorted vowels); prosodic excess (excess and equal stress, prolonged phonemes, prolonged intervals, slow rate); and phonatory-prosodic insufficiency (monoloudness, monopitch, harsh voice), which have served as a focus of subsequent studies of electromyography, kinematics, and speech acoustics in ataxic dysarthria.

Despite myriad motoric difficulties that are observable in AD, disturbances of *motor programming* do not appear to be the primary source of the speech movement abnormalities. The cortically programmed serial speech gestures are not disturbed in ataxic dysarthria although there are abnormalities in speech movement rate, range, and direction (Netsell, 1973). As noted by Netsell and Kent (1976):

> The preservation of the desired successional patterns in the face of conspicuous abnormalities in individual structural movements and speaking rate might be explained by assuming that the successional pattern for speech movements is programmed at the cortical level and that cerebellar dysfunction results in the delayed and inaccurate execution of the required submovements. In short, the coordination of articulatory movements is not destroyed, even though the overall movement pattern is slowed and individual movements may be misdirected (p. 106).

Respiration

Respiratory activity is compromised in ataxic speakers including vital capacity (Brown, Darley, & Aronson, 1970) and total lung capacity (Murdoch, Chenery, Stokes, & Hardcastle, 1991). Speech respiration is characterized by abnormal synchrony in the respiratory apparatus (Gilman & Kluin, 1984; Hiller, 1929). Abbs, Hunker, and Barlow (1983), in a kinematic study, described paradoxical respiratory activity in an ataxic speaker in which abdominal contributions to lung volume changes were inspiratory whereas rib cage contributions were expiratory. They suggested that the asynchrony of rib cage and abdomen could potentially interfere with lung volume control and subglottal pressure. Murdoch et al (1991), using strain gauge pneumographs, found "bizarre" movements of the abdomen and rib cage in a study of 12 ataxics. Abdominal paradoxing was found, with one exception, during the performance of sustained vowel and syllable repetition tasks. The paradoxing was most notable on demanding syllable repetition tasks compared with sustained vowels. Rib cage paradoxing (circumference of the rib cage increasing while the lung volume and circumference of the abdomen are decreasing) also was found in addition to motion jerks that originated from the rib cage and abdomen, and there were abrupt changes in the chest wall's contributions to lung volume displacements. The majority of the ataxics initiated reading and conversation below expected lung volume levels.

However, they expired through a large portion of their vital capacity on vowels and syllable repetitions.

Studies of respiratory kinematics suggest that ataxics have difficulty regulating the output of the respiratory apparatus for speech due to discoordinated rib cage/abdomen movements. Respiratory hypofunction in the form of subnormal vital capacity and forced expiratory volumes occurred in a significant minority of AD patients (Murdoch et al, 1991). Netsell (1973), however, found that a 60-year-old ataxic patient was able to maintain intraoral pressures of 5 cm H_2O and 10 cm H_2O and concluded that this subject did not have a respiratory component to her speech deficits. Deger, Ziegler, and Wessel (1999) investigated expiratory airflow control in 17 patients with ataxia and normal control subjects on hold and ramp-tracking tasks. In contrast to expected small-amplitude high-frequency corrections, the ataxic patients had fewer but more sweeping corrections and abrupt airflow stops, and showed no improvement in ramp-tracking precision over 15 learning trials. There is little doubt that the coordinated respiratory activity for speech in ataxia is compromised, but may be only weakly related to dysarthria severity. The effects of the incoordination of rib cage and abdomen on generation of sustained subglottal pressure for speech, however, have not been systematically investigated, a major research shortfall given the phonatory and prosodic abnormalities described as characteristic of the disorder.

Phonation

Early instrumental studies focused on the utility of acoustic analysis for differential diagnosis. Scripture (1916) utilized a phonoautograph, an instrument constructed of a mouthpiece that led to a metal tube covered with a flexible membrane. Movements of the membrane were recorded on a blackened cylinder. He reported that 20 patients with disseminated sclerosis, whether speech was affected or not, demonstrated waveforms consistent with jerky irregularities of tension of the vocal folds occurring at the beginning and end of a vowel. He interpreted these findings as a difficulty in the ability to make adjustments in laryngeal tension. Similarly, Janvrin (1933) and Janvrin and Worster-Drought (1932) utilized "sound tracks" to demonstrate upward jerks in the laryngeal waveform of a patient with disseminated sclerosis, which were interpreted as incoordination in laryngeal muscle function due to ataxia. Scripture (1933) believed waveform analysis was a reliable means of differential diagnosis, but Haggard (1969) demonstrated that there was significant overlap between multiple sclerosis and normal subjects in waveform variation, and noted that the claim of differential diagnosis should be viewed as a historical curiosity.

"Harshness" is most frequently used to describe phonatory function in ataxic dysarthria (Darley et al, 1969b; Gilman & Kluin, 1984; Joanette & Dudley, 1980). Kent and Netsell (1975) noted the frequent appearance of aperiodic vocal pulse striations in their ataxic speaker, which is typically believed to be due to hypotonia. Some patients may engage in excessive straining or squeezing in an attempt to compensate for weakened laryngeal function. Highly variable phonation with sudden bursts of loudness and irregular pitch and loudness increases might also be expected as a result of discoordination (Zwirner, Murry, & Woodson, 1991). Gentil (1990b) reported abnormally unsteady phonation of sustained vowels in terms of both fundamental frequency and intensity contours in all of his 14 Friedreich ataxia subjects. He concluded that this was due to respiratory-phonatory asynergy. Zwirner et al (1991) acoustically evaluated sustained vowel productions in terms of fundamental frequency, the standard deviation of fundamental frequency, jitter, shimmer, and signal-to-noise ratio in groups of parkinsonian, ataxic, and Huntington's subjects. They found a significant correlation between perceptual judgments of severity of dysphonia and all measures of phonatory variability for the cerebellar subjects. The cerebellar subjects differed significantly from normals on standard deviation of fundamental frequency and jitter, which may be respectively interpreted as indications of long-term and short-term variability in vocal fold vibration. However, the distributional overlap with the normal subjects on the acoustic measures was large. They concluded that as vocal instability increases, perceived severity of dysphonia increases for individuals with cerebellar lesions. Ackermann and Ziegler (1994), in a study of patients with either cerebellar atrophy or olivopontocerebellar atrophy, found increased jitter and pitch fluctuations for a subgroup of the patients that was not related to articulatory or nonspeech ataxia findings. Based on these earlier studies and acoustical analyses of prolonged vowel production in groups of ataxic speakers (Kent, Kent, Rosenbek, Vorperian & Weismer, 1997; Kent, et al, 2000) that found abnormalities in fundamental frequency fluctuations, shimmer, and peak amplitude variation, it can be concluded that phonatory irregularities are a dominant feature of voice quality in AD.

Articulation

Hypotonia is a primary neuromuscular characteristic of ataxia in speech musculature, although it may not account for all observed movement deficits (Netsell & Kent, 1976). Based on data from Abbs, Barlow, and Cole (1979) and Netsell and Abbs (1977), Netsell (1982) identified two types of electromyographic patterns in subjects with cerebellar lesions. One pattern is characterized by a gradual buildup of amplitude that approximates normal levels, but which then is prolonged with a corresponding increase in the duration of movement. A second pattern shows repetitive bursts of excitation and quieting, producing fluctuations in the degree of force between articulatory structures. Netsell summarized muscle function in ataxia as follows:

> In short, the cerebellar subject is slow, or slow plus irregular, in building up the requisite muscle force in the prime mover and, once the force is achieved, cannot rapidly suppress the activity... [and] ... cerebellar failure slows, or makes discontinuous, the normally phasic and precise muscle forces. As a consequence, all muscle contractions tend to have a uniformly long duration, yielding slow velocities to all movements and uniform duration to the syllables (pp. 43–44).

The finding of irregularity in muscle activation and suppression was demonstrated by Hirose, Kiritani, Ushijima, and Sawashima (1978), who found that EMG patterns in two ataxic patients were irregular in shape and timing, with a plateau of activity during a period of suppression with disturbed repetitive syllable production. Gentil (1990a), in an investigation of muscle function in antagonistic facial muscles plus the anterior belly of the digastric, observed increased reaction times between an auditory stimulus and the onset of muscular activity. There also was a loss of reciprocity between antagonistic muscles in eight of the 13 subjects studied, expanded mean durations of anticipatory muscle activity, and prolonged muscle activity on syllable segments, which he attributed to hypotonia. Interestingly, Forrest, Adams, McNeil, and Southwood (1991) did not find differences in the EMG between various neurogenic groups (including cerebellar lesion subjects) on the basis of co-contraction and reciprocal activity in antagonistic facial muscles.

The neuromuscular features of ataxic dysarthria, then, appear to be hypotonia associated with deficits in graded muscle force development and corresponding disruptions in the synchrony of muscle activation/suppression. Kent and Netsell (1975) suggested that hypotonia may be the primary source of speech abnormalities in ataxic dysarthria that produces delays in muscle force generation producing prolongation, reduced rates of muscular contraction causing slowed movement, and reduced range of movements producing telescoping. These observations are consistent with kinematic studies of ataxia.

Early speech movement studies in ataxia focused on case studies of paroxysmal ataxic dysarthria (Netsell & Kent, 1976) or generalized degeneration of the cerebellum (Kent & Netsell, 1975; Kent, Netsell, & Bauer, 1975). In these studies cinefluorography was used to measure displacements of the lip, jaw, and tongue during the production of sustained vowels and phrases. Primary findings included reduced articulatory velocities, prolongation of consonant constrictions and vowel steady states, inappropriate or missed articulatory targets, and poor tongue positioning for vowels. Microbeam-based measurement of lip and jaw movement (Hirose et al, 1978) also has revealed inconsistent velocities of lower lip movements and times when lip movement was dependent entirely on jaw movement. However, lip velocities, in contrast to Kent and Netsell's findings, were not markedly slowed for the ataxic subject. The authors concluded that ataxic dysarthria was characterized by "a difficulty in the initiation of purposeful movements and an inconsistency of articulatory movements, particularly in the repetitive production of a monosyllable" (p. 96). McNeil and Adams (1990) employed movement transducers affixed to the patients' lips and jaw, in conjunction with the co-occurring acoustic signal, to examine speech movement capabilities of four AD patients in comparison to normal controls and aphasic and apraxic subjects. The AD patients were significantly slower than normal on durations of opening and closing phases of a /b/ segment and time to peak velocity for the opening gesture. Using an optoelectric movement analysis system to examine lower lip movements during production of target words embedded in a carrier phrase,

Ackermann et al (1995) found increased prolongation of vocalic segments, but with durational contrasts suggesting preserved phonological vowel length specification. AD performance was characterized by a highly linear relationship between peak velocity and movement, but velocity-displacement ratios were decreased compared with normal subjects. In terms of lip movements, individuals with AD demonstrate reduced maximum velocities for a given amplitude of oral opening and closing (Ackermann, Hertrich, Daum, Scharf, & Spieker, 1997). These studies suggest that the primary movement characteristics of ataxia are reduced articulatory velocities and inaccuracy of movement.

Acoustical analysis has been the primary vehicle for inferences about movement-related deficits in ataxia and for examining the prosodic abnormalities characteristic of the disorder. Individuals with ataxic dysarthria demonstrate longer syllable durations, longer formant transitions, and, at times, longer voice onset times (VOTs) (Kent et al, 1979). Kent et al (1979) noted, however, that the slowed rate of the ataxic speaker may allow additional time to reach vowel targets. They also found that word durations for ataxic speakers were longer with a relative lengthening of both consonant clusters and word nuclei, and, in contrast to Ackermann et al (1995), noted a loss of durational distinctions between tense and lax vowels. Differences in variability of segment durations were not large, considering they were four to seven times longer than normal speakers', but there appeared to be highly variable lax vowels in the more severely involved patients. In the production of base words they demonstrated instances of lengthening, inconsistent reductions, and small reductions compared with normal speakers. Kent et al (1979) concluded that a fundamental feature of ataxia was the lengthening of segments, with some segments lengthened more than others, resulting in a disruption in the normal speech rhythm and timing. Duration appeared to reflect the severity of ataxia with longer segments reflecting more severe involvement. Gentil (1990b) examined the production of one-, two-, and three-syllable nonsense utterances to investigate variability. He found larger coefficients of variability in patients with Friedreich's ataxia, and concluded that inconsistency of segment duration was a feature of the speech disorder. Other findings included increased durations of single word and phrase productions, and reduced diadochokinetic rates. Keller (1990) also noted higher variability of vowels, occlusions, syllable durations, and VOTs in monosyllable repetition for three ataxic subjects. Ouellon, Ryalls, Lebeuf, and Joanette (1991) reported, in patients with Friedreich's ataxia, an increase in VOT variability resulting in a reduction of the voicing lead-lag differences for cognate pairs of French initial plosives (e.g., /p - b/), which in turn led to the percept of inconsistent substitution errors.

These findings were consistent, in part, with a study of seven subjects with Friedreich's ataxia (Ackermann & Hertrich, 1993). Twelve German sentences were produced from which target words were available for analysis. Syllable durations, with two exceptions, were outside the normal range. However, variation coefficients, with the exception of one syllable, were within the normal 95% confidence intervals for normal subjects. Duration ratios of stressed syllable to sentence duration were greater for the ataxic subjects. In spite of reduced stressed syllable duration, stress was marked by duration, suggesting that encoding of linguistic prosody was not impaired. No significant differences in intrasyllabic timing, as reflected in VOT, were observed for voiceless consonants, although variation coefficients were greater for the ataxic group. However, occlusion durations were increased. Primary findings, then, were increased syllable, vowel, and occlusion segment durations; normal or near-normal VOTs; and preservation of the timing of speech segments as reflected in variation coefficients.

Several studies have focused on diadochokinetic rates (Boutsen, Bakker, & Duffy, 1997; Ozawa, Shiromoto, Ishizaki, & Watamori, 2001; Tjaden & Watling, 2003) or differential performance as a function of speech task (e.g., Kent et al, 1997), and underscore the need for multiple levels of testing to capture a detailed picture of speech in AD. Ziegler and Wessel (1996) investigated syllable timing in 16 AD subjects during sentence production and rapid syllable repetition tasks. With one exception, rapid repetitive articulation, frequently irregularly paced, was slower than during sentence production and was a powerful predictor of dysarthria severity.

They ascribed the disproportionate slowing on the diadokokinetic task to the novel nature of a maximum performance repetition task compared with sentence production. Kent et al (1997) recorded six AD patients and normal middle-aged and older men during speech tasks that included vowel phonation, syllable repetition, monosyllabic word production, sentence repetition, and conversation. Acoustic analyses found increased segment duration variability, segment prolongations in syllable repetition and sentence recitations, and inflexibility to changes in speaking rate. The different tasks emphasized different aspects of the speech disorder in AD. The cerebellar patients demonstrated increased shimmer values and long-term fundamental frequency variability on the vowel prolongation task. However, word intelligibility was minimally informative in discriminating the two groups. Particular difficulty for the AD patients was noted in syllable repetition at a fast rate; sequences were slow and variable. The AD patients also demonstrated a slower speaking rate on sentences but did not differ on a derived scanning index. The authors emphasized that temporal regulation impairment was a primary component of AD, but manifestations of this impairment depended on the speaking task. In a subsequent study of 14 AD patients that included similar tasks, Kent et al (2000) concluded that AD is a global impairment of respiratory, laryngeal, and articulatory subsystems with some expected individual variability in the relative impairment of the systems. Evaluation of AD, based on these studies, requires use of varied speech tasks to identify the key features of the disorder and to capture individual variability.

Resonance

Variables related to resonance, an interactive acoustic byproduct of phonation and articulation, have not been well studied in AD. Oral resonances, or formants, appear to be normal if allowances are made for slowness in achieving target values and inconsistent overshoot and undershoot

(Kent & Netsell, 1975). Perceptual reports of hypernasal resonance relating to palatal function suggest that it is usually only minimally impaired (Darley, Aronson, & Brown, 1975; Enderby, 1983). Grunewell and Huskins (1979) reported inconsistent articulation errors (e.g., substitution of /b/ for /m/ or /m/ for /b/) associated with the phonetic feature of nasality in AD, which they interpreted to be due to coordination and timing difficulties. Yorkston and Beukelman (1981a) reported that, prior to treatment, one of their AD subjects was perceived to be significantly hypernasal, and this was supported by airflow and pressure measurements. However, the hypernasality proved to be attributable to discoordination of palatal movement with that of other articulators because it was eliminated in response to slowing of the speaking rate (Yorkston & Beukelman, 1981a).

Prosody

Perceptual impressions of pervasive dysprosody (e.g., scanning speech, prosodic excess, prosodic insufficiency) have dominated descriptions of AD. Studies have demonstrated that, unlike other forms of dysarthria, prosody and naturalness may be impaired independently of intelligibility in AD (Bunton, Kent, Kent, & Rosenbek, 2000; LeDorze Ryalls, Brassard, Boulanger, & Ratte, 1998; Linebaugh & Wolfe, 1984). Specific prosodic disturbances also may vary depending on the speaking task or linguistic domain in question (Kent et al, 1997). At the word level of analysis, aspects of word-level stress appear to be more intact. Odell, McNeil, Rosenbek, and Hunter (1991) perceptually examined vowel errors in speakers with AD. Although they reported a variety of segmental errors (e.g., more substitution than distortion errors, more errors in polysyllabic than monosyllabic words, and more error in noninitial positions of words), abnormal prosodic features at the single word level were not characteristic of AD subjects. Preserved abilities included perceptible marking of syllabic stress, and initiating and completing word productions. In contrast, acoustic analysis has demonstrated that AD subjects failed to shorten word stems when adding suffixes to words (Kent et al, 1979). Murry (1983a) suggested that ataxic dysarthrics use compensatory activity in the production of stress as a function of word position. Yorkston, Beukelman, Minifie, and Sapir (1984) examined sentence-level stress patterns in three AD patients using a combination of perceptual scaling and acoustical analyses of fundamental frequency, intensity, and duration. One patient exhibited inconsistent perceptible stress errors, one used exaggerated fundamental frequency differences to mark stress, and one used compensatory lengthening of stressed syllables.

At the phrase and sentence level of analysis, more marked occurrence of dysprosody has been consistently observed. Increased duration of syllables and segments and loss of durational distinctions between stressed and unstressed syllables, coupled with reduced control of fundamental frequency and intensity parameters, mark the prosodic abnormalities of ataxic speakers. Fewer words per tone group (Bunton et al, 2000) and occasional occurrence of unusually long pauses (Rosen, Kent, & Duffy, 2003) have also been reported. Attempts to acoustically quantify the percept of scanning speech based on syllable-duration measures have demonstrated increased syllable duration and increased syllable equalization within utterances for 14 cases with "pure cerebellar pathology" (Ackermann & Hertrich, 1994) and 14 cases of AD secondary to multiple sclerosis (Hartelius, Runmarker, Andersen, & Nord, 2000) in comparison to nondisabled control subjects. Hartelieus et al also demonstrated a greater than normal tendency toward isochrony, or uniformity of intervals between strongly stressed syllables in AD, which should also contribute to percepts of scanning or excess and equal stress. Paradoxically, both of these studies demonstrated abnormally increased coefficients of variation for syllable durations between utterances (Ackermann & Hertrich, 1994; Hartelius et al, 2000). Collectively, the findings suggest both inflexibility and instability of timing that may be indicative of a broader cerebellar movement timing disorder.

Kent et al (1979) described two fundamental frequency patterns characteristic of ataxics. One pattern was typified by fundamental frequency that falls within each syllable as if each syllable contained its own declarative form. A second pattern included a flat fundamental frequency contour like a monotone. Large sweeps in fundamental frequency (Gentil, 1990b; Kent & Netsell, 1975) also have been reported as characteristic of the disorder. Kent and Rosenbek (1979) employed descriptive spectrography to characterize ataxic dysprosody. They reported sweeping patterns with pronounced shifts in fundamental frequency accompanied by abnormalities in syllable durations, dissociated patterns with homogeneous intrasyllabic features characterized by segregated syllables of nearly uniform duration, and segregated syllabic patterns in which some prosodic cohesion is maintained as characteristic of AD. LeDorze et al (1998) reported abnormally reduced rate of speech as well as reduced variability of fundamental frequency in 10 speakers with AD secondary to Friedreich's ataxia based on quantitative acoustic analyses using a sentence repetition task. Five speakers with AD secondary to variable cerebellar pathology demonstrated abnormally increased word duration, and abnormally decreased variability of fundamental frequency and intensity based on quantitative acoustic analyses of conversational speech (Bunton et al, 2000).

In summary, all speech subsystems may be significantly deficient in AD. Speech is marked by hypotonia and discoordination with reduced velocities and inaccuracy of articulatory movements in the presence of grossly normal programming of speech sequences. Segments and syllables are variable and increased in duration, with a loss of durational distinctions between stressed and unstressed syllables. Slow rate and flat fundamental frequency contours, at times marked by wide sweeps or syllable specific declinations, characterize the prosody of these speakers.

♦ Assessment Considerations

The overall organization of the motor speech evaluation for AD does not differ conceptually from that of other types of dysarthria and need not be reiterated here (see Chapters 2 through 7). Some special considerations for assessing patients with AD are worth highlighting, however, because they feed directly into the planning, implementation, and monitoring of AD-specific treatment.

First, there are sufficient discrepancies in findings, across studies and between patients within studies, of the speech characteristics of AD to suggest the likelihood of differential subsystem impairments contributing to the variability of dysarthrias exhibited by different AD patients. This should not be surprising when dealing with a neural organ of the size, complexity, and connectivity of the cerebellum. (Consider for comparison the facetious proposition that all cerebral lesions should yield highly similar speech disturbances!) Functional localization and multiple somatotopic representation within the cerebellum have been established (Dichgans & Diener, 1984; Gilman, 1986; Thach, 1980). Behaviorally, outside of the speech mechanism, it is known that not all elements of possible cerebellar symptomatology (e.g., dysmetria, hypotonia, or tremor) will occur in a given patient; furthermore, distal versus proximal musculature, upper versus lower extremities, and left versus right sides may all be differentially affected (Gilman et al, 1981). By analogy, therefore, it is critical that each speech subsystem be evaluated for basic dysfunctions in the areas of muscular strength and tonus, coordination, speed, accuracy, and steadiness. Similarly, extremity functions should be examined, not only to support the diagnosis of ataxia but also to determine the extent to which they may be capitalized upon for treatment approaches that involve intersystemic reorganization (e.g., manual pacing) or other augmentation (e.g., alphabet board).

Second, the stereotype that AD speakers are intelligible, although often true, is not universally the case. Darley et al (1975) found AD to be the most intelligible of seven dysarthric subtypes, despite the fact that imprecise consonants and irregular articulatory breakdowns were among their most prominent deficiencies. Enderby (1983) observed her AD group to be the second most intelligible of five dysarthric subtypes. Mean intelligibility ratings on the nine-point interval scale used in the Frenchay Dysarthria Assessment were approximately two scale values below normal function, but were described as "abnormal but intelligible" (Enderby, 1983). As Enderby points out, however, it is also important to examine the standard deviations of such group ratings; AD patients falling near the −2 standard deviation benchmark would be characterized as 50% intelligible. Yorkston, Hammen, Beukelman, and Traynor (1990) report that the average percentage of sentence intelligibility (words that were actually understood) for a group of four AD patients at habitual speaking rate was approximately 41%. To achieve greater intelligibility, trade-offs in the form of compensatory slowing are usually necessary, which will affect the efficiency of information exchange (i.e., intelligible words per minute) and make AD speech sound peculiarly unnatural. Therefore, careful intelligibility assessments at different speaking rates using an instrument such as the Assessment of Intelligibility of Dysarthric Speech (Yorkston & Beukelman, 1981a) is routinely recommended.

Third, the evaluation of prosodic naturalness is particularly important in AD. Naturalness is the degree to which speech sounds acceptable and avoids bizarre behaviors. This is not to say that AD is the least natural sounding of the dysarthrias; it was in fact ranked second least bizarre by Darley et al (1975). The dilemma is that naturalness may be dramatically impaired in AD to an extent that would not be expected based on judgments of intelligibility or overall severity of deficit. Linebaugh and Wolfe (1984) demonstrated that, whereas naturalness, intelligibility, and rate were all interrelated in spastic dysarthria, these variables seem to operate independently in patients with AD. Similarly, Bunton et al (2000) demonstrated moderate degrees of prosodic impairment in AD in the presence of nearly normal intelligibility in AD, whereas the two variables were commensurately deficient in mixed (flaccid-spastic) dysarthria of amyotrophic lateral sclerosis. LeDorze et al (1998) also reported no correlation between intelligibility, rate, and prosody in speakers with AD. Perhaps this is because slowness as a motor symptom in cerebellar disease may be disassociated from other components such as dysmetria and directional inaccuracy, or because it occurs as a primary deficit in some patients and a compensatory strategy in others. Thus it cannot be assumed that a slow AD speaker is less natural-sounding than a fast one, or that more intelligible AD speakers use slower or faster rates than those who are less intelligible.

Fourth, abnormal prosodic factors including stress patterning, intonation, and pausal phenomena are particularly relevant in AD because they can lead both to decreased intelligibility and to decreased naturalness in the presence of relatively spared intelligibility (Yorkston et al, 1984). Moreover, for AD patients who are stimulable, the manipulation of prosodic variables can facilitate striking speech improvements (Yorkston & Beukelman, 1981b). Proper assessment of these variables requires careful integration of perceptual and instrumental methodology, particularly acoustic measures of fundamental frequency, intensity, and duration (Yorkston et al, 1984). Such measurements are increasingly available in everyday clinical settings with the growing utilization of commercial analysis systems, such as the Kay PENTAX (Pine Brook, NJ) Visipitch or IBM Speech Viewer, and viable clinical protocols for prosodic assessment are beginning to emerge (Seddoh & Robin, 2001).

♦ Treatment of Ataxic Dysarthria

As with other forms of dysarthria, treatment approaches for AD can be subdivided into those that maximize the physiological substrate for support of speech production versus those designed to affect compensated intelligibility (Rosenbek & LaPointe, 1985). Within the treatment sequence, improvement of underlying physiological support logically precedes speech-specific therapy activities. Exceptions to this principle can be made when trying to provide a patient with some functional communication strategies during the early stages of treatment. Maximization of physiological support includes such factors as surgical, pharmacological, and prosthetic interventions that improve the structure or function of the speech apparatus, as well as specific behavioral therapies to increase the strength, speed, stability, and accuracy of movement of component structures and muscles of the vocal tract. When the patient's underlying physiology has been improved to an appropriate extent, the patient is best able to learn compensatory speaking strategies. Compensated intelligibility, the primary goal of most dysarthria treatment, can be achieved through componential or symptomatic approaches that address specific aspects of respiration, phonation, resonation, articulation, and prosody; however, it can also be achieved through global approaches, wherein some strategic manipulation, often of a simplistic nature (e.g., slowing the speaking rate), may have beneficial consequences that reverberate throughout the speaking system. It is further recognized that enhancement of physiology may in itself improve intelligibility, and that speech or speech-like exercises might similarly ameliorate nonspeech muscle dysfunction. This section addresses the distinction between physiological enhancement versus compensated intelligibility, as well as the related issues of prosodic naturalness and augmentative facilitation as they apply to the treatment of AD.

Physiological Enhancement

Enhancement Through Medical Intervention

Unlike some other forms of dysarthria (e.g., flaccid velopharyngeal paralysis), there are no AD-specific surgical procedures that may be recommended to enhance vocal tract structure underlying speech. Similarly, specific pharmacological treatments for cerebellar ataxia have been unimpressive (Young & Penney, 1986). However, limited positive findings have been reported for the effects of isoniazid on limb intention tremor (Sabra, Hallett, Sudarsky, & Mullally, 1982) and physostigmine on ataxia (Kark, Budelli, & Wachsner, 1981). The beta-blockers clonazepam (Klonopin) and propranolol (Inderal) may also be helpful in controlling vocal intention tremor (Dworkin, 1991).

Appropriate medical interventions for the cerebellar disease states that have caused the dysarthria, which vary on the basis of etiology, may in many cases have a beneficial influence on speech. In *Disorders of the Cerebellum* (1981), Gilman et al discuss medical management of various pathologic states, providing illustrative case examples in which dysarthria and other communicative behavior improved following treatment. Surgical excision is an appropriate treatment for some forms of abscess, hemorrhages, and tumors; endarterectomy may be indicated in cases of complete arteriole occlusion, which results in emboli formation leading to recurrent transient ischemic attacks. Gilman et al (1981) report two cases in which significant dysarthria secondary to vascular lesions cleared completely following surgical decompression, with hematoma evacuation of the left cerebellar hemisphere. They also report the case of a 14-year-old girl in whom a medulloblastoma, filling the fourth ventricle and infiltrating part of the vermis, was removed and followed with radiotherapy. Six months postsurgery, her significant presurgical impairments in speech and mentation had improved to a normal level of functioning. Limb ataxia, which had affected handwriting, had also improved significantly.

According to Gilman et al (1981), several toxic and metabolic conditions that cause AD may respond favorably to nonsurgical interventions. Thallium poisoning may be corrected with removal of the toxin from the body; however, in severe cases this may require hemodialysis with cathartic agents and gastric lavage. Effects of alcohol-induced cirrhosis and hepatic disease may be reversed by reducing blood toxin levels while maintaining respiratory, cardiovascular, and renal support. AD and other related symptoms that developed in progressive systemic sclerosis patients who were fed histidine, resulting in zinc deficiency, experienced complete reversal when treated with zinc supplements. Nicotinamide deficiency is corrected by administration of that vitamin. AD associated with endocrine disorders results from diseases of the hormone-producing organs, and is correctable with correction of the endocrine disturbance. In some toxic conditions, early withdrawal of the offending substance may result in partial or complete reversal of ataxic symptoms. In a study of sway patterns in patients with chronic alcoholism and malnutrition, stance improved dramatically in patients who were abstinent, but continued to decline in those who were not (Dichgans & Diener, 1984). This is not always the case, however, as in some instances of long-term use of anticonvulsant medication (e.g., Dilantin), AD and other symptoms may persist after withdrawal and may continue to increase insidiously.

Enhancement Through Behavioral Therapy

This approach emphasizes direct physical exercise of specific muscles or muscle groups to improve the strength, accuracy, and timing of movements of the speech apparatus, while not targeting speaking per se as the treatment variable (Netsell & Daniel, 1979). Thus someone with weak respiratory musculature, for example, may exhibit short phrases and decreased loudness; it is assumed that by improving respiratory muscle function, phrase length, and loudness should also improve, or have greater potential for improvement (Rosenbek & LaPointe, 1985). It should be noted that exercises to enhance underlying physiological support for speech are not restricted to nonspeech motor activities. Many clinicians utilize speech-like stimuli (e.g., sustained vowels or repetitive monosyllables) during this phase of therapy; however, their intent is to improve function for a particular motoric process (e.g., steadiness) within a subsystem (e.g., respiration) rather than to perfect the production of individual speech sounds or teach specific compensatory speaking strategies. Throughout the implementation of a physical exercise approach, the careful use of baselining and charting procedures and routine probing for generalization to connected speech are strongly recommended. At present, there are no available data on the efficacy for AD of exercise regimens intended to enhance physiological substrates for support of speech. This discussion, therefore, is extrapolated from a combination of logical inferences based on known information about motor

system dysfunction in AD, treatment data available on other neuromotor disorders, and treatment suggestions offered by experienced clinicians in existing literature.

Strengthening exercises to improve *hypofunction* may be important in the treatment of some patients with AD. Hypotonia is a significant component of some ataxiogenic disorders, bearing in mind that weakness and fatigability are greatest in proximal musculature (Holmes, 1939). In addition, especially for the degenerative ataxias, less prominent spastic or flaccid weakness elements may be inextricably intermingled with the primary AD (see Gilman & Kluin, 1984). Hypotonia may negatively impact posture and respiratory, phonatory, and articulatory muscle function in AD. Hypotonic postural abnormalities of the trunk and head may interfere with effective speech production and should be managed accordingly (Murry, 1983b). Existing case study data for treatment of muscular hypofunction in other neuromotor disorders may provide a basis for experimental treatment in AD cases wherein hypofunction is found to be a significant variable. For example, Netsell and Daniel (1979) report the successful use of a U-tube manometer equipped with a "leak tube" as a visual feedback device for remediating flaccid respiratory hypofunction. The patient was trained to generate subglottal pressure levels over time that would be similar to those required for the production of phonated speech. The use of visual feedback from devices such as the Respitrace (Noninvasive Monitoring Systems Inc., Miami Beach, FL), which transduces rib cage and abdominal circumference, may provide a means to instruct hypofunctional AD patients to initiate speech at higher lung volumes. For AD patients with significant hypotonia or weakness of the articulatory musculature, specific strengthening exercises may be useful (Dworkin, 1991). For example, the use of tongue-strengthening exercises involving lingual pushing against resistance blocks has been described by Dworkin (1991) as part of a general exercise physiology sequence for hypofunctional articulation. In addition, EMG-derived electronic feedback signals, in the visual and auditory modalities, have been successfully employed to remediate facial weakness associated with flaccid dysarthria (Rubow, 1984).

Of even greater significance than hypofunction for the treatment of AD is the phenomenon of *decomposition of movement,* which includes problems with timing, stability, force development and termination, directional accuracy, and integration of motoric gestures. Kinematic analysis of AD patients' expiration during speech reveals frequent aberrations such as paradoxical breathing and intention tremor (Murdoch et al, 1991). Murry (1983b) suggests that steadiness of exhalation is a primary goal of respiratory training for AD, although this may be complicated by shallow expiration. He proposes three phases of treatment at the respiratory level. In the first stage, 3 to 4 seconds of steady exhalation is alternated with 3 to 4 seconds of rest. Expiration may be augmented by the use of manual self-monitoring by placing the palm of the hand on the abdomen and by using slight glottal friction to decrease the rate of expiratory airflow. In the second stage, steady vowel phonation is added to the expiration, which may be augmented by a visual feedback device. Part of the goal at this stage is to overcome inappropriate bursts of loudness, voicing interruptions, and initiation struggle. Once steady vowel phonation is habitual, the consistently steady and unexplosive production of individual one-syllable words is targeted. The third stage of treatment involves producing sequences of syllables on a single exhalation, moving gradually from repetitive monosyllables to multisyllabic words.

Ataxic dysphonia during speaking has been described perceptually as being monopitch, monoloud, and harsh (Brown et al, 1970); however, acoustical analyses have demonstrated increased variability of both fundamental frequency and intensity during sustained vowel, syllable, and sentence productions (Gentil, 1990a,b; Kent & Netsell, 1975; Zwirner et al, 1991). The precepts of excessive pitch changes and abnormal pitch fluctuations (Gilman & Kluin, 1984; Murry, 1983b) and excessive loudness variation (Brown et al, 1970) have also been described. Heterogeneity among AD patients and among observational methods may account for some apparent discrepancies. Nevertheless, decomposition of laryngeal movements often occurs, yielding marked aberrations in phonatory control. Phonatory dysmetria may well take the forms of pitch and loudness overshoot or undershoot in the same individuals saying the same thing at different times. Thus the goal of physiological therapy for the phonatory subsystem is to bring these aberrant mechanisms under greater volitional control. Basic phonatory steadiness is a natural outgrowth of the type of expiratory steadiness exercises described above (Murry, 1983b). In addition, timing and coordination of laryngeal movements may be developed through specific repetitive production drills. Murry (1983b), therefore, emphasizes pitch change exercises in which the patient learns to decrease and increase pitch differences voluntarily in real words and phrases in accordance with appropriate demands of meaning, and to smooth the pitch contour of any extreme or abrupt fluctuations. Visual biofeedback devices that depict fundamental frequency and intensity contours, such as the Kay PENTAX Visipitch or the IBM Speech Viewer, can be quite useful in this context.

The need for remediation of VOT abnormalities in AD has been suggested by Ouellon et al (1991), who argue that inconsistently perceived voicing substitution errors, resulting from the overlapping of VOT categories in AD, are in reality phonetic distortions related to laryngeal timing and coordination difficulties. They suggest, therefore, that phonological process remediation would be inappropriate, but favor exploiting the AD patient's intact knowledge of the voice-voiceless distinction to progressively move production toward more normal phonemic boundaries. Dworkin (1991) describes in detail a sequence of six exercises designed to improve laryngeal timing and coordination in AD that relies heavily on the use of an adaptation of the inexpensive Pro-Ed (Austin, TX) See Scape apparatus to visually monitor oral airflow during production drills. In steps 1 and 2, this program initially employs prolongation of the vowel for 3 seconds in repetitive consonant-vowel (CV) syllables, then alternating the prolonged CV syllables with 1-second glottal breath-holding pauses. Steps 3 and 4 involve the production of a vowel sequence (u: a: i: E: o: I:), which takes the form of a sustained vowel of changing resonance, wherein each

vowel target position is maintained for approximately 2 seconds. Subsequently, the durations of the component vowel targets are varied systematically. Step 5 involves prolonging the vowel duration of meaningful CV and CVCV words, while varying the duration of glottal breath-holding pauses between the words. Finally, in step 6, specific practice is incorporated as needed on producing sequences of words and sentences with progressively more normal voice quality.

Slowness and dysmetria of the articulatory subsystem have been reported by various investigators (Dworkin & Aronson, 1986; Gentil, 1990a; Kent & Netsell, 1975; McNeil & Adams, 1990). Murry (1983b) describes the phenomenon of *target velocity* as "the speed utilized in reaching the point of articulation, and then continuing on, through and away from the target once it has been reached" (p. 86). He suggests that target velocity, which is impaired in AD, is particularly important to articulatory precision. He further suggests the use of articulatory drills conducted at a speaking rate that is moderately faster than the patient's usual productions. These employ repetitive CV sequences, incorporating various consonants and vowels, initially with repetition of single monosyllables (e.g., /pi pi pi pi pi/) and subsequently with alternation of more complex syllable sequences exemplifying vowel or consonant contrasts (e.g., /pi pa pi pa pi pa/ or /pi ti pi ti pi ti/). Similar word and phrase level drills follow, systematically increasing in complexity. Augmentation by manual tapping or the use of a metronome is recommended to establish a rhythmical pattern for these exercises, and to develop in the patient a "metronomic sense" (p. 88) that should enhance conversational intelligibility. Finally, for significantly hypotonic patients, Murry recommends the use of vowel drills augmented with visual feedback using a mirror as a preliminary to the CV sequencing activities described above. These progress from sustained vowel productions, emphasizing visible features, to sequences of alternating vowel productions that maximize articulatory movements (e.g., /i a i a/) at increasing rates.

Dworkin (1991) presents a distinctive program of lingual, labial, and mandibular force physiology training as well as phonetic stimulation, which may be useful as treatments for the widespread incoordination deficits of the articulatory subsystem in AD. In his force physiology regimen, visual feedback is provided via a mirror, and auditory stimulation via a metronome is employed. In addition, special assistive devices, such as bite blocks (to decouple jaw movement from that of lip and tongue) and a crossbar apparatus constructed from tongue depressors, are used to present slight levels of resistance to the various articulators. Oral exercises, including such activities as raising/lowering the tongue tip, protruding/spreading the lips, and raising/lowering the mandible, are performed in time with metronome beats progressing from slow to fast and then variable rates. Specific efficacy data for force physiology treatment are provided for a flaccid dysarthria patient, who reportedly improved articulatory precision from a pretreatment score of 3.5 to a posttreatment score of 2.0 on a seven-point interval scale. Phonetic stimulation activities, described at length in Dworkin (1991), are an elaboration and extension of traditional phonetic placement techniques. Phonetic stimulation treatment is augmented with the use of simple positioning devices such as tongue depressors and cotton applicators for articulator positioning, as well as the Pro-ED See Scape apparatus, mirror feedback, and audio-recording.

Ultimately, the utility of exercise programs such as those described by Murry (1983b), Dworkin (1991), and others for treatment of AD must await confirmation through single-subject and group efficacy research designs. In the meantime, such programs appear to enjoy both face and content validity, and lend themselves well to accepted accountability procedures such as baselining, charting, and probing for generalization to connected speech. Thus, if AD patients demonstrate deficit areas such as hypotonia and dysmetria of the speech apparatus and have the ability to perform the requisite procedures, physiological enhancement exercises seem warranted to the extent that they continue to demonstrate measurable improvement within the task and on objective measures of connected speech (e.g., percent intelligibility). It should also be appreciated that the appropriate use of improvement of residual support for speech has an upper limit, and that there is a range beyond which it can be exaggerated to the detriment of the therapeutic process (Rosenbek & LaPointe, 1985).

Compensated Intelligibility and Prosodic Naturalness

Intelligibility

Although adjunctive treatment outcomes such as decreasing bizarre behaviors or improving prosodic naturalness are clearly legitimate objectives, most clinicians agree that the primary goal of speech therapy for dysarthria is to achieve a level of speech intelligibility that may be used for functional communicative purposes (which may vary depending on the specific needs and impairment severity of the individual patient). Assuming that physiological support has been enhanced through medical or behavioral interventions to an appropriate degree, it is crucial to assist the patient to make more optimal use of this available residual support when talking. This involves direct work on naturalistic connected speech production (i.e., words, phrases, sentences, and discourses) wherein respiratory, phonatory, resonatory, articulatory, and prosodic processes are integrated with one another and with linguistic, pragmatic, and emotional demands of communicative situations. Such work follows as a logical outgrowth of physical exercise programs that have incorporated speech-like stimuli of increasing complexity within their later stages (e.g., see Murry, 1983b).

In contrast to the physical exercise approaches, there now exists a published database of small sample studies of compensatory strategies for directly addressing the intelligibility of AD speech. All of these studies have emphasized the manipulation of suprasegmental variables (e.g., duration, pitch and loudness), but most typically speaking rate, as the preferred compensatory strategy for improving intelligibility (Berry & Goshorn, 1983; Caligiuri & Murry, 1983; Garcia & Dongilli, 1985; Sapir et al, 2003; Simmons, 1983; Yorkston & Beukelman, 1981b; Yorkston et al, 1990). Slowing of the speaking rate may, at first glance, seem counterintuitive as a treatment for AD; these patients are already using habitual rates that are markedly slower than characteristic values for normal adult speakers. However, attempts to increase speaking rate in AD subjects have resulted in markedly increased errors that negatively impact intelligibility (Gentil, 1990a; Yorkston & Beukelman, 1981a; Yorkston et al, 1984).

A variety of clinical techniques have been employed to control rate in the treatment of AD. For example, Rosenbek and LaPointe (1985) suggest that delayed auditory feedback may enhance articulation time, articulation adequacy, and prosody for some patients with AD. They indicate that delay intervals of 50 ms have been the most beneficial. Berry and Goshorn (1983) employed immediate visual feedback to enhance sentence production in a 60-year-old man with AD secondary to multiple cerebrovascular accidents. The patient was judged to be "overdriving" the speech mechanism by speaking too loudly and too rapidly. A four-channel storage oscilloscope provided a clinician model, an intensity target line, and a visual representation of the patient's own productions. Treatment was initiated wherein the patient was instructed to maintain intensity below the target line and fill up more than half the screen during the production of sentences. Sentence productions recorded before and after treatment, and at follow-up, were presented to 12 normal listeners in the presence of noise to evaluate intelligibility. Overall sentence intelligibility improved from pre- to posttreatment, from approximately 67 to 85% but declined to approximately 77% at follow-up. All three time intervals differed significantly from one another. Temporal acoustic measurements were obtained from oscillographic tracings for overall sentence duration, key word duration, and total pause time. For all three measures, there was a significant increase in duration from pre- to posttreatment, and a slight decrease in duration from posttreatment to follow-up. The durations at the follow-up recording session remained significantly longer than at pretreatment.

Garcia and Dongilli (1985) presented intelligibility data for short-term results of treatment of two AD patients using traditional, noninstrumented therapy techniques. The first patient was a 73-year-old woman with cerebellar dysfunction secondary to meningitis. Her treatment employed the use of slow rate via "syllable timed speech" with continuous phonation, and establishing appropriate stress patterns for polysyllabic words. Intelligibility was evaluated prior to and at 2 weeks following the onset of treatment by administering the Assessment of Intelligibility of Dysarthric Speech to two listeners. Although sentence intelligibility for this patient remained stable at about the 50% level before and after treatment, single-word intelligibility had increased from 31 to 70%. The second patient was an 84-year-old man with cerebellar dysfunction secondary to viral encephalitis. After 3 weeks of sentence level drills contrasting overall loudness levels, pitch, and stress patterns, his single-word intelligibility increased from 68 to 89% and sentence intelligibility increased from 70 to 95%. Liss and Weismer (1994) also demonstrated improved articulation in some AD speakers under conditions of contrastive stress in comparison with neutral sentence production using spectrographic analysis of formant transitions.

Yorkston and Beukelman (1981b) provide long-term treatment data on four AD patients who experienced ataxia secondary to acute nondegenerative etiologies. Each patient received a comprehensive treatment program consisting of rate control, development of self-monitoring skills, specific "point-place" assessment and treatment, and maximization of normal prosody. Rate control strategies included (1) the rigid imposition of rate using a manual pacing board or by pointing to the first letter of each word on an alphabet board; (2) rhythmic cuing by the clinician, who pointed to printed words for time intervals approximating normal speech rhythms; and (3) oscilloscopic feedback in the form of intensity tracings over time. All four patients were using habitual rates too rapid for their residual capabilities, and the optimum rate for enhancing intelligibility was initially established at approximately 60 to 65 words per minute. Self-monitoring skills were emphasized to enable the patient to generalize the slower speaking rate to nonclinical situations and to habituate the slower speaking rate. Point-place assessment and treatment was used as needed to address idiosyncratic difficulties such as context-specific vowel distortions in individual patients. Maximizing normal prosody involved the use of sentence-level contrastive stress drills to increase intelligibility and reduce bizarreness. This was accomplished by increasing the duration of stressed syllables while reducing extreme loudness peaks and fundamental frequency shifts. All four subjects improved dramatically from pre- to posttreatment measures of intelligibility, with a pretreatment mean of 18.5% and a posttreatment mean of 90.75%. However, only one subject was able to eventually achieve a speaking rate approximating the pretreatment value of 132 words per minute. The others continued to use extremely slow rates, of 60 to 74 words per minute.

Yorkston et al (1990) described the influence of computer-implemented rate control strategies on the intelligibility and naturalness of ataxic and hypokinetic dysarthric speech. Four dysarthric patients of each type were examined under four experimental rate conditions: (1) additive metered, in which one word at a time was added using equal durations for each word; (2) additive rhythmic, in which one word at a time was added with word durations approximating the patterns of normal speech; (3) cued metered, in which the entire passage was presented and each word successively underlined for equal durations; and (4) cued rhythmic, in which the entire passage was presented and each word underlined for durations approximating normal speech. These conditions were presented to each subject at 100%, 80%, and 60% of the speaker's habitual rate. For both dysarthric subgroups, intelligibility increased as speaking rate decreased. The AD patients' sentence intelligibility improved from a mean 40.9% at their habitual rates to a mean of 73.7% at 60% of the habitual rate. The additive conditions were more beneficial than the cued, and the metered conditions were more beneficial than the rhythmic (i.e., cued rhythmic was the least effective strategy). Although the results were impressive, it should be recognized that this was a single-shot experiment rather than an ongoing treatment efficacy study. A commercial software program replicating in part the pacing conditions used in this experiment is available for clinical application (Beukelman, Yorkston, & Tice, 1997).

Acoustic and physiological changes that underlie speech improvement using rate reduction treatment for AD appear to transcend merely increasing the duration of segments and utterances, yet the precise mechanisms remain poorly understood. Tjaden and Wilding (2004) demonstrated that reduced rate increased "vowel working space," effecting vocal track shapes in AD patients secondary to multiple sclerosis and in nondisabled speakers. It should be noted, however, that in this study intelligibility did not improve significantly. Hertrich and Ackermann (1998) used digital acoustic analysis and resynthesis of AD utterances to normalize durational and rhythmic aspects of AD speech. Improvement was noted on ratings of perceived slowness, disfluency, and rhythmic adequacy, but intelligibility ratings did not improve in response to artificial manipulation of duration. The authors suggest that articulatory dynamics and critical spectral target information may be the source of intelligibility deficits in AD rather than durational features alone. Consequently, to the extent that rate reduction improves AD intelligibility, it seems likely that prolonged duration provides the AD speaker with more time in which to approximate articulatory targets. Clinically, this suggests that having slowed an AD speaker's rate, attention in treatment may be needed on the statics and dynamics of articulatory accuracy.

Rate control also may be accomplished with the use of an alphabet board, with which the AD patient points to the initial letters of intended word productions (Beukelman and Yorkston, 1977). Although this method clearly provides the listener with signal-independent visual information to help disambiguate the distorted speech signal, studies have demonstrated that the use of an alphabet board that was not visible to listeners also significantly improved intelligibility of an AD patient's speech (Beukelman & Yorkston, 1977; Crow & Enderby, 1989). This benefit has been attributed to a "pacing effect" similar to rate reduction obtained with a pacing board. Intersystemic reorganization of speech either through manual pacing or gestures can be a viable treatment option for some dysarthric patients (Rosenbek, 1984). Preservation of upper extremity function in many AD patients (Gilman et al, 1981) provides an opportunity for the clinician to explore the use of manual strategies in managing AD.

An alternative to rate control therapy was explored by Sapir et al (2003), who administered the Lee Silverman Voice Treatment (LSVT) to a 48-year-old woman whose AD was associated with cerebellar dysfunction secondary to thiamine deficiency. The patient was noted to a have a weak and breathy voice in addition to other typical features of AD. The intensive 4-week LSVT program emphasized increasing vocal effort through the production of loud phonation. Speech improvement was noted in acoustic measures of vocal intensity, fundamental frequency, vowel formant frequencies, and consonant-to-vowel formant transitions. In addition, perceptual ratings of articulatory precision and pitch intonation also improved significantly. For this patient, all gains exhibited in speech measures except pitch intonation were maintained at 9-month follow up. Interestingly, the rate of speech also decreased from 198.5 words per minute before treatment to 161.4 words per minute following treatment. The extent to which rate changes, in addition to loudness, contributed to improved intelligibility is unclear. However, the findings suggests that the patient achieved widespread modifications of her customary speech production plan in response to LSVT. The authors caution, however, that LSVT should not be applied indiscriminately to all AD patients in that it may be indicated only for specific subtypes of AD (e.g., hypophonia). For example, Tjaden and Wilding (2004) demonstrated that, unlike speakers with hypokinetic dysarthria, speakers with AD secondary to multiple sclerosis did not improve in comparison to their habitual speech under a loud speech condition. In contrast these AD speakers benefited more from a slow speaking condition.

Naturalness

Yorkston et al (1990) also reported that both of their dysarthric subgroups sounded quite unnatural. The average naturalness rating for habitual rate of the AD group was three of seven scale values below normal. Differences in naturalness ratings between speaking rates and pacing conditions were negligible. These findings are consistent with the lack of relationship between naturalness and speaking rate reported by Linebaugh and Wolfe (1984). Yorkston et al (1990) concluded:

> Presumably dysarthric speech is already so unnatural that changing rate did not have a further detrimental effect. In the clinical setting a slight reduction in speech naturalness may be an acceptable price to pay for a substantial improvement in intelligibility (p. 558).

Some clinical research data have addressed prosodic naturalness in AD. Based on a perceptual-acoustic assessment protocol, Yorkston et al (1984) recommended a decision algorithm for implementing prosodic treatment: (1) Does the patient know where the stress should be located? If not, train stress locus recognition. (2) Does the patient adequately mark primary stress on target syllables? If not, identify and train strategies that can be reliably employed. (3) Do the strategies contribute to the naturalness of speech? If not, train to modify bizarre-sounding strategies. (4) Establish strategies that enhance naturalness in all speaking situations.

Simmons (1983) reported results of a year-long prosodic treatment program for a 26-year-old man with a closed head injury who exhibited severe ataxia, with primary speech characteristic of excess and equal stress, slowed rate, monoloudness, and monopitch. Prior therapy had enabled him to slow his rate and avoid slurring words; however, he complained of sounding "computer like." A four-phase treatment program was initiated that consisted of the following sequence: (1) training loudness and pitch variation; (2) altering word and sentence stress patterns by (a) inserting pauses prior to stressed units, (b) shortening unstressed syllables, and (c) decreasing loudness on unstressed syllables; (3) shortening syllable durations overall while maintaining stress patterns; (4) improving naturalness by (a) decreasing exaggerated pitch and loudness variations, (b) reducing the clipped and choppy quality caused by shortening words, and (c) smoothing out transitions between words. Ninety percent accuracy as judged by the clinician was the criterion for completion of each phase.

Spectrographic analysis of a standard sentence was employed to monitor the ongoing effects of treatment. At the initial baseline, spectrographic measurements confirmed that there was a flat fundamental frequency with relatively equal syllable durations and little variation in pause time, in addition to an overall slow rate of production (i.e., 136% of normal). Following phase 1, the patient's speech became markedly slower than at baseline (i.e., 203% of normal), presumably because more time was needed to make necessary changes in pitch and loudness. At completion of phase 2, speech was even more prolonged (i.e., 231% of normal). After phase 3, however, which targeted shortening duration, speech became less prolonged (i.e., 187% of normal). By the completion of the phase 4 it became even shorter, approaching pretreatment values (i.e., 144% of normal). The patient also had achieved a more normal distribution of syllable and pause durations. This study demonstrated that the patient's prosody became worse in treatment before it became better. Although this study does provide limited support for the potential efficacy of prosodic treatment in AD, the actual extent of improvement is difficult to evaluate in the absence of quantified perceptual judgments.

A perceptual study of prosodic treatment in AD has been provided by Caligiuri and Murry (1983), who presented immediate visual feedback to enhance prosodic control in two patients with AD. One patient was a 59-year-old man who exhibited AD secondary to cerebellar infarct, the other a 61-year-old man with a mixed dysarthria in which AD predominated secondary to multiple sclerosis. A storage oscilloscope was employed to provide a clinician model and visual feedback about word duration, vocal intensity, and intraoral air pressure associated with target stress. Speech production tasks progressed systematically from CV nonsense syllables through increasing levels of length and complexity to sentences varying with pragmatic intent. Contrastive stress techniques were employed at various stages. The 15-week treatment sequence involved an intensive visual feedback phase, a treatment withdrawal phase, and a no-visual-feedback treatment phase. Pre- to posttreatment changes in overall prosodic functioning in connected speech were evaluated by two reliable normal listeners using the perceptual method of paired comparison. The cerebellar infarct patient demonstrated 100% improvement in prosody following the visual feedback phase, but declined to 50% following the no-visual-feedback phases. The multiple sclerosis patient demonstrated 100% improvement following both the visual feedback and no-visual-feedback phases. Ratings of accuracy of word stress were found to improve following both treatment phases in the cerebellar infarct patient, and were associated with increased duration. The multiple sclerosis patient improved on word stress ratings, associated with pitch and intensity changes, only following the no-visual-feedback condition.

Bouglé, Ryalls, and Le Dorze (1995) also compared visual feedback to a no-visual-feedback condition for treating intonation in AD. Using the IBM Speech Viewer, both to provide visual feedback in the form of intonation contours and to perform quantitative acoustic analyses of patient responses, these authors examined two cases of AD subsequent to closed head trauma using multiple baseline single subject designs. Both patients exhibited equivalent gains resulting from treatment focusing on increasing variability and range of fundamental frequency while using the visual feedback device and during more traditional treatment using auditory modeling and verbal feedback provided by a clinician.

♦ Conclusion

This chapter has described the neural sensorimotor mechanisms and etiologies underlying AD, and reviewed the available literature pertaining to its characteristics and their remediation. Although substantial progress has occurred, there remain important questions facing speech clinicians working with these patients: Are there different AD subtypes stemming from differential subsystem impairments? Would such differential impairments lend themselves to differential treatment strategies? Can hypotonia be ameliorated through exercise programs to enhance underlying physiological support for speech? Does such enhancement influence intelligibility or naturalness of AD speech? There is today at least some hint from the literature that these questions may eventually be answered in the affirmative (see Boutsen, 1997; Sapir et al, 2003; Tjaden & Wilding, 2004). We continue to question what long-term strategies for rate control are most effective, and what factors govern the ability to eventually increase speaking rate toward a more naturalistic level? How much practical benefit may be ultimately derived from treatments focused on prosodic naturalness and augmentative facilitation (e.g., manual pacing or alphabet supplementation)? As with other types of dysarthria, there continues to be a need for randomized blind control studies to develop a higher-level evidence base for motivating clinical practice in this arena. It is hoped that the synthesis presented here will stimulate further research in these areas to improve the outlook for patients with AD.

References

Abbs J., Barlow, S., & Cole, K. (1979). Impairments of rapid muscle contraction as a physiologic feature of ataxic dysarthria. Presented to the American Speech-Language-Hearing Association, San Francisco

Abbs, J., Hunker, C., & Barlow, S. (1983). Differential speech motor subsystem impairments with suprabulbar lesions: neurophysiological framework and supporting data. In: W. Berry (Ed.), *Clinical Dysarthria* (pp. 21–56). San Diego: College-Hill Press

Ackermann, H., Graber, S., Hertrich, I., & Daum, I. (1999). Cerebellar contributions to the perception of temporal cues within the speech and non speech domain. *Brain and Language, 67,* 228–241

Ackermann, H. & Hertrich, I. (1993). Dysarthria in Friedreich's ataxia: Timing of speech segments. *Clinical Linguistics and Phonetics, 7,* 75–91

Ackermann, H. & Hertrich, I. (1994). Speech rate and rhythm in cerebellar dysarthria: an acoustic analysis of syllabic timing. *Folia Phoniatrica et Logopaedica, 46,* 70–78

Ackermann, H., Hertrich, I., Daum, I., Scharf, G., & Spieker, S. (1997). Kinematic analysis of articulatory movements in central motor disorders. *Movement Disorders, 12,* 1019–1027

Ackermann, H., Hertrich, I., & Scharf, G. (1995). Kinematic analysis of lower lip movements in ataxic dysarthria. *Journal of Speech and Hearing Research, 38,* 1252–1259

Ackermann, H. & Ziegler, W. (1994). Acoustic analysis of vocal instability in cerebellar dysfunctions. *Annals of Otology, Rhinology, and Laryngology, 103,* 98–104

Alexander G.E. & Delong, M. R. (1986). Organization of supraspinal motor system. In: A.K. Ansbury, G.M. McKhann, & W.I. McDonald (Eds.) *Diseases of the Nervous System: Clinical Neurobiology* (pp. 352–369). Philadelphia: W.B. Saunders

Beppu H., Suda, M., & Tanaka, R. (1983). Slow visuomotor tracking in normal man and in patients with cerebellar ataxia. In: J.E. Desmedt (Ed.), *Motor Control Mechanisms in Health and Disease* (pp. 889–895). New York: Raven Press

Berry, W.R. & Goshorn, E.L. (1983). Immediate visual feedback in the treatment of ataxic dysarthria: a case study. In: W.R. Berry (Ed.) *Clinical Dysarthria* (pp. 253–265). San Diego: College-Hill Press

Beukelman, D.R. & Yorkston, K. (1977). A communication system for the severely dysarthric speaker with an intact language system. *Journal of Speech and Hearing Disorders, 42,* 265–270

Beukelman, D.R., Yorkston, K., & Tice R. (1997). *Pacer/tally rate measurement software.* Lincoln, NE: Institute for Rehabilitation Science and Engineering, Madonna Rehabilitation Hospital

Blakemore, S., Frith, C.D., & Wolpert, D.M. (2001). The cerebellum is involved in predicting the sensory consequences of action. *Neuroreport, 12,* 1879–1884

Bouglé F., Ryalls, J., & Le Dorze, G. (1995). Improving fundamental frequency modulation in head trauma patients: a preliminary comparison of speech-language therapy conducted with and without IBM's SpeechViewer. *Folia Phoniatrica et Logopaedica, 47,* 24–32

Boutsen, F., Bakker, K. and Duffy, J. (1997). Subgroups in ataxic dysarthria. *Journal of Medical Speech-Language Pathology, 5,* 27–36

Bowman JP. (1971). *The Muscle Spindle and Neural Control of the Tongue: Implications for Speech.* Springfield, IL: Charles Thomas

Brooke, M., Uomoto, J.M., McLean, A. & Fraser, R.T. (1991). Rehabilitation of persons with traumatic brain injury: a continuum of care. In: Beukelman, DR & Yorkson, KM. (Eds) *Communication Disorders Following Traumatic Brain Injury: Management of Cognitive, Language, and Motor Impairments* (pp. 15–55). Austin: ProEd

Brooks, V.B. & Thach, W.T. (1981). Cerebellar control of posture and movement. In: V.B. Brooks (Ed.), *Handbook of Physiology, Section 1: The Nervous System, Vol. 2* (pp. 877–956). Bethesda: American Physiological Society

Brown, J.R., Darley, F.L., & Aronson, A.E. (1970). Ataxic dysarthria. *International Journal of Neurology, 7,* 302–318

Bunton, K., Kent, R.D., & Kent, J.F., Rosenbek, J.C. (2000). Perceptuo-acoustic assessment of prosodic impairment in dysarthria. *Clinical Linguistics and Phonetics, 14,* 13–24

Caligiuri, M. & Murry, T. (1983). The use of visual feedback to enhance prosodic control in dysarthria. In W. Berry (Ed.), *Clinical Dysarthria* (pp. 267–282). San Diego: College-Hill Press

Charcot, J.M. (1877). *Lectures on the Diseases of the Nervous System,* vol. 1. London: New Sydenham Society

Crow, E. & Enderby, P. (1989). The effects of an alphabet chart on the speaking rate and intelligibility of speakers with dysarthria. In: K.M. Yorkston, & D.R. Beukelman (Eds.), *Recent Advances in Clinical Dysarthria* (pp. 99–107). Boston: College-Hill

Darley, F.L., Aronson, A.E., & Brown, J.R. (1969a). Differential diagnostic patterns of dysarthria. *Journal of Speech and Hearing Research, 12*, 246–269

Darley, F.L., Aronson, A.E., & Brown, J.R. (1969b). Clusters of deviant speech dimensions in the dysarthrias. *Journal of Speech and Hearing Research, 12*, 462–496

Darley, F.L., Aronson, A.E., & Brown J.R. (1975). *Motor Speech Disorders.* Philadelphia: W.B. Saunders

Darley, F.L., Brown, J.R., & Goldstein, N. (1972). Dysarthria in multiple sclerosis. *Journal of Speech and Hearing Research, 15*, 229–245

Deger, K., Ziegler, W. & Wessel, K. (1999). Airflow tracking in patients with ataxic disorders. *Clinical Linguistics and Phonetics, 13*, 433–447

Dichgans, J. & Diener, H.C. (1984). Clinical evidence for functional compartmentalization of the cerebellum. In: J.R. Bloedel, J. Dichgans, & W. Precht (Eds.), *Cerebellar Functions* (pp. 126–147). Berlin: Springer-Verlag

Dworkin, J.P. (1991). *Motor Speech Disorders: A Treatment Guide.* St. Louis: Mosby Year Book.

Dworkin, J.P. & Aronson, A.E. (1986). Tongue strength and alternate motion rates in normal and dysarthric subjects. *Journal of Communication Disorders, 19*, 115–132

Eccles J. (1977). Cerebellar function in the control of movement (with special reference to the pioneer work of Sir Gordon Holmes). In: F.C. Rose (Ed.), *Physiological Aspects of Clinical Neurology* (pp 157–178). Oxford: Blackwell

Enderby, P.M. (1983). *Frenchay Dysarthria Assessment.* Austin: Pro-Ed

Farmakides, M. & Boone, D. (1960). Speech problems in patients with multiple sclerosis. *Journal of Speech and Hearing Disorders, 25*, 385–390

Forrest K., Adams, S., McNeil, M.R., & Southwood, H. (1991). Kinematic, electromyographic, and perceptual evaluation of speech apraxia, conduction aphasia, ataxic dysarthria, and normal speech production. In: C. A. Moore, & K. M. Yorkston & D. R. Buekelman (Eds). *Dysarthria and Apraxia of Speech: Perspectives on Management* (pp. 147–171). Baltimore: Paul. H. Brookes

French, L.A., Chou, S.N., Long, D.M. & Seljeskog, E.L. (1970). Clinical management of cerebellar neoplasms. In: W.S. Fields & W.D. Willis (Eds.), *The Cerebellum in Health and Disease* (pp 502–518). St. Louis: Warren H. Green

Garcia, J. & Dongilli, P. (1985). Ataxic dysarthria: case study reviews of treatment strategies. Presented to the American Speech-Language-Hearing Association, Washington, DC

Gentil M. (1990a). EMG analysis of speech production of patients with Friedreich disease. *Clinical Linguistics and Phonetics, 4*, 107–120

Gentil M. (1990b). Dysarthria in Friedreich disease. *Brain and Language, 38*, 438–448

Gilman, S. (1986). Cerebellum and motor dysfunction. In: A.K. Asbury, G.M. McKhann, & W.I. McDonald, (Eds.), *Diseases of the Nervous System: Clinical Neurobiology* (pp. 402–422). Philadelphia: W.B. Saunders

Gilman, S., Bloedel, J.R. & Lechtenberg, R. (1981). *Disorders of the Cerebellum.* Philadelphia: F.A. Davis.

Gilman, S. & Kluin, K. (1984). Perceptual analysis of speech disorders in Friedreich disease and olivopontocerebellar atrophy. In: J.R. Bloedel, J. Dichigans, & W. Precht (Eds.), *Cerebellar Functions* (pp. 148–163). Berlin: Springer Verlag

Gilman S. & Kluin, K. (1992). Speech disorders in cerebellar degeneration studied with positron emission tomography. In: A. Blitzer, M.F. Brin, C.T. Sasaki, S. Fahn, & K.S. Harris (Eds.), *Neurologic Disorders of the Larynx* (pp. 279–285). New York: Thieme

Granit R. (1977). Reconsidering the 'alpha-gamma switch' in cerebellar action. In: F.C. Rose (Ed.), *Physiological Aspects of Clinical Neurology* (pp. 201–213). Oxford: Blackwell

Grunwell. P. & Huskins, S. (1979). Intelligibility in acquired dysarthria—a neuro-phonetic approach: three case studies. *Journal of Communication Disorders, 12*, 9–22

Haggard M.P. (1969). Speech waveform measurements in multiple sclerosis. *Folia Phoniatrica, 21*, 307–312

Hallett, M., Shahani, B. & Young, R.R. (1975). EMG analysis of patients with cerebellar deficits. *Journal of Neurology, Neurosurgery and Psychiatry, 38*, 1163–1169

Hartelius, L., Runmarker, B., Andersen, O., & Nord, L. (2000) Temporal speech characteristics of individuals with multiple sclerosis and ataxic dysarthria: "Scanning Speech" revisited. *Folia Phoniatrica et Logopaedica, 52*, 228–238

Hertrich, I. & Ackermann, H. (1998). Auditory perceptual evaluation of rhythm-manipulated and resynthesized sentence utterances obtained from cerebellar patients and normal speakers: a preliminary report. *Clinical Linguistics and Phonetics, 12*, 427–437

Hertrich, I. & Ackermann, H. (1999). Temporal and spectral aspects of coarticulation in ataxic dysarthria: an acoustic analysis. *Journal of Speech, Language and Hearing Research, 42*, 367–381

Hiller, F. (1929). A study of speech disorders in Friedreich's ataxia. *Archives of Neurology and Psychiatry 2*, 75–90

Hirose, H., Kiritani, S., Ushijima, T. & Sawashima, M. (1978). Analysis of abnormal articulatory dynamics in two dysarthric patients. *Journal of Speech and Hearing Research, 43*, 96–105

Hogancamp, W.E., Rodriguez, M., Weinshenker, B.G. (1997). The epidemiology of multiple sclerosis. *Mayo Clinic Proceedings, 72*, 871–878

Holmes G. (1917). The symptoms of acute cerebellar injuries due to gunshot injuries. *Brain, 40*, 461–535

Holmes, G. (1939). The cerebellum of man. *Brain, 62*, 1–30

Ito, M. (1984). *The Cerebellum and Neural Control.* New York: Raven Press

Jankovic, J. & Fahn, S. (1980). Physiologic and pathologic tremors. *Annals of Internal Medicine, 93*, 460–465

Janvrin, F. (1933). Diagnosis of a nervous disease by sound tracks. *Nature, 132*, 642

Janvrin, F. & Worster-Drought, C. (1932). Diagnosis of disseminated sclerosis by graphic registration and film tracks. *Lancet, 2*, 1384

Joanette, Y. & Dudley, J. (1980). Dysarthric symptomatology of Friedreich's ataxia. *Brain and Language, 10*, 39–50

Kark, R.A., Budelli, M. & Wachsner, R. (1981). Double-blind, triple-crossover trial of low doses of oral physostigmine in inherited ataxias. *Neurology, 31*, 288–292

Keller, E. (1990). Speech motor timing. In: W.J. Hardcastle & A. Marchal (Eds.), *Speech Production and Speech Modeling* (pp. 343–364). Dordrecht: Kluwer

Kent, R. D., Kent, J. F., Duffy, J., Thomas, J., Weismer, G. & Stuntebeck, S. (2000). Ataxic dysarthria. *J Speech Lang Hear Research, 43*, 1275–1289

Kent, R.D., Kent, J. F., Rosenbek, J., Vorperian, H. & Weismer, G. (1997). A speaking task analysis of the dysarthria in cerebellar disease. *Folia Phoniatr Logopaedica, 49*, 63–82

Kent, R.D. & Netsell, R. (1975). A case study of an ataxic dysarthric: cineradiographic and spectrographic observations. *Journal of Speech and Hearing Disorders, 40*, 115–134

Kent, R.D., Netsell, R. & Abbs, J. (1979). Acoustic characteristics of dysarthria associated with cerebellar disease. *Journal of Speech and Hearing Research, 22*, 627–648

Kent, R.D., Netsell, R. & Bauer, L. (1975). Cineradiographic assessment of articulatory mobility in dysarthrias. *Journal of Speech and Hearing Disorders, 40*, 467–480

Kent, R.D. & Rosenbek, J. (1979). Prosodic disturbance and neurologic lesion. *Brain and Language, 15*, 259–291

Kornhuber, H. (1975). Cerebral cortex, cerebellum, and basal ganglia: an introduction to their functions. In E. Evarts (Ed.), *Central processing* (pp. 267–280). Cambridge: M.I.T. Press

Lam, R.L. & Ogura, J.H. (1952). An afferent representation of the larynx in the cerebellum. *Laryngoscope, 62,* 486–495

Le Dorze, G., Ryalls, J., Brassard, C., Boulanger, N., Ratte, D. (1998) A comparison of the prosodic characteristics of the speech of people with Parkinson's disease and Friedreich's ataxia with neurologically normal speakers. *Folia Phoniatrica et Logopaedica, 50,* 1–9

Lechtenberg, R. & Gilman, S. (1978). Speech disorders in cerebellar disease. *Annals of Neurology, 3,* 285–290

Leiner, H.C., Leiner, A.L. & Dow, R.S. (1991). The human cerebro-cerebellar system: its computing, cognitive, and language skills. *Behavioral Brain Research, 44,* 113–128

Linebaugh, C. & Wolfe, V. (1984). Relationships between articulation rate, intelligibility, and naturalness in spastic and ataxic speakers. In: M. McNeil, J. Rosenbek & A.E. Aronson (Eds.), *The Dysarthrias* (pp. 197–205). San Diego: College-Hill Press.

Liss, J.M. & Weismer, G. (1994). Selected acoustic characteristics of contrastive stress production in control geriatric, apraxic, and ataxic dysarthric speakers. *Clinical Linguistics and Phonetics, 8,* 45–66

Marsden, C.D., Merton, P.A., Morton H.B., Hallett, M., Adam, J. & Rushton, D.N. (1977). Disorders of movement in cerebellar disease in man. In: F.C. Rose (Ed.), *Physiological Aspects of Clinical Neurology* (pp. 179–199). Oxford: Blackwell

McNeil, M.R. & Adams, S. (1990). A comparison of speech kinematics among apraxic, conduction aphasic, ataxic dysarthric, and normal geriatric speakers. In: T. Prescott (Ed.), *Clinical Aphasiology,* vol. 19 (pp. 279 – 293). Austin: Pro-Ed

McNeil, M.R., Weismer, G., Adams, S. & Mulligan, M. (1990). Oral structure nonspeech motor control in normal, dysarthric, aphasic, and apraxic speakers: isometric force and static position control. *Journal of Speech and Hearing Research, 33,* 255–268

Mills, C.K. & Weisenburg, T.H. (1914). Cerebellar symptoms and cerebellar localization. *Journal of the American Medical Association, 63,* 1813–1818

Mortimer, J.A. (1975). Cerebellar responses to teleceptive stimuli in alert monkeys. *Brain Research, 83,* 369–390

Murdoch, B.E., Chenery, H., Stokes, P. & Hardcastle, W. (1991). Respiratory kinematics in speakers with cerebellar disease. *Journal of Speech and Hearing Research, 34,* 768–780

Murry, T. (1983a). The production of stress in three types of dysarthric speech. In: W. Berry (Ed.), *Clinical Dysarthria* (pp. 69–83). San Diego: College-Hill Press

Murry, T. (1983b). Treatment of ataxic dysarthria. In: W. Perkins (Ed.), *Current Therapy of Communication Disorders—Dysarthria and Apraxia* (pp. 79–89). New York: Thieme-Stratton

Netsell, R. (1973). Kinesiology studies of the dysarthrias. Unpublished paper, Speech Research Laboratory, University of Wisconsin, Madison

Netsell, R. (1982). Speech motor control and selected neurologic disorders. In: S. Grillner, B. Lindblom, J. Lubker & A. Persson (Eds.), *Speech Motor Control* (pp. 247–261). New York: Pergamon Press

Netsell, R. (1986). *A Neurobiologic View of Speech Production and the Dysarthrias.* San Diego: College-Hill Press

Netsell, R. & Abbs, J. (1977). Some possible uses of neuromotor speech disturbances in under-standing normal mechanism. In: M. Sawashima & F.S. Cooper (Eds.), *Dynamic Aspects of Speech Production: Current Results, Emerging Problems, and New Instrumentation: Proceedings* (pp 369–398). Tokyo: University of Tokyo Press

Netsell, R. & Daniel, B. (1979). Dysarthria in adults: physiologic approach to rehabilitation. *Archives of Physical Medicine and Rehabilitation, 60,* 502–508

Netsell, R. & Kent, R.D. (1976). Paroxysmal ataxic dysarthria. *Journal of Speech and Hearing Disorders, 41,* 93–109

Odell, K., McNeil, M., Rosenbek, J., Hunter, L. (1991). Perceptual characteristics of vowel and prosody production in apraxic, aphasic, and dysarthric speakers. *Journal of Speech and Hearing Research, 34,* 67–80

Ouellon, M., Ryalls, J., Lebeuf, J. & Joanette, Y. (1991). Le "Voice Onset Time" chez des dysarthriques de Friedreich. *Fonia Phoniatrica, 43,* 295–303

Ozawa, Y., Shiromoto, W., Ishizaki, F. & Watamori, T. (2001). Symptomatic differences in decreased alternating motion rates between individuals with spastic and with ataxic dysarthria: an acoustic analysis. *Folia Phoniatrica et Logopaedica, 53,* 67–72

Petersen, S.E., Fox, P.T., Posner, M.I., Mintun, M. & Raichle, M.E. (1989). Positron emission tomographic studies of the processing of single words. *Journal of Cognitive Neuroscience, 1,* 153–170

Portnoy, R.A. & Aronson A.E. (1982). Diadochokinetic syllable rate and regularity in normal and in spastic and ataxic dysarthric subjects. *Journal of Speech and Hearing Disorders, 47,* 324–328

Rondot, P., Jedynak, C.P. & Ferrey G. (1978). Pathological tremors: nosological correlates. *Clinical Neurophysioogyl, 5,* 95–113

Rosen, K.M., Kent, R.D. & Duffy, J.R. (2003) Lognormal distribution of pause length in ataxic dysarthria. *Clinical Linguistics and Phonetics, 17,* 469–486

Rosenbek J. (1984). Selected alternatives to articulation training for the dysarthric adult. In: H. Winitz (Ed.), *Treating Articulation Disorders for Clinicians by Clinicians* (pp. 249–262). Austin: Pro-Ed

Rosenbek, J.C. & LaPointe, L.L. (1985). The dysarthrias: Description, diagnosis and treatment. In: D.F. Johns (Ed.), *Clinical Management of Neurogenic Communication Disorders* (pp. 97–152). Boston: Little, Brown

Rubow, R. (1984). Role of feedback, reinforcement, and compliance on training and transfer in biofeedback-based rehabilitation of motor speech disorders. In: M.R. McNeil, J.C. Rosenbek, & A.E. Aronson (Eds.), *The Dysarthrias: Physiology, Acoustics, Perception, Management* (pp. 207–229). San Diego: College-Hill Press

Sabra, A.F., Hallett, M, Sudarsky L. & Mullally, W. (1982). Treatment of action tremor in multiple sclerosis with isoniazid. *Neurology, 32,* 912–913

Sapir, S., Spielman, J., Ramig, L., Hinds, S., Countryman, S., Fox, C., & Story, B. (2003) Effects of intensive voice treatment (the Lee Silverman Voice Treatment [LSVT]) on ataxic dysarthria: a case study. *American Journal of Speech-Language Pathology, 12,* 387–399

Sasaki, K. (1984). Cerebro-cerebellar interactions and organization of a fast and stable hand movement: cerebellar participation in voluntary movement and motor learning. In: J.R. Bloedel, J. Dichigans & W. Precht (Eds.), *Cerebellar Functions* (pp. 70–85). Berlin: Springer-Verlag

Seddoh, S.A. & Robin, D.A. (2001). Neurogenic disorders of prosody. In: D. Vogel & M.P. Cannito (Eds.), *Treating Disordered Speech Motor Control,* 2nd ed. (pp 277–320). Austin: Pro-Ed

Schell, G.R. & Strick, P.L. (1984). The origin of thalamic inputs to the arcuate premotor and supplementary motor areas. *Journal of Neuroscience, 4,* 539

Scripture, WE. (1916). Records of speech in disseminated sclerosis. *Brain, 39,* 455–477

Scripture, W.E. (1933). Diagnosis by sound tract. *Nature, 132,* 821–822

Simmons, N. (1983). Acoustic analysis of ataxic dysarthria: an approach to monitoring treatment. In: W. Berry (Ed.), *Clinical Dysarthria* (pp. 283–294). San Diego: College-Hill Press

Thach, W.T. (1975). Timing of activity in cerebellar dentate nucleus and cerebral motor cortex during prompt volitional movement. *Brain Research, 88,* 233–241

Thach, W.T. (1978). Correlation of neural discharge with pattern and force of muscular activity, joint position, and direction of the intended next movement in motor cortex and cerebellum. *Journal of Neurophysiology, 41(3),* 654–676

Thach, W.T. (1980). The cerebellum. In Mountcastle VB, ed. *Medical Physiology,* vol. I (pp. 722–746). St. Louis: C.V. Mosby

Tjaden, K. & Watling, E. (2003). Characteristics of diadochokinesis in multiple sclerosis and Parkinson's disease. *Folia Phoniatrica et Logopaedica, 55,* 241–259

Tjaden, K. & Wilding, G.E. (2004). Rate and loudness manipulations in dysarthria: acoustic and perceptual findings. *Journal of Speech, Language, and Hearing Research, 47,* 766–783

Victor, M. & Ferrendelli, J.A. (1970). The nutritional and metabolic diseases of the cerebellum. Clinical and pathological aspects. In: S.W. Fields & W.D. Willis (Eds.), *The Cerebellum in Health and Disease* (pp. 412–449). St. Louis: Warren H. Green

Vilis, T. & Hore J. (1981). Characteristics of saccadic dysmetria in monkeys during reversible lesions of medial cerebellar nuclei. *Journal of Neurophysiology, 46*, 828–838

Yorkston, K.M. & Beukelman D.R. (1981a). *Assessment of Intelligibility of Dysarthric Speech.* Austin: Pro-Ed

Yorkston K.M. & Beukelman, D.R. (1981b). Ataxic dysarthria: Treatment sequences based on intelligibility and prosodic considerations. *Journal of Speech and Hearing Research, 46*, 398–404

Yorkston, K.M., Beukelman, D.R., Minifie, F. & Sapir, S. (1984). Assessment of stress patterning. In: M.R. McNeil, J.C. Rosenbek, & A.E. Aronson (Eds.), *The Dysarthrias: Physiology, Acoustics, Perception, Management* (pp. 131–162). San Diego: College-Hill Press

Yorkston, K.M., Hammen, V., Beukelman, D.R. & Traynor C. (1990). The effect of rate control on the intelligibility and naturalness of dysarthric speech. *Journal of Speech and Hearing Disorders, 55*, 550–560

Young, A.B. & Penney, J.B. (1986). Pharmacologic aspects of motor dysfunction. In: A.K. Asbury, G.M. McKhann, & W.I. McDonald (Eds.) *Diseases of the Nervous System: Clinical Neurobiology,* vol. 1 (pp. 423–434). Philadelphia: W.B. Saunders

Ziegler, W. & Wessel, K. (1996). Speech timing in ataxic disorders: sentence production and rapid repetitive articulation. *Neurology, 47*, 208–214

Zwirner, P., Murry, T. & Woodson, G.E. (1991). Phonatory function of neurologically impaired patients. *Journal of Communication Disorders, 24*, 287–300

Chapter 10

Hyperkinetic Dysarthria

Richard I. Zraick and Leonard L. LaPointe

Neither from nor towards;
At still point there the dance is,
But neither arrest nor movement.
Words strain,
Crack and sometimes break, under the burden,
Under the tension, slip, slide, perish,
Decay with impressions, will not stay in place,
Will not stay still.

—T.S. Eliot, Burnt Norton, 1935

Eliot may not have intended it, but in this poem he captures aspects of disrupted movement and its subsequent effect on speech. The simple act of speaking, which often serves as the primary vehicle for expression of thought and emotion, actually results from a complex interaction of cognitive, linguistic, and motor processes. When the act of speaking is disrupted in some manner, it may be due to a breakdown in the generation of thought, the selection of words, or physical control of the speech act. In order for one to speak normally, three motor-related processes must occur: (1) motor planning, (2) motor programming, and (3) motor execution. It is during this latter process that disrupted movement can affect the act of speaking, and, as such, impede verbal communication.

This chapter describes the relationship of disrupted movement to disordered speech production, with a particular focus on hyperkinetic dysarthria. The extrapyramidal system and its role in movement control are briefly described, the clinical classification and definitions of hyperkinetic movement disorders are reviewed, and the evaluation and treatment of hyperkinetic dysarthria are described.

◆ The Extrapyramidal System

Clinicians have traditionally divided the motor system into two groups of circuits, generally referred to as the pyramidal system and the extrapyramidal system. The pyramidal system consists of the corticobulbar and corticospinal tracts. The extrapyramidal system includes all other structures that influence motor control, including the basal ganglia and the projection pathways from the brainstem to the spinal cord. Physiologically, the pyramidal and extrapyramidal systems interact, so separating them on this basis must be viewed as artificial. Nonetheless, diseases affecting these two systems present clinically with distinctive and separable signs.

The main elements of the extrapyramidal system are the basal ganglia, a collective name for large subcortical structures located near the lateral ventricles. The major components of the basal ganglia are the caudate and putamen (which together form the striatum), the globus pallidus (lateral and medial divisions), the substantia nigra (pars reticulata and pars compacta), and the subthalamic nuclei **(Fig. 10–1)**. There is a complex connectivity among basal ganglia–related structures, consisting of input to the basal ganglia, output from the basal ganglia, and direct and indirect pathways through the basal ganglia. The caudate and putamen (striatum) is generally considered the input side, and the medial globus pallidus and substantia nigra pars reticulata form the output side. The direct pathways through the basal ganglia facilitate movement because of increased thalamic activation of cortical motor areas; the indirect pathways inhibit movement because of decreased thalamic activation of cortical motor areas (Castro, Murchut, Neafsey, & Wurster, 2002). The basal ganglia control postural, automatic, reflex-like, involuntary movements, and muscle tone, and are believed to be especially important in the planning of slow, continuous movements. In addition to the basal ganglia, the cerebellum also influences motor control by regulating muscle tone, maintaining balance, and coordinating skilled movements.

Peripheral sensory feedback also plays a crucial role in the correct execution of a voluntary movement. Peripheral pathways conveying sensory information project to cortical motor areas, which use this information to assist with motor program execution. Abnormalities in the peripheral afferent input or in the brain response to sensory input may interfere with the processing of motor programs in the cortical motor areas. There is increasing evidence of sensory system involvement in the pathophysiology of certain movement disorders, such as Huntington's disease (HD), Parkinson's disease (PD), dystonia, and Tourette's syndrome (see Abbruzzese & Berardelli, 2003, for a thorough review of this topic).

Symptoms of basal ganglia dysfunction include either (1) *hypokinesia*, which is defined as a paucity of spontaneous movements; or (2) *hyperkinesia*, which is defined as excessive spontaneous movements. The etiologies of basal ganglia disorders include ischemic infarction, hemorrhage, or tumor in the striatum or subthalamic nuclei, or degenerative disorders such as PD (resulting in hypokinesia) and HD (resulting in hyperkinesia) (Castro et al, 2002).

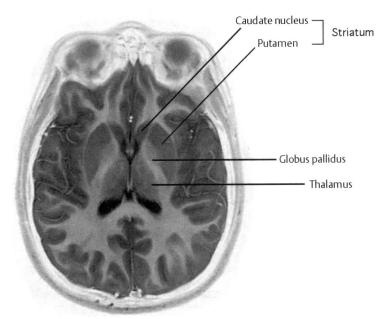

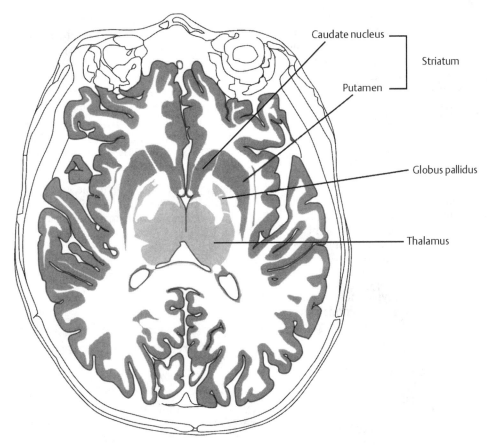

Figure 10–1 (A) Axial MRI of the brain through the cerebral hemispheres and **(B)** a drawing of the same, showing some of the main elements of the basal ganglia, the straitum (caudate nucleus and the putamen) and the globus pallidus. The basal ganglia are large subcortical structures that control postural, automatic, reflex-like involuntary movements and muscle tone by pathways that increase or decrease the thalamus's activation of cortical areas controlling these movements.

◆ Classification and Definition of Hyperkinetic Movement Disorders

Hyperkinetic syndromes can be classified into two general groups, quick forms and slow forms, which describe the speed of the involuntary abnormal movements. Salient features of the relatively quick forms are nonsustained involuntary movements, slowness of movement, and variable muscle hypertonus; features of the relatively slow forms are sustained involuntary movements, slowness of movement, and variable muscle hypertonus. Chorea, myoclonus, tic disorders, and ballismus are the most common of the quick forms, and athetosis, tardive dyskinesia, and dystonia are the most common of the slow forms. Tremor may co-occur with any of the aforementioned forms, or may be the principal sign of a movement disorder. Definitions of the more common hyperkinetic movement disorders (sometimes referred to as dyskinesias) are as follows (also see World-wide Education and Awareness for Movement Disorders, http://www.wemove.org/; and Movement Disorders Virtual University, http://www.mdvu.org/):

- *Chorea*: Jerky, irregular, relatively rapid involuntary movement that primarily involves muscles of the face or extremities. Choreic movements are relatively simple and discrete or highly complex in nature. Although involuntary and purposeless, these movements are sometimes incorporated into deliberate movement patterns. When several choreic movements are present, they often appear relatively slow, writhing, or sinuous, resembling *athetosis*.

- *Myoclonus*: Sudden, brief, shock-like movements. These movements may be positive or negative. Positive myoclonus results in contraction of a muscle or multiple muscles. In *asterixis*, or negative myoclonus, there is a brief loss of muscle tone and then the tightening (contraction) of other muscles; this results in a flapping-type motion. These movements, which cannot by stopped at will (nonsuppressible), often have a characteristic saw-tooth pattern, and they usually disappear during sleep.

- *Tics*: Involuntary, compulsive, stereotypic muscle movements or vocalizations that abruptly interrupt normal motor activities. These repetitive, purposeless motions (motor tics) or utterances (vocal tics) may be simple or complex in nature, may be temporarily suppressed, and are often preceded by a foreboding sensation or urge that is temporarily relieved following their execution. Simple tics include abrupt, isolated movements, such as repeated facial twitching, blinking, or shoulder shrugging, and simple sounds, including grunting, throat clearing, or sighing. Complex tics may involve more sustained, complex movements, such as deep knee bending or leg kicking, or complex vocalizations, including repeating another person's words or phrases (echolalia) or, rarely, explosive cursing (coprolalia).

- *Ballismus*: Uncontrolled, violent, flinging or actions of the proximal limbs. These movements may be sporadic or continuous and, in some patients, restricted to one side of the body (hemiballismus). Ballismus often occurs in association with other abnormal involuntary movements, including *athetosis*, *chorea*, and *dystonia*.

- *Athetosis*: Involuntary, relatively slow, writhing movements that essentially flow into one another. Athetotic and choreiform movements sometimes seem to combine with one another, hence the term *choreoathetosis*. Although athetosis may be most prominent in the face, neck, tongue, and hands, the condition may affect any muscle group.

- *Tardive dyskinesia*: Involuntary, rhythmic movements of the face, jaw, mouth, and tongue, such as lip pursing, chewing movements, or protrusion of the tongue. Facial movements are sometimes accompanied by involuntary, jerky or writhing motions (*choreoathetoid* movements) of the trunk, arms, and legs. It may result from extended therapy with certain antipsychotic medications such as haloperidol. In some patients, symptoms discontinue months or years after withdrawal of antipsychotic therapy. However, in others, the condition may not be reversible (see Chapter 56 for more information about this disorder).

- *Dystonia*: Sustained muscle contractions, usually producing twisting and repetitive movements or abnormal postures or positions. Almost all dystonic movements share a directional quality that is typically sustained, sometimes for an instant, as well as a consistency and predictability. Dystonic movements are directional, forcing the involved body part or region into an abnormal position, which is consistently present. Dystonic postures can be quite painful and severely affect life quality, as can most of the dyskinetic movement disorders described here.

- *Tremor*: Spontaneous, rhythmic, oscillatory movement of hands, limbs, head, or articulators. May occur at rest (resting tremor), while maintaining a position or posture against gravity (postural tremor), or while performing a movement (action tremor), or it may be accentuated toward the end of a movement (terminal tremor).

◆ Hyperkinetic Dysarthria Secondary to Disorders of Movement

As Hartman and Abbs (1988) state in their chapter on the dysarthrias of movement disorders, "The classification and description of movement disorders is broader than the motor speech changes that may accompany them. . . . It is important to note, however, that speech and oromotor control disturbances may be the first and occasionally the only signs and symptoms of a movement disorder" (p. 289). As noted by Duffy (1995), the effects of dyskinesia can be perceived during speech, seen during speech and oral mechanism examination, measured physiologically, and inferred from acoustic measurements.

Hyperkinetic dysarthria is difficult to define because it can be caused by many different disorders. In a Mayo Clinic study of a large number of patients with a primary speech-related diagnosis of dysarthria, 26% were classified as having hyperkinetic dysarthria (Duffy, 1995). Furthermore, the etiologies underlying hyperkinetic dysarthria included toxic/metabolic, degenerative, infectious, traumatic, vascular, multiple, or unknown. As Duffy points out, the distribution of etiologies of hyperkinetic dysarthria is quite different from that associated with most other dysarthria subtypes, noting "the elusive nature of the neuroanatomic bases of movement disorders" (p. 195) (see also, Kent, Duffy, Slama, Kent, & Clift, 2001; Kent, Kent, Duffy, & Weismer, 1998).

In the classic Mayo Clinic studies of Darley, Aronson, and Brown (1969a,b), it was reported that all basic motor-speech processes were disturbed in hyperkinetic dysarthria, perhaps as a direct result of the movement disorder, or as a result of anticipatory and compensatory behaviors (Duffy, 1995). From listener judgments, the eight most prominent auditory-perceptual features were imprecise consonants, prolonged intervals, variable speaking rate, monopitch, harsh voice quality, inappropriate silences, distortion of vowels, and excess and equal stress. Of these features, those that reflect prosodic disturbance (i.e., prolonged intervals, monopitch, inappropriate silences, and excess and equal stress) were most distinctive (see Kent & Rosenbek, 1982).

As Freed (2000) suggested, hyperkinetic dysarthria might best be thought of as a *group* of motor speech disorders, each being associated with one of the hyperkinetic movement disorders. With this construct in mind, it is perhaps most clinically useful to describe the hyperkinetic dysarthrias in the context of the underlying movement disorders causing the speech disturbance, according to Darley et al. (1969a,b) (see Kent & Rosen, 2004, for a discussion of the limitations to this approach).

◆ Hyperkinetic Dysarthria Associated with Chorea

Two of the most common choreiform disorders are Sydenham's chorea and HD. Sydenham's chorea occurs principally in children and adolescents, and HD occurs principally in adults. Both disorders are characterized by hyperkinesia, as well as speech, language, cognitive, and psychiatric disturbances.

Sydenham's Chorea

First described by Thomas Sydenham in 1686 as St. Vitus dance, Sydenham's chorea is characterized by adventitious choreic movements, muscle weakness, motor impersistence, and disturbances of speech, gait, and voluntary movements. Its etiology and pathophysiological mechanisms are still unclear, although its relation with a previous pathophysiological group A β-hemolytic streptococcus infection is well established (Goldenberg, Ferraz, Fonseca, Hilario, Bastos, & Sachetti, 1992). In approximately 30% of cases, Sydenham's chorea appears 2 to 3 months after an episode of rheumatic fever or polyarthritis (Simon, Aminoff, & Greenberg, 1999). The disorder may have an acute or insidious onset, usually subsiding within the following 4 to 6 months (Simon et al, 1999).

There has been very little research conducted on the hyperkinetic dysarthria associated with Sydenham's chorea. Nausieda, Grossman, Koller, Weiner, and Klawans (1980) conducted a retrospective study of 240 individuals with Sydenham's chorea and reported that 39% had dysarthria. Swedo and colleagues (1993) conducted comprehensive physical, neuropsychological, and psychiatric examinations on 11 moderately affected children, and reported that all were noted to be dysarthric, manifesting as "slurred or incoherent speech . . . with two children rendered mute" (p. 707); in all but two of the children, the dysarthria subsided within months of initiating medical treatment and was not present at 18-month follow-up. Additional studies reporting the presence of dysarthria in Sydenham's chorea were conducted by Kulkarni and Anees (1996), who examined 60 children in India, and Goldenberg et al (1992), who examined 187 children in Brazil.

Huntington's Disease

Huntington's disease is an inherited neurodegenerative illness associated with the early degeneration of the basal ganglia motor control circuitry (Hallett, 1993). The inheritance is via an autosomal dominant trait, which means that each child of an affected parent has a 50% risk of developing the disease (Conneally, 1984). Prevalence is reported to be 4 to 7/100,000 in the United States (Qin & Gu, 2004). Over 30,000 people in North America are afflicted with HD, with an additional 150,000 unaffected individuals considered to be at an immediate risk for developing the disease by having an affected parent (Conneally, 1984). Clinically, great variation in age at onset, duration of illness, and course of disease is seen (Mayeux, Stern, Herman, Greenbaum, & Fahn, 1986; Roos, Hermans, Vegter-van der Vlis, van Ommen, & Bruyn, 1993). Most individuals with HD develop symptoms in their 40s and 50s, although there may be subtle changes much earlier (Bonelli, Wenning, & Kapfhammer, 2004; Su, Conneally, & Foroud, 2001; Rosenblatt, Ranen, Nance, & Paulsen, 1999; Rothlind, Bylsma, Peysner, Folstein, & Brandt, 1993). According to Rosenblatt et al (1999) the average survival time after diagnosis is approximately 15 to 20 years, although some patients have lived 30 or 40 years with the disease. Sialorrhea (drooling), hyperkinetic dysarthria, and dysphagia invariably develop as the patient deteriorates to a rigid, akinetic state followed by death (Hamilton, Wolfson, Peavy, Jacobson, & Corey-Bloom, 2004; Imbriglio, 1992; Kagel & Leopold, 1992; Kent, Kent, Duffy, & Weismer, 1998; Yorkston, Miller, & Strand, 1995).

Several studies have been conducted on the hyperkinetic dysarthria associated with HD. In the Mayo Clinic studies of 30 adult subjects with chorea (Darley et al, 1969a,b), it was reported that all basic motor-speech processes were disturbed. From listener judgments, the five most prominent dysarthric features included imprecise consonants, prolonged intervals, variable speaking rate, monopitch, and harsh voice quality. Of the four general clusters of features that were identified (resonatory incompetence, articulatory incompetence, prosodic insufficiency, and prosodic excess), the prosodic deviations proved to be the most distinctive features. Caligiuri and Murray (1984), in their acoustic-perceptual study of five individuals with HD, found no correlation between limb chorea and the presence or severity of dysarthria, with their findings attributed to generalized pathophysiological changes associated with basal ganglia disease rather than a manifestation of underlying chorea. Ramig (1986) studied the acoustic-speech characteristics of speakers with HD and found that during sustained vowel production, abrupt drops in fundamental frequency, adductor and abductor phonatory arrests, and reduced vowel durations were noted. Ramig, however, attributed her findings to the choreiform movements of the laryngeal musculature.

Ludlow, Connor, and Bassich (1987) examined performance of individuals with HD and normal speakers on speech timing tasks. They reported that speech reaction time was unimpaired, whereas changes in the duration of syllables, of pauses between phrases, and of sentences were all reduced in speakers with HD. The HD speakers also had reduced syllable repetition rates. The ratios of word to phrase time, and of phrase to sentence time, remained constant across regular and fast speaking rates and did not differ from normal in either patient group. Their results suggested that PD and HD patients were not impaired in speech planning or initiation, but had poor control over the duration of speech events. Zwirner, Murry, and Woodson (1991) compared the vocal tract steadiness of individuals with HD to that of normal speakers and found that affected speakers displayed greater fundamental frequency variability and formant frequency variability. Zwirner and Barnes (1992) evaluated the relationship between laryngeal and articulomotor stability in individuals with HD and normal speakers. Significantly higher values were found for the variability in fundamental frequency and format frequency of patients who had HD compared with normal speakers. No significant correlations were found between format frequency variability and the variability of the fundamental frequency for the HD speakers.

Hertrich and Ackermann (1994) examined syllable lengths, vowel durations, and voice onset time (VOT) in individuals with HD and in normal control speakers. These investigators reported that all HD speakers presented with increased variability of utterance duration or VOT; a subgroup had reduced speech tempo concomitant with lengthening of short vowels; and durational parameters of phonetic timing, e.g., stress contrast, were largely unimpaired. Hartelius, Carlstedt, Ytterberg, Lillvik, and Laakso (2003) characterized the presence and nature of dysarthria in speakers with mild and moderate HD. They reported that significant speech deviations were found in all areas of speech production tested: respiration, phonation, oral motor performance, articulation, prosody, and intelligibility. The most severe deviations were in phonation, oral motor performance including oral diadochokinesis, and prosody. No correlation was found between age or gender and severity of dysarthria, but a significant difference in the severity of dysarthria was found between the group with mild HD

Table 10–1 Primary Perceptual Speech Characteristics of the Hyperkinetic Dysarthria Associated with Chorea

Process	Characteristic(s)
Phonation-respiration	Sudden forced inspiration-expiration; voice stoppages; transient breathiness; strained-harsh voice quality; excess loudness variations
Resonance	Intermittent hypernasality
Articulation	Distortions and irregular breakdowns; slow and irregular alternate motion rates
Prosody	Prolonged intervals and phonemes; variable rate; inappropriate silences; excessive inefficient-variable patterns of stress

From the work of Darley et al (1969b). Adapted from Duffy, J.R. (1995). *Motor Speech Disorders—Substrates, Differential Diagnosis, and Management* (pp. 189–221). St. Louis: Mosby.

and the group with moderate HD. The most frequently occurring perceptual deviations found in continuous speech were mainly related to speech timing and phonation and were hypothesized to reflect the underlying excessive and involuntary movement pattern. **Table 10–1** presents the primary perceptual speech characteristics of the hyperkinetic dysarthria associated with chorea.

◆ Hyperkinetic Dysarthria Associated with Myoclonus

As described by Simon et al (1999), myoclonic jerks can be classified according to their distribution, relationship to precipitating stimuli, or etiology. Generalized myoclonus has a widespread distribution, whereas focal myoclonus is restricted to a particular part of the body. Myoclonus may occur as a normal phenomenon in healthy persons, as an isolated abnormality, as a manifestation of epilepsy, or as a feature of a variety of degenerative, infectious, and metabolic disorders (Sperling & Herrmann, 1985).

The soft palate, larynx, and diaphragm may all exhibit myoclonus. Palatal myoclonus, which can occur rhythmically at a rate of 1 to 4 Hz, may result in temporary hypernasality and articulatory imprecision. Laryngeal myoclonus frequently occurs in combination with palatal myoclonus (Drysdale, Ansell, & Adeley, 1993) and can have the additional effect of temporarily interrupting phonation. Diaphragmatic myoclonus can be detected during sustained phonation, and can result in slight interruptions of airflow. A relationship may exist between palatal-pharyngeal-laryngeal myoclonus and essential tremor. The two conditions share several perceptual and physical characteristics, including intermitted voice arrests during contextual speech, rhythmical voice arrest during vowel prolongation, movements of the pharynx and larynx beneath the skin, and abnormal adduction/abduction of the vocal folds (Aronson, 1980). In

Table 10–2 Primary Perceptual Speech Characteristics of the Hyperkinetic Dysarthria Associated with Palatopharyngolaryngeal Myoclonus

Process	Characteristic(s)
Phonation-respiration	Often no apparent abnormality; when severe, there may be momentary voice arrests during contextual speech; during vowel prolongation, voice arrests or myoclonic beats at 60–240 Hz
Resonance	Usually normal, but occasional intermittent hypernasality
Articulation-prosody	Usually normal, but brief silent intervals if myoclonus interrupts inhalation or initiation of exhalation, phonation, or articulation

From the work of Darley et al (1969b). Adapted from Duffy, J.R. (1995). *Motor Speech Disorders—Substrates, Differential Diagnosis, and Management* (pp. 189–221). St. Louis: Mosby.

Table 10–3 Primary Perceptual Speech Characteristics of the Hyperkinetic Dysarthria Associated with Gilles de la Tourette Syndrome

Process	Characteristic(s)
Phonation-respiration	Coughing, grunting, throat clearing, screaming, moaning, etc.
Resonance	Sniffing
Articulation-prosody	Humming, whistling, lip smacking, echolalia, palilalia, coprolalia

From the work of Darley et al (1969b). Adapted from Duffy, J.R. (1995). *Motor Speech Disorders—Substrates, Differential Diagnosis, and Management* (pp. 189–221). St. Louis: Mosby.

addition to problems with speech, individuals with acquired palatal myoclonus may have problems with auditory processing (Kurauchi, Kaga, & Shindo, 1996). **Table 10–2** presents the primary perceptual speech characteristics of the hyperkinetic dysarthria associated with palatopharyngolaryngeal myoclonus.

◆ Hyperkinetic Dysarthria Associated with Tic Disorders

As described by Simon et al (1999), tics can be classified into four groups depending on whether they are simple or multiple and transient or chronic. Transient simple tics are very common in children, usually terminate spontaneously within 1 year, and generally require no treatment. Chronic simple tics can develop at any age but often begin in childhood, and treatment is unnecessary in most cases. Persistent simple or multiple tics of childhood or adolescence generally begin before age 15 years. There may be single or multiple motor tics—often vocal tics—but complete remission occurs by the end of adolescence. The syndrome of multiple motor and vocal tics is generally referred to as Gilles de la Tourette's syndrome.

Tourette's syndrome was first described by Frenchman Gilles de la Tourette in 1885. The first signs of Tourette's consist of motor tics in 80% of cases, and vocal tics in 20% (Alsobrook & Pauls, 2002; Simon et al, 1999). When the initial sign is a motor tic, it most commonly involves the face, taking the form of sniffing, barking, blinking, or forced eye closure. Vocal tics commonly consist of grunts, barks, hisses, throat clearing, or coughing, and sometimes inappropriate verbal utterances emerge (Serra-Mestres, Robertson, & Shetty, 1998). Such utterances may take the form of coprolalia (vulgar or obscene speech, e.g., "Fuck you," "Up yours"); echolalia (parroting speech, e.g., Examiner: "Touch

your nose." Patient: "Touch your nose"); and palilalia (repetition of self-generated words or phrases). These speech disturbances have been shown to occur in pauses, before and after clauses, and on typically de-emphasized words (Frank, 1978). In many cases, these speech disturbances have been linked to attention deficit disorder, learning disabilities, and obsessive-compulsive disorder (Baer, 1994; Pauls, Leckman, & Cohen, 1993). Fortunately, the incidence of Tourette's syndrome is less than 1 in 100,000 (Friedhoff, 1982), and drug therapy utilizing antidopaminergic agents has been shown to be effective in many cases. **Table 10–3** presents the primary perceptual speech characteristics of the hyperkinetic dysarthria associated with Tourette's syndrome.

◆ Hyperkinetic Dysarthria Associated with Athetosis

Athetosis is a minor subcategory of cerebral palsy (Morris, Grattan-Smith, Jankelowitz, Fung, Clouston, & Hayes, 2002; Srivastava, Laisram, & Srivastava, 2002) and is rarely used to describe movement disorders acquired in adulthood. As a result, the literature on the dysarthria of athetosis is based almost exclusively on studies of children or adults with cerebral palsy. The articulatory abnormalities noted in individuals with athetosis include wide-ranging jaw movements, inappropriate tongue placement, intermitted velopharyngeal closure, retrusion of the lower lip, and prolonged transition time for articulatory movements (Kent & Netsell, 1978). Intelligibility of connected speech has been reported to be markedly decreased, though phonemic competence is intact, suggesting that athetoid individuals lack the neuromuscular control for articulatory precision (Platt, Andrews, & Howie, 1980; Platt, Andrews, Young, & Quinn, 1980). Neilson and O'Dwyer (1984) and O'Dwyer and Neilson (1988) have reported that involuntary movements typically occur between, rather than during, production of syllables, suggesting that the dysarthria observed in persons with athetoid cerebral palsy may be attributed to abnormal control of voluntary movements, not to involuntary movement.

◆ Hyperkinetic Dysarthria Associated with Tardive Dyskinesia

Tardive syndromes are a group of delayed-onset abnormal involuntary movement disorders induced by a dopamine receptor blocking agent (Fernandez & Friedman, 2003). There are several phenomenologically distinct types of TS. The term *tardive dyskinesia* (TD) has been used to refer to the tardive syndrome that presents with rapid, repetitive, stereotypic movements mostly involving the oral, buccal, and lingual areas. The term *tardive* describes two features of the disorder: (1) that it occurs after chronic therapy with these drugs, and (2) that the disorder is persistent. TD occurs in approximately 20% of patients treated with neuroleptic medications, and the incidence of new cases increases with increasing duration of therapy (Fernandez, Krupp, & Friedman, 2001; Jeste, 2000; Weiner & Goetz, 1999). Early detection of hyperkinetic dysarthria in patients who have chronically ingested neuroleptic agents may play a critical role in preventing TD (Gabbert, Schwade, & Tobey, 2002; Portnoy, 1979; see Chapter 56 for more information about this disorder).

TD primarily involves the tongue, lips, and jaw, and, to a lesser degree, the larynx and respiratory musculature (Faheem, Brightwell, Burton, & Struss, 1982; Feve, Angelard, & Lacau St. Guily, 1995; Weiner, Goetz, Nausieda, & Klawans, 1979). A combination of tongue twisting and protrusion, lip smacking and puckering, and chewing movements in a repetitive and stereotypic fashion is often observed (Jankovic, 1995). The involuntary mouth movements in TD may be suppressed by patients when they are asked to do so. It can also be suppressed by voluntary actions such as putting food in the mouth or talking, and thus is not commonly disabling. In the Mayo Clinic studies (Darley at al, 1969a,b) articulatory deviations were reported to be the most prominent features noted in individuals with TD. Other studies have reported that temporal, prosodic, and phonatory deviations, as well as articulatory deviations, may occur (Gerratt, 1983; Gerratt, Goetz, & Fischer, 1984).

◆ Hyperkinetic Dysarthria Associated with Dystonia

Dystonia is a collective term for a variety of neurogenic disorders of posture and movement characterized by abnormal muscle contractions, which may be accompanied by irregular repetitive movements. Dystonia may affect most of the body or specific body parts, and a common classification of the disorder is by body distribution. Classification by body distribution includes *generalized dystonia*, affecting at least one or both legs plus another area of the body; *segmental dystonia*, affecting two or more contiguous areas of the body; and *focal dystonia*, affecting only one part or area of the body (Fahn, 1988). Focal dystonias that may affect

Table 10–4   Primary Perceptual Speech Characteristics of the Hyperkinetic Dysarthria Associated with Dystonia

Process	Characteristics
Phonation-respiration	Strained-harsh voice quality; voice stoppages; audible inspiration; excess loudness variations; alternating loudness; voice tremor
Resonance	Hypernasality
Articulation	Distorted vowels; irregular break downs; slow, irregular alternate motion rates
Prosody	Inappropriate silences; excess loudness variation; excessive-inefficient-variable stress patterns

From the work of Darley et al (1969b). Adapted from Duffy, J.R. (1995). *Motor Speech Disorders—Substrates, Differential Diagnosis, and Management* (pp. 189–221). St. Louis: Mosby.

speech and voice include orolingual-mandibular dystonia, laryngeal dystonia, and cervical dystonia (also known as spasmodic torticollis). These focal dystonias result in unique speech and voice profiles, which bear closer examination. **Table 10–4** presents the primary perceptual speech and voice characteristics of the hyperkinetic dysarthria associated with dystonia.

Individuals with orolingual-mandibular dystonia have abnormal movements of the vocal tract, including sustained tongue movements, clenched jaw, or forced jaw opening (Schulz & Ludlow, 1991; Yoshida, & Iizuka, 2003; Yoshida, Kaji, Shibasaki, & Iizuka, 2002). These signs often occur with blepharospasm (uncontrolled eye blinks), and this complex has been referred to as focal cranial dystonia or Meige syndrome (Jankovic, 1988a,b). Phonation, prosody, and articulation all are disturbed (Darley, Aronson, & Brown, 1975), and slow speech rate, inappropriate silences and pauses, abnormal stress, and imprecise consonants have been documented (Golper, Nutt, Rau, & Coleman, 1983; Tolosa, 1981).

The voice disorder resulting from laryngeal dystonia is referred to as spasmodic dysphonia (SD), reflecting the phenomenon of laryngospasm during phonation. There are three subtypes of SD—adductor, abductor, and mixed—so labeled to reflect which aspect of vocal fold movement is impaired. Adductor SD occurs most commonly by far, followed by the abductor and mixed types (Blitzer & Brin, 1992). Three syllable-level adductor SD signs have been identified by researchers as being key to the classification of the adductor SD voice: (1) pitch shift (Ludlow, Naunton, Sedory, Schulz, & Hallett, 1988; Sapienza, Walton, & Murry, 1999, 2000), (2) phonatory break (Davidson & Ludlow, 1996; Langeveld, Drost, Frijns, Zwinderman, & Baatenburg de Jong, 2000; Ludlow, et al, 1988), and (3) aperiodicity (Ludlow et al, 1988; Sapienza et al, 1999, 2000). These three signs have been shown to differentiate adductor SD speakers from control speakers (Sapienza et al, 1999) and also to differentiate adductor SD speakers from those with muscular tension dysphonia (Sapienza et al, 2000). Glottal fry has been shown to help

Table 10–5 Primary Perceptual Speech Characteristics of the Hyperkinetic Dysarthria Associated with Spasmodic Dysphonia

Process	Characteristics
Phonation-respiration	*Adductor:* Continuous or intermittent strained, jerky, squeezed, effortful quality with voice arrests when severe; if tremor-based, voice tremor may be apparent during vowel prolongation at higher pitches
	Abductor: Brief, breathy or aphonic segments, most obvious at beginning of utterances or in voiceless consonant environments
Resonance	*Adductor:* Usually normal
	Abductor: Usually normal, but occasional intermittent hypernasality and nasal air emission
Articulation-prosody	*Adductor:* Inappropriate silences; silent articulatory movements; sound repetitions; slow rate and slow alternate motion rates
	Abductor: Phrases may be short

From the work of Darley et al (1969b). Adapted from Duffy, J.R. (1995). *Motor Speech Disorders—Substrates, Differential Diagnosis, and Management* (pp. 189–221). St. Louis: Mosby.

Table 10–6 Acoustic Speech-Voice Characteristics of the Hyperkinetic Dysarthria Associated with Spasmodic Torticollis

Parameter	Gender
Lower habitual fundamental frequency	Females
Lower ceiling fundamental frequency	Females
Restricted frequency range	Females
Shorter /s/ maximum duration	Both
Shorter /z/ maximum duration	Both
Shorter /ah/ maximum phonation duration	Both
Slower sequential articulatory movement rates	Both
Slower alternate articulatory movement rates	Both
Longer phonatory reaction time	Both
Slower reading rate (in words per minute)	Both
Lower overall intelligibility rating	Both
Increased jitter	Both
Increased shimmer	Both
Increased harmonic-to-noise ratio	Females

From the work of Case, LaPointe, and Duane (1990), LaPointe, Case, and Duane (1993), and Zraick, LaPointe, Case, and Duane (1993).

characterize adductor SD speakers as well (Davidson & Ludlow, 1996; Langeveld et al, 2000). Sign expression in adductor SD has been reported by Erickson (2003) to be more frequent in predominantly voiced sentences than in predominantly voiceless sentences, regardless of level of syntactic complexity. Erickson further reported that center-embedded sentences comprising predominantly voiced consonants were found to evoke the greatest number of adductor SD signs. Erickson's findings confirmed the report of Barkmeier, Case, and Ludlow (2001) that expert listeners typically perceived voice breaks, a symptom of adductor SD, in voiced environments, and typically perceived breathy breaks, a symptom of abductor SD, in voiceless environments. **Table 10–5** presents the primary perceptual speech and voice characteristics of persons with SD.

Individuals with spasmodic torticollis (ST), sometimes called cervical dystonia, have tonic or intermittent hyper-contractions of their neck muscles that typically cause involuntary deviation of the head from its normal position. Until the early 1990s, very little was known about speech and voice characteristics associated with ST. Much of what is known about the speech and voice of persons with ST comes from an 8-year collaboration between the Arizona Dystonia Institute and Arizona State University, where more than 300 subjects with a variety of dystonic impairments were evaluated. Detailed reports of the speech characteristics of individuals with ST have been presented in several sources (Case, LaPointe, & Duane, 1990; LaPointe, Case, & Duane, 1993; Zraick, LaPointe, Case, & Duane, 1993). **Table 10–6** presents the distinguishing acoustic speech-voice characteristics of persons with ST.

◆ Hyperkinetic Dysarthria Associated with Voice Tremor

Essential tremor (ET) is a hyperkinetic movement disorder that most often affects the head, arms, or hands. It is the most common of the movement disorders, with approximately 50% of cases being familial and most of the rest being idiopathic (Duffy, 1995). Although ET has been referred to as a benign disorder, symptoms are typically progressive and potentially disabling, often forcing patients to change jobs or seek early retirement (Koller, Biary, & Cone, 1986). The age- and gender-adjusted prevalence of ET is 305.6 per 100,000, with an annual incidence of 23.7 per 100,000 (Rajput, Offord, & Beard, 1984). The age of onset is bimodal and peaks in early adulthood (early 20s) and again in later adulthood in the sixth decade. The disease prevalence increases with increasing age, but there is currently no evidence that ET increases an individual's risk of mortality (Sullivan, Hauser, & Zesiewicz, 2004).

Essential tremor is a heterogeneous condition with variable clinical expression (Hubble, Busenbark, & Pahwa, 1997; Louis, Ford, Wendt, & Cameron, 1998; Louis, Marcer, & Cote, 1995). Ninety percent of patients have an upper extremity tremor, whereas 50% have a head tremor, 30% have a voice tremor, and 15% have a leg or chin tremor (Hsu, Chang, & Sung, 1990). During contextual speech, essential (i.e., organic) voice tremor may not be apparent, especially when it is mild. Vowel prolongation is typically the best task for eliciting voice tremor (Aronson, 1990), which can be heard as rhythmical frequency modulations of 4 to 7 Hz, sometimes accompanied by fluctuations in loudness. Sometimes essential voice tremor can coexist in the presence of other cranial tremors (Kent, Duffy, Vorperian, & Thomas, 1998).

Table 10–7   Primary Perceptual Speech Characteristics of the Hyperkinetic Dysarthria Associated with Voice Tremor

Process	Characteristic(s)
Phonation-respiration	Quavering, rhythmic, waxing and waning tremor, most evident on vowel prolongation, at a rate of approximately 4–7 Hz; voice arrests may occur in severe forms
Resonance	Normal
Articulation	Usually normal, but rate may be slowed
Prosody	Normal pitch and loudness variability may be restricted or altered

From the work of Darley et al (1969b). Adapted from Duffy, J.R. (1995). *Motor Speech Disorders—Substrates, Differential Diagnosis, and Management* (pp. 189–221). St. Louis: Mosby.

Table 10–7 presents the primary perceptual speech and voice characteristics of persons with essential voice tremor.

♦ Evaluation of Hyperkinetic Dysarthria

Evaluation of dysarthric speech is often undertaken with the eventual goal of differential description and diagnosis of dysarthria subtypes. Historically, classification systems such as the Mayo Clinic system (Darley et al, 1969a,b) have been taught in college courses, have been widely used clinically, and have been used to describe participants in research studies (Kent, 1994). However, issues regarding the reliability of the Mayo Clinic system have been raised (Kent, 1994, 1996; Simmons & Mayo, 1997; Zyski & Weisiger, 1987), with many of these issues revolving around the reliance on perceptual methods to describe and classify disordered speech production. As reviewed by Kent (1994), perceptually based instruments such as rating scales have many shortcomings, including poor reliability for some rated dimensions, uncertain definition of rated dimensions, psychometric unsuitability, and limited analytic potential. What may be required for the future development of sensitive and effective clinical evaluation is an integration of human perceptual judgment with instrumental evaluation (Collins, 1984; Kent, 1994).

There have been efforts to establish task-based profiles of some dysarthria subtypes (see Kent & Kent, 2000). Typical tasks include sustained vowel phonation, syllable repetition, and production of connected speech. Connected speech can be obtained from reading of a passage, description of a picture, rote utterances, or spontaneous conversation. Specific tasks are often chosen based on their utility in (1) helping classify type of dysarthria, (2) describing subgroups and individual variations within dysarthria subtype, and (3) indicating pathophysiology in the subsystems of speech production (Kent & Kent, 2000). In the absence of a task-based profile for hyperkinetic dysarthria, a useful overall

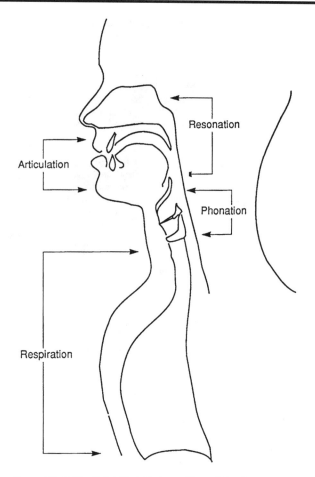

Figure 10–2 The Point-Place System of Speech Production

scheme for evaluation of the speech production system is the "functional component" or "point-place" system **(Fig. 10–2)**. This means of viewing speech production components has been outlined in many sources (LaPointe, & Katz, 1994; Netsell, 1986; Rosenbek & LaPointe, 1985). Briefly, the point-place system calls for examination of the speech processes of respiration, phonation, resonance, articulation, and prosody. The Dysarthria Examination Battery (Drummond, 1993) is an easy-to-administer standardized instrument based on the point-place system, and it contains many tasks **(Table 10–8)** that appear to be sensitive to the nature of the deficits noted in hyperkinetic dysarthria.

The effect of speaking task on the expression of hyperkinetic dysarthria is unknown from a review of the literature, as is the effect of speaking task on listeners' perception of the features of this dysarthria subtype. There is an established literature reporting speech task effects in normal speakers (for an overview, see Lowit-Leuschel & Docherty, 2001), and there is an emerging literature that suggests speech task effects in certain other types of dysarthria (Brown & Docherty, 1995; Kempler & Van Lancker, 2002; Kent, Kent, Rosenbek, Vorperian, & Weismer, 1997; Lowit-Leuschel & Docherty, 2001), as well oral, nonspeech task effects in dysarthria and acquired apraxia of speech (Ackermann, Konczak, & Hertrich, 1997; Kent, Kent, Duffy, Thomas, Weismer,

Table 10–8 Potential Speech Tasks for the Assessment of Hyperkinetic Dysarthria

Speech Process	Task
Respiration	Rate and type of respiration
	Vital capacity
	Maximum phonation time
	s/z ratio
	Words per exhalation
Phonation	Habitual pitch and habitual loudness
	Pitch range
	Optimal pitch
	Loudness range
	Optimal loudness
	Vocal quality
Resonation	Velar movement
	Nasal emission of air
	Nasality
Articulation	Speech intelligibility
	Labial movements
	Mandibular movement
	Lingual movements (speech)
	Lingual active resistance
Prosody	Reading rate
	Stress and intonation (perceptual)
	Stress and intonation (acoustic)

Adapted from Drummond, S.S. (1993). *Dysarthria Examination Battery*. Tucson, AZ: Communication Skill Builders.

& Stuntebeck, 2000; Portnoy & Aronson, 1982; Ziegler, 2002; Ziegler, Hartmann, & Hoole, 1993). This latter literature, combined with literature confirming task effects for nonoral motor acts (e.g., Connor & Abbs, 1991; Teasdale & Stelmach, 1988), may provide some basis for expecting speaking task effects in hyperkinetic dysarthria.

The reliability with which experts can rate hyperkinetic dysarthria has recently been investigated. Zraick, Davenport, Tabbal, Hicks, Hutton, and Patterson (2004) examined the reliability of perceptual ratings made by medical experts and expert speech-language pathologists using the Unified Huntington's Disease Rating Scale (UHDRS), a comprehensive instrument developed by the Huntington Study Group (1996) to assess the relevant clinical features of HD, including speech impairment (Marder, Zhao, Myers, Cudkowicz, Kayson, & the Huntington Study Group, 2000; Siesling, van Vugt, Zwinderman, Kieburtz, & Roos, 1998; Siesling, Zwinderman, van Vugt, Kieburtz, & Roos, 1997; Zraick, Dennie, Tabbal, Hutton, Hicks, & O'Sullivan, 2003). Thirteen individuals with mild to moderate HD produced a standard speech protocol, which included sustained vowel phonation, description of a standard picture, reading of a standard passage, and recitation of the numbers 1 to 10. Using a nine-point equal-appearing interval scale, the experts rated speech severity from audiotape. For the sample of mildly dysarthric speech obtained, interrater reliability for both the medical experts and the speech-language pathologists was reported to be greater than 0.80, whereas the mean intrarater reliability for the

medical experts was 0.95, and for the speech-language pathologists it was 0.97. Zraick et al (2004) concluded that "with the use of a standardized speech protocol and modified rating criteria, the Speech item in the Motor Examination subscale of the UHDRS can be used reliably by medical experts and speech-language pathologists to describe the speech of patients with mild-moderate HD" (p. 31).

◆ General Treatment Principles for Hyperkinetic Dysarthria

Precise clinical and physiological determination of the nature and extent of motor-speech subsystem disturbances is the basis of an effective treatment plan for hyperkinetic dysarthria. Once a differential diagnosis has been made, objective therapy goals can be set, procedures for achieving those goals can be chosen, and measures for testing the efficacy of the treatment plan can be employed. In many cases, medical management, either surgical or pharmacological, is a vital first order of treatment.

Therapy for hyperkinetic dysarthria follows the same basic therapy principles as that of other dysarthria subtypes, and communication disorders in general. That is, short-term goals are set, treatment objectives are determined, and treatment techniques are chosen. A short-term goal is a statement about what the patient and others will do within a mutually agreed upon time frame; usually there is a short-term goal for each affected speech subsystem. Treatment objectives are operationally defined, measurable objectives that the clinician creates in an effort to gauge whether or not the short-term goals have been met. Treatment techniques are specific activities designed to facilitate reaching the treatment objective(s), and ultimately, the short-term goal(s).

General short-term therapy goals by speech subsystem might include the following:

- *Respiration*: Improve respiratory support and the use of respiration for speech.

- *Phonation*: Maximize use of phonation to improve communication skills.

- *Resonance*: Reduce the amount of perceived hypernasality/nasal air emission to increase intelligibility of speech.

- *Articulation*: Improve articulation to increase intelligibility.

- *Prosody*: Improve use of prosody to increase intelligibility/naturalness.

- *Environment*: Patient and listener will improve the environment in which communication takes place.

Specific treatment objectives for hyperkinetic dysarthria might include the following:

- *Respiration*: Work on timing and phrasing of breathing for speech.

- *Phonation*: Work on reducing the effects of increased muscle tone and weakness.

- *Resonance*: Work on better control and efficiency of the velopharyngeal mechanism.

- *Articulation*: Work on the precision of oromotor movements. Improve patient's place of articulation.

- *Prosody*: Work on the use of stress to convey meaning. Improve use of intonation.

- *Environmental*: Work to eliminate environmental obstacle to communication.

Specific treatment techniques for hyperkinetic dysarthria might include the following (largely taken from Dworkin, 1991; Rosenbek & LaPointe, 1985; Yorkston, Beukelman, Strand, & Bell, 1999):

- *Respiration*: Muscle relaxation and postural adjustment. Air pressure generation. Prolonged inhalations/exhalation. Quick breathing. Inhalatory/exhalatory synchronization. Isolated sound production. Connected speech breathing.

- *Phonation*: For hyperadduction: relaxation of laryngeal musculature, yawn-sigh phonation, and vowel prolongations. For hypoadduction: holding the breath, nonspeech vocal fold valving, phonatory vocal fold valving, and hard attack phonation. For fluctuating valving: voice motor planning and laryngeal timing and coordination (see also Boone, McFarlane, & Von Berg, 2002; Case, 2000).

- *Resonance*: Behavioral: isometric contraction, continuous positive airway pressure (CPAP). Prosthetic: palatal lift. Surgical: pharyngeal flap, pharyngoplasty.

- *Articulation*: Muscle tone reduction, muscle strengthening, force physiology training, and phonetic stimulation in various contexts.

- *Prosody*: Direct and indirect attention to speech naturalness, e.g., rate control, modified prosodic patterning.

As with nearly all communication disorders, the effects of intervention can and should be measured and documented. Many systems exist for documenting the course of behavioral or instrumental treatment. Baseline and periodic audio and video recordings can be used throughout a course of treatment, and computer-based analysis systems such as the Multi-Dimensional Voice Program™ (Kay Elemetrics, Pine Brook, NJ, 1993) can be used to document a patient's pre- and posttherapy status (Kent, Vorperian, & Duffy, 1999; Kent, Vorperian, Kent, & Duffy, 2003; Yiu, Worrall, Longland,

& Mitchell, 2000), and integrated with perceptual judgments (Collins, 1984; Weismer, 1984). The use of an instrument like the Base-10 Response Form (LaPointe, 1991) can also be useful in recording and evaluating treatment change in hyperkinetic dysarthria. This system is used to clearly specify, score, and plot countable communication behaviors of clients enrolled in treatment programs. The reality of third-party reimbursement and the increasing recognition of the importance of quality assurance and accountability of services underscored the development of this approach to documenting aspects of treatment efficacy.

Additionally, other components of sensitive and humanistic clinical management are an integral part of intervention for hyperkinetic dysarthria. This includes adequate client and family counseling. Throughout the course of treatment, families and individuals need to be provided with information as few know or are familiar with the professional jargon and restricted and esoteric vernacular of medical conditions (e.g., "Your father has an idiopathic spasmodic torticollis that affects his jitter and shimmer"). Translations need to be made, explanations have to be given, participation needs to be enlisted, and assurance and encouragement need to be an intimate part of the rehabilitation challenge. Individualism and humanism need to guide all intervention efforts, and the medical caregiver blunder of viewing the human being as a disorder needs to be avoided at all costs. Careful sensitive clinical management interweaves all of these humanistic elements and principles into the tapestry of the special skills and knowledge required to understand and treat these unfamiliar and alien conditions.

◆ Conclusion

Hyperkinetic dysarthria is a challenging neuromotor speech disorder. It arises from and is associated with disorders of movement, including chorea, myoclonus, tic disorders, athetosis, tardive dyskinesia, dystonia, and tremor. These conditions are believed to result from neuropathology in the extrapyramidal system, more specifically the basal ganglia and their major pathways, which are important components in the planning and programming of learned movements. Hyperkinetic dysarthria can be intrusive, disruptive, and disabling, and can affect all of the major components of speech production. We are in the embryonic stages of understanding these disorders, but the efforts of science and enlightened clinical hypothesis testing, as well as the emergence and refinement of technology, bode well for the future.

References

Abbruzzese, G. & Berardelli, A. (2003). Sensorimotor integration in movement disorders. *Movement Disorders, 18,* 231–240

Ackermann, H., Konczak, J., & Hertrich, I. (1997). The temporal control of repetitive articulatory movements in Parkinson's disease. *Brain and Language, 56,* 312–319

Alsobrook, J.P. & Pauls, D.L. (2002). A factor analysis of tic symptoms in Gilles de la Tourette's syndrome. *American Journal of Psychiatry, 159,* 291–296

Aronson, A. (1980). *Clinical Voice Disorders: An Interdisciplinary Approach.* New York: Thieme-Stratton

Baer, L. (1994). Factor analysis of symptom subtypes of obsessive compulsive disorder and their relation to personality and tic disorders. *Journal of Clinical Psychiatry, 55,* 18–23

Barkmeier, J.M., Case, J.L., & Ludlow, C.L. (2001). Identification of symptoms for spasmodic dysphonia and vocal tremor: a comparison of expert and nonexpert judges. *Journal of Communication Disorders, 34,* 21–37

Blitzer, A., & Brin, M. F. (1992). The dystonic larynx. *Journal of Voice, 6,* 294–297

Bonelli, R.M., Wenning, G.K., & Kapfhammer, H.P. (2004). Huntington's disease: present treatments and future therapeutic modalities. *International Clinical Psychopharmacology, 19,* 51–62

Boone, D.R., McFarlane, S., & Von Berg, S. (2004). *The Voice and Voice Therapy,* 7th ed. Engelwood Cliffs, NJ: Prentice-Hall

Brown, A. & Docherty, G. (1995). Phonetic variation in dysarthric speech as a function of sampling task. *European Journal of Communication Disorders, 30,* 17–35

Caligiuri, M. & Murry, T. (1984). Identification of a performance deficit in dysarthria associated with Huntington's disease. Presented at the Clinical Dysarthria Conference, Tucson, AZ

Case, J. (2002). *Clinical Management of Voice Disorders,* 4th ed. Austin: Pro-Ed

Case, J., LaPointe, L., & Duane, D. (1990). Speech and voice characteristics in spasmodic torticollis. Presented at the International Congress of Movement Disorders, Washington, DC. (*Abstract in Movement Disorders, 5,* 84.)

Castro, A.J., Murchut, M.P., Neafsey, E.J., & Wurster, R.D. (2002). *Neuroscience: An Outline Approach.* St. Louis: Mosby

Collins, M. (1984). Integrating perceptual and instrumental procedures in dysarthria assessment. *Journal of Communication Disorders, 5,* 159–170

Conneally, P.M. (1984). Huntington disease: genetics and epidemiology. *American Journal of Human Genetics, 36,* 506–526

Connor, A.P. & Abbs, J. (1991). Task-dependent variations in parkinsonian motor impairments. *Brain, 114,* 321–332

Darley, F., Aronson, A., & Brown, J. (1969a). Differential diagnostic patterns of dysarthria. *Journal of Speech and Hearing Research, 12,* 246–269

Darley, F., Aronson, A., & Brown, J. (1969b). Clusters of deviant speech dimensions in the dysarthrias. *Journal of Speech and Hearing Research, 12,* 462–496

Darley, F., Aronson, A., & Brown, J. (1975). *Motor Speech Disorders.* Philadelphia: W.B. Saunders

Davidson, B.J., & Ludlow, C.L. (1996). Long-term effects of botulinum toxin injections in spasmodic dysphonia. *Annals of Otology, Rhinology, and Laryngology, 105,* 33–42

Drummond, S.S. (1993). *Dysarthria Examination Battery.* Tucson, AZ: Communication Skill Builders

Drysdale, A.J., Ansell, J., & Adeley, J. (1993). Palato-pharyngo-laryngeal myoclonus: an unusual cause of dysphagia and dysarthria. *Journal of Laryngology and Otology, 107,* 746–747

Duffy, J.R. (1995). *Motor Speech Disorders—Substrates, Differential Diagnosis, and Management* (pp. 189–221). St. Louis: Mosby

Dworkin, P. (1991). *Motor Speech Disorders: A Treatment Guide.* St. Louis: Mosby

Erickson, M. (2003). Effects of voicing and syntactic complexity on sign expression in adductor spasmodic dysphonia. *American Journal of Speech-Language Pathology, 12,* 416–424

Faheem, A., Brightwell, D., Burton, G., & Struss, A. (1982). Respiratory dyskinesia and dysarthria from prolonged neuroleptic use: Tardive dyskinesia? *American Journal of Psychiatry, 139,* 517–518

Fahn, S. (1988). Concept and classification of dystonia. In S. Fahn, C. Marsden, & B. Calne (Eds.), *Advances in Neurology,* vol. 50 (p. 4). New York: Raven Press

Fernandez, H.H., & Friedman, J.H. (2003).Classification and treatment of tardive syndromes. *Neurologist, 9,* 16–27

Fernandez, H.H., Krupp, B., & Friedman, J.H. (2001). The course of tardive dyskinesia and parkinsonism in psychiatric inpatients: 14-year follow-up. *Neurology, 56,* 805–807

Feve, A., Angelard, B., Lacau St. Guily, J. (1995). Laryngeal tardive dyskinesia. *Journal of Neurology, 242,* 455–499

Frank, S. (1978). Psycholinguistic findings in Gilles de la Tourette syndrome. *Journal of Communication Disorders, 11,* 349–363

Freed, D. (2000). *Motor Speech Disorders: Diagnosis and Treatment.* San Diego: Singular Thomson Learning

Friedhoff, A. (1982). Gilles de la Tourette syndrome. *Advances in Neurology, 35,* 335–339

Gabbert, G., Schwade, N., & Tobey, E.A. (2002). A tutorial on speech production sequelae associated with psychotropic and antiepileptic treatment of mental illness. *Journal of Medical Speech-Language Pathology, 10,* 87–99

Gerratt, B.R. (1983). Formant frequency fluctuation as an index of motor steadiness in the vocal tract. *Journal of Speech & Hearing Research, 26,* 297–304

Gerratt, B., Goetz, C., & Fischer, H. (1984). Speech abnormalities in tardive dyskinesia. *Archives of Neurology, 41,* 273–276

Goldenberg, J., Ferraz, M.B., Fonseca, A.S., Hilario, M.O., Bastos, W., & Sachetti, S. (1992). Sydenham chorea: clinical and laboratory findings. Analysis of 187 cases. *Revista Paulista de Medicina, 110,* 152–157

Golper, L., Nutt, J., Rau, M., & Coleman, R. (1983). Focal cranial dystonia. *Journal of Speech and Hearing Disorders, 48,* 128–134

Hallett, M. (1993). Physiology of basal ganglia disorders: an overview. *Canadian Journal of Neurological Sciences, 20,* 177–183

Hamilton, J.M., Wolfson, T., Peavy, G.M., Jacobson, M.W., Corey-Bloom, J. (2004). Rate and correlates of weight change in Huntington's disease. *Journal of Neurology, Neurosurgery, and Psychiatry, 75,* 209–212

Hartelius, L., Carlstedt, A., Ytterberg, M., Lillvik, M., & Laakso, K. (2003). Speech disorders in mild and moderate Huntington disease: results of dysarthria assessments of 19 individuals. *Journal of Medical Speech-Language Pathology, 11,* 1–14

Hartman, D. & Abbs, J. (1988). Dysarthria of movement disorders. In: J. Jankovic & E. Tolosa (Eds.), *Advances in Neurology: Facial Dyskinesias,* vol. 49 (pp. 289–306). New York: Raven Press

Hertrich, I. & Ackermann, H. (1994). Acoustic analysis of speech timing in Huntington's disease. *Brain and Language, 47,* 182–196

Hsu, Y.D., Chang, M.K., & Sung, S.C. (1990). Essential tremor: Clinical, electromyographical and pharmacological studies in 146 Chinese patients. *Zhonghua Yi Xue Za Zhi (Taipei), 45,* 93–99

Hubble, J.P., Busenbark, K.L., & Pahwa, R. (1997). Clinical expression of essential tremor: effects of gender and age. *Movement Disorders, 12,* 969–972

Imbriglio, S. (1992). Huntington's disease at mid-stage. *Clinical Management, 12,* 62–72

Jancovic, J. (1988a). Cranial-cervical dysarthrias: an overview. In J. Jankovic & E. Tolosa (Eds.), *Advances in Neurology: Facial Dyskinesias,* vol. 49 (pp. 289–306). New York: Raven Press

Jankovic, J. (1988b). Etiology and differential diagnosis of belpharospasm and oromandibular dystonia. In J. Jankovic & E. Tolosa (Eds.), *Advances in Neurology: Facial Dyskinesias,* vol. 49 (pp. 103–116). New York: Raven Press

Jankovic J. (1995). Tardive syndromes and other drug-induced movement disorders. *Clinical Neuropharmacology, 18,* 197–214

Jeste, D.V. (2000). Tardive dyskinesia in older patients. *Journal of Clinical Psychiatry, 61* (suppl 4), 27–32

Kagel, M.C., & Leopold, N.A. (1992). Dysphagia in Huntington's disease: a 16-year retrospective study. *Dysphagia, 7,* 106–114

Kempler, D. & Van Lancker, D. (2002). Effect of speech task on intelligibility in dysarthria: a case study of Parkinson's disease. *Brain and Language, 80,* 449–464

Kent, R.D. (1994). The clinical science of motor speech disorders: a personal assessment. In: J. Till, K. Yorkston, & D. Beukleman (Eds.), *Motor Speech Disorders: Assessment and Treatment* (pp. 3–18). Baltimore: Paul H. Brookes

Kent, R.D. (1996). Hearing and believing: some limits to the auditory-perceptual assessment of speech and voice disorders. *American Journal of Speech-Language Pathology, 7,* 7–23

Kent, R.D., Duffy, J.R., Slama, A., Kent, J.F., & Clift, A. (2001). Clinicoanatomic studies in dysarthria: review, critique, and directions for research. *Journal of Speech and Hearing Research, 44,* 535–551

Kent, R.D., Duffy, J.R., Vorperian, H.K., & Thomas, J.E. (1998). Severe essential vocal and oromandibular tremor: a case report. *Phonoscope, 4,* 237–253

Kent, R.D. & Kent, J.F. (2000). Task-based profiles of the dysarthrias. *Folia Phoniatrica et Logopaedica, 52,* 48–53

Kent, R.D., Kent, J.F., Duffy, J., Thomas, J.E., Weismer, G., & Stuntebeck, S. (2000). Ataxic dysarthria. *Journal of Speech, Language and Hearing Research, 43,* 1275–1289

Kent, R.D., Kent, J.F., Duffy, J., & Weismer, G. (1998). The dysarthrias: speech voice profiles, related dysfunctions, and neuropathology. *Journal of Medical Speech Language Pathology, 6,* 165–211

Kent, R.D., Kent, J.F., Rosenbek, J.C., Vorperian, H.K., & Weismer, G. (1997). A speaking task analysis of the dysarthria in cerebellar disease. *Folia Phoniatrica et Logopaedica, 49,* 63–82

Kent, R.D. & Netsell, R. (1978). Articulatory abnormalities in the athetoid cerebral palsy. *Journal of Speech and Hearing Disorders, 43,* 353–373

Kent, R.D. & Rosen, K. (2004). Motor control perspectives on motor speech disorders. In: B. Maassen, R.D. Kent, H. Peters, P. van Lieshout, & W. Hulstijn (Eds.), *Speech Motor Control in Normal and Disordered Speech* (pp. 285–311). New York: Oxford University Press

Kent, R.D. & Rosenbek, J. (1982). Prosodic disturbance and neurologic lesion. *Brain and Language, 15,* 259–291

Kent, R.D., Vorperian, H.K., & Duffy, J.R. (1999). Reliability of the Multi-Dimensional Voice Program™ for the analysis of voice samples of subjects with dysarthria. *American Journal of Speech-Language Pathology, 8,* 129–136

Kent, R.D., Vorperian, H.K., Kent, J.F., & Duffy, J.R. (2003). Voice dysfunction in dysarthria: application of the Multi-Dimensional Voice Program.™ *Journal of Communication Disorders, 36,* 281–306

Koller, W.C., Biary, N., & Cone, S. (1986). Disability in essential tremor: effect of treatment. *Neurology, 36,* 1001–1004

Kulkarni ,M. & Anees, S. (1996). Sydenham's chorea. *Indian Pediatrics, 33,* 112–115

Kurauchi, T., Kaga, K., & Shindo, M. (1996). Abnormalities of ABR and auditory perception test findings in acquired palatal myoclonus. *International Journal of Neuroscience, 85,* 273–283

Langeveld, T.P.M., Drost, H.A., Frijns, J.H.M., Zwinderman, A.H., & Baatenburg de Jong, R.J. (2000). Perceptual characteristics of adductor spasmodic dysphonia. *Annals of Otology, Rhinology, and Laryngology, 109,* 741–748

LaPointe, L. (1991). *Base-10 Response Form* (revised manual). San Diego: Singular

LaPointe, L., Case, J., & Duane, D. (1993). Perceptual-acoustic speech and voice characteristics of subjects with spasmatic torticollis. In: J. Till, K. Yorkston, & D. Beukleman (Eds.), *Motor Speech Disorders: Assessment and Treatment* (pp. 40–45). Baltimore: Paul H. Brookes

LaPointe, L. & Katz, R. (1994). Neurogenic disorders of speech. In G. Shames, E. Wiig, & W. Secord (Eds.), *Human Communication Disorders: An Introduction,* 4th ed. (pp. 480–518). New York: Macmillan

Lowit-Leuschel, A. & Docherty, G. (2001). Prosodic variation across sampling tasks in normal and dysarthric speakers. *Logopedics, Phonetics, and Vocology, 26,* 151–164

Louis, E.D., Ford, B., Wendt, K.J., & Cameron, G. (1998). Clinical characteristics of essential tremor: data from a population-based cohort. *Movement Disorders, 13,* 803–808

Louis, E.D., Marcer, K., & Cote, K., (1995). Differences in the prevalence of essential tremor among elderly African-Americans, Caucasians and Hispanics in northern Manhattan. *Archives of Neurology, 52,* 1201–1205

Ludlow, C.L., Connor, N., & Bassich, C. (1987). Speech timing in Parkinson's and Huntington's disease. *Brain and Language, 32,* 195–214

Ludlow, C.L., Naunton, R.F., Sedory, M.A., Schulz, G.M., & Hallett, M. (1988). Effects of botulinum toxin injections on speech in adductor spasmodic dysphonia. *Neurology, 38,* 1220–1225

Marder, K., Zhao, H., Myers, R.H., Cudkowicz, M., Kayson, E., & the Huntington Study Group. (2000). Rate of functional decline in Huntington's disease. *Neurology, 54,* 452–458

Mayeux, R., Stern, Y., Herman, A., Greenbaum, L., & Fahn, S. (1986). Correlates of early disability in Huntington's disease. *Annals of Neurology, 20,* 727–731

Morris, J.G., Grattan-Smith, P., Jankelowitz, S.K., Fung, V.S., Clouston, P.D., & Hayes, M.W. (2002). Athetosis II: the syndrome of mild athetoid cerebral palsy. *Movement Disorders, 17,* 1281–1287

Nausieda, P., Grossman, B., Koller, W., Weiner, W., & Klawans, H. (1980). Sydenham chorea: an update. *Neurology, 30,* 331–334

Neilson, P., & O'Dwyer, N. (1984). Reproducibility and variability of speech muscle activity in athetoid dysarthria of cerebral palsy. *Journal of Speech and Hearing Research, 27,* 502–517

Netsell, R. (1986). *A Neurobiological View of Speech Production and the Dysarthrias.* San Diego, CA: College-Hill Press

O'Dwyer, N.J., & Neilson, P.D. (1988). Voluntary muscle control in normal and athetoid dysarthric speakers. *Brain, 111* (pt 4), 877–899

Pauls, D.L., Leckman, J.F., & Cohen, D.J. (1993). Familial relationship between Tourette's disorder, attention deficit disorder, learning disabilities, speech disorders, and stuttering. *Journal of the American Academy of Child and Adolescent Psychiatry, 32,* 1044–1050

Platt, L., Andrews, G., & Howie, P. (1980). Dysarthria of adult cerebral palsy: II. Phonemic analyses of articulation errors. *Journal of Speech and Hearing Research, 23,* 41–45

Platt, L., Andrews, G., Young, M., & Quinn, P. (1980). Dysarthria of adult cerebral palsy: I. Intelligibility and articulatory impairment. *Journal of Speech and Hearing Research, 23,* 28–40

Portnoy, R. (1979) Hyperkinetic dysarthria as an early indicator of impending tardive dyskinesia. *Journal of Speech and Hearing Disorders, 44,* 214–219

Portnoy, R.A., & Aronson, A.E. (1982). Diadochokinetic syllable rate. *Journal of Speech and Hearing Disorders, 47,* 324–328

Qin, Z. & Gu, Z. (2004). Huntington processing in pathogenesis of Huntington disease. Acta Pharmacologica Sinica, *25,* 1243–1249.

Rajput, A.H., Offord, K.P., & Beard, C.M., (1984). Essential tremor in Rochester, Minnesota: a 45-year study. *Journal of Neurology, Neurosurgery and Psychiatry, 47,* 466–470

Ramig, L. (1986). Acoustic analysis of phonation in patients with Huntington's disease. *Annals of Otology, Rhinology and Larygology, 95,* 288–293

Roos, R.A., Hermans, J., Vegter-van der Vlis, M., van Ommen, G.J., & Bruyn, G.W. (1993). Duration of illness in Huntington's disease is not related to age at onset. *Journal of Neurology, 56,* 98–100

Rosenbek, J. & LaPointe, L. (1985). The dysarthrias: Description, diagnosis and treatment. In: D. Johns (Ed.), *Clinical Management of Neurogenic Communication Disorders* (pp. 97–157). Boston: Little, Brown

Rosenblatt, A., Ranen, N., Nance, M., & Paulsen, J. (1999). *A Physician's Guide to the Management of Huntington's Disease.* New York: Huntington's Disease Society of America.

Rothlind, J.C., Bylsma, F.W., Peysner, C., Folstein, S.E., & Brandt, J. (1993). Cognitive and motor correlates of everyday functioning in early Huntington's disease. *Journal of Nervous and Mental Disease, 181,* 194–199

Sapienza, C.M., Walton, S., & Murry, T. (1999). Acoustic variations in adductor spasmodic dysphonia as a function of speech task. *Journal of Speech, Language, and Hearing Research, 42,* 127–140

Sapienza, C.M., Walton, S., & Murry, T. (2000). Adductor spasmodic dysphonia and muscular tension dysphonia: acoustic analysis of sustained phonation and reading. *Journal of Voice, 14,* 502–520

Schulz, G., & Ludlow, C. (1991). Botulinum treatment for orolingual-mandibular dystonia: speech effects. In: C. Moore, K. Yorkston, & D. Beukelman (Eds.), *Dysarthria and Apraxia of Speech: Perspectives on Management* (pp. 227–241). Baltimore: Paul H. Brookes

Serra-Mestres, J., Robertson, M.M., & Shetty, T. (1998). Palicoprolalia: an unusual variant of palilalia in Gilles de la Tourette's syndrome. *Journal of Neuropsychiatry and Clinical Neurosciences, 10,* 117–118

Siesling, S., van Vugt, J., Zwinderman, K., Kieburtz, K., & Roos, R. (1998). Unified Huntington's Disease Rating Scale: a follow up. *Movement Disorders, 13,* 915–919

Siesling, S., Zwinderman, K., van Vugt, J., Kieburtz, K., Roos, R. (1997). A shortened version of the motor section of the Unified Huntington's Disease Rating Scale. *Movement Disorders, 12,* 229–234.

Simmons, K.C. & Mayo, R. (1997). The use of the Mayo Clinic System for differential diagnosis of dysarthria. *Journal of Communication Disorders, 30,* 117–132

Simon, R., Aminoff, M., & Greenberg, D. (1999). *Clinical Neurology,* 4th ed. Stamford, CT: Appleton and Lange

Sperling, M. & Herrmann, C. (1985). Syndrome of palatal myoclonus and progressive ataxia: two cases with magnetic resonance imaging. *Neurology, 35,* 1212–1214

Srivastava, V.K., Laisram, N., & Srivastava, R,K. (1992). Cerebral palsy. *Indian Pediatrics, 29,* 993–996

Sullivan, K.L., Hauser, R.A., & Zesiewicz, T.A. (2004). Essential tremor: epidemiology, diagnosis, and treatment. *The Neurologist, 10,* 250–258

Swedo, S., Leonard, H., Schapiro, M., Casey, B., Mannheim, G., Lelane, M., & Rattew, D. (1993). Sydenham's chorea: physical and psychological symptoms of St. Vitus dance. *Pediatrics, 91,* 706–713

Teasdale, N., & Stelmach, G.E. (1988). Movement disorders: the importance of the movement context. *Journal of Motor Behavior, 20,* 258–264

Tolosa, E. (1981). Clinical features of Meige's disease (idiopathic orofacial dystonia): a report of 17 cases. *Archives of Neurology, 38,* 147–151

Weiner, W., & Goetz, C. (1999). *Neurology for the Non-Neurologist,* 4th ed. Philadelphia: Lippincott Williams & Wilkins

Weiner, W., Goetz, C., Nausieda, P., & Klawans, H. (1979). Respiratory dyskinesias: Extrapyramidal dysfunction and dyspnea. *Annals of Internal Medicine, 88,* 327–331

Weismer, G. (1984). Acoustic description of dysarthric speech: perceptual correlates and physiological inferences. *Seminars in Speech and Language, 5,* 293–314

Yiu, E., Worrall, L., Longland, J., & Mitchell, C. (2000). Analyzing vocal quality of connected speech. *Clinical Linguistics and Phonetics, 14,* 295–305

Yorkston, K., Beukleman, D., Strand, E., & Bell, K. (1999). *Management of Motor Speech Disorders in Children and Adults,* 2nd ed. Austin: Pro-Ed

Yorkston, K.M., Miller, R.M., & Strand, E.A. (1995). *Management of Speech and Swallowing in Degenerative Diseases.* Tucson, AZ: Communication Skill Builders

Yoshida, K., Iizuka, T. (2003). Jaw deviation dystonia evaluated by movement-related cortical potentials and treated with muscle afferent block. *Cranio—The Journal of Craniomandibular Practice, 21,* 295–300

Yoshida, K., Kaji, R., Shibasaki, H., & Iizuka, T. (2002). Factors influencing the therapeutic effect of muscle afferent block for oromandibular dystonia and dyskinesia: implications for their distinct pathophysiology. *International Journal of Oral and Maxillofacial Surgery, 31,* 499–505

Ziegler, W. (2002). Task-related factors in oral motor control: speech and oral diadochokinesis in dysarthria and apraxia of speech. *Brain and Language, 80,* 556–575

Ziegler, W., Hartmann, E., & Hoole, P. (1993). Syllabic timing in dysarthria. *Journal of Speech and Hearing Research, 36,* 683–693

Zraick, R.I., Davenport, D.J., Tabbal, S.D., Hicks, G.S., Hutton, T.J., & Patterson, J. (2004). Reliability of speech intelligibility ratings using the Unified Huntington's Disease Rating Scale. *Journal of Medical Speech-Language Pathology, 12,* 31–40

Zraick, R.I., Dennie, T.M., Tabbal, S.D., Hutton, T.J., Hicks, G.S. & O'Sullivan, P. (2003). Reliability of speech intelligibility ratings using the Unified Parkinson's Disease Rating Scale. *Journal of Medical Speech-Language Pathology, 11,* 227–240

Zraick, R., LaPointe, L., Case, J., & Duane, D. (1993). Acoustic correlates of vocal quality in spasmodic torticollis. *Journal of Medical Speech-Language Pathology, 1,* 261–269

Zwirner, P. & Barnes, G. (1992). Vocal tract steadiness: A measure of phonatory and upper airway motor control during phonation in dysarthria. *Journal of Speech & Hearing Research, 35,* 761–768

Zwirner, P., Murry, T., & Woodson, G. (1991). Phonatory function of neurologically impaired patients. *Journal of Communication Disorders, 24,* 287–300

Zyski, B. J. & Weisiger, B. E. (1987). Identification of dysarthria types based on perceptual analysis. Journal of Communication Disorders, 20, 367-378.

Chapter 11

Hypokinetic Dysarthria

Scott G. Adams and Allyson Dykstra

The term *hypokinetic dysarthria*, first introduced by Darley, Aronson, and Brown (1969a), refers to the speech characteristics observed in patients with Parkinson's disease (PD) (Darley, Aronson, & Brown, 1969a,b). Darley et al (1969a,b, 1975) called this motor speech disorder *hypokinetic*, based on their view that the physiological basis of the dysarthria involved a reduction in the mobility of movements for speech. This reduced mobility is primarily reflected in speech movements that are abnormally smaller and less forceful. Hypokinetic dysarthria gives one the impression that the articulation, intensity, and emotional expressiveness of speech have become compressed or attenuated.

Unlike most of the other dysarthrias, the characteristics of hypokinetic dysarthria were identified by a systematic analysis of patients with one specific disease: idiopathic PD (Darley et al, 1969a,b). As a result, hypokinetic dysarthria is generally considered to be essentially synonymous with the dysarthria of (idiopathic) PD. As Duffy (2005) concisely states "hypokinetic dysarthria is the dysarthria of Parkinson's disease" (p. 190).

The vast majority (78%) of individual's with hypokinetic movement disorders have idiopathic PD (Stacey & Jankovic, 1992). A smaller percentage (22%) of hypokinetic disorders are associated with other forms of parkinsonism such as progressive supranuclear palsy, Wilson's disease, multisystem atrophy, postencephalitic parkinsonism, drug-induced parkinsonism, and atherosclerotic parkinsonism. The speech characteristics of these forms of parkinsonism have not been well studied, but they typically have hypokinetic features plus features of other types of dysarthria (i.e., a mixed type of dysarthria). Whereas few studies have examined the speech manifestations of these less common forms of parkinsonism (Darley et al, 1975; Grewel, 1957; Metter & Hanson, 1991), there is an extensive literature on speech in idiopathic PD. In addition, it has been suggested that PD accounts for 98% of cases with hypokinetic dysarthria seen in speech pathology practices (Berry, 1983; Duffy, 1995). As such, this chapter focuses exclusively on the nature and treatment of the hypokinetic dysarthria associated with idiopathic PD. In particular, this chapter summarizes the perceptual, acoustic, and physiological data related to speech production in PD, and describes several behavioral, instrumental, and prosthetics approaches that have been used in the treatment of hypokinetic dysarthria in PD. The reader is referred to a separate chapter on Parkinson's disease for a discussion of the pathophysiology and nonspeech diagnostic symptoms associated with PD as well as a description of surgical and pharmacological treatments for PD.

◆ Presenting Perceptual, Acoustic, and Physiological Speech Signs and Symptoms in Parkinson's Disease

Perceptual Findings

It is estimated that between 60% and 80% of PD patients develop speech symptoms as the disease progresses (Atarashi & Uchida, 1959; Uziel et al, 1975; Mutch, Strudwick, Roy, et al, 1986; Selby, 1968; Streifler & Hofman, 1984). In the early stages of PD, many patients complain of a reduction in speech intensity, or "hypophonia." Patients with hypophonia can become extremely frustrated by the increasingly frequent requests that they receive to speak louder and repeat themselves. In addition to reduced speech intensity, several clinical reports have noted that patients with PD demonstrate reduced stress and intonation patterns, abnormal voice qualities, distorted consonantal sounds, and abnormally rapid or slow speaking rates. See Canter (1963, 1965a,b) for reviews of the early literature, which was based largely on individual clinical impressions of speech in PD.

Over the past 30 years, several researchers have conducted systematic perceptual studies of speech in PD. These perceptual studies have verified many of the earlier clinical impressions, and have added several new dimensions to the clinical profile of hypokinetic dysarthria in PD.

Loudness Level

Although reduced loudness is generally recognized as one of the major speech symptoms in PD, it has rarely been examined in systematic perceptual studies. In Darley et al's (1975) extensive perceptual study of seven dysarthria groups, they found that in the 15 patients with PD that they examined, the average perceived speech loudness levels were lower than those of the other dysarthric groups. This finding suggests that reduced speech loudness is a distinctive characteristic of speech in PD and, as such, may have a useful role in the differential diagnosis of hypokinetic dysarthria.

Nevertheless reduced speech loudness does not appear to be present in all dysarthric PD patients. Ludlow and Bassich (1984) reported that only 42% (5/12) of their dysarthric patients with PD were perceived as having reduced speech loudness. Similarly, another study found that only 49% of dysarthric patients with PD (20/41) self-reported that they had developed hypophonia (Gamboa, et al, 1997). However, these values may underestimate the actual proportion of dysarthric patients with PD who are hypophonic, given that many PD patients appear to be able to compensate for their hypophonia during formal speech testing. It also has been suggested that patients with PD may have perceptual deficits that make it difficult for them to accurately identify hypophonia in their own speech (Ho, Bradshaw, & Iansek, 2000).

Pitch and Loudness Variation

Reduced pitch and loudness variation were among the most prominent speech deficits observed in Darley et al's (1969a,b, 1975) perceptual studies of speech in PD. Based on their average perceptual rating scale scores, the following hierarchy of deviant dimensions was observed in 32 patients with PD: (1) monopitch, (2) reduced stress, (3) monoloudness, (4) imprecise consonants.

The first three of the above dimensions were judged to be more deviant in patients with PD than in any of the other six neurological groups examined. The authors summarized their results as follows: "Characteristics most distinctive of hypokinetic dysarthria comprise significantly reduced variability in pitch and loudness, reduced loudness level overall, and decreased use of all vocal parameters for achieving stress and emphasis" (Darley et al, 1975, p. 195).

Ludlow and Bassich (1984) reported that within their sample of 12 patients with PD, most were judged to have significant prosodic abnormalities including monopitch, monoloudness, pitch breaks, inappropriate silences, and reduced stress. Specifically, 67% of the patients with PD were perceived as being abnormally monopitch, whereas 58% were perceived as monoloud.

Voice Quality

It appears that many patients with PD experience changes in voice quality. Logemann and Fisher (Logemann, Boshes, & Fisher, 1973; Logemann, Fisher, Boshes, et al, 1978) found that voice disorders such as breathiness, hoarseness, roughness, and tremor were among the most frequent speech symptoms, occurring in 89% of their sample of 200 patients with PD. Moreover, in approximately 45% of these patients, a voice disorder was the only symptom of dysarthria.

Darley et al (1975) reported that the voice of many patients with PD was perceived as either harsh or breathy, and that these characteristics occurred with about an equal degree of severity. In contrast, Ludlow and Bassich (1984) found that 83% of their patients with PD had abnormally harsh voices, whereas only 17% were judged to have abnormally breathy voices. Similarly, Logemann et al (1978) found that only 15% of their patients with PD had abnormally breathy voices. One explanation for this apparent inconsistency may be related to the observation that individuals with PD often demonstrate a co-occurrence of breathy and harsh voice quality. In one study of 20 individuals with PD, perceptual ratings of hoarseness and breathiness were found to be highly correlated (0.65–0.95) (Baumgartner, Sapir, & Ramig, 2001). The frequent co-occurrence of a breathy and harsh voice quality may have created inconsistencies in the rating of these voice qualities across previous perceptual studies.

Primary or true vocal tremor is infrequently perceived in PD. Logemann et al (1973) found that 14% of their 200 patients with PD had vocal tremor. An important consideration in the assessment of vocal tremor is that vocal tremor often can be secondary and caused by tremor in regions of the body that are quite distant from the larynx. For example, tremor of the trunk, head, or upper limb can sometimes lead to the perception of a secondary vocal tremor. A final consideration is that primary vocal tremor may be related to the progression and severity of PD. One study reported some cases of vocal tremor in late-stage PD but none in early-stage PD (Holmes, Oates, Phyland, et al, 2000). This result may be related to the finding that as PD progresses, as many as 50% of patients with PD may develop a moderate action tremor in addition to the traditional resting tremor of PD (Louis et al, 2001a).

Consonant Articulation

In an early description of imprecise consonant articulations in PD, Cramer (1940) noted that plosives appeared to lack precision and were produced almost like fricatives. Logemann and Fisher (Logemann et al, 1973, 1978) reported that in the 200 patients with PD they examined, 45% demonstrated articulatory disorders. In a later study, Logemann and Fisher (1981) provided a detailed description of the speech articulation errors in PD, based on phonetic transcriptions of 90 patients' speech. Their analysis revealed that stops, affricates, and fricatives were often distorted, and that these distortions appeared to be the result of an inadequate narrowing of the vocal tract. That is, stops and affricates became more fricative-like, and fricatives showed a general reduction in frication energy.

Logeman and Fisher (Logemann et al, 1973, 1978) hypothesized that in PD there is a relationship between the severity of an articulatory disorder and the predominant place of the articulation errors. For example, patients with PD with the mildest articulatory disorders had difficulties primarily with consonants involving placement of the tongue dorsum (/k/ and /g/), whereas the articulatory errors of the more severe patients with PD involved more anterior vocal tract placements such as the tongue blade, lips, and tongue tip. These authors further suggest that there may be a progression of dysfunction in PD, beginning with the laryngeal system and subsequently involving the posterior tongue, more anterior portions of the tongue, and finally the labial articulators. They suggested that this progression, from more posterior vocal tract (voice) deficits, to deficits involving more anterior portions of the vocal tract, may be related to a predictable pattern of neural degeneration in the somatotopic representations of the speech articulators in PD. Recent evidence of very early neuropathology in the motor nuclei of the vagus nerve in PD appears to provide some support for this vocal tract degeneration hypothesis (Braak et al, 2003).

Although this progressive vocal tract degeneration hypothesis is intriguing, other interpretations are possible. It is conceivable that the capacity of two different vocal tract structures to produce the movements necessary for speech could be differentially reduced by an equivalent motor impairment. For example, a 50% increase in both laryngeal and lip rigidity may severely disrupt the normal patterns of vocal fold vibration but have relatively minor effects on lip movements required for speech. Similarly, equivalent motor impairments may have differential effects on articulatory precision and the perceived clarity of speech. For example, a 50% reduction in the range of tongue tip movements may have a more dramatic impact on perceived speech clarity than an equivalent 50% reduction in the range of jaw movements.

Imprecise consonant articulation is probably the primary cause of intelligibility deficits in hypokinetic dysarthria. Darley et al (1969a) found a very high correlation between ratings of reduced intelligibility and imprecise consonants (0.92). In addition, 78% (25/32) of their patients with PD were perceived to have *reduced intelligibility*. Similarly, Duffy's (2005) retrospective review of 125 individuals with hypokinetic dysarthria found that 77% had reduced intelligibility. A potentially important consideration in the assessment of intelligibility in PD is the nature of the speech task. Kempler and Van Lancker (2002) found a dramatic difference in the intelligibility for spontaneous speech (29%) and reading aloud (78%) in one subject with PD. This example highlights the common observation that small changes in the demands of a task can have powerful effects on motor performance in PD.

Rate of Speech

Several previous studies have indicated that PD patients can demonstrate abnormal speaking rates (Forrest, Nygaard, Pisoni, & Siemers, 1998; Nishio & Niimi, 2001). In his review of the early studies of PD speech, Canter (1963) observed that although some authors reported abnormally rapid speech in PD, a more common observation was that PD patients had "slow rates of speaking." Logemann and Fisher (1978) found that the proportion of PD patients who demonstrated either an abnormally rapid or slow speech rate was only approximately 20%. Darley et al (1975) noted that although slow speech is a common feature of most dysarthric groups, rapid speech only occurred in the patients with PD. This suggests that rapid speech can be a useful diagnostic sign in PD; however, it appears that the proportion of patients with PD who demonstrate rapid speech is relatively small. An examination of the results from several previous studies suggests that between 6% and 13% (mean 10.5%) of PD patients may demonstrate an abnormally rapid rate of speech (Canter, 1963 [6%]; Darley et al, 1975 [13%]; Logemann et al, 1978 [11%]; Ludlow & Bassich, 1984 [8%]).

In contrast to the finding that only a small proportion of patients with PD demonstrate a rapid "habitual" speaking rate, it appears that a large percentage of patients with PD

have difficulty making adjustments in their rate of speech. For example, Ludlow and Bassich (1984) found that 83% of their patients with PD had difficulty increasing their rate of speech when asked to speak rapidly. This difficulty in modifying speaking rate was found to be one of the most frequent and severe speech characteristics in their patients with PD.

Dysfluencies

Some individuals with PD experience dysfluent speech. Early studies have noted that 16 to 44% of patients with PD demonstrate *phoneme repetitions* (Darley et al, 1975; Logemann et al, 1973). In most cases these repetitions represent a relatively mild dysfluency. The prevalence of moderate-to-severe dysfluency is probably less than 5% in PD. The typical dysfluencies observed in PD can be characterized as rapid and blurred repetitions of phonemes occurring at the beginning of utterances or following a pause (Duffy, 1995). However, in some individuals with PD and reemergent dysfluencies following a history of developmental stuttering, the characteristics of their childhood dysfluencies are retained but in a more severe form (Shahed & Jankovic, 2001). It has been suggested that similar mechanisms may be involved in childhood stuttering and in reemergent dysfluencies associated with PD (Shahed & Jankovic, 2001). A study by Leder (1996) suggested that the emergence of acute adult-onset stuttering in PD may be indicative of extrapyramidal disease. The underlying mechanisms contributing to dysfluent speech in PD is poorly understood, however. Louis, Winfield, Fahn, and Ford (2001) suggested that alterations in central dopaminergic activity may be associated with dysfluencies, palilalia, and freezing in PD. Anderson, Hughes, Rothi, Crucian, and Heilman (1999) found that in an individual with PD and developmental dysfluencies, dopaminergic therapy (carbidopa-levodopa) was associated with more severe stuttering characterized by an increased number of sound repetitions, blocks, and fillers during "on" periods than during the "off" period of treatment. Duffy (1995) suggested that dysfluencies in PD may be analogous to limb motor symptoms such as difficulty with the initiation of motor movements and festination of gait observed in walking.

Acoustic Findings

Intensity Level and Intensity Decay

As discussed in the previous section, perceptual studies have suggested that patients with PD are perceived as speaking with decreased loudness and a reduced range of loudness. Interestingly, the acoustic correlates of these perceptual features have sometimes been difficult to find. For example, various authors have reported no differences between patients with PD and normals on measures of average peak speech intensity (Canter, 1963; Ludlow & Bassich, 1984), and average peak intensity range (Canter,

1963) or relative speech intensity (Metter & Hanson, 1986) obtained during connected speech. In contrast, several studies have been able to document reduced speech intensity in PD (Adams, Haralabous, Dykstra, Abrams, & Jog, 2005; Fox & Ramig, 1997; Ho, Iansek, & Bradshaw, 1999b). In general, these studies indicate that subjects with PD have speech intensities that are, on average, 2 to 4 dB lower than normal. This reduced speech intensity has been observed across most speech tasks; however, it does appear that the type of speech task can have important effects on speech intensity (Fox & Ramig, 1997). For example, relative to normal, Moon, Adams, Jog (2006) found that subjects with PD had a greater reduction in speech intensity for conversational speech than reading passages or memorized sentences. Part of this task effect may be related to the greater attentional demands of conversational speech relative to other speech tasks. This is supported by a finding that when attention is divided, such as during a concurrent manual tracking task, reduced speech intensity can become further exacerbated in PD (Ho, Iansek, & Bradshaw, 2002).

Another consideration is the role of speech context in the assessment of speech intensity in PD. A few studies have examined the effect of speaking contexts (i.e., background noise, interlocuter distance) that are known to have an effect on normal speech intensity regulation. Increasing levels of background noise and increasing interlocuter distances are associated with systematic increases in speech intensity in normals. Subjects with PD show similar and parallel increases in speech intensity across these contexts but at consistently lower levels (2 to 4 dB lower) than normals (Adams et al, 2005, 2006; Ho et al, 2001). In general, these findings suggest that individuals with PD show a normal pattern of intensity regulation but with an "overall gain reduction" for intensity (see Ho et al, 1999, for an exception to these general findings). These results appear to be analogous to the reduced range of movement and overall scale reduction that is found for limb movements in PD.

Intensity (loudness) decay also has been suggested as important and possibly a distinctive feature of hypokinetic dysarthria (Ho et al, 2001). Compared with normal control subjects (N), Ho et al (2001) observed a significantly greater intensity decay (negative slope) for subjects with PD during production of prolonged vowels (PD = −0.78; N = −0.41 dB/s) and paragraph reading (PD = −4; N = −2 dB/sec). In contrast, Rosen, Kent, and Duffy (2005) failed to find a significant difference between subjects with PD and normal control subjects for intensity decay in prolonged vowels or conversational speech. But they did observe a significantly greater intensity decay for subjects with PD during a diadochokinetic task. These inconsistent intensity decay results further highlight the potentially powerful influence that the speech task can have on assessment results in hypokinetic dysarthria.

As a final assessment consideration, patients with PD may not use their habitual speech intensity levels in the unnatural context of the laboratory or speech clinic. Therefore, methods for obtaining acoustic measures of speech intensity outside of the clinical setting may need to be developed to establish valid estimates of hypophonia in PD.

Fundamental Frequency Level & Variability

Canter (1963) reported that fundamental frequency (F0) was significantly higher in patients with PD than in normal speakers. Several later studies reported similar elevations in F0 (Doyle, Raade, St. Pierre, & Desai, 1995; Gamboa et al, 1997; Kent, Vorperian, Kent, & Duffy, 2003). In contrast, a few studies have reported no differences in the F0 levels of PD and normal subjects (Metter & Hanson, 1986; Zwirner, Murry, & Woodson, 1991). The reason for these discrepancies is unclear. It has been suggested that levodopa medication levels may have an effect on F0 levels (Sanabria, Ruiz, Gutierrnez, Marquez, Escobar, Gentil, & Cenjor, 2001). It has also been suggested that F0 may increase with the clinical severity of PD (Metter & Hanson, 1986).

Acoustic studies of F0 variation have been consistent with the numerous perceptual studies demonstrating that monopitch is a feature of the dysarthria in PD speech. That is, patients with PD have been found to have a reduced range of F0 in connected speech (Canter, 1963; Gamboa et al, 1997; Kent et al, 2003; Ludlow & Bassich, 1984) and on tests of maximum F0 range (Bunton, Kent, Kent, & Duffy, 2001; Canter, 1965; Gamboa et al, 1997; Ludlow & Bassich, 1984), when compared with normal speakers. In addition, it appears that there may be a gradual reduction in the range of F0 in connected speech as the severity of PD increases (Metter & Hanson, 1986). One concern with regard to measures of F0 variability is that although it is assumed that reduced F0 variability is causally linked to the perception of monopitch, the few studies that have attempted to clearly demonstrate this association have been relatively unsuccessful (Adams, Reynoe-Briscoe, & Hutchinson, 1998; Ludlow & Bassich, 1984). On the other hand, one study has demonstrated a relatively strong association (−0.69) between the slope of F0 declination (PD = −0.56; N = −6.17 Hz/sec) and the perception of monopitch in PD (Adams et al, 1998).

Voice Quality/Phonatory Function

Maximum Phonation Time   The results of studies of maximum phonation time (MPT) in PD have been inconsistent. Although some studies have indicated that patients with PD have reduced MPTs (Boshes, 1966; Canter, 1965a; Yuceturk, Yilmaz, Egrilmez, & Karaca, 2002), others have suggested that patients with PD have MPT values similar to those of age-equivalent normal subjects (Buck & Cooper, 1956; Fox & Ramig, 1997; Gamboa et al, 1997; Ho et al, 2001; Kreul, 1972; Ramig, Horii, & Bonitati, 1991). Although these inconsistencies may reflect differences in the characteristics of the patient populations that were studied (i.e., severity level, symptom profiles, etc.), it is also likely that the methods of testing MPT influenced these results. Previous reports suggest that MPT values are highly variable, and significantly influenced by the testing procedures, and the amount of practice that subjects receive (Kent, Kent, & Rosenbek, 1987).

Standard Deviation of F0   Standard deviation of F0 (SDF0) is one of several acoustic measures of voice quality that has been examined in PD. Unlike measures of F0 variation over phrase-length or sentence-length utterances, SDF0 is a measure of F0 variation over a short period (1 to 3 seconds) of steady phonation (i.e., prolonged vowels). SDF0 values have been found to be higher and more variable in patients with PD than in normal speakers (Doyle et al, 1995; Ramig, Scherer, Titze, et al, 1988; Zwirner et al, 1991). In addition, SDF0 is correlated significantly with perceptual judgments of dysphonia in PD (Zwirner et al, 1991).

Jitter and Shimmer   These acoustic measures reflect cycle-to-cycle variations in the duration (jitter) and amplitude (shimmer) of the voice signal. Patients with PD have been found to have significantly higher and more variable (across patient) jitter values than normal speakers (Gamboa et al, 1997; Kent et al, 2003; Ramig et al, 1988; Zwirner et al, 1991). Shimmer values have been reported to be either higher than or equal to those of normal speakers (Kent et al, 2003; Zwirner et al, 1991). In addition, when repeated measures were obtained over a period of several hours, patients with PD were found to demonstrate more variable jitter and shimmer values than age-equivalent normal speakers (Winckel & Adams, 1992).

Signal-to-Noise Ratio   The acoustic voice signal contains a certain amount of noise energy. Normal voices have low levels of noise, whereas many abnormal voices show greater noise levels (Colton & Casper, 1990). Signal/noise ratio (S/N) is a measure of the relative amount of noise energy that is present in the voice signal. S/N was originally developed as an acoustic measure of vocal hoarseness (Yumoto, 1983). S/N values have been found to be either higher than (Ramig et al, 1988) or not significantly different from those of normal subjects (Kent et al, 2003; Zwirner et al, 1991).

Vocal Tremor   Tremor, in the range of 3 to 7 Hz, has been observed in the acoustic voice signals of patients with PD (Ludlow, Bassich, Connor, & Coulter, 1986; Ramig, Scheror, Titze, 1998; Philippbar, Robin, & Luschei, 1989). When present, the tremor is more likely to affect the frequency domain than the amplitude domain of the acoustic voice signal (Ludlow, Bassich, Connor, & Coulter, 1986; Philippbar, Robin, & Luschei, 1989).

Imprecise Consonant Articulation

Several acoustic studies have provided information regarding the potential acoustic correlates of imprecise consonant articulation in PD speech. Three such acoustic correlates are spirantization, spectral tilt, and the timing of vocal onsets and offsets. Spirantization is the presence of fricative-like, aperiodic noise during stop closures. Patients with PD have been found to produce an abnormal amount of spirantization particularly during bilabial stops (Weismer, 1984b). Spectral tilt refers to the relative distribution of energy (i.e., high versus low frequencies) in the spectra of stop and fricative consonants. Patients with PD appear to produce fricatives such as /s/ and /sh/ with an abnormal distribution of spectral energy. In particular, the fricative spectra obtained from patients with PD can show an overall tilt toward the lower frequencies (Uziel, Bohe, Cadilhac, et al, 1975; Weismer, 1984a). It is possible that both spirantization and low frequency spectral tilt are the acoustic correlates of the stop and fricative distortions that have been described in previous perceptual studies (Cramer, 1940; Logemann et al, 1978). Future studies are required to further elucidate the relationship between these perceptual and acoustic variables.

Weismer (1984b) reported that patients with PD produce a significant amount of voicing during the normally voiceless closure interval of voiceless stops. Consistent with this, Ackermann and Ziegler (1991) showed that sound intensity levels during stop closures are significantly higher in patients with PD than in normal speakers (presumably due to voicing into closure). Furthermore, these higher intensity levels during stop closures were significantly correlated ($r = .64$) with perceptual ratings of the PD patients' severity of articulatory imprecision (Ackermann & Ziegler, 1991).

Forrest, Weismer, and Turner (1989) reported longer voice onset times (VOTs) in patients with PD, relative to normal subjects, and suggested that this may reflect a movement initiation problem (a classic movement deficit in PD) at the level of the larynx. Similarly, Ludlow and Bassich (1984) and Kreul (1972) found that patients with PD were impaired significantly on vowel repetition tasks that required the rapid repetition of on-off phonations. An alternate explanation is that abnormal VOTs in PD are related to a basic coarticulation problem. Support for a mild coarticulation abnormality in PD has been indicated in a couple of studies (Tjaden, 2000b; Tjaden, 2003).

The acoustics of vowels has received limited attention in PD because they have been judged to be less severely impaired relative to consonants (Darley et al, 1975). Some acoustic studies indicate that vowel distortions contribute to intelligibility deficits in PD through reductions in F1 frequencies of low vowels and reductions in the vowel space of the vowel quadrilateral (Bunton & Weismer, 2001; Weismer, Jeng, Laures, Kent, & Kent, 2001).

Diadochokinetics   Studies of diadochokinesis (DDK) provide additional information about consonant articulations in PD. Several studies have examined the DDK rate of stop consonant syllables in PD (Canter, 1965; Kreul, 1972; Ludlow, Connor, & Bassich, 1987). Two of these studies found no differences between patients with PD and normal speakers for DDK involving the voiceless plosives /p/, /t/, and /k/ (Kreul, 1972; Ludlow et al, 1987). In contrast, a third study found that patients with PD had significantly reduced repetition rates for DDK involving the voiced plosives /b/, /d/, and /g/, relative to normal speakers (Canter, 1965). Several factors could have given rise to these discrepant results, including the use of voiced versus voiceless DDKs, and other factors related to DDK testing procedures (for further discussion see Kent et al, 1987).

Rate of Speech

Consistent with the results of perceptual studies, acoustic studies have indicated that a small proportion of patients with PD produce speech segments that are shorter in duration and therefore more rapid than those of normal speakers. For example, Canter (1963) found that although patients with PD as a group had median phrase and syllable durations that were no different from those of normal speakers, one of 17 patients with PD examined had abnormally short segment durations. Both short segment and transition durations have been reported in the speech of a small proportion of patients with PD (Forrest, Weismer, & Turner, 1989; Uziel et al, 1975; Weismer, 1984b; Weismer, Kimelman, & Gorman, 1985).

As mentioned previously, patients with PD have difficulty modifying their speech rate when they are requested to speak more rapidly. However, when patients with PD do achieve faster rates of speech, the relative timing of words within phrases is preserved and remains equivalent to that of normal speakers (Ludlow, Connor, & Bassich, 1987; Volkmann, Hefter, Lange, et al, 1992).

An important consideration with regard to the measurement of speech rate is that acoustic and perceptual values often do not show perfect agreement. For example, Torp and Hammen (2000) found that when PD patients and controls have an acoustically equivalent speech rate the PD patients' speech rate will be perceived to be faster than the controls' speech rate. It has been hypothesized that the imprecise consonants in PD speech may produce a kind of phonetic blurring that causes speech to be perceived as faster than normal (Weismer, 1984b). This suggests that when attempting to obtain a measure of speech rate in PD, it may be important to use both perceptual and acoustic procedures.

Physiological Findings

Respiratory/Aerodynamic

Respiratory dysfunction appears to be a common cause of death in PD (De Pandis et al, 2002). Therefore, it is not surprising that patients with PD have been reported to show reduced values on many measures of aerodynamic function including (1) a reduction in the total amount of air expended during maximum phonation tasks (Mueller, 1971); (2) reduced intraoral air pressure during consonant-vowel (CV) productions (Marquardt, 1973; Mueller, 1971; Solomon & Hixon, 1993); and (3) reduced vital capacity (Cramer, 1940; De la Torre, Mier, & Boshes, 1960; Laszewski, 1956). It has been suggested that patients with PD may fail to generate

sufficient aerodynamic energy necessary for normal speech (Mueller, 1971).

In addition to overall reductions in aerodynamic function, there is also evidence of increased aerodynamic variability and abnormal airflow patterns in PD (Schiffman, 1985; Vincken, Gauthier, Dollfuss, et al, 1984). For example, Vincken et al (1984) identified two types of airflow abnormalities in patients with PD during maximal inspiratory and expiratory tasks: type A involved regular, tremor-like oscillations (4 to 8 Hz) in airflow, whereas type B was characterized by an irregular, rapidly changing pattern of airflow and brief periods of zero airflow. Vincken et al (1984) suggested that these airflow abnormalities may reflect variations in airflow resistance caused by abnormal movements of glottic and supraglottic structures. However, respiratory kinematic and electromyograph (EMG) studies suggest that these airflow abnormalities also may be the result of irregularities in chest wall movement and respiratory muscle activation patterns (Estenne, Hubert, & Troyer, 1984; Murdoch, Chenery, Bowler, et al, 1989). For example, Murdoch et al (1989) noted that patients with PD demonstrated highly unusual chest wall kinematics including marked irregularities in the rate and amplitude of individual respiratory excursions, and "paradoxical" inspiratory events during sustained vowels and syllable repetitions. Solomon and Hixon (1993) noted that at the initiation of speech breath groups, patients with PD had relatively smaller rib cage volumes and larger abdominal volumes than normal subjects. It was suggested that this may reflect a relative reduction in the compliance of the rib cage in PD. Increases in abdominal excursions were suggested to reflect the PD patient's attempt to compensate for this reduction in rib cage compliance. Interestingly, Solomon and Hixon found little variation in the PD patients' respiratory patterns across different points in the levodopa drug cycle. They suggested that drug-cycle–related fluctuations in motor performance may not have a substantial effect on speech breathing in PD.

Laryngeal

Several physiological studies have examined laryngeal function in PD. Hanson, Gerratt, and Ward (1984) observed abnormal laryngeal signs in 30 of 32 patients with PD who underwent laryngoscopic examinations. The most prominent sign was bowed vocal folds, which occurred to varying degrees in 30 of the 32 patients with PD examined. During phonation, the bowed vocal folds were noted to vibrate with a greater width and a greater amount of glottic aperture than is normally observed. Bowed vocal folds and incomplete vocal fold adduction has frequently been observed in several subsequent studies of PD (Blumin, Pcolinsky, & Atkins, 2004; Perez, Ramig, & Smith, 1996; Smith, Ramig, Dromey, Perez, & Samandari, 1995; Yuceturk et al, 2002). Two very different explanations for bowed vocal folds have been presented. The first hypothesis is that reduced muscular effort, reduced muscle activation, or weakness causes bowing and incomplete adduction (underactivation hypothesis) (Baker, Ramig, Luschei, & Smith, 1998; Fox Morrison, Ramig, & Sapir, 2002; Ramig, 1995). The second hypothesis is that vocal fold bowing is caused by laryngeal muscle rigidity and excessive laryngeal muscle activity that disrupts the normal reciprocal balance between vocal fold muscles (overactivation hypothesis) (Gallena, Smith, Zeffiro, & Ludlow, 2001; Hanson et al, 1984). Preliminary laryngeal EMG evidence has been obtained for both of these hypotheses (Baker et al, 1998; Gallena et al, 2001; Luschei, Ramig, Baker, & Smith, 1999).

Hanson et al (1984) observed a laryngeal asymmetry in 26 of their 30 patients with PD. This asymmetry was frequently associated with one side showing (1) a more posterior position of the vocal process, (2) a more posterior and lateral position of the apex of the arytenoids, and (3) a more contracted ventricular fold than is seen in normal speakers. The side demonstrating these laryngeal signs consistently corresponded to the side of the body that was most affected by the disease. With disease progression, it is known that patients with PD experience an increasing degree of bilateral limb impairment, and this tendency toward bilateral involvement appears to be paralleled in the laryngeal system. A small number of studies have reported bilateral vocal fold paralysis, particularly in the late stages of PD (Holinger, Holinger, & Holinger, 1976; Huppler, Schmidt, & Devine, 1955; Plasse & Liberman, 1981; Schley, Fenton, & Niimi, 1982).

Electroglottographic (EGG) studies have reported that subjects with PD have abnormally large speed quotient values (opening/closing ratio: PD = 2.9; N = 1), and a poorly defined closing period, suggesting that the vocal folds were opening slowly, relative to the rate of closure, and that there may have been inadequate or incomplete closure of the vocal folds (Hanson & Metter, 1983; Jiang, Lin, Wang, & Hanson 1999). In Uziel et al's (1975) study of 18 patients with PD, EGG waveforms were reported to be reduced in amplitude relative to those of normal speakers. It was hypothesized that these reduced EGG signals reflected reduced laryngeal movements caused by a hypertonia (i.e., overactivation hypothesis) of the laryngeal musculature.

Velopharyngeal

Aerodynamic and kinematic studies have indicated that the amplitudes of velopharyngeal movements are reduced in PD (Hirose, Kiritani, Ushijima, et al, 1981; Hoodin & Gilbert, 1989a,b). Furthermore, the degree of velopharyngeal impairment appears to be positively correlated with disease severity (Hoodin & Gilbert, 1989a,b). Perceptual studies indicate that approximately 10 to 40% of patients with PD have a mild degree of hypernasality (Chenery, Murdoch, & Ingram, 1988; Darley et al, 1975; Hoodin & Gilbert, 1989b; Logemann et al, 1978). On the other hand, one physiological (accelerometric) study has found that 71% of patients with PD had nasality values that were more than one standard deviation above those of normal control subjects (Theodoros, Murdoch, & Thompson, 1995).

Orofacial

Jaw Kinematics   Several studies have described abnormalities in the lip and jaw movements of patients with PD

during speech and nonspeech tasks (Caligiuri, 1987, 1989b; Connor & Abbs, 1991; Connor, Abbs, Cole, et al, 1989; Forrest et al, 1989; Hirose, 1986; Hirose et al, 1981; Hunker, Abbs, & Barlow, 1982). Studies of jaw movement have consistently reported that, relative to normal speakers, patients with PD show a significant reduction in the size and peak velocity of jaw movements during speech (Connor et al, 1989; Forrest et al, 1989). Forrest et al (1989) indicated that the jaw movements of patients with PD were, on average, approximately half the size of the jaw movements observed in normal subjects. Interestingly, the durations of jaw movements during speech produced by patients with PD and normal speakers were not significantly different. Thus, the PD group exhibited normal speed of speech-related jaw movements. This finding is of interest in comparison to data reported by Connor and Abbs (1991). When patients with PD were asked to produce visually guided, nonspeech jaw movements, their jaw movements were significantly slower than those of normal subjects. Taken together, the studies by Forrest et al and Connor and Abbs suggest the possibility that certain kinematic impairments in PD, in this case bradykinesia, may be task-dependent. The potential importance of the task-dependent nature of PD oral motor impairments has been further emphasized in a recent study of jaw and finger motor tracking in PD (Adams et al, 2004). These authors found that for nonspeech tracking tasks, oral (jaw) motor impairments were equivalent or parallel to limb (finger) motor impairments. This notion of task specificity in PD impairments may help to explain the clinical observation that patients with PD with significant limb and oral nonspeech bradykinesia frequently demonstrate speech rates that are within normal limits.

Lip Kinematics   Studies of lip movements in PD have been somewhat inconsistent. Although reduced amplitude and peak velocity of lower lip movements during speech have been reported in PD (Caligiuri, 1987, 1989a,b; Forrest et al, 1989; Hirose et al, 1981; Hunker et al, 1982), normal lower lip kinematic patterns for speech also have been observed (Connor et al, 1989). This inconsistency may reflect the fact that different experimental approaches have been employed across studies, including bite-block versus non–bite-block speech, connected speech versus syllable repetitions, and jaw-referenced versus non–jaw-referenced lower lip movements. The type of speech task may have also played a role. As an example, Dromey (2000) found that instructions to speak loudly or hyperarticulate were both associated with a significant increase in the size of lip movements in PD. Ackermann, Konczak, and Hertrich (1997) also showed an effect of speech rate on the size of lip movements in PD.

Other movement abnormalities of the lower lip that have been noted in PD include (1) an increase in the ratio of movement amplitude to peak velocity (Forrest et al, 1989), (2) reductions in the deceleration phase of movements (Forrest et al, 1989), and (3) reversals in the normal sequencing of lower lip and jaw movements (Connor et al, 1989).

Two studies have examined the relationship between reduced size of lower lip movements and rigidity in PD, by measuring passive lip stiffness (Caligiuri, 1987, 1989a; Hunker et al, 1982). Whereas Hunker et al (1982) reported a significant positive relationship between passive lip stiffness and labial hypometria (i.e., decreased movement amplitude), Caligiuri (1987, 1989a) failed to observe a relationship. Taken together, these findings support the view that although rigidity and hypometria may co-occur in PD, the two variables do not appear to be causally related.

Force Control and Strength Measures Studies of orofacial force control have found that patients with PD produce decreased maximum voluntary lip and tongue closing forces (Solomon, Robin, & Luschei, 2000; Solomon, Lovell, Robin, Luschei, 1995; Ward, Theodoros, Murdoch, & Cahill, 1999; Wood, Hughes, & Hayes et al, 1992), slower rate of development of lip and tongue forces (Gentil, Perrin, Tournier, & Pollak, 1999), and increased instability on isometric oral force tasks (Abbs, Hartman, & Vishwanat, 1987; Barlow & Abbs, 1983; Gentil, Tournier, Pollak, Benabid, 1999). In contrast to these results, McAuliffe, Ward, Murdoch, and Farrell (2005) failed to find a difference between PDs and older normal controls on measures of tongue strength, rate of force change, and endurance.

Increases in force instability appear to become more pronounced when patients with PD were required to produce increasingly higher levels of isometric force. Furthermore, the degree of force instability differs across various orofacial structures. For example, Abbs et al (1987) reported that for a given target isometric force, the tongue showed greater force instability than the lip, which in turn showed greater instability than the jaw (Abbs et al, 1987; Barlow & Abbs, 1983). Although these isometric force studies have been interpreted as showing differential force impairments across orofacial structures in PD, it also has been suggested that force instability measures may be differentially affected by the degree of tremor present in each structure (Abbs, 1990; Weismer, 1990). This possibility is supported by the results of a study by Philippbar et al (1989) that found that in PD patients with tremor in two or more structures, there was a different dominant tremor frequency in each structure. Based on this finding, the authors suggest that a peripheral mechanism, as opposed to a central mechanism, may play an important role in the generation of PD postural tremor (see Rack and Ross, 1986, for a further discussion of peripheral mechanisms in PD tremor). In contrast, Hunker and Abbs examined orofacial resting tremor, and reported that patients with PD showed similar resting tremor frequencies across different orofacial structures. They interpreted the finding as an indication that PD resting tremor may be caused by a central mechanism possibly involving an aberrant neural oscillator (Hunker & Abbs, 1984).

Electromyograph Findings Orofacial EMG studies of speech in PD have reported two major abnormalities: (1) increased levels of tonic resting and background EMG activity in both lip and jaw muscles (Hunker & Abbs, 1984; Leanderson, Meyerson, & Persson, 1971, 1972; Moore & Scudder, 1989; Netsell, Daniel, & Celesia, 1975); and (2) loss of reciprocity with increased EMG coactivation patterns in functionally antagonistic lip and jaw muscle groups (Hirose, 1986; Hirose et al, 1981; Hunker & Abbs, 1984; Leanderson et al, 1971, 1972; Moore & Scudder, 1989). Some authors have suggested that these abnormal EMG patterns are associated with the parkinsonian symptom of rigidity. In addition, there is evidence that these abnormal EMG patterns become more apparent as the disease progresses (Netsell et al, 1975). Levodopa medication is reported to produce a reduction in these abnormal EMG patterns in some patients with PD (Netsell et al, 1975).

Another finding to emerge from EMG studies is that there may be deficits in orofacial reflex function in PD. Caligiuri and Abbs (1987) measured lower lip EMG activity (orbicularis oris inferior) and found that the magnitude of the short-latency component of the perioral reflex was greater in patients with PD than in normal speakers. They suggested that this apparent increase in the sensitivity of the perioral reflex may be related to a more generalized impairment in oral sensorimotor function in PD (Caligiuri & Abbs, 1987; Caligiuri, Heindel, & Lohr, 1992).

Sensorimotor, Sensory, and Perceptual Impairments

Whereas PD traditionally has been viewed as primarily a disease of motor output, there has been increasing evidence of sensorimotor, sensory, and perceptual deficits in PD (Koller, 1984; Lewis & Byblow, 2002; Schneider, Diamond, & Markham, 1986; Schneider & Lidsky, 1987; Snider, Fahn, Isgreen, et al, 1976; Tamburin et al, 2003; Tatton, Eastman, Bedingham, et al, 1984). Tatton et al (1984) originally proposed a causal link between sensorimotor impairment and the major motor symptoms of PD. More specifically, they hypothesized that bradykinesia, rigidity, and decreased movement repertoire in PD are related to an abnormal processing of the mechanoreceptor sensory inputs used in the generation and execution of movements. Subsequent studies in the orofacial system have provided support for this sensorimotor hypothesis (Schneider et al, 1986; Schneider & Lidsky, 1987). Relative to normal speakers, patients with PD have been found to produce a greater number of errors on tests of orofacial sensorimotor integration such as jaw proprioception, lingual localization, and motor tracking of orofacial stimuli (Schneider et al, 1986). Additional studies are required to determine what impact these sensorimotor deficits have on orofacial motor performance in PD.

Of potential importance to our understanding of PD speech disorders is the investigation of auditory-motor integration deficits in PD. Early studies of auditory function in PD indicate that patients with PD exhibit a hyperactive stapedial reflex (Murofushi, Yamane, & Osanai, 1992) and deficits in the temporal discrimination of auditory stimuli (Artieda, Pastor, & Lacruz, 1992). Later speech perception studies found that patients with PD demonstrate abnormalities in speech intensity perception (Ho et al, 1999, 2000; but not found in Dromey & Adams, 2000), reactions to shifts in vocal pitch (Kiran & Larson, 2001), perception of word medial silent cues for voicing (t/d contrast) (Graber, Hertrich,

Daum, Spieker, & Ackermann, 2002) and phoneme identification in slow speech (Forrest et al, 1998), perception of speech rate (Breitenstein, Van Lancker, Daum, & Waters, 2001; Tjaden, 2000a), and the perception of emotional tone or prosody of speech (Breitenstein et al, 2001; Pell & Leonard, 2003). The relationship between these abnormalities in auditory/speech perception and the speech production deficits associated with PD remains poorly understood. Several early reports attempted to address the relationship between PD patients' speech prosody deficits and their perception of speech prosody (Blonder, Gur, & Ruben, 1989; Caekebeke, Jennekens-Schinkel, van der Linden, et al, 1991; Darkins, Fromkin, & Benson, 1988; Hartman & Abbs, 1985; Scott & Caird, 1984, 1985; Scott, Caird, & Williams, 1984), but no clear relationship has emerged.

Related to the proposed perception of prosody deficit is the suggestion that some individuals with PD have difficulty in the recognition of facial expressions (Dujardin, Blairy, Defebvre, Duhem, Noël, Hess, et al, 2004; Jacobs, Shuren, Bowers, & Heilman, 1995; Kan, Kawamura, Hasegawa, Mochizuki, & Nakamura, 2002; Sprengelmeyer, Young, Mahn, Schroeder, Woitalla, Büttner, et al, 2003). There is an emerging literature that basal ganglia pathology may be associated with difficulties in the recognition of selective facial expressions that include disgust (Dujardin et al, 2004; Kan et al, 2002; Pell & Leonard, 2005; Sprengelmeyer et al, 2003), anger (Dujardin et al, 2004; Spengelmeyer et al, 2003), and fear (Kan et al, 2002).

Given the increasing evidence suggesting sensorimotor, sensory, and perceptual deficits in PD, it would seem important for future treatment studies to examine the influence of sensory manipulations on speech performance in PD.

◆ Treatment of Hypokinetic Dysarthria in Parkinson's Disease

A variety of methods have been employed in attempts to improve the speech of patients with PD including traditional, perceptually based behavioral speech therapy, instrumentally based biofeedback therapy, and prosthetic or assistive speech devices. Regardless of the method of choice, treatment typically has aimed at one or several of the following: (1) increasing speech intensity, (2) improving speech prosody (i.e., monotonous/monoloud speech), (3) reducing rapid speech, and (4) increasing articulatory mobility and precision.

Behavioral Treatments

Prior to 1980, very few studies addressed the use of behavioral speech therapy in PD (Allan, 1970; Sarno, 1968). Those that did typically did not provide detailed descriptions of the treatment methods and the measures of treatment outcome employed. For example, Sarno (1968) reported on the treatment of over 300 patients with PD who had received 6 months of biweekly behavioral speech therapy focused on intensity control, facial mobility, and speech articulator mobility. However, the specific treatment protocol was not described, and treatment outcome was limited to general clinical impressions. Sarno (1968) suggested that the patients with PD showed some improvements in speech production during the treatment sessions but failed to transfer these changes to situations outside the clinical setting. Although Sarno did not provide evidence in support of this conclusion, the problem of transfer of treatment has been addressed by several other investigators and appears to be one of the most important issues in the treatment of PD speech. This issue is discussed in more detail in the next section.

During the 1980s, several treatment studies provided brief descriptions of the speech therapy procedures and measures of treatment outcome employed with patients with PD (Perry & Das, 1981; Robertson & Thomson, 1984; Scott & Caird, 1981, 1983). For example, Robertson and Thomson (1984) reported on 12 patients with PD who received 2 weeks (30 to 40 hours) of intensive group speech therapy focused on improving (1) respiratory control and capacity; (2) control of pitch variation and vocal loudness; (3) range, strength, and speed of speech and nonspeech oral movements; and (4) control of speech rate. A perceptual rating (0 to 4 scale) of eight dysarthric speech parameters was used to measure treatment outcome. Each patient's speech was rated in the clinic, prior to therapy, immediately following therapy, and at 3 months posttherapy. The results of the study suggested that these patients with PD showed significant improvements on all eight speech parameters immediately following therapy and at 3 months posttreatment. It should be noted that this study has been criticized with regard to ease of replication and psychometric adequacy (Yorkston, Spencer, & Duffy, 2003). Since the late 1980s there have been a substantial number of behavioral treatment studies that demonstrate good replicability, psychometric adequacy, and acceptable experimental controls (Yorkston et al, 2003). Most of these more recent efficacy studies have focused on the Lee Silverman Voice Treatment (LSVT) program (Ramig, Fox, & Sapir, 2004).

Lee Silverman Voice Treatment

The LSVT was developed by Ramig and colleagues (Ramig, Bonitati, Lemke, & Horii, 1994; Ramig et al, 1988) to address the problem of low speech intensity in patients with PD. LSVT is an intensive, high-effort treatment that focuses primarily on the vocal/laryngeal system. It is based on the hypothesis that reduced amplitude of motor drive to the laryngeal (and respiratory) muscles is the primary cause of low speech intensity or hypophonia in PD (Ramig et al, 2004). This reduction in motor/neural drive is also believed to be linked to a basic problem in the "sensory perception of effort" (Ramig et al, 2004). This impaired sense of effort is thought to cause a scaling down in the magnitude of the motor output that controls speech intensity. The goals of LSVT are to (1) increase phonatory effort and vocal fold adduction, (2) increase respiratory support, and (3) recalibrate the sense of effort required to achieve appropriate levels of speech intensity (Ramig et al, 2004). Throughout the treatment, patients are encouraged to "think loud." LSVT involves an intensive, 16-session (four sessions per week for

4 weeks) program with clearly specified exercises, progression criteria, and quantification procedures. The treatment procedures are considered highly replicable because of a detailed manual and workshops that are available for clinician training and certification (Ramig, Countryman, Thompson, & Horii, 1995a; Yorkston et al, 2003).

Over the past 10 years, there have been more than a dozen studies directed toward systematically establishing the efficacy of LSVT through a wide range of outcome measures and study designs. This efficacy evidence has been carefully reviewed in several sources (Duffy, 2005; Ramig et al, 2004; Yorkston et al, 2003). Early LSVT efficacy studies involving single-subject designs, uncontrolled group studies, and nonrandomized designs (Countryman, Ramig, & Pawlas, 1994; Ramig et al, 1991, 1994) led to later studies that used randomized untreated controls, randomized comparison treatment groups, placebo controls, blinded evaluation procedures, and long-term (12 and 24 month) outcome measures (Ramig, Countryman, O'Brien, Hoehn, & Thompson, 1996; Ramig, Sapir, Fox, & Countryman, 2001b; Ramig et al, 1995a, 2001a; Sapir et al, 2002). The cumulative result of this impressive programmatic effort has led to a substantial amount of efficacy evidence. This section focuses on four of the main LSVT efficacy results. First, in-clinic evaluations that were conducted immediately after LSVT demonstrate significant improvements in perceptual and acoustic measures of loudness and intensity (Ramig et al, 1994, 1995, 1996, 2001a,b). Second, post-LSVT evaluations demonstrate significant improvements on a wide range of additional perceptual, acoustic aerodynamic, and physiological measures of speech and oral motor performance as well as patient self-ratings. Some of these additional improved measures include MPT (Ramig et al, 1994b), F0 variability in sentences (Ramig et al, 1994, 1996, 2001b), subglottic air pressure (Ramig & Dromey, 1996), vocal fold adduction (Smith et al, 1995), speech quality and intelligibility ratings (Ramig et al, 1994, 1995; Sapir et al, 2002; Ward et al, 2000), voice quality (Baumgartner et al, 2001), maximum tongue strength (Ward, Theodoros, & Murdoch, 2000), swallowing function (Sharkawi, Ramig, Logemann, Pauloski, Rademaker, Smith, Pawlas, Baum, & Werner, 2002), and facial expressiveness (Spielman, Borod, & Ramig, 2003). Third, in-clinic measures of speech intensity (as well as other measures) generally indicate maintenance of improvements at both 12- and 24-month posttreatment follow-up (Ramig et al, 1994, 2001a). Fourth, LSVT demonstrates superior improvement in measures of speech intensity (and other measures) when compared with either untreated patients or patients who received an alternative treatment that only focused on respiratory function (Ramig et al, 1995, 1996, 2001).

Although LSVT represents an uncommon and impressive effort at establishing efficacy evidence in the field of motor speech disorders, there are a couple of criticisms and concerns. First, the primarily laryngeal/intensity focus of treatment may be regarded as too narrow to be applicable to most hypokinetic dysarthrics and patients with PD. In many hypokinetic dysarthrics nonlaryngeal processes such as oral articulation, velopharyngeal control, respiratory function, and postural control may play a greater role in producing reduced speech intensity than the laryngeal processes. In addition, for many hypokinetic dysarthrics, low speech intensity is just one of several abnormal speech parameters (imprecise consonants, hypernasality, dysfluency, rapid speech, etc.) that should be addressed in treatment. Additional research is required to determine the types of patients that are most likely to benefit from LSVT and also to compare the effects of LSVT and to more multidimensional methods of treatment for hypokinetic dysarthria (see Sullivan, Brune, & Beukelman, 1996, for an example of an effective multidimensional method). A second concern is that most of the efficacy evidence for LSVT has been obtained from measures obtained in the speech clinic. None of the previous LSVT efficacy studies has obtained objective measures of improvements in speech intensity in ecologically valid situations outside of the speech clinic. Because of this limitation, there is very little evidence that LSVT is effective in addressing the transfer of treatment problem in PD. As previously mentioned, the transfer of treatment problem is arguably the most important concern in the treatment of hypokinetic dysarthria in PD (Rubow & Swift, 1985; Sarno, 1968).

To illustrate the potential problem of in-clinic measures and the transfer of treatment problem, imagine the following fictitious example. A new treatment for hypophonia is developed that is called Request to Speak Louder (RSL). It is developed to be fast-acting and simply involves asking subjects to speak much louder one time. Pretreatment measures of speech intensity are made in the clinic from a prolonged vowel and a reading passage. After applying this rapid, one-time RSL treatment, the subject's speech intensity is again measured (posttreatment). It is quite likely that for many patients with PD there will be a significant increase in speech intensity as a result of this simple fictitious RSL treatment. This is because most patients with PD can produce louder speech for at least a short period of time as soon as they are requested to do so. On the other hand, it is very unlikely that this fictitious RSL treatment would lead to a continuation of loud speech outside of the speech clinic or the training context. However, until we examine speech intensity outside of the clinic (and outside of the specific training context) the in-clinic measures of intensity will give the impression that this one-time RSL is an effective treatment for hypophonia.

In summary, the literature on behavioral speech treatment in PD indicates that significant improvements in speech can be obtained on a wide variety of measures within the speech clinic setting. What remains unclear, however, is the extent to which patients with PD are able to transfer these improvements to situations outside of the clinic.

Instrumental Biofeedback Treatments

Several reports have examined the effectiveness of biofeedback for the treatment of PD speech disorders (Hand, Burns, & Ireland, 1979; Johnson & Pring, 1990; Netsell & Cleeland, 1973; Rubow & Swift, 1985; Scott & Caird, 1981, 1983; Yorkston, Beukelman, & Bell, 1988). Many of the speech dimensions that are most impaired in PD, such as pitch variation, speech loudness, and speech rate, can be easily transduced and displayed using a variety of simple laboratory

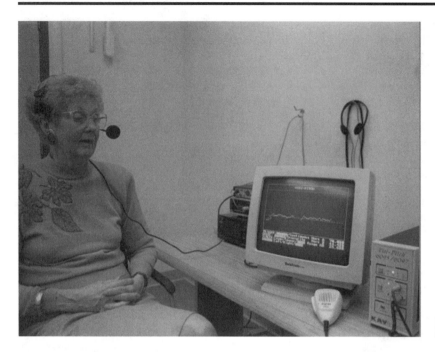

Figure 11–1 Kay Elemetrics' Visipitch (http://www. kayelemetrics.com/).

instruments. These include pitch meters, sound pressure meters, and oscilloscopes. In addition, a variety of relatively inexpensive computer-based programs that provide real-time displays of pitch and loudness, such as Kay Elemetrics' (Pine Brook, NJ) Visipitch **(Fig. 11–1)**, are becoming standard instruments in the clinical setting.

Scott and Caird (1983) compared the effectiveness of speech therapy with and without visual biofeedback. The therapy involved an intensive period of prosodic exercises (10 one-hour sessions in 2 weeks) aimed at improving pitch and loudness variation. A voice-operated light source (Vocalite) provided visual biofeedback about these prosodic dimensions. Ratings of the patients' prosodic abnormality (0 to 7 scale), obtained before and after treatment indicated that patients who received prosodic exercises alone showed a 33% improvement, whereas patients who received prosodic exercises plus visual biofeedback demonstrated a 45% improvement on ratings of speech prosody.

Johnson and Pring (1990) used intensive visual biofeedback therapy in attempts to modify abnormal speech prosody and reduced speech intensity in six patients with PD. Patients received 10 one-hour therapy sessions over a 4-week period. Biofeedback was provided through a computer program (Visispeech), and audio recordings of the patients' speech, before and after therapy, were used to obtain perceptual ratings (Frenchay Dysarthria Scale) and acoustic measures. Following therapy, the patients with PD showed significant improvements on the perceptual ratings and on several acoustic measures including maximum intensity level and range, intensity during conversation and reading, and maximum pitch range.

These studies suggest that (1) improvements in the speech of PD patients can be achieved through biofeedback therapy, (2) these improvements can be measured in the clinical setting through the use of both perceptual and acoustic procedures, and (3) improvements achieved

through behavioral therapy plus biofeedback are greater than improvements achieved with behavioral therapy alone. As in the case of the behavioral treatment studies discussed previously, reports on the use of biofeedback generally have not demonstrated that improvements in speech are transferred beyond the clinical setting (Yorkston et al, 2003). One exception is a study by Rubow and Swift (1985) in which objective, instrumental measures of PD speech outside of the clinic following treatment were provided. Rubow and Swift (1985) used intensive visual biofeedback therapy to treat one patient with PD whose speech was characterized by low speech intensity. The patient received 18 sessions of visual biofeedback regarding his speech intensity and progressed through a hierarchy of structured tasks until he demonstrated improved speech intensity within the clinical setting. To obtain measures of speech outside of the clinic, the patient was fit with a small portable computer that recorded his speech intensity throughout the day. Out-of-clinic measures of speech intensity were obtained before and after the period of intensive biofeedback therapy. Rubow and Swift (1985) reported that intensive biofeedback therapy produced little improvement in the patient's speech intensity outside of the clinical setting. Although this study was limited to the examination of only one patient with PD, it is extremely important because it provides the first objective, instrumental evidence that patients with PD may be experiencing significant difficulty transferring the beneficial effects of speech therapy into speaking situations outside of the clinical setting.

With the recent development of devices such as the voice accumulator and voice dosimeter for monitoring long-term speech performance in everyday conversational situations, it should now be relatively easy to obtain objective out-of-clinic measures for the evaluation of treatment transfer in PD (Beukers, Blenens, Kingma, Marres, 1995; Popolo, Svec, Rogge-Miller, Titze, 2003; Popolo, Svec, & Titze, 2005; Ryu,

Komiyama, Kanee, & Watanabe, 1983; Szabo, Hammarberg, Hakansson, & Sodersten, 2001). Determining that there has been a transfer of treatment to conversational situations outside of the clinic is a common concern in the treatment of most communication disorders. However, some of the cognitive and sensorimotor deficits associated with PD suggest that the generalization of new speech strategies into habitual speech may be particularly difficult for these patients (McNamara, Obler, Durso, et al, 1992; Saint-Cyr, Taylor & Lang, 1988; Schneider et al, 1986). For example, Saint-Cyr et al (1988) found that PD is characterized by a specific cognitive deficit wherein the patient has difficulty learning new procedures or "habits." It is possible that this "procedural learning deficit" is part of the reason that many patients with PD have difficulty generalizing new speech behaviors into situations outside the clinic. If this is the case, then the use of traditional, behaviorally oriented speech therapy techniques that rely on the patient's ability to independently establish new habitual patterns of speech may need to be reconsidered. In contrast to this evidence of a procedural learning deficit, it appears that persons with PD can demonstrate a normal pattern of speech motor learning during some learning procedures. For example, Adams, Page, and Jog (2002) found that patients with PD showed a normal pattern of speech motor learning and retention when they were given different types of summary feedback in a study involving the acquisition of a novel, slower rate of speech.

Another potentially important consideration for behavioral speech therapy programs is that patients with PD may have a much higher degree of context-dependency with respect to motor learning and the establishment of new motor behaviors. For example, Onla-Or (2001) found that motor learning for rapid goal-directed arm movements in individuals with PD showed abnormally greater context-dependency. That is, in order for performance of the movement task to be comparable to control subjects, both the context of the practice task and the retention task needed to be the same (Onla-Or, 2001). This excessive context-dependency in motor learning may play an important causal role in the transfer of treatment problem in PD. If so, future therapy programs may need to incorporate extensive simulations of natural conversational environments and contexts during speech therapy sessions. One example would be to use multitalker background noise while training increased speech intensity. This type of simulated environment may carry more meaning for individuals with PD and increase their motivation to speak at increased speech intensities inside and outside of the clinic setting. In addition, the experience of using appropriate speech intensities in the simulated environment may facilitate the use of these same speech intensities when experiencing similar multitalker noise situations outside of the speech clinic.

Prosthetic and Assistive Device Treatments

One means of circumventing the transfer of treatment problem in PD is through the use of assistive speech devices. Like other prosthetic devices (e.g., eye glasses, hearing aids), assistive speech devices can provide an immediate benefit to the patient's communication, and the devices often remain effective for as long as the patient continues to wear them. In addition, most assistive devices require a minimum amount of patient instruction and training. This means that the patient is not required to establish new habitual patterns of behavior. Because of this, assistive devices may prove to be particularly effective forms of treatment for parkinsonian speech disorders.

One of the most commonly prescribed assistive devices used in the treatment of speech deficits associated with PD is the portable voice amplifier (**Fig. 11–2**) (Armstrong, Jans, & MacDonald, 2000). In spite of their widespread use, very

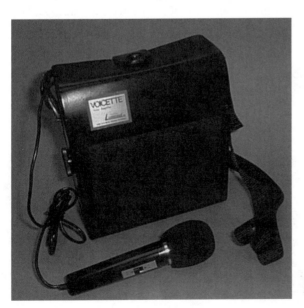
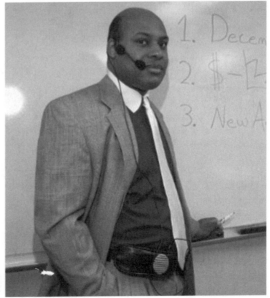

A   B

Figure 11–2 Voice amplifiers. **(A)** Voicette Amplifier (http://www.luminaud.com/). **(B)** Chattervox Amplifier (http://chattervox.com/).

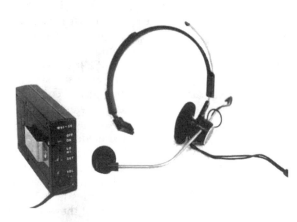

Figure 11–3 Wintronix's Voice Intensity Indicator, Model WVI-55 (P.O. Box 384, Eastlake, Colorado, 80614).

little data are available on the prevalence of voice amplifier use among patients with PD or on the relative effectiveness of the various voice amplifiers that are currently being recommended to patients with PD (Greene & Watson, 1968; Yorkston et al, 2003). Yorkston et al (1988) described one PD patient with low voice intensity who was provided with a voice amplifier after he failed to transfer the gains made in therapy to situations outside of the speech clinic. Although this case report suggests that the voice amplifier may have provided a solution to this patient's transfer of treatment difficulties, no data regarding the patient's effective use of this device were presented. In patients with PD who have been fit with voice amplifiers, it would be useful to examine (1) the amount of time that the amplifier is worn each day, (2) the average level of speech intensity that is produced, and (3) the level of communicative success (i.e., the number of requests to repeat or clarify) that is attained while wearing the amplification device (McCormick & Roy, 2002).

Rubow and Swift (1985) used a portable assistive (biofeedback) device with one patient with PD in order to facilitate the transfer of increased speech intensity into situations outside of the clinic setting. The assistive device monitored the patient's conversational speech and provided a warning tone, through a miniature earphone, whenever his intensity level fell below a predetermined (60 dB) intensity level. The authors monitored the patient's out-of-clinic conversations through the use of a portable microcomputer, and determined the amount of time that his speech intensity fell below the target level (60dB). Out-of-clinic measures made before and after fitting the assistive biofeedback device demonstrated a significant improvement in the patient's out-of-clinic speech intensity when he was wearing the assistive device. Although this study was limited to a single patient, the development of a commercially available portable intensity biofeedback device by Wintronix (Eastlake, CO) **(Fig. 11–3)** makes it relatively easy for clinicians to evaluate the efficacy of this type of assistive device on a larger number of patients with PD. Recently, Kay Pentax (Morristown, NJ; www.kaypentax.com) has developed a portable Ambulatory Phonation Monitor (model 3200) for obtaining long-term measures related to vocal intensity and other vocal parameters. This device, which is worn on a waist belt, can also provide real-time feedback about ongoing speech intensity via an additional vibrotactile feedback warning device.

Masking noise has been found to cause patients with PD to significantly increase their speech intensity (Adams & Lang, 1992; Adams et al, 2005). It has been suggested that a portable voice-activated masker (e.g., Edinburgh Masker) should be investigated as a possible assistive device for the treatment of hypophonia in PD (Adams & Lang, 1992; Dewar, Dewar, Austin, & Brash, 1979).

Another assistive speech device that has been used in treating the rapid speech that is associated with PD is the portable delayed auditory feedback (DAF) device **(Fig. 11–4)** (Adams, 1993; Downie, Low, & Lindsay, 1981a,b; Dagenais, Southwood, & Lee, 1998; Hanson & Metter, 1983; Yorkston

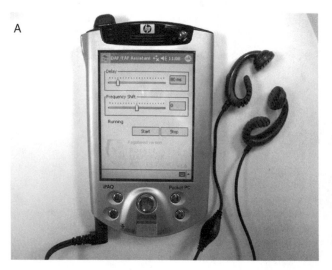

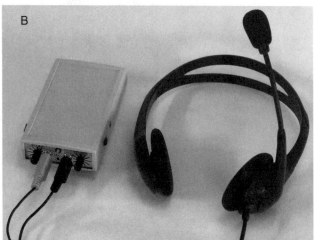

Figure 11–4 Delayed auditory feedback devices. **(A)** Artifactsoft DAF running on a Pocket PC (HP iPAQ 5550) with Platronics stereo microphone headset (model M100i) (http://www.artefactsoft.com). **(B)** Casafutura School DAF (http://casafutura.com/).

et al, 1988, 2003). Auditory feedback delays in the range of 50 to 150 ms have been shown to produce a dramatic slowing of speech rate. For example, Hanson and Metter (1983) examined the effects of DAF (150 ms delay) in two patients with PD with rapid speech. Measures of speech rate, speech intensity, and intelligibility (rated on a 1 to 7 scale) were obtained four times over a 3-month interval. Across the 3 months of testing, DAF produced consistent and significant reductions (25 to 30%) in the patients' speech rates and also improved the patients' speech intensity and intelligibility. As with behavioral and biofeedback approaches to speech therapy, out-of-clinic measures of the effect of the DAF device are needed. However, those reports that have included PD patients' personal accounts suggest that the benefits of DAF can be maintained outside of the clinic for periods of at least 2 years (Adams, 1993; Downie et al, 1981b).

Delayed auditory feedback appears to require little patient instruction beyond the procedures for fitting and operating the device. Yorkston et al (1988) have suggested that in order to maximize the effectiveness of DAF, patients should be instructed to (1) produce the first word of a sentence with relatively strong intensity, (2) speak in full sentences rather than single words, and (3) avoid trying to "overdrive" the effects of DAF. This third point refers to the observation that some patients may attempt to compensate for the DAF by speaking more rapidly. Although this initial resistance to DAF is usually brief, some patients may need to be instructed to "allow" the DAF to slow their speech. In one of the few group studies of DAF in PD, Adams (1998) found that all 20 patients with PD shifted to a slower rate of speech under 80 ms of DAF; however, only the 10 patients with fast speech showed a significant increase in their speech intelligibility while using DAF **(Fig. 11–5).**

Several other assistive devices have been offered as alternatives to DAF for the treatment of rapid speech in PD (Beukelman & Yorkston, 1977; Hammen, Yorkston, & Beukelman, 1989; Helm, 1979; Lang & Fishbein, 1983; Yorkston et al, 1988; Yorkston, Hammen, Beukelman, et al, 1990). Helm (1979) reported improvements in one PD patient's rapid speech and palilalia when he employed a pacing board. The pacing board consisted of a narrow board with seven dividers equally spaced along its 1-foot length. The patient tapped from left to right between the dividers as he spoke each syllable. This syllable-by-syllable tapping caused a significant reduction in the patient's speaking rate. The pacing board has the advantage of being less expensive than DAF devices (Lang & Fishbein, 1983).

Further studies are required to compare the relative effectiveness of these rate reduction techniques. As an example, the intelligibility scores for one patient's speech were obtained while using either a DAF device or a pacing board (Adams, 1997). DAF was associated with significantly higher intelligibility scores. This appeared to be related to the patient's production of rapid and festinating finger tapping movements, which interfered with his consistent use of the pacing board.

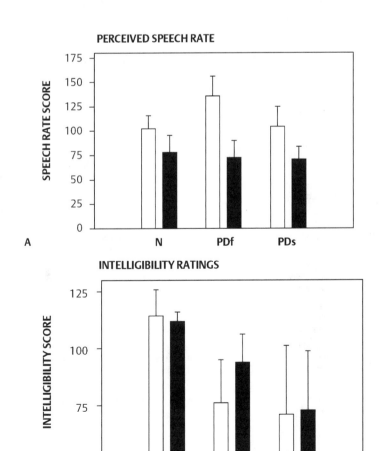

Figure 11–5 Effects of DAF (80 ms) on **(A)** speech rate and **(B)** intelligibility in 10 normals (N), 10 fast rate (PDf), and 10 slow/normal rate (PDs) patients with Parkinson's disease (PD).

Another pacing technique involving finger tapping while speaking is the paced alphabet board technique (Beukelman & Yorkston, 1977; Yorkston et al, 1988, 2003). In this technique, the patient must touch the first letter of each word on a small portable alphabet board before it is spoken. The time taken to find and move to each new letter produces a significant reduction in speaking rate. Crow and Enderby (1989) reported on one patient with PD who used an alphabet board (and first letter pointing) to slow speech by more than 50%. This slower paced speech was associated with a 17% increase in the intelligibility of patient's conversational speech. This pacing procedure also may be useful for PD patients who demonstrate both rapid speech and festinating limb movements.

A final rate reduction technique that has been used in attempts to reduce speaking rate in PD involves the use of computer-generated pacing procedures (Hammen & Yorkston, 1996; Yorkston et al, 1988, 1990). In this technique, patients with PD read aloud sentences as they are presented on a computer screen. Yorkston et al (1990) examined several methods of sentence presentation and found that in the four hypokinetic dysarthric patients they examined, the most effective method was an additive metered presentation. In the additive metered procedure, a sentence was presented word by word across the computer screen, with each word receiving an equal presentation duration. This pacing procedure resulted in significant reductions in speaking rate and increased speech intelligibility scores. A current version of this Pacer software is commercially available (http://www.madonna.org/res_software. htm). Because this assistive device relies on a computer-generated pacer, it is unlikely that it can be incorporated into a portable assistive device. Therefore, its application will largely be restricted to the clinical setting, or possibly to a home computer for the purpose of extended practice. The extent to which patients with PD can generalize the gains achieved through this rate reduction procedure to out-of-clinic settings remains to be determined.

◆ Conclusion

Hypokinetic dysarthria, which is essentially synonymous with the dysarthria of Parkinson's disease, is caused by damage to specific basal ganglia subsystems and their associated sensorimotor processes. Hypokinetic dysarthria is characterized primarily by imprecise consonants, low speech intensity, reduced prosody (i.e., monotone), harsh and breathy voice quality, and fast or inconsistent speech rate (i.e., short rushes). A variety of neurosurgical and dopamine-related drug therapies have been developed to treat the major limb symptoms of Parkinson's disease. These medical therapies have been found to have limited or inconsistent effects on hypokinetic dysarthria. On the other hand, there is growing evidence that several behavioral programs, instrumental procedures, and assistive devices are relatively effective in the treatment of hypokinetic dysarthria. There has been a substantial amount of efficacy evidence provided for the LSVT program, which focuses on the laryngeal system and the problem of low speech intensity. Additional research is required to strengthen the efficacy evidence of other more multidimensional and instrumentally based treatment programs. It is also essential that future efficacy studies address the very important transfer of treatment problem in hypokinetic dysarthria and Parkinson's disease.

References

Abbs, J.H. (1990). Orofacial impairment in Parkinson's disease: reply from the author. *Neurology, 40,* 192–193

Abbs, J.H., Hartman, D.E., & Vishwanat, B. (1987). Orofacial motor control impairment in Parkinson's disease. *Neurology, 37,* 394–398

Ackermann, H., Konczak, J., & Hertrich, I. (1997). The temporal control of repetitive articulatory movements in Parkinson's disease. *Brain and Language, 56,* 312–319

Ackermann, H. & Ziegler, W. (1991). Articulatory deficits in parkinsonian dysarthria: an acoustic analysis. *Journal of Neurology, Neurosurgery, and Psychiatry, 54,* 1093–1098

Adams, S.G. (1993). Accelerating speech in a case of hypokinetic dysarthria: descriptions and treatment. In: J.A. Till, D.R. Beukelman, & K.M. Yorkston (Eds.), *Motor Speech Disorders: Advances in Assessment and Treatment.* Baltimore: Paul H. Brookes

Adams, S.G. (1997). Hypokinetic dysarthria in Parkinson's disease. In: M. R. McNeil (Ed.), *Clinical Management of Sensorimotor Speech Disorders.* New York: Thieme

Adams, S.G. (1998). Effect of delayed auditory feedback on fast Parkinsonian speech. Paper presented at the Conference on Motor Speech, Tucson, Arizona

Adams, S.G., Haralabous, O., Dykstra, A., Abrams, K., & Jog, M.S. (2005). Effects of multi-talker background noise on the intensity of spoken sentences in Parkinson's disease. *Canadian Acoustics, 33,* 94–95

Adams, S.G., Jog, M., Eadie, A., Dykstra, A., Gauthier, G., & Vercher, J.L. (2004). Jaw and finger movements during visual and auditory motor tracking in Parkinson's disease. *Journal of Medical Speech-Language Pathology, 11,* 215–222

Adams, S.G. & Lang, A.E. (1992). Can the Lombard effect be used to improve low voice intensity in Parkinson's disease? *European Journal of Disorders of Communication, 27,* 121–127

Adams, S.G., Moon, B., Dykstra, A., Abrams, K., Jenkins, M. & Jog, M. (2006). Effects of multi-talker noise on conversational speech in Parkinson's disease. Conference on Motor Speech, Austin, Texas

Adams, S.G., Page, A.D. & Jog M.S. (2002). Summary feedback schedules and speech motor learning in Parkinson's disease. *Journal of Medical Speech-Language Pathology, 10,* 215–220

Adams, S.G., Reyno-Briscoe, K., & Hutchinson, L. (1998). Acoustic correlates of monotone speech in Parkinson's disease. *Canadian Acoustics, 26,* 86–87

Allan, C.M. (1970). Treatment of non fluent speech resulting from neurological disease—treatment of dysarthria. *British Journal of Disorders of Communication, 5,* 3–5

Anderson, J.M., Hughes, J.D., Rothi, L.J.G., Crucian, G.P., & Heilman, K.M. (1999). Developmental stuttering and Parkinson's disease: the effects of levodopa treatment. *Journal of Neurology, Neurosurgery, and Psychiatry, 66,* 776–778

Armstrong, L., Jans, D., & MacDonald, A. (2000). Parkinson's disease and aided AAC: Some evidence from practice. *International Journal of Language and Communication Disorders, 35,* 377–389

Artieda, J., Pastor, M.A., & Lacruz, F. (1992). Temporal discrimination is abnormal in Parkinson's disease. *Brain, 115,* 199–210

Baker, K.K., Ramig, L.O., Luschei, E.S., & Smith, M.E. (1998). Thyroarytenoid muscle activity associated with hypophonia in Parkinson disease and aging. *Neurology, 51,* 1592–1598

Barlow, S.M. & Abbs, J.H. (1983). Force transducers for the evaluation of labial, lingual, and mandibular motor impairments. *Journal of Speech and Hearing Research, 26,* 616–621

Baumgartner, C.A., Sapir, S., & Ramig, L.O. (2001). Voice quality changes following phonatory-respiratory effort treatment (LSVT(r)) versus respiratory effort treatment for individuals with Parkinson's disease. *Journal of Voice, 15,* 105–114

Berry, W.R. (1983). *Clinical Dysarthria.* San Diego: College-Hill

Beukelman, D.R. & Yorkston, K.M. (1977). A communication system for the severely dysarthric speaker with an intact language system. *Journal of Speech and Hearing Disorders, 42,* 265–270

Blonder, L.X., Gur, R.E., & Ruben, C.G. (1989). The effects of right and left hemiparkinsonism on prosody. *Brain and Language, 36,* 193–207

Blumin, J.H., Pcolinsky, D.E., & Atkins, J.P. (2004). Laryngeal findings in advanced Parkinson's disease. *Annals of Otology, Rhinology and Laryngology, 113,* 253–258

Boshes, B. (1966). Voice changes in parkinsonism. *Journal of Neurosurg, 21,* 286–288

Braak, H., Del Tredici, K., Rub, U., de Vos, R.A.I., Jansen Steur, E.N.H., & Braak, E. (2003). Staging of brain pathology related to sporadic Parkinson's disease. *Neurobiology of Aging, 24,* 197–211

Braak, H., Rub, U., Jansen Steur, E.N.H., Del Tredici, K., & de Vos, R.A.I. (2005). Cognitive status correlates with neuropathologic stage in Parkinson disease. *Neurology, 64,* 1404–1410

Breitenstein, C., Van Lancker, D., Daum, I., & Waters, C.H. (2001). Impaired perception of vocal emotions in Parkinson's disease: influence of speech time processing and executive functioning. *Brain and Cognition, 45,* 277–314

Buck, J.F. & Cooper, I.S. (1956). Speech problems in parkinsonian patients undergoing anterior choroidal artery occlusion or chemopallidectomy. *Journal of the American Geriatrics Society, 4,* 1285–1290

Buekers, R., Blenens, E., Kingma, H., Marres, E.H.M.A. (1995). Vocal loads as measured by the voice accumulator. *Folia Phoniatrica et Logopaedica, 47,* 252–261

Bunton, K., Kent, R.D., Kent, J.F., & Duffy, J.R. (2001). Effects of flattening fundamental frequency contours on sentence intelligibility in speakers with dysarthria. *Clinical Linguistics and Phonetics, 15,* 181–193

Bunton, K. & Weismer, G. (2001). The relationship between perception and acoustics for a high-low vowel contrast produced by speakers with dysarthria. *Journal of Speech, Language, and Hearing Research, 44,* 1215–1228

Caekebeke, J.F.V., Jennekens-Schinkel, A., van der Linden, M.E., et al. (1991). The interpretation of dysprosody in patients with Parkinson's disease. *Journal of Neurology, Neurosurgery, and Psychiatry, 54,* 145–148

Caligiuri, M.P. (1987). Labial kinematics during speech in patients with parkinsonian rigidity. *Brain, 110,* 1033–1044

Caligiuri, M.P. (1989a). Short-term fluctuations in orofacial motor control in Parkinson's disease. In: K.M. Yorkston & D.R. Beukelman (Eds.), *Recent Advances in Clinical Dysarthria* (pp. 199–212). Boston: College-Hill Press

Caligiuri, M.P. (1989b). The influence of speaking rate on articulatory hypokinesia in parkinsonian dysarthria. *Brain and Language, 36,* 493–502

Caligiuri, M.P. & Abbs, J.H. (1987). Response properties of the perioral reflex in Parkinson's disease. *Experimental Neurology, 98,* 563–572

Caligiuri, M.P., Heindel, W.C., & Lohr, J.B. (1992). Sensorimotor disinhibition in Parkinson's disease: effects of levodopa. *Annals of Neurology, 31,* 53

Canter, G.J. (1963). Speech characteristics of patients with Parkinson's disease: I. Intensity, pitch, and duration. *Journal of Speech and Hearing Disorders, 28,* 221–229

Canter, G.J. (1965a). Speech characteristics of patients with Parkinson's disease: II. Physiological support for speech. *Journal of Speech and Hearing Disorders, 30,* 44–49

Canter, G.J. (1965b). Speech characteristics of patients with Parkinson's disease: III. Articulation, diadochokinesis, and over-all speech adequacy. *Journal of Speech and Hearing Disorders, 30,* 217–224

Chenery, H.J., Murdoch, B.E. & Ingram, J.C.L. (1988). Studies in Parkinson's disease: perceptual speech analyses. *Australian Journal of Human Communication Disorders, 16,* 17–29

Colton, R.H. & Casper, J.K. (1990). *Understanding Voice Problems: A Physiological Perspective for Diagnosis and Treatment.* Baltimore: Williams & Wilkins

Connor, N.P. & Abbs, J.H. (1991). Task-dependent variations in parkinsonian motor impairments. *Brain, 114,* 321–332

Connor, N.P., Abbs, J.H., Cole, K.J., et al. (1989). Parkinsonian deficits in serial multiarticulate movements for speech. *Brain, 112,* 997–1009

Countryman, S., Ramig, L.O. & Pawlas, A.A. (1994). Speech and voice deficits in parkinsonian plus syndromes: can they be treated? *Journal of Medical Speech language Pathology, 2,* 211–226

Cramer, W. (1940). De spaak bij patienten met Parkinsonisme. *Logopaedica Phoniatrica, 22,* 17–23

Crow, E. & Enderby, P. (1989). The effects of an alphabet chart on the speaking rate and intelligibility of speakers with dysarthria. In: K.M. Yorkston, D.R. Beukelman (Eds.), *Recent Advances in Clinical Dysarthria* (pp. 99–108). Boston: College-Hill

Dagenais, P.A., Southwood, M.H., & Lee, T.L. (1998). Rate reduction methods for improving intelligibility of dysarthric speakers with Parkinson's disease. *Journal of Medical Speech-Language Pathology, 6,* 143–157

Darkins, A.W., Fromkin, V.A., & Benson, D.F. (1988). A characterization of the prosodic loss in Parkinson's disease. *Brain and Language, 34,* 315–327

Darley, F.L., Aronson, A.E., & Brown, J.R. (1969a). Clusters of deviant speech dimensions in the dysarthrias. *Journal of Speech and Hearing Research, 12,* 462–496

Darley, F.L., Aronson, A.E., & Brown, J.R. (1969b). Differential diagnostic patterns of dysarthria. *Journal of Speech and Hearing Research, 12,* 246–269

Darley, F.L., Aronson, A.E., & Brown, J.R. (1975). *Motor Speech Disorders* (pp. 192–297). Philadelphia: W. B. Saunders

De la Torre, R., Mier, M., & Boshes, B. (1960). Evaluation of respiratory function—preliminary observation. *Quarterly Bulletin of Northwestern Universiy Medical School, 34,* 232–236

De Pandis, M.F., Starace, A., Stefanelli, F., Marruzzo, P., Meoli, I., De Simone, G., Prati, R., & Stocchi, F. (2002). Modification of respiratory function parameters in patients with severe Parkinson's disease. *Neurological Science, 23,* 69–70

Dewar, A., Dewar, A.D., Austin, W.T.S., & Brash, H.M. (1979). The long term use of an automatically triggered auditory feedback masking device in the treatment of stammering. *British Journal of Disorders of Communication, 14,* 219–229

Downie, A.W., Low, J.M., & Lindsay, D.D. (1981a). Speech disorder in parkinsonism: use of delayed auditory feedback in selected cases. *Journal of Neurology, Neurosurgery, and Psychiatry, 44*, 852–853

Downie, A.W., Low, J.M., & Lindsay, D.D. (1981b). Speech disorder in parkinsonism: usefulness of delayed auditory feedback in selected cases. *British Journal of Disorders of Communication, 16*, 135–139

Doyle, P.C., Raade, A.S., St. Pierre, A., & Desai, S. (1995). Fundamental frequency and acoustic variability associated with production of sustained vowels by speakers with hypokinetic dysarthria. *Journal of Medical Speech-Language Pathology, 3*, 41–50

Dromey, C. (2000). Articulatory kinematics in patients with Parkinson disease using different speech treatment approaches. *Journal of Medical Speech-Language Pathology, 8*, 155–161

Dromey, C. & Adams, S. (2000). Loudness perception and hypophonia in Parkinson disease. *Journal of Medical Speech-Language Pathology, 8*, 255–259

Duffy, J.R. (1995). *Motor Speech Disorders*. Toronto, ON: Mosby

Duffy, J.R. (2005). *Motor Speech Disorders*, 2nd ed. Toronto, ON: Mosby

Dujardin, K., Blairy, S., Defebvre, L., Duhem, S., Noël, Y., Hess, U., et al. (2004). Deficits in decoding emotional facial expressions in Parkinson's disease. *Neuropsychologia, 42*, 239–250

Estenne, M., Hubert, M., & Troyer, A.D. (1984). Respiratory-muscle involvement in Parkinson's disease. *New England Journal of Medicine, 311*, 1516–1517

Forrest, K., Nygaard, L., Pisoni, D.B., & Siemers, E. (1998). Effects of speaking rate in word recognition in Parkinson's disease and normal aging. *Journal of Medical Speech-Language Pathology, 6*, 1–12

Forrest, K., Weismer, G., & Turner, G.S. (1989). Kinematic, acoustic, and perceptual analyses of connected speech produced by parkinsonian and normal geriatric adults. *Journal of the Acoustical Society of America, 85*, 2608–2622

Fox, C.M., Morrison, C.E., Ramig, L.O, & Sapir, S. (2002). Current perspectives on the Lee Silverman Voice Treatment (LSVT) for individuals with idiopathic Parkinson disease. *American Journal of Speech-Language Pathology*, 11:111-123

Fox, C. & Ramig, L. (1997). Vocal sound pressure level and self-perception of speech and voice in men and women with idiopathic Parkinson disease. *American Journal of Speech-Language Pathology, 6*, 85–94

Gage, H. & Storey, L. (2004). Rehabilitation for Parkinson's disease: a systematic review of available evidence. *Clinical Rehabilitation, 18*, 463–482

Gallena, S., Smith, P.J., Zeffiro, T., & Ludlow, C.L. (2001). Effects of Levodopa on laryngeal muscle activity for voice onset and offset in Parkinson disease. *Journal of Speech, Language, and Hearing Research, 44*, 1284–1299

Gamboa, J., Jimenez-Jimenez, F.J., Nieto, A., Montojo, J., Orti-Pareja, M., Molina, J.A., Garcia-Albea, E., & Cobeta, I. (1997). Acoustic voice analysis in patients with Parkinson's disease treated with dopaminergic drugs. *Journal of Voice, 11*, 314–320

Gentil, M., Perrin, S., Tournier, C.L., & Pollak, P. (1999). Lip, tongue and forefinger force control in Parkinson's disease. *Clinical Linguistics and Phonetics, 13*, 45–54

Gentil, M., Tournier, C.L., Pollak, P., Benabid, A.L. (1999). Effect of bilateral subthalamic nucleus stimulation and dopatherapy on oral control in Parkinson's disease. *European Neurology, 42*, 136–140

Graber, S., Hertrich, I., Daum, I., Spieker, S., & Ackermann, H. (2002). Speech perception deficits in Parkinson's disease: underestimation of time intervals compromises identification of durational phonetic contrasts. *Brain and Language, 82*, 65–74

Greene, M.C.L & Watson, B.W. (1968). The value of speech amplification in Parkinson's disease patients. *Folia Phoniatrica, 20*, 250–257

Grewel, F. (1957). Dysarthria in post-encephalitic parkinsonism. *Acta Psychiatrica Neurologica Scandinavica, 32*, 440–449

Hammen, V.L & Yorkston, K.M. (1996). Speech and pause characteristics following speech rate reduction in hypokinetic dysarthria. *Journal of Communication Disorders, 29*, 429–445

Hammen, V.L., Yorkston, K.M., & Beukelman, D.R. (1989). Pausal and speech duration characteristics as a function of speaking rate in normal and parkinsonian dysarthric individuals. In: K.M. Yorkston & D.R. Beukelman (Eds.), *Recent Advances in Clinical Dysarthria* (pp. 213–224). Boston: College-Hill

Hand, C.R., Burns, M.O., & Ireland, E. (1979). Treatment of hypertonicity in muscles of lip retraction. *Biofeedback and Self-Regulation, 4*, 171–181

Hanson, D.G., Gerratt, B.R., & Ward, P.H. (1984). Cinegraphic observations of laryngeal function in Parkinson's disease. *Laryngoscope, 94*, 348–353

Hanson, W.R. & Metter, E.J. (1983). DAF speech rate modification in Parkinson's disease: a report of two cases. In: W.R. Berry (Ed.), *Clinical Dysarthria* (pp. 231–251). San Diego: College-Hill

Hartman, D.E. & Abbs, J.H. (1985). The response of the apparent receptive speech disorder of Parkinson's disease to speech therapy [letter to the editor]. *Journal of Neurology, Neurosurgery, and Psychiatry, 48*, 606

Helm, N.A. (1979). Management of palilalia with a pacing board. *Journal of Speech and Hearing Disorders, 44*, 350–353

Hirose, H. (1986). Pathophysiology of motor speech disorders (dysarthria). *Folia Phoniatrica, 38*, 61–88

Hirose, H., Kiritani, S., Ushijima, T., et al. (1981). Patterns of dysarthric movements in patients with parkinsonism. *Folia Phoniatrica, 33*, 204–215

Ho, A.K., Bradshaw, J.L., & Iansek, R. (2000). Volume perception in parkinsonian speech. *Movement Disorders, 15*, 1125–1131

Ho, A.K., Iansek, R., & Bradshaw, J.L. (2001). Motor instability in parkinsonian speech intensity. *Neuropsychiatry, Neuropsychology, and Behavioural Neurology, 14*, 109–116

Ho, A.K., Iansek, R., & Bradshaw, J.L. (2002). The effect of a concurrent task on Parkinsonian speech. *Journal of Clinical Experimental Neuropsychology, 24*, 36–47

Holinger, L.D., Holinger, P.C., & Holinger, P.H. (1976). Etiology of bilateral vocal cord paralysis: review of 389 cases. *Annals of Otology, Rhinology, and Laryngology, 85*, 428–436

Holmes, R.J., Oates, J.M., Phyland, D.J., & Hughes, A.J. (2000). Voice characteristics in the progression of Parkinson's disease. *International Journal of Language and Communication Disorders, 35*, 407

Hoodin, R.B. & Gilbert, H.R. (1989a). Nasal airflows in parkinsonian speakers. *Journal of Communication Disorders, 22*, 169–180

Hoodin, R.B. & Gilbert, H.R. (1989b). Parkinsonian dysarthria: an aerodynamic and perceptual description of velopharyngeal closure for speech. *Folia Phoniatrica, 41*, 249–258

Hunker, C.J. & Abbs, J.H. (1984). Physiological analyses of parkinsonian tremors in the orofacial system. In: M.R. McNeil, J.C. Rosenbek, & A.E. Aronson (Eds.), *The Dysarthrias: Physiology, Acoustics, Perception, Management* (pp. 69–100). San Diego: College-Hill Press

Hunker, C.J., Abbs, J.H., & Barlow, S.M. (1982). The relationship between parkinsonian rigidity and hypokinesia in the orofacial system: a quantitative analysis. *Neurology, 32*, 749–754

Huppler, E.G., Schmidt, H.W., & Devine, K. (1955). Causes of vocal cord paralysis. *Mayo Clinic Proceedings, 30*, 518–521

Jacobs, D.H., Shuren, J., Bowers, D., Heilman, K.M. (1995). Emotional facial imagery, perception, and expression in Parkinson's disease. *Neurology, 45*, 1696–1702

Jiang, J., Lin, E., Wang, J., & Hanson, D.G. (1999). Glottographic measures before and after Levodopa treatment in Parkinson's disease. *Laryngoscope, 109*(8), 1287–1294

Johnson, J.A. & Pring, T.R. (1990). Speech therapy and Parkinson's disease: a review and further data. *British Journal of Disorders of Communication, 25*, 183–194

Kan, Y., Kawamura, M., Hasegawa, Y., Mochizuki, S., Nakamura, K.(2002). Recognition of motion from facial, prosodic and written verbal stimuli in Parkinson's disease. *Cortex, 38*, 623–30

Keller, E., Vigneux, P., & Laframboise, M. (1991). Acoustic analysis of neurologically impaired speech. *British Journal of Disorders of Communication, 26*, 75–94

Kempler, D. & Van Lancker, D. (2002). Effect of speech task on intelligibility in dysarthria: A case study of Parkinson's disease. *Brain and Language, 80,* 449–464

Kent, R.D. & Kent, J.F. (2000). Task-based profiles of the dysarthrias. *Folia Phoniatrica et Logopaedica, 52,* 1–3

Kent, R.D., Kent, J.F., & Rosenbek, J.C. (1987). Maximum performance tests of speech production. *J Speech and Hearing Disorders, 52,* 367–387

Kent, R.D., Vorperian, H.K., Kent, J.F., & Duffy, J.R. (2003). Voice dysfunction in dysarthria: application of the multi-dimensional voice program. *Journal of Communication Disorders, 36,* 281–306

King, J.B., Ramig, L.O., Lemke, J.H., et al. (1993). Parkinson's disease: longitudinal changes in acoustic parameters of phonation. *Journal of Medical Speech-Language Pathology, 4,* 135–149

Kiran, S. & Larson, C.R. (2001). Effect of duration of pitch-shifted feedback on vocal responses in patients with Parkinson's disease. *Journal of Speech, Language, and Hearing Research, 44,* 975–987

Koller, W.C. (1984). Sensory symptoms in PD. *Neurology, 34,* 957–959

Kreul, E.J. (1972). Neuromuscular control examination (NMC) for parkinsonism: vowel prolongations and diadochokinetic and reading rates. *Journal of Speech and Hearing Research, 15,* 72–83

Lang, A.E. & Fishbein, B. (1983). The "pacing board" in selected speech disorders of Parkinson's disease. *Journal of Neurology, Neurosurgery, and Psychiatry, 46,* 789

Laszewski, Z. (1956). Role of the department of rehabilitation in preoperative evaluation of parkinsonian patients. *Journal of the American Geriatric Society, 4,* 1280–1284

Leanderson, R., Meyerson, B.A., & Persson, A. (1971). Effect of l-dopa on speech in Parkinsonism an EMG study of labial articulatory function. *Journal of Neurology, Neurosurgery and Psychiatry, 43,* 679–681

Leanderson, R., Meyerson, B.A., & Persson, A. (1972). Lip muscle function in parkinsonian dysarthria. *Acta Otolaryngologica, 74,* 350–357

Leder, S.B. (1996). Adult onset of stuttering as a presenting sign in a parkinsonian-like syndrome: a case report. *Journal of Communication Disorders, 29,* 471–478

Le Dorze, G., Dionne, L., Ryalls, J., Julien, M., & Ouellet, L. (1992). The effects of speech and language therapy for a case of dysarthria associated with Parkinson's disease. *European Journal of Disorders of Communication, 27,* 313–324

Lewis, G.N. & Byblow, W.D. (2002). Altered sensorimotor integration in Parkinson's disease. *Brain, 125,* 2089–2099

Liotti, M., Ramig, L.O., Vogel, D., New, P., Cook, C.I., Ingham, R.J., Ingham, J.C., & Fox, P.T. (2003). Neural correlates of voice treatment revealed by PET. *Neurology, 60,* 432–440

Lloyd, A.J. (1999). Comprehension of prosody in Parkinson's disease. *Cortex, 35,* 389–402

Logemann, J., Boshes, B., & Fisher, H. (1973). The steps in the degeneration of speech and voice control in Parkinson's disease. In: J. Siegfried (Ed.), *Parkinson's Diseases: Rigidity, Akinesia, Behavior* (pp. 101–112). Vienna: Hans Huber

Logemann, J.A. & Fisher, H.B. (1981). Vocal tract control in Parkinson's disease: Phonetic feature analysis of misarticulations. *Journal of Speech and Hearing Disorders, 46,* 348–352

Logemann, J.A., Fisher, H.B., Boshes, B., et al. (1978). Frequency and co-occurrence of vocal tract dysfunctions in the speech of a large sample of Parkinson patients. *Journal of Speech and Hearing Disorders, 43,* 47–57

Louis, E.D., Levy, G., Cote, L.J., Mejia, H., Fahn, S., & Marder, K. (2001a). Clinical correlates of action tremor in Parkinson disease. *Archives of Neurology, 58,* 1630–1634

Louis, E.D., Winfield, L., Fahn, S., & Ford, B. (2001b). Speech Dysfluency Exacerbated by Levodopa in Parkinson's disease. *Movement Disorders, 16*(3), 562–565

Ludlow, C.L. & Bassich, C.J. (1984). Relationships between perceptual ratings and acoustic measures of hypokinetic speech. In: M.R.

McNeil, J.C. Rosenbek, & A.E. Aronson (Eds.), *The Dysarthrias: Physiology, Acoustics, Perception, Management* (pp. 163–192). San Diego: College-Hill

Ludlow, C.L., Bassich, C.J., Connor, N.P., & Coulter, D.C. (1986). Phonatory characteristics of vocal fold tremor. *Journal of Phonetics, 14,* 509–515

Ludlow, C.L., Connor, N.P., & Bassich, C.J. (1987). Speech timing in Parkinson's and Huntington's disease. *Brain and Language, 32,* 195–214

Luschei, E.S., Ramig, L.O., Baker, K.L., & Smith, M.E. (1999). Discharge characteristics of laryngeal single motor units during phonation in young and older adults and in persons with Parkinson disease. *Journal of Neurophysiology, 81,* 2131–2139

Marquardt, T.P. (1973). *Characteristics of Speech in Parkinson's Disease: Electromyographic, Structural Movement, and Aerodynamic Measurements.* Unpublished doctoral dissertation, University of Washington, Seattle

McAuliffe, M.J., Ward, E.C., Murdoch, B.E., & Farrell, A.M. (2005). A non-speech investigation of tongue function in Parkinson's disease. *Journal of Gerontology [A] Biological Science and Medical Science, 60A,* 667–674

McCormick, C.A. & Roy, N. (2002). The ChatterVox portable voice amplifier: a means to vibration dose reduction? *Journal of Voice, 16,* 502–508

McNamara, P., Obler, L.K., Durso, R., et al. (1992). Speech monitoring skills in Alzheimer's disease, Parkinson's disease, and normal aging. *Brain and Language, 42,* 38–51

Metter, E.J. & Hanson, W.R. (1986). Clinical and acoustic variability in hypokinetic dysarthria. *Journal of Communication Disorders, 19,* 347–366

Metter, E.J. & Hanson, W.R. (1991). Dysarthria in Progressive Supranuclear Palsy. In: C.A. Moore, K.M. Yorkston, & D.R. Beukleman (Eds.), *Dysarthria and Apraxia of Speech: Perspectives on Management* (pp. 127–136). Baltimore: Paul H. Brookes

Mlcoch, A.G. (1987). Diagnosis and Treatment of Parkinsonian Dysarthria. In: W.C. Koller (Ed.). *Handbook of Parkinson's Disease* (pp. 181–207). New York: Marcel Dekker

Moon, B., Adams, S.G., Jog, M. (2006). Effects of background noise, listener context, speech task, and requests for clarification on speech intensity in Parkinson's disease. *Stem-Sprak-, en Taalpathologie, 14:84*

Moore, C.A. & Scudder, R.R. (1989). Coordination of jaw muscle activity in parkinsonian movement: description and response to traditional treatment. In: K.M. Yorkston & D.R. Beukelman (Eds.), *Recent Advances in Clinical Dysarthria* (pp. 147–163). Boston: College-Hill

Moretti, R., Torre, P., Antonello, R.M., Capus, L., Gioulis, M., Zambito Marsala, S., Cazzato, G., & Bava, A. (2003). Speech initiation hesitation following subthalamic nucleus stimulation in a patient with Parkinson's disease. *European Neurology, 49,* 251–253

Mueller, P.B. (1971). Parkinson's disease: motor-speech behavior in a selected group of patients. *Folia Phoniatrica, 23,* 333–346

Murdoch, B.E., Chenery, H.J., Bowler, S., et al. (1989). Respiratory function in Parkinson's subjects exhibiting a perceptible speech deficit: A kinematic and spirometric analysis. *Journal of Speech and Hearing Disorders, 54,* 610–626

Murofushi, T., Yamane, M., & Osanai, R. (1992). Stapedial reflex in Parkinson's disease. *Journal of Otology, Rhinology, and Laryngology, 54,* 255–258

Mutch, W.J., Strudwick, A., Roy, S.K., et al. (1986). Parkinson's disease: disability review and management. *British Medical Journal, 293,* 675–677

Nakashima, K., Maeda, M., Tabata, M., Adachi, Y., Kusumi, M., & Ohshiro, H. (1997). Prognosis of Parkinson's disease in Japan. Tottori University Parkinson's disease epidemiology (TUPDE) study group. *European Neurology, 38,* 60–63

Netsell, R., Cleeland, C.S. (1973). Modification of lip hypertonia in dysarthria using EMG feedback. *Journal of Speech and Hearing Disorders, 38,* 131–140

Netsell, R., Daniel, B., & Celesia, G.G. (1975). Acceleration and weakness in parkinsonian dysarthria. *Journal of Speech and Hearing Disorders, 40,* 170–178

Nishio, M. & Niimi, S. (2001). Speaking rate and its components in dysarthric speakers. *Clinical Linguistics and Phonetics, 15*, 309–317

Onla-Or, S. (2001). *Motor Skill Learning in Individuals with Parkinson's Disease: Consideration of Cognitive and Motor Demands.* A dissertation presented to the Faculty of the Graduate School for the degree of Doctor of Philosophy (Biokinesiology), University of Southern California

Pell, M.D. & Leonard, C.L. (2003). Processing emotional tone from speech in Parkinson's disease: a role for the basal ganglia. *Cognitive, Affective, and Behavioral Neuroscience, 3*, 275–288

Pell, M.D., Leonard, C.L. (2005). Facial expression decoding in early Parkinson's disease. *Brain Research, Cognitive Brain Research, 23*, 327–340

Perez, K.S., Ramig, L.O., & Smith, M.E., et al. (1996). The Parkinson larynx: tremor and videostroboscopic findings. *Journal of Voice, 10*, 354–361

Perry, A.R. & Das, P.K. (1981). Speech assessment of patients with Parkinson's disease. In: F.C. Rose & R. Capildeo (Eds.), *Research Progress in Parkinson's Disease* (pp. 373–383). Kent: Pitman

Philippbar, S.A., Robin, D.A., & Luschei, E.S. (1989). Limb, jaw, and vocal tremor in Parkinson's patients. In: K.M. Yorkston & D.R. Beukelman (Eds.), *Recent Advances in Clinical Dysarthria* (pp. 165–197). Boston: College-Hill

Pinto, S., Gentil, M., Fraix, V., Benabid, A.L., Pollak, P. (2003). Bilateral sub-thalamic stimulation effects on oral force control in Parkinson's disease. *Journal of Neurology, 250*, 179–187

Pinto, S., Ozsancak, C., Tripoliti, E., Thobois, S., Limousin-Dowsey, P., & Auzou, P. Treatments for dysarthria in Parkinson's disease. *Lancet Neurology, 3*, 547–556

Pinto, S., Thobois, S., Costes, N., Le Bars, D., Benabid, A., Broussolle, E., Pollak, P., & Gentil, M. (2004). Subthalamic nucleus stimulation and dysarthria in Parkinson's disease: a PET study. *Brain, 127*, 602–615

Plasse, H.M. & Liberman, A.N. (1981). Bilateral vocal cord paralysis in Parkinson's disease. *Arch Otolaryngology, 107*, 252–253

Popolo, P., Svec, J., Rogge-Miller, K., Titze, I.R. (2003). Technical considerations in the design of a wearable voice dosimeter. *Acoustical Society of America*, Cancun

Popolo, P.S., Svec, J.G., & Titze, I.R. (2005) Adaptation of a pocket PC for use as a wearable voice dosimeter. *Journal of Speech, Language, and Hearing Research, 48*, 780–791

Putnam, A.H.B. (1988). Review of research in dysarthria. In: H. Winitz (Ed.), *Human Communication and Its Disorders: A Review* (pp. 107–223). Norwood: Ablex

Rack, P.M.H. & Ross, H.F. (1986). The role of reflexes in the resting tremor of Parkinson's disease. *Brain, 109*, 115–141

Ramig, L.O. (1995). Speech therapy for patients with Parkinson's disease. In: W.C. Koller & G. Paulson (Eds.), *Therapy of Parkinson's disease*, 2nd ed. (pp. 539–550). New York: Marcel Dekker

Ramig, L.O. (1998). Treatment of speech and voice problems associated with Parkinson's disease. *Topics in Geriatric Rehabilitation, 14*, 28–43

Ramig, L.O., Bonitati, C.M., Lemke, J.H. & Horii, Y. (1994). Voice treatment for patients with Parkinson's disease: development of an approach and preliminary efficacy data. *Journal of Medical Speech Language Pathology, 2*, 191–210

Ramig, L.O., Countryman, S., O'Brien, C., Hoehn, M., & Thompson, L. (1996). Intensive speech treatment for patients with Parkinson's disease: short- and long-term comparison of two techniques. *Neurology, 47*, 1496–1504

Ramig, L.O., Countryman, S., Thompson, L.L., & Horii, Y. (1995a). Comparison of two forms of intensive speech treatment for Parkinson disease. *Journal of Speech and Hearing Research, 38*, 1232–1251

Ramig, L.O. & Dromey, C. (1996). Aerodynamic mechanisms underlying treatment-related changes in vocal intensity in patients with Parkinson disease. *Journal of Speech & Hearing Research, 39*, 798–807

Ramig, L.O., Fox, C., & Sapir, S. (2004). Parkinson's disease: Speech and voice disorders and their treatment with the Lee Silverman Voice Treatment. *Seminars in Speech and Language, 25*, 169–180

Ramig, L.O., Horii, Y., & Bonitati, C.M. (1991). The efficacy of voice therapy for patients with Parkinson's disease. *NCVS Status and Progress Report, 1*, 61–86

Ramig, L.O., Pawlas, A.A., & Countryman, S. (1995b). *The Lee Silverman Voice Treatment.* Iowa City, IA: National Center for Voice and Speech

Ramig, L.O., Sapir, S., Countryman, S., Pawlas, A.A., O'Brien, C., Hoehn, M., & Thompson, L.L. (2001a). Intensive voice treatment (LSVT®) for patients with Parkinson's disease: a 2 year follow up. *Journal of Neurology, Neurosurgery, and Psychiatry, 71*, 493–498

Ramig, L.O., Sapir, S., Fox, C., & Countryman, S. (2001b). Changes in vocal loudness following intensive voice treatment (LSVT) in individuals with Parkinson's disease: a comparison with untreated patients and normal age-matched controls. *Movement Disorders, 16*, 79–83

Ramig, L.O., Scherer, R.C., Titze, I.R., et al. (1988). Acoustic analysis of voices of patients with neurologic disease: rationale and preliminary data. *Annals of Otology, Rhinology, and Laryngology, 97*, 164–172

Ramig, L.O. & Verdolini, K. (1998). Treatment efficacy: voice disorders. *Journal of Speech, Language, and Hearing Research, 41*, S101–S116

Robertson, S.J. & Thomson, F. (1984). Speech therapy in Parkinson's disease: a study of the efficacy and long term effects of intensive treatment. *British Journal of Disorders of Communication, 19*, 213–224

Rosen, K.M., Kent, R.D., & Duffy, J.R. (2005). Task-based profile of vocal intensity decline in Parkinson's disease. *Folia Phoniatrica et Logopaedica, 57*, 28–37

Rousseaux, M., Krystkowiak, P., Kozlowski, O., Ozsancak, C., Blond, S., & Destee, A. (2004). Effects of subthalamic nucleus stimulation on Parkinsonian dysarthria and speech intelligibility. *Journal of Neurology, 251*, 327–334

Rubow, R. & Swift, E. (1985). A microcomputer-based wearable biofeedback device to improve transfer of treatment in parkinsonian dysarthria. *Journal of Speech and Hearing Disorders, 50*, 178–185

Ryu, W., Komiyama, S., Kanee, S., & Watanabe, H. (1983). A newly devised speech accumulator. *ORL Journal of Otorhinolaryngology and Its Related Specialties, 45*, 108–111

Saint-Cyr, J.A., Taylor, A.E., & Lang, A.E. (1988). Procedural learning and neostriatal dysfunction in man. *Brain, 111*, 941–959

Sanabria, J., Ruiz, P.G., Gutierrez, R., Marquez, F., Escobar, P., Gentil, M., & Cenjor, C. (2001). The effect of Levadopa on vocal function in Parkinson's disease. *Clinical Neuropharmacology, 24*(2), 99–102

Sapir, S., Ramig, L.O., Hoyt, P., Countryman, S., O'Brien, C., & Hoehn, M. (2002). Speech loudness and quality 12 months after intensive voice treatment (LSVT®) for Parkinson's disease: a comparison with an alternative speech treatment. *Folia Phoniatrica et Logopaedica, 54*, 296–303

Sarno, M.T. (1968). Speech impairment in Parkinson's disease. *Archives of Physical Medicine and Rehabilitation, 49*, 269–275

Sathyaprabha, T.N., Kapavarapu, P.K., Pall, P.K., Thennarasu, K., & Raju, T.R. (2005). Pulmonary functions in Parkinson's disease. *Indian Journal of Chest Diseases and Allied Sciences, 47*, 251–257

Schiffman, P.L. (1985). A "saw-tooth" pattern in Parkinson's disease. *Chest, 87*, 124–126

Schley, W.S., Fenton, E., & Niimi, S. (1982). Vocal symptoms in Parkinson disease treated with levodopa: a case report. *Annals of Otology, 91*, 119–121

Schneider, J.S., Diamond, S.G., & Markham, C.H. (1986). Deficits in orofacial sensorimotor function in Parkinson's disease. *Annals of Neurology, 19*, 275–282

Schneider, J.S. & Lidsky, T.I. (1987). *Basal Ganglia and Behavior: Sensory Aspects of Motor Functioning.* Toronto: Hans Huber

Schulz, G.M. & Grant, M.K. (2000). Effects of speech therapy and pharmacologic and surgical treatments on voice and speech in Parkinson's disease: a review of the literature. *Journal of Communication Disorders, 33*, 59–88

Scott, S. & Caird, F.I. (1981). Speech therapy for patients with Parkinson's disease. *British Medical Journal, 283*, 1088

Scott, S. & Caird, F.I. (1983). Speech therapy for Parkinson's disease. *Journal of Neurology, Neurosurgery, and Psychiatry, 46*, 140–144

Scott, S. & Caird, F.I. (1984). The response of the apparent receptive speech disorder of Parkinson's disease to speech therapy. *Journal of Neurology, Neurosurgery, and Psychiatry, 47*, 302–304

Scott, S. & Caird, F.I. (1985). The response of the apparent receptive speech disorder of Parkinson's disease to speech therapy [response to letter to the editor]. *Journal of Neurology, Neurosurgery, and Psychiatry, 48,* 606

Scott, S., Caird, F.I., & Williams, B. (1984). Evidence for an apparent sensory speech disorder in Parkinson's disease. *Journal of Neurology, Neurosurgery, and Psychiatry, 47,* 840–843

Scott, S., Caird, F.I., & Williams, B.O. (1985). *Communication in Parkinson's Disease* (pp. 1–113). Rockville: Aspen

Selby, G. (1968). Parkinson's disease. In: P.J. Vinken & G.W. Bruyn (Eds.), *Handbook of Clinical Neurology,* vol. 6. Amsterdam: North Holland

Shahed, J. & Jankovic, J. (2001). Re-emergence of childhood stuttering in Parkinson's disease: a hypothesis. *Movement Disorders, 16,* 114–118

Sharkawi, A., Ramig, L., Logemann, J.A., Pauloski, B.R., Rademaker, A.W., Smith, C.H., Pawlus, A., Baum, S., & Werner, C. (2002). Swallowing and voice effects of Lee Silverman Voice Treatment (LSVT): a pilot study. *Journal of Neurology, Neurosurgery & Psychiatry, 72*(1), 31–36

Smith, M.E., Ramig, L.O., Dromey, C., Perez, K.S., & Samandari, R. (1995). Intensive voice treatment in Parkinson disease: laryngostroboscopic findings. *Journal of Voice, 9,* 453–459

Snider, S.R., Fahn, S., Isgreen, W.P., et al. (1976). Primary sensory symptoms in parkinsonism. *Neurology, 26,* 423–429

Solomon, N.P. & Hixon, T.J. (1993). Speech breathing in Parkinson's disease. *Journal of Speech and Hearing Research, 36,* 294–310

Solomon, N.P., Lorell, D.M., Robin, D.A., Rodnitzky, R.L., & Luschei, E.S. (1995). Tongue strength and endurance in mild to moderate Parkinson's disease. *Journal of Medical Speech-Language Pathology, 3,* 15–26

Solomon, N.P., Robin, D.A., & Luschei, E.S. (2000). Strength, endurance, and stability of the tongue and hand in Parkinson disease. *Journal of Speech, Language, and Hearing Research, 43,* 256–267

Spielman, J.L., Borod, J.C., & Ramig, L.O. (2003). The effects of intensive voice treatment on facial expression in Parkinson disease. *Cognitive and Behavioural Neurology, 16,* 177–188

Spitzer, S.M., Liss, J.M., Caviness, J.N., & Adler, C. (2000). An exploration of familiarization effects in the perception of hypokinetic and ataxic dysarthric speech. *Journal of Medical Speech-Language Pathology, 8,* 285–293

Sprengelmeyer, R., Young, A.W., Mahn, K., Schroeder, U., Woitalla, D., Büttner, T., et al.(2003). Facial expression recognition in people with medicated and unmedicated Parkinson's disease. *Neuropsychologia, 41,* 1047–1057

Stacy, M. & Jankovic, J. (1992). Differential diagnosis of Parkinson's disease and the parkinsonism plus syndromes. *Neurologic Clinics, 10*(2), 341-359

Stewart, C., Winfield, L., Hunt, A., Bressman, S.B., Fahn, S., Blitzer, A., & Brin, M.F. (1995). Speech dysfunction in early Parkinson's disease. *Movement Disorders, 10,* 562–565

Streifler, M. & Hofman, S. (1984). Disorders of verbal expression in parkinsonism. In: R.G. Hassler, & J.F. Christ (Eds.), *Advances in Neurology* (pp. 385–393). New York: Raven Press

Sullivan, M.D., Brune, P.J., & Beukelman, D.R. (1996). Maintenance of speech changes following group treatment for hypokinetic dysarthria of Parkinson's disease. In: D.A. Robin, K.M. Yorkston, & D.R. Beukelman (Eds.), *Disorders of Motor Speech: Assessment, Treatment, and Clinical Characterization* (pp. 287–307). Baltimore: Paul H. Brookes

Szabo, A., Hammarberg, B., Hakansson, A., & Sodersten, M.A. (2001). Voice accumulator device: evaluation based on studio and field recordings. *Logopaedica Phoniatrica Vocologica, 26,* 102–117

Tamburin, S., Fiaschi, A., Idone, D., Lochner, P., Manganotti, P., & Zanette, G. (2003). Abnormal sensorimotor integration is related to disease severity in Parkinson's disease: a TMS study. *Movement Disorders, 18,* 1316–1324

Tatton, W.G., Eastman, M.J., Bedingham, W., et al. (1984). Defective utilization of sensory input as the basis for bradykinesia, rigidity and decreased movement repertoire in Parkinson's disease: a hypothesis. *Canadian Journal of Neurological Sciences, 11,* 136–143

Theodoros, D.G., Murdoch, B.E., & Thompson, E.C. (1995). Hypernasality in Parkinson disease: a perceptual and physiological analysis. *Journal of Medical Speech-Language Pathology, 3,* 73–84

Thompson, A.K. (1978). A clinical rating scale of speech dysfunction in Parkinson's disease. *South African Journal of Communication Disorders, 25,* 39–52

Tjaden, K. (2000a). A preliminary study of factors influencing perception of articulatory rate in Parkinson disease. *Journal of Speech, Language, and Hearing Research, 43,* 997–1010

Tjaden, K. (2000b). An acoustic study of coarticulation in dysarthric speakers with Parkinson disease. *Journal of Speech, Language, and Hearing Research, 43,* 1466–1480

Tjaden, K. (2003). Anticipatory coarticulation in multiple sclerosis and Parkinson's disease. *Journal of Speech, Language, and Hearing Research, 46,* 990–1008

Torp, J.N. & Hammen, V.L. (2000). Perception of Parkinsonian speech rate. *Journal of Medical Speech-Language Pathology, 8,* 323–329

Turner, R.S. & Anderson, M.E. (2005). Context-dependent modulation of movement-related discharge in the primate globus pallidus. *Journal of Neuroscience, 25,* 2965–2976

Uziel, A., Bohe, M., Cadilhac, J., et al. (1975). Les troubles de la voix et de la parole dans les syndromes parkinsoniens. *Folia Phoniatrica, 27,* 166–176

Vincken, W.G., Gauthier, S.G., Dollfuss, R.E., et al. (1984). Involvement of upper-airway muscles in extrapyramidal disorders, a cause of airflow limitation. *New England Journal of Medicine, 311*), 438–442

Volkmann, J., Hefter, H., Lange, H.W., et al. (1992). Impairment of temporal organization of speech in basal ganglia diseases. *Brain and Language, 43,* 386–399

Wang, E., Kompoliti, K., Jiang, J.J., & Goetz, C.G. (2000). An instrumental analysis of laryngeal responses to apomorphine stimulation in Parkinson disease. *Journal of Medical Speech-Language Pathology, 8,* 175–186

Ward, E.C., Theodoros, D.G., & Murdoch, B.E. (2000). Changes in maximum capacity tongue function following the Lee Silverman Voice Treatment program. *Journal of Medical Speech-Language Pathology, 8,* 331–335

Ward, E.C., Theodoros, D.G., Murdoch, B.E., & Cahill, L.M. (1999). The use of a miniature lip transducer system in the assessment of patients with Parkinson's disease. *Journal of Medical Speech-Language Pathology, 7,* 175–179

Weismer, G. (1984a). Acoustic descriptions of dysarthric speech: Perceptual correlates and physiological inferences. *Seminars in Speech and Language, 5,* 293–314

Weismer, G. (1984b). Articulatory characteristics of parkinsonian dysarthria: segmental and phrase-level timing, spirantization, and glottal-supraglottal coordination. In: M.R. McNeil, J.C. Rosenbek, & A.E. Aronson (Eds.), *The Dysarthrias: Physiology, Acoustics, Perception, Management* (pp. 101–130). San Diego: College-Hill

Weismer, G. (1990). Orofacial impairment in Parkinson's disease [letter to the editor]. *Neurology, 40,* 191–192

Weismer, G., Jeng, J.Y., Laures, J.S., Kent, R.D., & Kent, J.F. (2001). Acoustic and intelligibility characteristics of sentence production in neurogenic speech disorders. *Folia Phoniatrica et Logopaedica, 53,* 1–18

Weismer, G., Kimelman, M.D.Z., & Gorman, S. (1985). More on the speech production deficit associated with Parkinson's disease. *Journal of the Acoustical Society of America, 78*(suppl 1), S55

Weismer, G., Yunusova, Y., & Westbury, J.R. (2003). Interarticulator coordination in dysarthria: an x-ray microbeam study. *Journal of Speech, Language, and Hearing Research, 46,* 1247–1261

Whitehill, T.L., Ma, J.K.Y., & Lee, A.S.Y. (2003). Perceptual characteristics of Cantonese hypokinetic dysarthria. *Clinical Linguistics and Phonetics, 17,* 265–271

Winckel, J. & Adams, S.G. (1992). Drug-cycle related voice changes in Parkinsonian patients. *Journal of the American Speech and Hearing Association, 34,* 158

Winholtz, W.S. & Ramig, L.O. (1992). Vocal tremor analysis with the vocal demodulator. *Journal of Speech and Hearing Research, 2,* 119–137

Wood, L.M., Hughes, J., Hayes, K.C., et al. (1992). Reliability of labial closure force measurements in normal subjects and patients with CNS disorders. *Journal of Speech and Hearing Research, 35,* 252–258

Yorkston, K.M. (1996). Treatment efficacy: dysarthria. *Journal of Speech and Hearing Research, 39,* S46–S57

Yorkston, K.M., Beukelman, D.R., & Bell, K.R. (1988). *Clinical Management of Dysarthric Speakers.* Boston: College-Hill

Yorkston, K.M., Hammen, V.L., Beukelman, D.R., et al. (1990). The effect of rate control on the intelligibility and naturalness of dysarthric speech. *Journal of Speech and Hearing Disorders, 55,* 550–560

Yorkston, K.M., Spencer, K.A., & Duffy, J.R. (2003). ANCDS Bulletin Board: behavioral management of respiratory/phonatory dysfunction from dysarthria: a systematic review of the evidence. *Journal of Medical Speech-Language Pathology, 11,* xiii–xxxviii

Yuceturk, A.V., Yilmaz, H., Egrilmez, M., & Karaca, S. (2002). Voice analysis and videolaryngostroboscopy in patients with Parkinson's disease. *European Archives of Otorhinolaryngology, 259,* 290–293

Yumoto, E. (1983). The quantitative evaluation of hoarseness: a new harmonics to noise ratio method. *Archives of Otolaryngology, 109,* 48–52

Zia, S., Cody, F., & O'Boyle, D. (2000). Joint position sense is impaired by Parkinson's disease. *Annals of Neurology, 47,* 218–228

Zwirner, P., Murry, T., & Woodson, G.E. (1991). Phonatory function of neurologically impaired patients. *Journal of Communication Disorders, 24,* 287–300

Chapter 12

Spastic Dysarthria

Bruce E. Murdoch, Elizabeth C. Ward, and Deborah G. Theodoros

The term *spastic dysarthria* was first used by Darley, Aronson, and Brown (1969a,b) to describe the speech disturbance seen in association with damage to the upper motor neurons that convey nerve impulses from the motor areas of the cerebral cortex to the lower motor neurons originating from the bulbar cranial nerve nuclei. The lesions associated with spastic dysarthria can involve either the cortical motor areas from which the descending motor pathways originate (primarily the precentral gyrus and premotor cortex) or the descending tracts themselves as they pass through the internal capsule, cerebral peduncles or the brainstem. The speech characteristics of spastic dysarthria are presumed to reflect the effects of hypertonicity (spasticity) and weakness of the bulbar musculature in a way that slows movement and reduces its range and force (Murdoch, Thompson, & Theodoros, 1997). The reference to "spastic" in the term *spastic dysarthria* is therefore a reflection of the clinical signs of upper motor neuron damage, which include spastic paralysis or paresis of the involved muscles, hyperreflexia (e.g., hyperactive jaw-jerk), little or no muscle atrophy (except for the possibility of some atrophy associated with disuse), and the presence of pathological reflexes (e.g., sucking reflex).

◆ Pathophysiology

Neurological Disorders Associated with Upper Motor Neuron Lesions

Two major syndromes can be attributed to upper motor neuron damage: pseudobulbar palsy (supranuclear bulbar palsy) and spastic hemiplegia. Both are characterized by spasticity and impairment or loss of voluntary movements. Pseudobulbar palsy takes its name from its clinical resemblance to bulbar palsy (pseudo = false) and is associated with a variety of neurological disorders that bilaterally disrupt the upper motor neuron connections to the bulbar cranial nerves. In this condition, the bulbar muscles, including the muscles of articulation, the velopharynx, and the larynx are hypertonic and exhibit hyperreflexia. In addition, there is a reduction in the range and force of movement of the bulbar muscles as well as slowness of individual and repetitive movements. The rhythm of repetitive movements, however, is regular and the direction of movement normal. Symptoms of pseudobulbar palsy include bilateral facial paralysis, dysarthria, dysphonia, bilateral hemiparesis, incontinence, and bradykinesia. Drooling from the corners of the mouth is common and many of these patients exhibit excessive emotional responses (e.g., uncontrolled outbursts of laughing or crying) to otherwise normal emotional and environmental stimuli. A hyperactive jaw reflex and positive sucking reflex are also evident. Swallowing problems are also a common feature, and there is a definite danger of choking in the more severe cases.

The etiology of pseudobulbar palsy varies, but may include multiple strokes, brain damage sustained as the result of head injuries acquired in accidents, extensive brain tumors, multiple sclerosis, cerebral palsy of infancy, or progressive degeneration of the brain. In childhood, the most common cause of pseudobulbar palsy is hypoxic ischemic encephalopathy. In most cases this is associated with intrapartum asphyxia, although severe anoxic brain damage at any stage can cause the same disorder. Brainstem ischemia with infarction resulting from embolization in association with congenital heart disease can also cause pseudobulbar palsy in children. Pseudobulbar palsy and associated spastic dysarthria may also be seen in children who have suffered head injuries with elevated intracranial pressure and a midbrain or upper brainstem shearing injury. Although a common cause of pseudobulbar palsy in adolescents and young adults, multiple sclerosis is not a common cause of spastic dysarthria in prepubertal children. Degenerative disorders such as metachromatic leukodystrophy can also cause childhood pseudobulbar palsy. Cerebral palsy encompasses a whole range of developmental neuromuscular pathologies, occurring in three major forms: spastic, athetoid, and atactic. Consequently, speech disturbances associated with cerebral palsy are variable, reflecting differing involvement of cortical, subcortical, cerebellar, and nuclear structures. This chapter focuses on pseudobulbar palsy associated with acquired brain lesions rather than on congenital conditions such as cerebral palsy.

Although lesions that cause spastic dysarthria can be located in several different regions of the brain, including the cerebral cortex, the internal capsule, cerebral peduncles, or brainstem, for such lesions to produce a persistent spastic dysarthria they need to disrupt the upper motor neuron connections bilaterally. To understand the need for bilateral lesions, an understanding of the neuroanatomy of the upper motor neuron pathways is required. The neuroanatomy of the upper motor neuron system is described in the next section.

Unilateral upper motor neuron lesions produce spastic hemiplegia, a condition in which the muscles of the lower face and extremities on the opposite side of the body are primarily affected. The bulbar muscles are not greatly affected (for reasons explained in the next section), with weakness being confined to the contralateral lips, lower half of the face, and tongue. The forehead, palate, pharynx, and larynx are largely unaffected. Consequently, unlike pseudobulbar palsy, spastic hemiplegia is not associated with problems in mastication, swallowing, velopharyngeal function, or laryngeal activity. The tongue appears normal in the mouth but deviates to the weaker side on protrusion. Only a transitory dysarthria composed of a mild articulatory imprecision rather than a persistent spastic dysarthria is present.

◆ Neuroanatomy of the Upper Motor Neuron System

Two major components compose the upper motor neuron system: direct and indirect. The direct component, also known as the pyramidal system, is composed of neurons that project their axons from their cell bodies located in the cortical motor areas directly to the level of the lower motor neurons without synapsing along the way. In contrast, the indirect component (previously referred to as the extrapyramidal system) involves multisynaptic pathways that originate from the motor cortex but then pass to the level of the lower motor neurons via multisynaptic connections that involve structures such as the basal ganglia, various brainstem nuclei, the reticular formation, cerebellum, and thalamus. For instance, many of the extrapyramidal fibers descend from the motor cortex in the internal capsule and cerebral peduncles to the pons and are then relayed to the cerebellum from which projections then pass to either the brainstem or back of the cerebral cortex via the thalamus. Many other extrapyramidal fibers descend from the motor cortex via the internal capsule to the basal ganglia where they are relayed by a variety of pathways to the excitatory and inhibitory centers of the brainstem. Overall, the extrapyramidal system is said to compose all of those tracts, besides the pyramidal system, that transmit motor signals from the cortical motor areas to the lower motor neurons. The final pathways for transmission of extrapyramidal signals to the lower motor neurons include the vestibulospinal tracts, the tectospinal tracts, the rubrospinal tracts, and the reticulospinal tracts. The extrapyramidal system is thought to be primarily responsible for postural arrangements and the orientation of movement in space, whereas the pyramidal system is chiefly responsible for controlling the far more discrete and skilled voluntary aspects of a movement.

Anatomically the pyramidal and extrapyramidal systems lie in close proximity to one another. Consequently, acquired brain lesions that affect one system also usually involve the other, and disorders restricted to only one component of the upper motor neuron system are rarely seen in clinical neurology. Pseudobulbar palsy is thought to result from combined damage to the pyramidal and extrapyramidal systems, the damage to the extrapyramidal system presumably leading to the hypertonus and hyperreflexia, and the pyramidal lesions to the loss of skilled movements.

Based on their projections to the midbrain, bulbar region of the brainstem, or spinal cord, three major fiber groups are recognized as composing the pyramidal system: the corticomesencephalic tracts, the corticobulbar tracts, and the corticospinal tracts (pyramidal tracts proper). In that they terminate by synapsing with lower motor neurons in the nuclei of cranial nerves V, VII, IX, X, XI, and XII, the corticobulbar tracts are the most important component of the pyramidal system with regard to the occurrence of spastic dysarthria. The clinical outcome of lesions that disrupt the corticobulbar tracts, however, depends very much on whether the lesion is unilateral or bilateral. This is particularly the case with respect to the effect on speech production, with permanent spastic dysarthria resulting only from bilateral corticobulbar lesions. The reason for this lies in the nature of the upper motor neuron innervation of the bulbar cranial nerve nuclei. Although there is a predominance of corticobulbar fibers that cross to innervate cranial nerve motor nuclei on the contralateral side, there is also considerable ipsilateral (uncrossed) innervation. To state this another way, most of the motor nuclei of the cranial nerves in the brainstem receive bilateral upper motor neuron connections. Based on the clinical signs observed in cases of unilateral upper motor neuron lesions, it would appear that the ipsilateral upper motor neuron connection is adequate to maintain near-normal function in most muscles controlled by the bulbar cranial nerves, with the exception of the tongue and muscles in the lower half of the face. Consequently, unilateral corticobulbar lesions are not associated with spasticity or weakness in the forehead, muscles of mastication, soft palate (i.e., no hypernasality), pharynx (i.e., no swallowing problems), or larynx (i.e., no dysphonia). There is, however, demonstrable weakness in the lower face, lips and tongue on the opposite side as well as weakness in the extremities of the opposite side. Although unilateral upper motor neuron lesions, therefore, may be associated with a mild transient dysarthria due to weakness of the contralateral orbicularis oris and tongue, the weakness is too mild to impair speech permanently.

◆ Clinical Features of Spastic Dysarthria

Four major symptoms of muscular dysfunction subsequent to disruption of the upper motor neuron supply to the speech musculature have been identified: spasticity, weakness, limited range of movement, and slowness of movement. It is these physiological features that are characteristically identified as the underlying basis of the majority of the deviant speech behaviors observed in persons with spastic dysarthria.

Perceptual and Acoustic Features

All aspects of speech production including respiration, phonation, resonation, and articulation are affected in pseudobulbar palsy but to varying degrees. Overall spastic dysarthria is characterized by slow, dragging, labored speech that is produced with much effort.

On the basis of a perceptual analysis, the deviant speech characteristics of spastic dysarthria have been reported to cluster primarily in the areas of articulatory-resonatory incompetence and prosodic insufficiency (Darley et al, 1969a,b). In particular, Darley and coworkers identified the following features to be the most prominent perceptible deviant speech dimensions exhibited by persons with pseudobulbar palsy: imprecise consonants, monopitch, reduced stress, harsh voice quality, monoloudness, low pitch, slow rate, hypernasality, strain-strangled voice quality, short phrases, distorted vowels, pitch breaks, continuous breathy voice, and excess and equal stress. Chenery, Murdoch, and Ingram (1992) identified a similar set of deviant perceptual features in their group of subjects with pseudobulbar palsy, whereas Thompson and Murdoch (1995a) reported a similar speech profile in a group of nonpseudobulbar palsy subjects with mild to moderate spastic dysarthria subsequent to cerebrovascular accident.

Oromotor examinations of persons with spastic dysarthria also reveal a characteristic pattern of deficits. Specifically, oromotor examination usually reveals the presence of weakness in the muscles of the lip and tongue with movement of the tongue in and out of the mouth usually performed slowly. The extent of tongue movement is often very limited, such that the patient may be unable to protrude his/her tongue beyond the lower teeth. Lateral movements of the tongue are also restricted, although the tongue is of normal size. Voluntary lip movements are also usually slow and restricted in range. These findings are consistent with the consonant imprecision and slow articulation rate noted in perceptual studies of spastic dysarthria noted above. Using the Frenchay Dysarthria Assessment (Enderby, 1983), Enderby (1986) identified the major aspects of spastic dysarthria (in decreasing order of frequency of occurrence): poor movement of the tongue in speech, slow rate of speech, poor phonation and intonation, poor intelligibility in conversation, reduced alternating movements of the tongue, poor lip movements in speech, reduced maintenance of palatal elevation, poor intelligibility of description, hypernasality, and lack of control of volume.

In support of the findings of Darley et al (1969a,b), other groups of researchers have also identified a slow rate of speech in spastic dysarthric speakers based on their performance when reading a standard passage (Linebaugh & Wolfe, 1984; Ziegler & Von Cramon, 1986). As a measure of articulation rate, Linebaugh and Wolfe (1984) used the mean syllable duration, which was obtained by dividing the audible speech emission time by the number of syllables produced during a standard reading passage. Using this method they found that spastic dysarthric speakers had significantly longer mean syllable durations than normal speakers and that the mean syllable duration significantly correlated with both intelligibility and naturalness for spastic dysarthric speakers. In an attempt to make Darley and coworkers' (1969a,b) concepts of slow rate, imprecise consonants, and distorted vowels more precise and quantifiable, Ziegler and Von Cramon (1986), using a computerized signal processing technique, reported spastic dysarthric

speakers to have increased word and syllable durations (indicative of a slow rate), a reduction of sound pressure level contrast in consonant articulation (indicative of imprecise consonants), and centralization of vowel formants (indicative of distorted vowels). In addition to a slower rate of speech, spastic dysarthric speakers have also been reported to have significantly slower syllable repetition rates than normal subjects (Dworkin & Aronson, 1986; Portnoy & Aronson, 1982).

Physiological and Acoustic Features

Although perceptual analysis remains the foundation of day-to-day dysarthria assessment, the inherent inadequacies of this approach casts serious doubts over the suitability of perceptual analysis as the primary tool in the differential diagnosis and treatment of dysarthria. Orlikoff (1992) proposed that the identification of abnormal perceptual features through perceptual analysis merely defines the presence of the disorder and documents the overall speech disability. It does not, however, define the nature of the underlying pathophysiological dysfunction. Murdoch et al (1997) proposed that dysarthria treatment should be based on a thorough pathophysiological assessment to determine the status of muscular impairment in each of the speech production subsystems. Physiological assessment should be used not only to explain and quantify speech impairments but also to help parse the subsystems of the speech mechanism that are disordered. Understanding the underlying pathophysiological deficits contributing to the speech disorder, through a combined perceptual, acoustic, and physiological approach, can lead to more efficient and effective treatment strategies by enabling clinicians first to better define the loci of the speech deficits (i.e., articulatory, velopharyngeal, laryngeal, or respiratory), and second to identify those features of the speech disorder whose improvement would lead to the greatest gains with treatment. Roy, Leeper, Blomgren, and Cameron (2001) used a combined perceptual, acoustic, and physiological approach to plot the recovery of an individual with severe spastic dysarthria, and confirmed the benefits of this approach to diagnosis and treatment and for tracking the effects of interventions. The following sections provide a summary of the major findings from the relatively few physiological and acoustic investigations of subjects with spastic dysarthria reported to date.

Articulatory Function

Instrumental studies have confirmed a reduced range of articulatory movement and a slowing down in the rate of speech in patients with pseudobulbar palsy. Hirose (1986) used a range of different instrumental techniques, including cineradiography and x-ray microbeam systems, fiberoptic and photoglottographic recording, ultrasonic techniques, position-sensitive detector, and electromyographic assessment to investigate a variety of dysarthria patients. A reduced range of articulatory movements and a slow rate of speech were observed in subjects with pseudobulbar palsy. However, the consistency of the dynamic pattern of articulatory movements as observed in syllable repetition tasks tended to be preserved. This latter finding is consistent with the perceptual findings of Darley et al (1969a,b) that spastic dysarthric patients have regular rhythm of syllable repetition.

In support of the findings of Darley et al (1969a,b), researchers have also identified a slow rate of speech in spastic dysarthric speakers based on their performance when reading a standard passage (Linebaugh & Wolfe, 1984). As a measure of articulation rate, Linebaugh and Wolfe used the mean syllable duration, which was obtained by dividing the audible speech emission time by the number of syllables produced during a standard reading passage. Using this method they found that spastic dysarthric speakers had significantly longer mean syllable duration than normal speakers and that the mean syllable duration significantly correlated with both intelligibility and naturalness for spastic dysarthric speakers.

Ziegler and Von Cramon (1986) attempted to quantify speech rate and articulatory mobility of the speech of 10 patients with spastic dysarthria using acoustic evaluation. The results of their investigation revealed increased word and consonant-vowel (CV) syllable durations in the speech of all dysarthric patients, again quantifying the perception of a reduced speech rate in subjects with spastic dysarthria. Ziegler and Von Cramon attributed the presence of increased word and syllable durations to reduced movement velocity of the tongue, lips, jaw, and velum. Reduced syllable repetition rates in subjects with spastic dysarthria have also been reported by Dworkin and Aronson (1986).

In addition to an altered rate of speech production, a marked reduction in sound pressure level contrast in consonant articulation and centralization of vowel formants have been noted in the speech of subjects with spastic dysarthria (Ziegler & Von Cramon, 1986). These findings represent acoustic evidence to support the perception of imprecise consonants and imprecise vowels in the speech of these subjects. Acoustic investigations of a short segment of speech from a subject with spastic dysarthria have also revealed several other acoustic correlates of the perceptual features of imprecise articulation, including relative weak frication intensity noise and a shift in aperiodic energy during the production of the sounds "s" and "sh" (Weismer, 1984). The characteristic perceptual feature of distorted vowels was also found to have several acoustic correlates, including unusually short or long vowel durations, inappropriate target formant frequencies, or aberrant formant transitions (Weismer, 1984).

Electropalatography has also been used to examine the articulatory movements of dysarthric subjects. Hardcastle, Morgan-Barry, and Clark (1985) examined the lingual movements of three subjects, one dyspraxic and two dysarthric, one of whom had moderate spastic dysarthria. The results of this investigation revealed that the dysarthric subjects produced distortions in target configurations for consonant sounds, manifest mainly by a reduction in spatial goals (e.g., incomplete closures for stops). The subject with spastic dysarthria also demonstrated overshoot of target goals. On the basis of these findings it was concluded that the dysarthric subjects demonstrated inadequate control over muscular tension requirements for consonant articulation.

From these investigations it can be determined that the presence of imprecise consonants in the speech of subjects with spastic dysarthria appears to be the result of physiological impairments in the function of the articulators. Indeed, investigations of articulatory function have revealed specific strength and motor control deficits in subjects with spastic dysarthria. Dworkin and Aronson (1986) used a semiconductor strain-gauge force transducer to assess tongue strength in a group of 18 dysarthric subjects, including three with spastic dysarthria. They found that the dysarthric group had weaker tongue strength, as well as reduced and unsustained levels of maximum tongue strength effort, compared with normal controls during sustained effort tasks.

An investigation of the lingual function of a group of 16 subjects with spastic dysarthria similarly revealed deficits in maximum tongue pressure following upper motor neuron damage (Thompson, Murdoch, & Stokes, 1995a). In addition, these assessments revealed an impaired rate of repetitive tongue movement in the dysarthric group as well as evidence of fatigue during sustained effort tasks, in comparison with the performance of a group of age-matched control subjects (Thompson et al, 1995a). Similarly, impairments in maximum force, repetition rate and endurance capabilities were also observed in the labial function of subjects with upper motor neuron damage (Thompson, Murdoch, & Stokes, 1995b).

In addition to reductions in the maximum force/pressures generated by the articulators of subjects with spastic dysarthria, several investigations have also identified deficits in force control (Abbs, Hunker, & Barlow, 1983) and a reduction in the rate of force change (Barlow & Abbs, 1986) of the articulators of these subjects. Abbs et al (1983) detailed the results of articulatory function in a subject with congenital spasticity. Assessment revealed force control deficits in the lips, tongue, and jaw of this subject, with the lips and tongue having the most instability at maximum force levels, whereas jaw instability was greatest at very low force levels. The reduced capacity to recruit muscle forces at normal rates is also recognized as a fundamental pathophysiological feature of orofacial control in patients with the upper motor neuron syndrome (Barlow & Abbs, 1986). Barlow and Abbs examined fine force and position control in six normal males and in five adults with congenital cerebral palsy of a predominantly spastic form, and the results of their investigation revealed reductions in the average rate of force change in the lips, tongue, and jaw of these dysarthric subjects.

One theory proposed to explain the presence of articulatory deficits in subjects with spastic dysarthria suggested that the impaired motor performance of the articulators was the outcome of hypertonus in the articulatory musculature. There is now evidence, however, to suggest that this theory may be invalid and that hypertonus may not be causally related to abnormal motor performance (Barlow & Abbs, 1984). Barlow and Abbs analyzed articulatory force control in six male subjects with congenital spasticity. Their investigation was designed to assess the theory that if hypertonus was the basis for articulatory impairment observed in these subjects, then the impairments of the lips, tongue, and jaw should be relative to the number of muscle spindles known to be present in these muscles. The results of their investigation revealed that the motor performance deficits of the subjects with spasticity were not disproportionately severe in motor systems with dense spindle innervation. In fact, it was noted that impairments of the tongue, which has only relatively few muscle spindles, were greater than the lip or jaw impairments. On the basis of these findings, Barlow and Abbs contend that in the cranial motor system, aberrant actions of the stretch reflex mechanisms do not underlie impairments of voluntary motor control. Determination of the exact nature of the physiological mechanisms underlying the impairments identified in the articulators of subjects with spastic dysarthria is an area in need of further investigation.

Velopharyngeal Function

Velopharyngeal function is also usually compromised in spastic dysarthria. Although symmetrical, elevation of the soft palate during phonation appears to be slow and may be incomplete. Consequently, hypernasality is a usual finding in pseudobulbar palsy. As pointed out by Darley, Aronson, and Brown (1975), however, the degree of hypernasality associated with upper motor neuron lesions tends to be less than in conditions such as bulbar palsy that involved damage to the lower motor neurons. The movement pattern of the velopharyngeal musculature in the spastic dysarthric group has been described as symmetrical, with the rate of elevation of the soft palate during phonation slow and sometimes incomplete. The palate usually responds reflexively when stimulated with a tongue depressor.

Thompson and Murdoch (1995b) investigated the presence of nasality disturbances in a group of 18 dysarthric subjects with upper motor neuron damage following a cerebrovascular accident (CVA). They used the accelerometric assessment technique to indirectly evaluate the functioning of the velopharyngeal component of the speech mechanism in these subjects. The results of their investigation revealed that the CVA subjects, as a group, produced a significantly higher degree of nasality on the production of nonnasal speech tasks than the control subjects. No significant difference, however, was observed between the two groups on the production of nasal utterances. Consequently, the results of the instrumental investigation confirmed the presence of hypernasal resonance in the group of subjects with spastic dysarthria. The results of the individual evaluation of each subject, however, revealed that less than half of the subjects presented with disorders of nasal resonance, indicating a relatively low incidence of nasality disorders in subjects with predominantly mild and mild to moderate degrees of spastic dysarthria. No subject was found to have hyponasality on the basis of the instrumental assessment.

The presence of hypernasality in the speech of subjects with spastic dysarthria has been attributed to the presence of slow and incomplete evaluation of the soft palate (Chenery et al, 1992). Based on personal observations made during cineradiography, Aten (1983) reported that following initial evaluation, there is progressive failure of velar closure in spastic dysarthric patients when counting or during production of serial speech. In subjects with more severe resonance disorders, Aten describes an "inertia in initiating

speech activities" (p. 70), which is not actually weakness but rather "a rapid onset of increased resistance to stretch" (p. 70), which blocks the normal movement of the velum (Aten, 1983).

Hirose, Kiritani, and Sawashima (1982) used an x-ray microbeam system to analyze the articulatory dynamics of two patients with pseudobulbar palsy and two with amyotrophic lateral sclerosis (ALS). In their observations of articulatory movements during repetition of the word *ten,* it was found that the degree of velum elevation during the /t/ section of the utterance became lowered with repetition of the utterance. The tendency toward lowering of the velum during the repetition was determined to be indicative of the effects of fatigue, and the underlying basis for the presence of hypernasal voice quality in these patients. This observed pattern of behavior is consistent with the personal observations of Aten (1983) noted previously.

At present it is assumed that the noted reduction in speed and range of movements of the palate, such as those reported by Aten (1983), are the product of spasticity in the muscles responsible for palatal elevation. Unfortunately, however, there has been a lack of systematic, direct investigations of palatal movement in subjects with spastic dysarthria. Consequently, to more fully understand the mechanisms underlying the hypernasality identified in this subject group, there is a need for more detailed physiological investigations of velopharyngeal function to be conducted, incorporating endoscopic, x-ray microbeam, and electromyographic investigations of the velar mechanism both at rest and during connected speech.

Laryngeal Function

Since the descriptions of the perceptual features of spastic dysarthria provided by Darley et al (1969a,b), it has been assumed that bilateral upper motor neuron lesions are manifest at the laryngeal level primarily by increased tone of the laryngeal muscles leading to narrowing of the laryngeal aperture. This narrowing is supposedly the result of hyperadduction of the vocal cords. Hypertonic changes in the vocal cords, however, cannot be easily visualized, so that laryngoscopy of pseudobulbar cases often does not reveal any obvious abnormality in their structure and function. The presence of hypertonicity in the laryngeal adductor muscles is suggested, however, by the observed harsh voice quality and strained-strangled sound of the voice in pseudobulbar palsy.

These features are thought to be caused by the exhaled breath stream during speech being squeezed through the stenosed laryngeal valve. Aerodynamically, stenosis of the laryngeal aperture would be expected to manifest as increased glottal resistance, increased subglottal pressure, decreased laryngeal airflow during phonation, and a decrease in ab/adduction rate of the vocal folds (Hillman, Holmberg, Perkell, Walsh, & Vaughan, 1989; Smitheran & Hixon, 1981). Investigations of the vocal fold vibratory cycle have also indicated that increased vocal fold tension associated with laryngeal hypofunction results in increased fundamental frequency and corresponding decreases in the duty cycle and closing times. Consequently, electroglottographic investigation of the laryngeal function of spastic dysarthria would be expected to identify increased fundamental frequency and a decreased duty cycle and closing time.

In an investigation of laryngeal function of subjects with predominantly mild to moderate spastic dysarthria following cerebrovascular accidents, Murdoch, Thompson, and Stokes (1994) were able to only partly confirm the presence of these laryngeal parameters. Using both electroglottographic and aerodynamic techniques, they reported that only 50% of their group of spastic dysarthric speakers exhibited a predominance of features classically associated with hyperfunctional laryngeal activity, including increased resistance, elevated pressures, and decreased laryngeal airflow. Even then, not all of these features were always evident in the same dysarthric speaker. The remaining 50% of their spastic dysarthric group exhibited hypofunctional laryngeal features demonstrating lower than normal resistance and higher than normal airflow during phonation. One explanation for this unexpected finding provided by Murdoch et al was that, as a result of hypertonus, the movements of the vocal cords to the midline during phonation are sufficiently slowed to allow some air wastage. Alternatively, it was suggested that the hypofunctional laryngeal parameters is the result of the speaker adopting compensatory laryngeal behaviors to reduce the muscular effort needed to produce speech against hypertonic vocal cords. Murdoch et al noted the need for replication of their study and for further physiological investigation of laryngeal function in spastic dysarthria.

Respiratory Function

Impaired respiratory support for speech has been identified as one of the predominant perceptual features of speech disorders associated with upper motor neuron damage (Darley et al, 1975; Enderby, 1983). As in the case of laryngeal function, few quantitative instrumental studies have been reported on speech respiration in pseudobulbar palsy. Murdoch, Noble, Chenery, and Ingram (1989) investigated speech breathing in patients with pseudobulbar palsy following CVAs. They reported that four of their five pseudobulbar palsy cases had below normal vital capacities. In addition, their pseudobulbar palsy subjects had irregularities in their chest wall movements during vowel and syllable production tasks, which they speculated could possibly be attributed to spasticity and weakness of the muscles of the chest wall. In a later study (Thompson & Murdoch, 1995c), the respiratory function and speech breathing abilities of a group of 18 subjects with mild to moderate spastic dysarthria following CVA were investigated. Analysis of the kinematic patterns during production of maximum effort speech tasks (e.g., vowel prolongations) identified reduced lung volumes in the spastic dysarthria group consistent with the findings of Murdoch et al (1989). Particularly during the production of maximum effort tasks, there was evidence to suggest that the reduced lung volumes observed in the subjects with spastic dysarthria were contributed to by reduced rib cage and abdominal expansion during inspiration as well as reduced abdominal contraction during expiration, possibly as a result of the

presence of spasticity or weakness of the chest wall muscles. Spirometric analysis also confirmed reduced lung volumes and capacities in the dysarthric subject group (Thompson & Murdoch, 1995c).

It would appear, therefore, that a decrease in the excursion of the chest wall muscles during both the inspiratory and expiratory phases of respiration contributes to a reduction in the volumes exchanged during maximum respiratory efforts in spastic dysarthric speakers. At this point, without the benefits of electromyographic investigations of the chest wall musculature of these subjects, it is assumed that the reduced chest wall movement is the result of spasticity and weakness. Further investigation of the actual physiological mechanisms influencing the muscular movements of the respiratory systems of persons with spastic dysarthria, however, is required.

Summary of the Perceptual, Physiological, and Acoustic Investigations

In general, the acoustic and physiological studies that have been performed tend to support the perceptual analysis of spastic dysarthria reported by Darley et al (1969a,b). These studies have shown that spastic dysarthric speakers have a slow rate of speech most probably caused by longer durations of syllables and perhaps longer pauses within and between words. There is evidence that the articulators move through a reduced range, and that tongue strength in spastic dysarthria is reduced compared with normal. Although observations made during cineradiography of spastic dysarthric speakers suggest that velopharyngeal function is impaired, objective instrumental validation is needed. Those instrumental studies reported to date have indicated that impairments in speech breathing may contribute to the overall speech problem in spastic dysarthria. Although it is thought that the disturbed functioning of the various components of the speech mechanism is the product of the spasticity associated with bilateral upper motor neuron lesions, this interpretation remains speculative. and further objective validation of this hypothesis is required.

♦ Treatment

Currently patients with spastic dysarthria receive treatment procedures based on the assumption that the perceived speech deficits are a result of spasticity in the various components of the speech mechanism. As is evident from the previous section, however, few studies based on objective physiological assessment of the speech mechanism in spastic dysarthric speakers have been reported in the literature. To enable the design of specific treatments for various forms of dysarthria, information regarding their physiological basis is required. As stated by Abbs and DePaul (1989) "The quality of clinical treatment for dysarthria generally is related to the degree of knowledge of the pathophysiology and extent to which reliable assessment procedures can be devised to exploit that knowledge" (p. 207). It follows, then, that the efficiency and effect (such as the generalization of skills to untrained tasks) of dysarthria treatment can only be improved when the therapy techniques are selected to remediate specific physiological deficits. As Orlikoff (1992) stated, "a custom made assessment leads to a custom fit therapy program" (p. 37). One outcome, therefore, of the dearth of physiological data relating to the speech mechanism in spastic dysarthria is that few authors have developed programs designed specifically for remediation of the speech disorder in this population.

This section discusses therapy techniques that have either been effectively used in intervention with subjects with spastic dysarthria or that have been used with other dysarthric groups but could have high applicability for the intervention of spastic dysarthria. It is unfortunate that the majority of studies that have assessed dysarthria treatment and management using a variety of treatment procedures have often had limited subject numbers and have included subjects with a variety of types of dysarthria resulting from different etiologies. A true evaluation of the use of certain therapy techniques for subjects with spastic dysarthria, therefore, is difficult at this time.

Several the treatment strategies for the functional components of the motor speech system have already been well discussed in the literature (Halpern, 1986; Netsell & Rosenbek, 1986; Rosenbek & La Pointe, 1978); however, it is hoped that this chapter can highlight some of the new instrumental techniques available for the therapist and how these techniques may be useful in the treatment of patients with spastic dysarthria.

Prognostic Issues

Predicting the prognosis of a patient is often difficult due to the wide range of variables that can influence progress. Authors have listed factors such as neurological status and history, time since onset, age, motivation, personality, intelligence, associated language, cognitive and sensory problems, severity of the dysarthric involvement, skill of the clinician, type of treatment, and home environment, as just some of the points to be considered (Kearns & Simmons, 1990; Rosenbek & La Pointe, 1978).

One of the most influential of the prognostic factors is the clinician's ability to implement the most appropriate and efficient therapy approach to ensure a better outcome for the patient. Netsell and Rosenbek (1986) discussed six main factors that can influence the treatment decisions the clinician can make, with reference to treating the dysarthrias in general: (1) the severity of neurological insult, (2) the underlying pathophysiology, (3) the medical status, (4) available methods and tools, (5) time available, and (6) the patient's need to communicate. Several of these factors have a great influence over the treatment decisions that need to be made for subjects with spastic dysarthria. In particular, the severity of the insult and the underlying pathophysiology of the dysarthria can greatly influence treatment decisions. Langworthy and Hesser (1940) noted that subjects with pseudobulbar palsy show varying abnormalities in their speech depending on the amount of strength of voluntary control lost and the condition of either increased or decreased

tone in the muscles. Treatment, therefore, must be based on a thorough pathophysiological assessment to determine the status of the muscular impairment, whether it be increased or decreased tone, in each of the speech subsystems. Therapy techniques must then be selected to correspond to this physiological state. As therapy techniques that can effect change in severely spastic muscle groups, such as the larynx, are limited, the severity of impairment in each subsystem also dictates the availability of techniques that can be the most effective for the patient.

At the more detailed level of planning and scheduling of therapy sessions, there are still more factors that the clinician must consider in order for therapy to be efficient and effective for the patient. In their chapter on the dysarthrias, Rosenbek and La Pointe (1978) provide an excellent summary of therapy level planning considerations. Factors such as scheduling of sessions, use of drill work, the decision of individual versus group therapy, the hierarchical organization of symptoms, the setting of the specific treatment goals, and how to help the person to be a productive patient are well discussed. Such factors, however, are relevant to the treatment of all dysarthric patients and therefore do not require further specific evaluation here.

Treatment of Specific Speech Processes

Rosenbek and La Pointe (1978) state that the goal of dysarthria therapy is not to enable the patient to achieve normal speech, but rather, through therapy, to enable the patient to achieve *compensated intelligibility*. Several different approaches to the treatment of motor speech disorders can be utilized by clinicians, including behavioral techniques, instrumental therapy techniques, and surgical or prosthetic types of intervention; a pragmatic approach to the treatment of dysarthria (Kearns & Simmons, 1988) has also been discussed. These approaches allow therapists treating motor speech disorders to modify structure, increase function, and teach the patients new compensatory behaviors (Caligiuri & Murry, 1983).

The behavioral approach to dysarthria management includes teaching patients new skills, compensations, or adjustments that utilize traditional treatment techniques involving stimulus presentation, patient response, and response contingencies (Kearns & Simmons, 1990). Some of the difficulties with using the behavioral therapy techniques, however, include the lack of sensitivity, calibration, and quantitative nature of the data obtained. For this reason, much of the recent research interest into therapy for dysarthria has been focused on studies investigating the use of instrumental approaches involving biofeedback techniques.

The growth of commercially available instrumentation designed to provide feedback on several different physiological parameters is increasing. Netsell and Daniel (1979) note that most adult dysarthric patients can actually improve the function of their individual speech components when given biofeedback. Biofeedback instrumentation transforms covert physiological processes of speech production into precisely expressed signals via auditory, visual, or tactile pathways (Nemec & Cohen, 1984), and thereby allows the patient to focus on the key elements of a specific problem through instantaneous and simplified comparison between their muscle actions and normal muscle control (Netsell & Daniel, 1979). Research has shown that therapy using biofeedback can assist with the return of function even after subject performance has plateaued using traditional therapy techniques (Nemec & Cohen, 1984). Consequently, the use of biofeedback techniques provides a promising approach for the remediation of a variety of aspects of speech disorders.

Rubow (1980) discussed the need for research focusing on the development of reliable, valid instrumental technology and the need for greater understanding of biofeedback methodology (i.e., in what order should the components be treated, does nonspeech training generalize to speech tasks, and which tasks can be learned through training and for which types of dysarthrias?). Although research to date has done much to validate the importance of biofeedback, there still exists a need for efficacy studies to be undertaken, based on greater subject numbers and focusing on specific dysarthric groups to establish reliable and effective biofeedback techniques that can help effect change in the clinical setting.

Specific details of the behavioral, instrumental, and prosthetic therapy techniques available for the intervention of disorders of respiration, articulation, phonation, resonance, and prosody in subjects with spastic dysarthria are detailed below.

Classifying therapy techniques as pragmatic approaches is relatively new. The treatment procedures in this category include those therapy techniques that involve helping the patient to maximize communication within situations and contexts of daily life (Kearns & Simmons, 1990). Kearns and Simmons note that taking a pragmatic approach requires the clinician to work closely with patients and their families to evaluate environmental obstacles to communication and find solutions. The focus, therefore, of this type of approach is to develop strategies to help the client, and that will generalize into their communicative environment.

In the pragmatic approach, treatment does not focus on the dysarthric impairment but rather on the patient as a communicator in various contexts (Kearns & Simmons, 1988). Kearns and Simmons outlined some examples of pragmatic treatments: (1) *Environmental manipulation* involves the alteration of the communicative environment to enhance communication. Examples of this are strategies such as avoiding communication in dark or noisy places; reducing the distance between dysarthric speaker and listener to compensate for volume deficits; and learning to maximize situational, nonverbal, and gestural cues to aid the listener. (2) *Utterance length* involves modifying the length of utterances. (3) *Repair strategies* involve teaching effective repair strategies, such that a request for clarification by the listener is not met by the dysarthric speaker's simply repeating the utterance without modifications. (4) *Self-monitoring* is linked with the repair strategies and involves teaching patients to listen to their output and learn to monitor the need to make adjustments. (5) *Topic and attention getting* involves teaching the dysarthric speaker to ensure that the listener is oriented to the topic at hand, which can help improve the conversational situation.

Effective treatment of patients with spastic dysarthria, therefore, is dependent on the skills of the clinician in thoroughly assessing the physiological bases of the presenting speech deficit and then in selecting and combining treatment approaches that are best suited to effect change in the patient. The next several subsections discuss those techniques that are available for the therapist, for disorders of respiration, phonation, articulation, resonance, and prosody.

Respiration

Physiological investigations of the speech breathing abilities of subjects with spastic dysarthria have found deficits in the speech breathing process that could conceivably contribute to the perceived respiratory deficits of these patients (Murdoch et al, 1989; Thompson & Murdoch, 1995c). In a study conducted in the Motor Speech Research Centre at the University of Queensland, kinematic and spirometric assessments of 18 subjects with dysarthria due to upper motor neuron damage following CVA revealed that the dysarthric group had reduced lung volumes and capacities compared with the controls as well as reduced lung volume excursions during speech tasks (Thompson & Murdoch, 1995c). In addition, on comparison to the control group, the CVA group demonstrated reduced contributions of the abdominal muscles during speech production.

Traditionally, regardless of the type of approach taken (e.g., behavioral, instrumental), therapy for respiratory deficits has been directed toward increasing the subjects' vital capacity, and generally improving strength and coordination of the lungs (Robertson & Thompson, 1986). The results of our study (Thompson & Murdoch, 1995c) indicate that while the dysarthric subject group may benefit from a component that concentrates on strengthening and coordinating the rib cage and abdominal muscles, a particular emphasis should be placed on improving the contributing role of the abdominal muscles in the respiratory process for speech. Indeed, this study emphasizes the important role instrumental evaluations play in determining the nature of the physiological impairment, and directing therapy specifically to the underlying bases for the perceived respiratory deficits in each subject.

Traditional Therapy　　Speech production requires the controlled, sustained, and smooth flow of a sufficient air supply (Kearns & Simmons, 1990). Consequently, the main aim of respiratory therapy is to help the patient achieve controlled exhalation for speech (Boone, 1977; Eisenson, 1985; Kearns & Simmons, 1990; Robertson & Thompson, 1986; Rosenbek & La Pointe, 1978). Some of the specific treatment goals that can help the patient achieve improved breath support for speech, include increasing breath control, increasing the depth of inspiration, and improving breath control and air wastage during speech production (Moncur & Brackett, 1974).

Several researchers have suggested a variety of techniques that may help improve the breath support and control for speech. Shimizu, Watanabe, and Hirose (1992) discussed the use of the accent method with seven subjects with motor speech disorders. Five of these subjects had pseudobulbar type speech disorders and two had ataxic speech. Training took place during 30-minute sessions over 14 to 20 months, during which time the emphasis in therapy was to make the patient relax his neck, shoulders, and upper chest and to transfer the respiratory effort to the abdominal level during breathing. After 4 months an improvement in speech was noted, and by the end of therapy it was found that phonation time had extended, oral diadochokinetic rate for /pa/ had increased, duration of syllables were shorter and more stable, and speech intelligibility had improved (Shimizu et al, 1992). Although it is difficult to evaluate Shimizu et al's procedure based on the information provided in the conference proceedings alone, it would appear that focusing respiratory therapy on improving the role of the abdominal muscles during speech can be beneficial for subjects with spastic dysarthria. This finding supports the suggestions by Thompson and Murdoch (1995c) that the respiratory process of subjects with spastic dysarthria could benefit from therapy specifically designed to improve the abdominal contribution to the speech breathing process.

Netsell and Hixon (1992) described the use of another technique, inspiratory checking, that is designed to help breath control, with six head injured, dysarthric subjects. The technique consists of a two-part instruction to "take a deep breath" and "now let the air out slowly," which effectively trains the patient to regulate the flow of air and volume loss during speech. By following the instruction, the subject inhales more air and, therefore, can make use of the passive recoil pressures available for speech. The task of letting the air out slowly also then forces the subjects to use the inspiratory muscles forces to maintain a relatively constant subglottal air pressure. Of the six subjects taking part in the trials, three showed improvement using this technique. Consequently, Netsell and Hixon concluded that the technique of inspiratory checking was a viable method for some individuals with speech breathing dysfunction.

Aten (1983) specifically outlined the use of breathy sighs with subjects with spastic dysarthria to help establish an easy airflow. The intent of this technique is that, once established, the breathy sigh can be shaped into breath support for voice. Aten describes the technique as using "the least amount of breath possible to allow the subjects to produce a briefly sustained relaxed phonation that is audible but essentially voiceless" (p. 73).

Other behavioral techniques that may benefit subjects with spastic dysarthria are the adjustment of posture and the self-monitoring of their respiratory supply. Netsell and Rosenbek (1986) note that some patients experience increases in loudness either when lying or sitting, or in supine or prone positions. Consequently, adjusting the posture of the patient into a position that makes respiratory control easiest, can be very beneficial, especially for patients who are not ambulatory. Relaxation of the head, neck, and shoulders can also help decrease tension and improve respiration.

Providing abdominal support by pushing on the abdominal muscles during exhalation is a simple but useful technique to improve respiratory support for speech (Rosenbek & La Pointe, 1978). By pushing on the abdominal muscles, the pressure provides a means of passive breath release and, therefore, can further help a subject with spastic dysarthria

increase respiratory support while at the same time reduce tension in the respiratory musculature.

Instrumental Therapy   Some of the better known of the instrumental techniques for increasing respiratory support for speech include the use of an air pressure transducer coupled to an oscilloscope, and the U-tube water manometer; these devices and their construction are described in detail elsewhere (Rosenbek & La Pointe, 1978). Both techniques are based on the principle of encouraging the patient to produce consistent low-pressure exhalation over a period of time. Daniel-Whitney (1989) reported the successful use of the U-tube manometer to provide biofeedback of interoral air pressure for a child with dysarthria following traumatic brain injury. Using this technique, the child was able to progress from being able to sustain 1 cm H_2O for no more than 1 second, to achieve 5 cm H_2O for 2.5 seconds with the help of visual feedback. The biofeedback technique, therefore, helped the child achieve almost normal performance on this task, as people are considered to have adequate respiratory support for speech when they can generate 5 cm H_2O and maintain this at a steady level of 3 to 5 seconds (Netsell & Daniel, 1979).

Although the use of instrumental devices such as the U-tube manometer may be beneficial for some patients, there may also be the tendency for these tasks to actually increase tension in subjects with spastic dysarthria, due to the nature of the task. It has been noted that taking in too much air in inspiration can actually exaggerate tension of the thorax and the throat (Froschels & Jellinek, 1941). Consequently, tasks such as these that encourage taking deep breaths may actually trigger an increase in tension, and therefore their use may need to be monitored closely with the spastic dysarthric patient. It is important that the therapist adequately assesses the point at which taking in a deep breath may trigger an increase in tension, and then encourage the patient to breathe as deeply as possible without exerting past this point. Additionally, the presence of other factors such as oral weakness, incoordination, abnormal reflexes, or involuntary movements may also contraindicate the use of these techniques with some spastic patients.

Hixon, Goldman, and Mead (1973), in their study of the chest wall kinematics of normal subjects, noted that "subjects given feedback in the form of a storage oscilloscope display of a relative motion diagram could voluntarily trace out a wide variety of prescribed motion pathways while speaking, including those where they used either all rib cage or all abdomen when instructed to do so" (p. 108). There is the potential, therefore, for respiratory kinematics to be modified into a feedback treatment. Using an ABAB design, the current authors examined the efficacy of traditional therapy and kinematic biofeedback therapy on two subjects with mixed dysarthrias (spastic-flaccid, spastic-ataxic) following closed head injury. The results of the study revealed that while both the traditional and the instrumental methods were effective in remediating abnormal respiratory patterns in the two subjects, the biofeedback method effected a greater and more consistent change in the respiratory parameters under treatment in both subjects.

Surgical/Prosthetic Therapy   Prosthetic techniques for improving respiratory support for speech in subjects with spastic dysarthria concentrate on improving and enhancing the abdominal contribution to the exhaled breath stream. Aten (1983) reported that some patients with spastic dysarthria benefit greatly from providing a more natural posture for speech by supporting or "girdling" (Rosenbek & La Pointe, 1978) the abdominal musculature with an elastic bandage. Through the use of this technique, subjects with spastic dysarthria have been noted to produce better airflow with less effort as well as having reduced strained-strangled phonation (Aten, 1983). Aten, however, reported that caution must be taken not to restrict thoracic movement with the girdle as this may disturb the natural pattern of breathing. Consequently, Aten suggests as a preferable method the use of a thick leather belt 2 to 3 inches in diameter positioned and stabilized around the waist beneath the ribs.

Rosenbek and La Pointe (1978) also suggested the use of a board that could be attached to the patient's wheelchair at the level of the abdominal muscles that the patient could lean into to help force the airflow. The use of this technique, however, has been reported to be less than successful with subjects with spastic dysarthria (Aten, 1983). One other prosthetic approach that may prove beneficial with subjects with spastic dysarthria involves elevating the arms with the use of slings thus allowing the patient to initiate and sustain breath with less overall effort (Aten, 1983; Rosenbek & La Pointe, 1978).

Phonation

Arguably, the strained-strangled voice quality of patients with spastic dysarthria is often the least responsive of the motor speech subsystems to therapeutic intervention. Therefore, there is a need for a better understanding of the motor physiology at the laryngeal level for subjects with spastic dysarthria, in addition to a greater number of efficacy studies reporting trialed treatments for this population. Unfortunately, though, reviews of the voice research literature by Moore (1977), Perkins (1985), and Hillman, DeLassus Gress, Hargrave, Walsh, and Bunting (1990) have concluded that over the years there has been very little change in the practices of voice therapy. Additionally, there have been few published reports of research evaluating the efficacy of intervention for voice disorders (Hillman et al, 1990). The following subsection on treatment of the phonatory deficits for patients with spastic dysarthria reflects the need for research to provide the therapist with more knowledge about the physiological functioning of the larynx and a greater number of therapy options on which they can base their therapy.

Traditional Therapy   Behavioral techniques that can contribute to reducing laryngeal hyperadduction in subjects with spastic dysarthria include general body and specific head and neck relaxation exercises, specific vocal exercises to decrease laryngeal tension in the vocal cords, and techniques designed to decrease tension in the laryngeal musculature by altering the focus of voice production. Moncur and Brackett (1974) recommended several relaxation techniques, both general and specific, that can be applied to reduce whole body, head, and neck tension in voice-disordered patients. Theoretically, it is believed that incorporating relaxation techniques into the therapy program for subjects with spastic dysarthria may help decrease some of the muscle tension in these patients. Training patients to achieve a state of relaxation by themselves can be beneficial to help them counteract periods of spasticity when they occur.

One of the most widely used techniques to reduce hyperadduction at the level of the vocal folds is breathy onset phonation. Aten (1983) reported that initiating phonation after a breathy sigh is a useful technique for decreasing the perceived strain-strangled quality in the voice of subjects with spastic dysarthria. With this technique, therapy begins with producing a relaxed, breathy sigh of short duration that can be gradually shaped into a relaxed /a/ vowel, which then can progress to the production of single-syllable consonant-vowel-consonant (CVC) words. Aten suggested that the CVC words begin with the letter *h* and are followed by open mouth vowels and a nasal consonant or continuants (e.g., "harm," "halt") while avoiding the use of plosives and affricates due to the excess pressure and musculature movement required. It is also important to encourage the patient to produce all movements in a relaxed and slow manner, without force or excess effort, to avoid triggering the spastic contractions. Chewing and yawning techniques have been discussed in the literature as beneficial in reducing laryngeal tension in subjects with hyperfunctional laryngeal activity (see Moncur & Brackett, 1974, and Boone, 1977, for more detail). Their application with subjects with spastic dysarthria, however, may be restricted by the musculature effort involved in the chewing and yawning, which may trigger an increase in tension in the musculature rather than relaxation.

Possibly one other important behavioral technique that patients must learn is the ability to use their auditory skills to monitor their own voice production. Having the ability to effectively listen and evaluate the quality of the vocal productions can enable patients to recognize examples of the desired voice quality when it is produced. Being able to make judgments about voice production and knowing techniques that can be used to modify the production provides patients with the ability to generalize this quality to other speech tasks and to settings outside the clinic.

Instrumental Therapy   One instrumental therapy technique that may be applicable for disorders of phonation in subjects with spastic dysarthria is the use of electromyograph (EMG) biofeedback techniques to reduce laryngeal tension. Stemple, Weiler, Whitehead, and Komray (1980) discussed the use of EMG biofeedback with seven subjects who had vocal nodules due to increased laryngeal tension, and found that these subjects could reduce tension levels with EMG biofeedback training. Prosek, Montgomery, Walden, and Schwartz (1978) also investigated using the EMG technique on decreasing laryngeal tension for subjects with functional voice disorders, and reported some success with the technique with half of their subject group. Although the subjects in these EMG studies did not have the same underlying physiological deficits as subjects with spastic dysarthria, EMG biofeedback to reduce hypertonia in other aspects of the speech mechanism (Nemec & Cohen, 1984) has been successful for subjects with spastic dysarthria. Consequently, there is enough evidence to advocate the use of the EMG technique to help decrease laryngeal tension for spastic dysarthric patients.

Other instrumental assessment techniques that could have beneficial application as therapy tools include the VisiPitch (Kay Elemetrics, Pine Brook, NJ) and the laryngograph. As a feedback system, the VisiPitch computer system provides instantaneous visual feedback for several target behaviors including fundamental frequency and intensity, average fundamental frequency and intensity, pertubation, and voice onset time. Using this system, the patient can receive visual feedback of performance as well as compare performance with the clinicians' model. The laryngograph is an electroglottographic technique that utilizes electrical impedance to estimate vocal cord contact during phonation. Again, the patient can receive visual feedback through observing the glottal wave recorded by the equipment and displayed on the computer screen. Hard glottal attacks are represented in the waveforms as a short steep closing phase as opposed to more breathy onsets of phonation that are represented by a more gradual gentle slope. The combination of this technique of feedback with behavioral therapy for breathy onsets could possibly be a beneficial therapy technique. There are no reports in the literature of treatment using the VisiPitch or the laryngograph as biofeedback tools; however, there are certainly opportunities for them to be incorporated as a therapeutic method for subjects with spastic dysarthria.

Surgical/Prosthetic Therapy Surgical management is not an intervention approach that is regularly taken for hyperfunctional voice disorders. The possibility of reducing severe spastic dysphonic conditions, however, through reducing laryngeal innervation unilaterally may warrant investigation. The induction of unilateral vocal cord paralysis through the reduction of innervation is a technique that has been used for subjects with spastic dysphonia (Dedo & Shipp, 1980). Injections of botulinum toxin into the laryngeal muscles have been used to temporarily paralyze one of the vocal cords in the attempt to relieve the symptoms of strangled phonation in subjects with spastic dysphonia (Blitzer & Brin, 1992; Zwirner, Murry, Swenson, & Woodson, 1991, 1992). There are no reports in the literature, however, to support the effectiveness of either of these surgical procedures in reducing the strained-strangled phonation of subjects with spastic dysarthria.

Articulation

Rosenbek and La Pointe (1978) stated that the aim of articulation treatment is "to improve the patients volitional-purposive control of speech sound production to the limits imposed by his physiologic support for speech" (p. 295). In the case of subjects with spastic dysarthria, Aten (1983) redefined this goal as "achieving modest improvements in articulatory precision without overflow of tension into the oral or laryngeal/

respiratory musculature" (p. 75). The patient with spastic dysarthria is described as having labored jaw closure, restricted tongue movements (particularly isolated velar contacts) and lip closures which "at best are crude with very limited flexibility" (p. 75). The articulatory abilities of patients with spastic dysarthria, therefore, are often quite impaired, due in part to both the compromised function of the articulators and the coexisting deficits of impaired respiration, phonation, and resonance. Consequently, articulation therapy for subjects with spastic dysarthria must be preceded by therapy for disorders of voice onset and voice control, and by improving oral flow through the reduction of nasal resonance and emission prior to successful intervention work with the articulators (Aten, 1983).

Traditional Therapy Although several authors have discussed orofacial treatment procedures in great detail (Netsell & Rosenbek, 1986; Rosenbek & La Pointe, 1978) much of the information discussed by the authors has been concentrated on training procedures that increase tone, and the speed, range, and accuracy of the articulatory muscles. Due, however, to the already existing increased tone in the articulators of subjects with spastic dysarthria, work on speed, rate, and force is not appropriate for these subjects, as abrupt transitions and quick articulatory movements tend only to increase tension and trigger difficulties (Aten, 1983). Aten outlined treatment strategies designed to improve intelligibility for subjects with spastic dysarthria that involved stressing the concepts of gentle approximation of consonants and emphasizing clear vowel productions with a minimum of constriction and tension. The hierarchy of tasks involves beginning with open mouth vowels, and then progressing to high tongue-jaw vowels (e.g., /i/). Following this, the patient is encouraged to produce CVC words beginning with the letter *h* and initially only containing continuant or liquid sounds; then later, when these have been produced successfully, more demanding sounds including voiced and then unvoiced plosives and finally affricates can be included. In each case, Aten states that approximation of sound production is the realistic objective for these patients.

Instrumental Therapy The most popular instrumental technique for modifying the function of the articulators is EMG feedback of muscle function and tone. The use of EMG biofeedback techniques has been discussed in the literature as providing beneficial intervention for modifying tone in orofacial muscles. Daniel-Whitney (1989) reported the successful use of EMG biofeedback to increase tone in the orbicularis oris muscle of a child with severe spastic-ataxic dysarthria. The child presented with weak lips and poor lip closure, and the results of EMG recordings of the lip muscles demonstrated no evidence of spasticity. Therapy using the EMG biofeedback was focused on increasing lip muscle tone and was successful in helping the child attain lip closure.

EMG biofeedback techniques have also been successful in reducing tension in subjects with spastic dysarthria. Nemec and Cohen (1984) used EMG biofeedback techniques with a male subject with spastic dysarthria to increase awareness of generalized tension in the facial muscles involved in elevation and depression of the mandible. Training focused on generalized reduction of tension in the facial muscles and gaining conscious control over the desired response. Speech intelligibility for the subject was noted to improve due to appropriate lingual postures accompanying mandibular closure, and follow-up assessments revealed good generalization of the newly acquired skills.

The movement of the articulators in subjects with spastic dysarthria is often restricted by increased tone. Another approach to reduce this tone other than EMG is the use of vibration therapy to improve the state of relaxation of the muscles. Daniel-Whitney (1989) discussed the use of vibration therapy for a child with severe spastic ataxic dysarthria. The child presented with reduced jaw opening and trials with prosthetic management only achieved some increased jaw opening. Relaxation of the masseter using bilateral vibration for periods of 20 minutes was found to be successful in further increasing jaw opening from 12 to 25 mm (Daniel-Whitney, 1989).

Another instrumental technique that may have therapeutic application for subjects with spastic dysarthria is the electropalatograph. The technique of electropalatography (EPG) involves the use of an artificial palate that contains several electrodes exposed to the lingual surface. When the artificial palate is in place, it can provide details of the timing and location of the tongue with the hard palate during continuous speech. By using the artificial palate as a training tool, it can help provide patients with visual feedback of the location of their tongue during articulation and how this positioning needs to be adjusted to achieve a closer approximation of the sound. One possible detrimental factor to this technique, however, is the cost and time involved in constructing the palate. An article by Hardcastle, Gibbon, and Jones (1991) provides a good description of the electropalate and its functions.

Surgical/Prosthetic Therapy   Types of prosthetic management for articulation disorders discussed in the literature for use with all types of dysarthria include items such as jaw slings, which can help maintain jaw closure (Kearns & Simmons, 1988), and bite blocks, which stabilize the jaw and effectively force the patient to make lip and tongue movements without assistance from the jaw (Netsell & Rosenbek, 1986; Rosenbek & La Pointe, 1978). Daniel-Whitney (1989) outlined a case study of a child with severe spastic-ataxic dysarthria following traumatic brain injury for whom improving jaw opening was an important treatment goal. Using increasing numbers of tongue depressors inserted between the teeth, they reported success with increasing jaw opening from 2 to 12 mm. Following this technique a bite block was also trialed in the attempt to obtain additional opening; however, this was unsuccessful as the child demonstrated extensor spasm on insertion of the block. Although prosthetic management was useful to some extent, this case study report demonstrates that the increased tone in subjects with spastic dysarthria may often prevent or at least restrict the use of some types of treatment.

Resonance

Disorders of resonance in the dysarthrias can result from abnormal tongue positioning, an increase or lack of tension in the articulatory muscles, or an impairment in coordination of the velopharyngeal mechanism (Rosenbek & La Pointe, 1978). Subjects with spastic dysarthria, therefore, may have disorders of resonance as a result of spasticity or weakness in any one or all of these muscle groups. Disruptions of resonance stemming from deficits in articulatory posturing or tension can be remediated using techniques discussed in the above section on articulatory deficits. This section, therefore, addresses the intervention strategies useful in remediating disruptions of velopharyngeal function.

The most prominent disorder of resonance associated with spastic dysarthria is hypernasality. Hypernasality in spastic dysarthria results from spasticity and weakness of the velopharyngeal muscles, which in turn may result in the subject having either an inconsistent or an incomplete closure of the velopharyngeal port during speech. In his chapter on treatment in spastic dysarthria, Aten (1983) reported that, in his experience of observing the velum of spastic dysarthric subjects using cineradiography, the initial elevation of the velum in these patients is soon followed by a progressive failure of the velum to elevate during serial speech activities. In subjects with a more severe resonance disorder, Aten describes an "inertia in initiating speech activities" (p. 70). Aten accounts for these velar movements as not actually weakness, but rather "a rapid onset of increased resistance to stretch" (p. 70), which results in blocking the movement pattern.

Determining the need for therapeutic intervention for velopharyngeal dysfunction is often difficult due to coexisting deficits in other aspects of the speech production mechanism. A thorough assessment of the velopharyngeal muscles' structure and function, as well as determining the degree to which the hypernasality is disrupting speech production in subjects with spastic dysarthria, is therefore critical to accurate therapeutic intervention. Although the therapy decisions for the more mild and more severe cases can be made with relative confidence, Netsell and Rosenbek (1986) suggested some guidelines are needed to help make the decisions for those patients who fall into what they describe as the "gray area." The decision to treat these cases can be aided by considering the following factors: (1) the relative severity of involvement in the other functional components, (2) whether the treatment of the velopharynx would enhance function in other areas (e.g., tax the respiratory system less), and (3) whether the velopharyngeal function would benefit from treating other components first or simply having the patient speak more slowly and with greater effort (Netsell & Rosenbek, 1986).

Traditional Therapy   Many of the traditional approaches to the treatment of hypernasality have been based on the principles of increasing velopharyngeal muscle strength, learning to direct airflow, and increasing patient awareness of velopharyngeal function. Pushing techniques that involve the patient's attempting velopharyngeal closure while simultaneously pushing with the hands against an object or simply tensing other muscles, and tasks that encourage the patient to control and modify the airstream using balls, whistles, candles, fluff, powder, paper, bubbles, straws, etc., have been discussed at length elsewhere (Halpern, 1986). However, there have been reports that such therapy techniques, on the whole, are not effective (Powers & Starr, 1974), possibly because they do not provide the patient with information on the timing of articulatory gestures during speech (Künzel, 1982). The relevance of these techniques with subjects with spastic dysarthria has not been specifically assessed; however, if, as Aten (1983) suggests, the problems with velopharyngeal control is a progressive failure of the velum to elevate as the resistance to stretch increases, single sound tasks and nonspeech tasks may be of little benefit for these patients. Pushing techniques that effectively increase tension may also adversely affect the patient with spastic dysarthria for whom the aim is to decrease the amount of tension in the speech system.

Another behavioral approach for modifying disorders of resonance is oral resonance therapy. Having a raised mandible and retracted tongue during speech can actually enhance nasal resonance. Consequently, speech exercises that emphasize increased jaw widening and tongue movements can help to open the oral cavity as a resonator and provide additional reduction in the perceived levels of hypernasality.

Examples and specific tasks for oral resonance therapy can be found elsewhere in vocal therapy texts such as Moncur and Brackett (1974).

Instrumental Therapy A major contributing factor to the problem of treating hypernasality, however, stems from the inability of the subject to perceive velopharyngeal movements and receive adequate feedback. Due to the difficulties of receiving feedback about the muscle functioning using traditional therapy approaches, the use of biofeedback techniques for hypernasality therapy has proven to be very beneficial for patients. Over the past years, several different instrumental systems have been designed and trialed with a variety of patients to provide the dysarthric speaker with feedback on velopharyngeal functioning during speech and nonspeech tasks. In the literature to date, however, there are very few reports of the efficacy of biofeedback techniques with dysarthric subjects. As a result, we can again only speculate on the effectiveness of such therapy techniques for spastic dysarthric subjects.

In the late 1970s and early 1980s, several researchers introduced some of the first instrumental biofeedback techniques for velopharyngeal dysfunction. Shelton, Paesani, McClelland, and Bradfield (1975) and Shelton, Beaumont, Trier, and Furr (1978) discussed the use of an endoscope with visual feedback of the movements of the lateral pharyngeal walls provided on a closed circuit monitor. Siegel-Sadewitz and Shprintzen (1982) and Witzel, Tobe, and Salyer (1988) used flexible fiberoptic nasopharyngoscopes to obtain close observations of the velopharyngeal sphincter during connected speech. Velographs, palatal training appliances (Tudor & Selly, 1974), and displacement transducers (Moller, Path, Werth, & Christiansen, 1973) have also been demonstrated to be effective in increasing palatal movements during phonation.

Although these instrumental methods have been found to effect change in the velopharyngeal function of several different speech disordered patients, mainly cleft palate subjects, generalization and long-term maintenance of the skills acquired using these techniques have not been documented. In addition, the ability to use this equipment in a clinical setting is restricted by factors such as cost, complexity of equipment, and in some cases, such as nasoendoscopy and endoscopy, the need for a physician to be present.

There are some instrumental techniques, however, that are less invasive and more easily incorporated into clinical use. One such system is the Nasometer (Kay Elemetrics), which provides an indirect measure of velopharyngeal function through measuring acoustic energy output. The Nasometer is a microcomputer-based instrument designed for the assessment and treatment of patients with disorders of nasality, and unlike many of the instrumental techniques previously discussed, this program is simple to use, comparatively inexpensive, and has applications for both children and adults. The equipment consists of two directional microphones set onto a horizontal sound separator plate that rests against the patient's top lip, creating a shelf between the nose and the mouth. During speech production, information regarding the relative amount of nasal acoustic energy in a patient's speech is then displayed on the computer screen expressed as a "nasalance" score. In addition to evaluating the degree of nasality, the Nasometer program also provides visual displays such as bar displays and real-time screen displays of the degree of nasalance the person produces during speech. This provides the patient with feedback about the degree of nasal acoustic output during tasks and consequently allows the patient to attempt to monitor and control velopharyngeal functioning. Studies of the effectiveness of the system as a therapy tool, however, are still required.

The accelerometer is another assessment tool based on indirectly measuring velopharyngeal function, which also has applications as a system to provide feedback. Horii and Monroe (1983) outlined the use of accelerometers coupled with visual feedback via an oscilloscope display and auditory feedback through a microphone/headset as a simple and cost-effective feedback tool for velopharyngeal therapy.

One other possible biofeedback aid that has been mentioned in the literature is the Exeter Bio-Feedback Nasal Anemometer (EBNA) (Bioinstrumentation Ltd., Exeter, UK) (Hutters & Brondsted, 1992). This system consists of a flow-sensing device that contains a electrically heated bead that works on the same principles as a hot wire anemometer that is then placed in a mask that is positioned over the nose. The EBNA system is reported to be much less expensive and more convenient than other airflow systems (Hutters & Brondsted, 1992). Its efficacy as a clinical tool, however, remains undetermined.

Surgical/Prosthetic Therapy The decision to use invasive, prosthetic intervention to remediate hypernasality must be based on several general factors: (1) the severity of the hypernasality, (2) the degree to which hypernasality is affecting other aspects of the speech mechanism, (3) attempts at therapeutic intervention using behavioral and instrumental methods have been unsuccessful, and (4) the absence of contraindicating factors for surgery or postsurgical therapy. Indeed, although there have been no specific criteria lists compiled that predict the success of prosthetic management, investigations into palatal lift prosthetic intervention have indicated that it is a successful method for subjects with severe velopharyngeal dysfunction (Lotz & Netsell, 1984, cited in Netsell & Rosenbek, 1986). How long the lift is effective, though, is a matter that requires investigation, as Aten (1983) reported that the positive effects of palatal lifts with severely spastic dysarthric patients do tend to dissipate over time due to increased tension in the hypopharyngeal and laryngeal musculature. Subjects with less severe deficits, however, have been found to benefit over a longer period of time, and may not require the lift after a few months (Aten 1983).

A palatal lift prosthesis is designed to help compensate for reduced or incoordinated movement of the velopharyngeal muscles. Consequently, subjects with severe spastic dysarthria, which is affecting the functioning of the velopharyngeal musculature, may involve the use of a palatal lift prosthesis. The lift is usually designed to attach to the teeth, and consists of a hard plastic shelf attached to the posterior section of the plate that projects posteriorly under the soft palate and maintains elevation. The aim of using a palatal lift is to allow the lateral pharyngeal walls to move toward the midline and contact with the velum that is being artificially raised by the prosthesis. Individual differences in velopharyngeal anatomy, muscle action, and patterns of velopharyngeal closure mean that prosthetic management of velopharyngeal incompetence must be based on a thorough instrumental observation of muscle function. Construction of a palatal lift is discussed elsewhere (Schweiger, Netsell, & Sommerfeld, 1970; Spratley, Chenery, & Murdoch, 1988); however, in general, the lift is designed so that when the prosthesis is in place, the velum is continually raised, yet the subject can breath comfortably through the nose when the lateral edges of the lift have been extended maximally (Netsell & Daniel, 1979).

Gonzalez and Aronson (1970) investigated the use of the palatal lift prosthesis for the treatment of both anatomical and neurological velopharyngeal insufficiency. Of the 19 patients in the neurological subgroup investigated, 10 had spastic paresis of the velopharyngeal musculature resulting from upper motor neuron damage, five had flaccid paresis, and four had mixed spastic-flaccid paresis. All patients at the immediate, 3-month, and 1-year assessments showed moderate to marked improvements in the reduction of hypernasality and nasal emission, as well as an increase in speech intelligibility due to the improved ability to build intraoral pressure. In addition to this finding, reassessment at 2 years after the initial fitting of the prosthesis of four (three neurological and one anatomical) of the original patients showed improved palatopharyngeal efficiency with the prosthesis removed. This finding demonstrated that, in addition to being used to correct and improve palatopharyngeal closure, the prosthesis may in fact stimulate palatopharyngeal musculature, and function as a supportive type of prosthesis until the muscles gain strength and activity to effect palatopharyngeal closure (Gonzalez & Aronson, 1970). Unfortunately, as Lotz and Netsell (1984, cited in Netsell & Rosenbek, 1986) reported, the long-term effects of palatal lifts have not been documented, and therefore further research into the long-term effects of palatal lift prosthetic management is required to evaluate the role it has in stimulating palatopharyngeal movement.

Gonzalez and Aronson (1970) noted several selection criteria to be considered to optimize successful prosthetic intervention. In their study, subjects were selected for the lift prosthesis after oral and cineradiographic examinations determined the residual muscular activity in the palatopharyngeal region and the presence of adequate retention for the prosthesis. Physiological, psychological, or financial status was also considered. Based on their experience, Lotz and Netsell (1984, cited in Netsell & Rosenbek, 1986) suggested some physiologically based selection criteria for successful prosthetic intervention: (1) If nasal air flow on oral sounds is consistently above 200 cc/s, successful treatment of the velopharynx should increase speech intelligibility. (2) If nasal flows are in the range of 100 cc/s, they do not have a major impact on intelligibility if intraoral pressures for oral sounds are 5 to 10 cm H_2O and orofacial articulation is reasonable. (3) If intraoral pressures are below 4 cm H_2O for oral sounds, nasal flows of 100 cc/s can be clinically significant and treatment of the velopharynx may be necessary.

There are also several other factors to be taken into consideration that contraindicate the fitting of a palatal lift, especially for subjects with spastic dysarthria. Daniel (1982) found that hypersensitivity of the gag reflex is another factor to be considered, after noting that some patients, even following successful desensitization of the gag reflex, could not tolerate the prosthesis. As a possible solution to this problem, Aten (1983) discussed the use of a palatal lift with spastic dysarthric patients that has flexible twin wire extensions from the denture acrylic that can easily be adjusted in the anterior-posterior and vertical planes to allow graduated support to the velum. The flexibility of the structure of this lift thus allowed patients to gradually become accustomed to the lift and help extinguish the gag reflex. Gonzalez and Aronson (1970) also noted that a palatal lift should not be used when a person has a very spastic or stiff soft palate that does not tolerate elevation. Strong velar, palatoglossus, or pharyngeal contractions can also inhibit the subject from retaining the device (Netsell & Rosenbek, 1986).

Prosody

Disruptions of the suprasegmental and prosodic features of speech may result in affected intelligibility. Consequently, prosodic features should receive equal attention in dysarthria treatment and management. It is often the case, however, that prosodic intervention is initiated in the final stages of therapy or not at all. The three prosodic features—rhythm, stress, and intonation—are the result of the interaction of suprasegmental factors such as pitch, loudness, articulation time, and pause time (Rosenbek & La Pointe, 1978). Rhythm is defined as "the perception of the time program applied to the phonetic events" (Netsell, 1973, p. 224), whereas stress is considered to be "the perception of syllable emphasis, relative to the emphasis perceived on other syllables in the same sentences or phrase" (p. 224). Rosenbek and La Pointe suggest that the treatment of rhythm and stress can be achieved using a common method, as stress is a result of changes in pitch, loudness, articulation time, and pause time, whereas rhythm is considered the timing of speech, which also results, in part, from changes in pause time. Intonation, which is defined as "the perception of changes in the fundamental frequency of vocal fold vibration during speech production" (p. 244), in contrast, requires separate intervention strategies.

The prosodic features of subjects with spastic dysarthria are often impaired due to the combination of characteristic low, monotonous pitch, monotony of loudness, shortness of phrases, and a slow rate of speech characterized by labored articulation.

Traditional Therapy The variables that affect the elements of prosody are complex and interrelated (Kearns & Simmons, 1988). Consequently, many of the behavioral therapy techniques discussed previously in the articulation, phonation, and respiration subsections have some effect on the prosodic elements of speech (e.g., increased respiratory support with relaxed phonation may have a carryover effect to increase phrase length). There are some specific intervention techniques, however, that can be applied to modify aspects such as stress and intonation.

Aten (1983) reported that therapy involving stress and contrast exercises may be useful toward the end of treatment for patients with less severe spastic dysarthria.

Contrastive stress drills involve the production of the same sentence each time, however, and the focus of the stress is changed such that the meaning of the sentence changes (e.g., "Bob bit *Bill*"; "*Bob* bit Bill"). These drills can also be effectively combined with rate control and articulation work to improve intelligibility. Therapy tasks that target intonation patterns include reading aloud text that has been marked with the natural intonation patterns and pause times that are appropriate for the passage. Moncur and Brackett (1974) have written an excellent chapter on therapy for prosodic disruption that outlines several treatment techniques and stimuli.

Aten (1983) reported little success eliminating monotony or increasing rate in the moderate to severely involved spastic dysarthric patients. The use of a pacing technique to regulate the rhythm of speech has been suggested as a possible technique to improve rate and intelligibility in spastic dysarthria (Nailling & Horner, 1979). Other more simplified techniques involve instructing the patient to speak at a slower rate. Articulating at a slower rate and pausing between words can often prevent triggering of increased spasticity in the speech system and, therefore, improve intelligibility. Unfortunately such techniques often result in producing equalized stress patterns that differ from normal speech production (Barnes, 1983).

Monotonous quality in speech is often perceived as a deficit in fundamental frequency variation. However, it has been suggested in the literature that attempting to reduce a monotonous voice quality through the modification pitch and intonation alone may be insufficient. Soloman, Ludolph, and Thompson (1984, cited in Bellaire, Yorkston & Beukelman, 1986) acoustically analyzed the fundamental frequency of speech samples of normal subjects and subjects defined as having monotonous speech, and found that the range of fundamental frequency excursion for each group was not different. Bellaire et al reported that therapy to improve breath patterning in a subject with mild dysarthria following closed head injury resulted in a reduction of the patient's monotonous voice quality. Bellaire et al, therefore, concluded that the perception of monotony must include factors other than fundamental frequency. From the results of the investigation, it appeared that the speech of the patient Bellaire et al had investigated was judged to be

monotonous, at least in part as a consequence of his short, regular breath groups. These results emphasize the need to assess the breath patterns of speech and the role of the breath group as a unit of prosody that requires intervention. Specific tasks and exercises for breath patterning can be found in Moncur and Brackett (1974).

Instrumental Therapy There have been reports in the literature on the use of biofeedback techniques for the intervention of prosodic disturbances. Caligiuri and Murry (1983) demonstrated the effectiveness of biofeedback training on articulatory precision, speaking rate, and prosody for three subjects with dysarthria. In their study, Caligiuri and Murry displayed intensity and duration information as well as interoral air pressure information on a four-channel storage oscilloscope. Results of nine weeks of visual feedback therapy revealed improvements in speaking rate, prosodic control, and a reduction in the overall severity of the speech disorder (Caligiuri & Murry, 1983).

The VisiPitch (Kay Elemetrics) is a commercially available biofeedback tool that can provide the patient with performance feedback on several target behaviors including pitch, range, vocal intensity, speech rate, intonation, and stress patterns. Through the computer system the clinician can demonstrate the target behavior and then have the patient practice the task with the aid of the visual feedback on the screen. There have been no reports cited in the literature of the effectiveness of this equipment in the treatment of prosody for subjects with spastic dysarthria; therefore, its application for this population can only be assumed.

♦ Conclusion

Spastic dysarthria results from bilateral disruption of the upper motor neuron connections to the bulbar cranial nerves. The resulting speech disturbance has been described as slow, dragging, labored speech that is produced with some effort. To date, few specific treatments for spastic dysarthria have been proposed, largely reflecting a lack of published reports concerning the physiological functioning of the various components of the speech production mechanism in spastic dysarthric speakers. It is thought that the deviant speech dimensions perceived to be present in spastic dysarthria are the products of spasticity in the speech musculature. Although some confirmatory studies have been reported in the case of many components of the speech production system, this interpretation remains speculative. Until such time as comprehensive studies of the physiological functioning of the speech production mechanism of spastic dysarthric speakers are reported, further development of effective treatment procedures for this condition will be hampered. This chapter discussed the application of techniques used in dysarthria treatment in general to the rehabilitation of disordered speech in spastic dysarthria. In addition, the few reported treatments that have been trialed with spastic dysarthric speakers were reviewed.

References

Abbs, J.H. & De Paul, R. (1989). Assessment of dysarthria: a critical prerequisite to treatment. In M.M. Leahy (Ed.), *Disorders of Communication: The Science of Intervention.* London: Taylor & Francis

Abbs, J.H., Hunker, C.J., & Barlow, S.M. (1983). Differential speech motor subsystem impairments with suprabulbar lesions: neurophysiological framework and supporting data. In: W.R. Berry (Ed.), *Clinical Dysarthria* (pp. 21–56). San Diego: College-Hill Press

Aten, J.A. (1983). Treatment of spastic dysarthria. In: W. Perkins (Ed.), *Dysarthria and Apraxia* (pp. 69–77). New York: Thieme-Stratton

Barlow, S.M. & Abbs, J.H. (1986). Fine force and position control of select orofacial structures in the upper motor neurone syndrome. *Experimental Neurology, 94,* 699–713

Barlow, S.M. & Abbs, J.H. (1984). Orofacial fine motor control impairments in congenital spasticity: evidence against hypertonus-related performance deficits. *Neurology, 34,* 145–150

Barnes, G.J. (1983). Suprasegmental and prosodic considerations in motor speech disorders. In: W. Berry (Ed.), *Clinical Dysarthria* (pp. 57–68). San Diego: College-Hill Press

Bellaire, K., Yorkston, K., & Beukelman, D.R. (1986). Modification of breath patterning to increase naturalness of a mildly dysarthric speaker. *Journal of Communication Disorders, 19,* 271–280

Blitzer, A. & Brin, M.F. (1992). Treatment of spasmodic dysphonia (laryngeal dystonia) with local injections of botulinum toxin. *Journal of Voice, 6,* 365–369

Boone, D.R. (1977). *The Voice and Voice Therapy.* Englewood Cliffs, NJ: Prentice-Hall

Caligiuri, M.P. & Murry, T. (1983). The use of visual feedback to enhance prosodic control in dysarthria. In: W.R. Berry (Ed.), *Clinical Dysarthria.* San Diego: College-Hill Press, 267–282

Chenery, H.J., Murdoch, B.E., & Ingram, J.C.L. (1992). The perceptual speech characteristics of persons with pseudobulbar palsy. *Australian Journal of Human Communication Disorders, 20,* 21–31

Daniel, B. (1982). A soft palate desensitization procedure for patients requiring a palatal life prosthesis. *Journal of Prosthetic Dentistry, 48,* 565–566

Daniel-Whitney, B. (1989). Severe spastic-ataxic dysarthria in a child with traumatic brain injury: questions for management. In: K.M. Yorkston & D.R. Beukelman (Eds.), *Recent Advances in Clinical Dysarthria.* Boston: Little, Brown, 129–137

Darley, F.L., Aronson, A.E., & Brown, J.R. (1969a). Differential diagnostic patterns of dysarthria. *Journal of Speech and Hearing Research, 12,* 246–269

Darley, F.L., Aronson, A.E., & Brown, J.R. (1969b). Clusters of deviant speech dimensions in the dysarthrias. *Journal of Speech and Hearing Research, 12,* 462–496

Darley, F.L., Aronson, A.E., & Brown, J.R. (1975). *Motor Speech Disorders.* Philadelphia: W.B. Saunders

Dedo, H. & Shipp, T. (1980). *Spastic Dysphonia.* Houston: College-Hill Press

Dworkin, J.P. & Aronson, A.E. (1986). Tongue strength and alternate motion rates in normal and dysarthric subjects. *Journal of Communication Disorders, 19,* 115–132

Eisenson, J. (1985). *Voice and Diction. A Program for Improvement,* 5th ed. New York: Macmillan

Enderby, P. (1983). *Frenchay Dysarthria Assessment.* San Diego: College-Hill Press

Enderby, P. (1986). Relationships between dysarthric groups. *British Journal of Disorders of Communication, 21,* 189–197

Froschels, E. & Jellinek, A. (1941). *Practice of Voice and Speech Therapy.* Boston: Expression Company

Gonzalez, J.B. & Aronson, A.E. (1970). Palatal lift prosthesis for treatment of anatomic and neurologic palatopharyngeal insufficiency. *Cleft Palate Journal, 7,* 91–104

Halpern, H. (1986). Therapy for agnosia, apraxia and dysarthria. In: R. Chapey (Ed.), *Language Intervention Strategies in Adult Aphasia.* Baltimore: Williams & Wilkins, 97–116

Hardcastle, W.J., Gibbon, F.E., & Jones, W. (1991). Visual display of tongue-palate contact: electropalatography in the assessment and remediation of speech disorders. *British Journal of Disorders of Communication, 26,* 41–74

Hardcastle, W.J., Morgan-Barry, R.A., & Clark, C.J. (1985). Articulatory and voicing characteristics of adult dysarthric and verbal dyspraxic speakers: an instrumental study. *British Journal of Disorders of Communication, 20,* 249–270

Hillman, R.E., DeLassus Gress, C., Hargrave, J., Walsh, M., & Bunting, G. (1990). The efficacy of speech-language pathology intervention: voice disorders. *Seminars in Speech and Language, 11,* 297–309

Hillman, R.E., Holmberg, E.B., Perkell, J.S., Walsh, M., & Vaughan, C. (1989). Objective assessment of vocal hyperfunction: an experimental framework and initial results. *Journal of Speech and Hearing Research, 32,* 373–392

Hirose, H. (1986). Pathophysiology of motor speech disorders (dysarthria). *Folia Phoniatrica, 38,* 61–68

Hirose, H., Kiritani, S., & Sawashima, M. (1982). Patterns of dysarthric movement in patients with amyotrophic lateral sclerosis and pseudobulbar palsy. *Folia Phoniatrics, 34,* 106–112

Hixon, T.J., Goldman, M., & Mead, J. (1973). Kinematics of the chest wall during speech production: volume displacement of the rib cage, abdomen, and lung. *Journal of Speech and Hearing Research, 16,* 78–115

Horii, Y. & Monroe, N. (1983). Auditory and visual feedback of nasalization using a modified accelerometric method. *Journal of Speech and Hearing Research, 26,* 472–475

Hutters, B. & Brondsted, K. (1992). A simple nasal anemometer for clinical purposes. *European Journal of Disorders of Communication, 27,* 101–119

Kearns, K.P. & Simmons, N.N. (1988). Motor speech disorders: The dysarthrias and apraxia of speech. In: N.J. Lass, I.V. McReynolds, J.L. Northern & D.E. Yoder (Eds.), *Handbook of Speech-Language Pathology and Audiology.* Toronto: B.C. Decker

Kearns, K.P. & Simmons, N.N. (1990). The efficacy of speech-language pathology intervention: motor speech disorders. *Seminars in Speech and Language, 11,* 273–295

Künzel, H.J. (1982). First applications of a biofeedback device for the therapy of velopharyngeal incompetence. *Folia Phoniatrica, 34,* 92–100.

Langworthy, O.R. & Hesser, F.H. (1940). Syndrome of pseudobulbar palsy: an anatomic and physiologic analysis. *Archives of Internal Medicine, 65,* 106–121

Linebaugh, C.W. & Wolfe, V.E. (1984). Relationships between articulation rate, intelligibility and naturalness in spastic and ataxic speakers. In: M.R. McNeil, J.C. Rosenbek, & A.E. Aronson (Eds.), *The Dysarthrias: Physiology, Acoustics, Perception, Management.* San Diego: College-Hill Press, 197–205

Moller, K.T., Path, M., Werth, L., & Christiansen, R. (1973). The modification of velar movement. *Journal of Speech and Hearing Disorders, 38,* 323–334

Moncur, J.P. & Brackett, I.P. (1974). *Modifying Vocal Behaviour.* New York: Harper & Row

Moore, G.P. (1977). Have the major issues in voice disorders been answered by research in speech science? A fifty year retrospective. *Journal of Speech and Hearing Disorders, 42,* 152–160

Murdoch, B., Noble, J., Chenery, H., & Ingram, J. (1989). A spirometric and kinematic analysis of respiratory function in pseudobulbar palsy. *Australian Journal of Human Communication Disorders, 17,* 21–35

Murdoch, B.E., Thompson, E.C., & Stokes, P.D. (1994). Phonatory and laryngeal dysfunction following upper motor neurone vascular lesions. *Journal of Medical Speech-Language Pathology, 2,* 177–189

Murdoch, B.E., Thompson, E.C., & Theordoros, D.G. (1997). Spastic dysarthria. In: M.R. McNeil (Ed.), *Clinical Management of Sensorimotor Speech Disorders* (pp. 287–310). New York: Thieme

Nailling, K. & Horner, J. (1979). Reorganizing neurogenic articulation disorders by modifying prosody. Paper presented at the Convention of the American Speech-Language-Hearing Association, Atlanta

Nemec, R.E. & Cohen, K. (1984). EMG biofeedback in the modification of hypertonia in spastic dysarthria: case report. *Archives of Physical Medicine and Rehabilitation, 65*, 103–104

Netsell, R. (1973). Speech physiology. In: F. Minifie, T. Hixon, & F. Williams (Eds.), *Normal Aspects of Speech, Hearing and Language.* Englewood Cliffs, NJ: Prentice-Hall

Netsell, R. & Daniel, B. (1979). Dysarthria in adults: physiologic approach to rehabilitation. *Archives of Physical and Medical Rehabilitation, 60*, 502–508

Netsell, R. & Hixon, T.J. (1992). Inspiratory checking in therapy for individuals with speech breathing dysfunction. *American Speech-Language-Hearing Association, 34*, 152

Netsell, R. & Rosenbek, J. (1986). Treating the dysarthrias. In: R. Netsell (Ed.), *A Neurobiologic View of Speech Production and the Dysarthrias* (pp. 123–152). San Diego: College-Hill Press

Orlikoff, R.F. (1992). The use of instrumental measures in the assessment and treatment of motor speech disorders. *Seminars in Speech and Language, 13*, 25–37

Perkins, W. (1985). Assessment and treatment of voice disorders: state of the art. In: J. Costello (Ed.), *Speech Disorders in Adults.* San Diego: College-Hill Press, 111–179

Portnoy, R.A. & Aronson, A.E. (1982). Diadochokinetic syllable rate and regularity in normal and in spastic and ataxic dysarthric subjects. *Journal of Speech and Hearing Disorders, 47*, 324–328

Powers, G. & Starr, C.D. (1974). The effects of muscle exercises on velopharyngeal gap and nasality. *Cleft Palate Journal, 11*, 28–35

Prosek, R.A., Montgomery, A.A., Walden, B.E., & Schwartz, D.M. (1978). EMG biofeedback in the treatment of hyperfunctional voice disorders. *Journal of Speech and Hearing Disorders, 43*, 282–294

Robertson, S.J. & Thompson, F. (1986). *Working with Dysarthrics: A Practical Guide to Therapy for Dysarthria.* Oxon: Winslow Press

Rosenbek, J.D. & La Pointe, L.L. (1978). The dysarthrias: description, diagnosis and treatment. In: D. Johns (Ed.), *Clinical Management of Neurogenic Communicative Disorders* (pp. 251–310). Boston: Little, Brown

Roy, N., Leeper, H.A., Blomgren, M., & Cameron, R.M. (2001). A description of phonetic, acoustic and physiological changes associated with improved intelligibility in a speaker with spastic dysarthria. *American Journal of Speech-Language Pathology, 10*, 274–288

Rubow, R. (1980). Biofeedback in the treatment of speech disorders. Speech Motor Control Laboratories Preprints (Autumn), Waisman Center, University of Wisconsin, Madison

Schweiger, J., Netsell, R., & Sommerfield, R. (1970). Prosthetic management and speech improvement in individuals. *Journal of American Dental Association, 80*, 1348–1353

Shelton, R.L., Beaumont, K., Trier, W., & Furr, M. (1978). Videoendoscopic feedback in training velopharyngeal closure. *Cleft Palate Journal, 15*, 6–12

Shelton, R.L., Paesani, A., McClelland, K., & Bradfield, S. (1975). Panendoscopic feedback in the study of voluntary velopharyngeal movements. *Journal of Speech and Hearing Disorders, 40*, 232–244

Shimizu, M., Watanabe, Y., & Hirose, H. (1992). Use of the Accent method in training for patients with motor speech disorders. *Folia Phoniatrica, 44*, 73

Siegel-Sadewitz, V.L. & Shprintzen, R.J. (1982). Nasopharyngoscopy of the normal velopharyngeal sphincter: an experiment of biofeedback. *Cleft Palate Journal, 19*, 194–200

Smitheran, J.R. & Hixon, T.J. (1981). A clinical method for estimating laryngeal airway resistance during vowel production. *Journal of Speech and Hearing Disorders, 46*, 138–146

Spratley, M.H., Chenerey, H.J., & Murdoch, B.E. (1988). A different design of palatal lift appliance: review and case reports. *Australian Dental Journal, 33*, a491–495

Stemple, J.C., Weiler, E., Whitehead, W., & Komray, R. (1980). Electromyographic biofeedback training with patients exhibiting a hyperfunctional voice disorder. *Laryngoscope, 90*, 471–476

Thompson, E.C. & Murdoch, B.E. (1995a). Interpreting the physiological bases of dysarthria from perceptual analyses: an examination of subjects with UMN type dysarthria. *Australian Journal of Disorders in Communication, 23*, 1–23

Thompson, E.C. & Murdoch, B.E. (1995b). Disorders of nasality in subjects with upper motor neurone type dysarthria following cerebrovascular accident. *Journal of Communication Disorders, 28*, 261–276

Thompson, E.C. & Murdoch, B.E. (1995c). Respiratory function associated with dysarthria following upper motor neurone damage. *Australian Journal of Disorders in Communication, 23*, 61–87

Thompson, E.C., Murdoch, B.E., & Stokes, P.D. (1995a). Tongue function in subjects with upper motor neurone type dysarthria following cerebrovascular accident. *Journal of Medical Speech-Language Pathology, 3*, 27–40

Thompson, E.C., Murdoch, B.E., & Stokes, P.D. (1995b). Lip function in subjects with upper motor neurone type dysarthria following cerebrovascular accident. *European Journal of Disorders of Communication, 30*, 451–466

Tudor, C., & Selly, W. (1974). A palatal training appliance and a visual aid for use in the treatment of hypernasal speech. *British Journal of Disorders of Communication, 9*, 117–123

Weismer, G. (1984). Acoustic descriptions of dysarthric speech: Perceptual correlates and physiological inferences. *Seminars in Speech and Language, 5*, 293–313

Witzel, M.A., Tobe, J., & Salyer, K. (1988). The use of nasopharyngoscopy biofeedback therapy in the correction of inconsistent velopharyngeal closure. *International Journal of Pediatric Otorhinolaryngology, 15*, 137–142

Ziegler, W., & Von Cramon, D. (1986). Spastic dysarthria after acquired brain injury: an acoustic study. *British Journal of Disorders of Communication, 21*, 173–187

Zwirner, P., Murry, T., Swenson, M., & Woodson, G.E. (1991). Acoustic changes in spasmodic dysphonia after botulinum toxin injection. *Journal of Voice, 5*, 78–84

Zwirner, P., Murry, T., Swenson, M., & Woodson, G.E. (1992). Effects of botulinum toxin therapy in patients with adductor spasmodic dysphonia: Acoustic, aerodynamic, and videoendoscopic findings. *Laryngoscope, 102*, 400–406

Additional Reading

Murdoch, B.E. (1998). *Dysarthria: A Physiological Approach to Assessment and Treatment.* Cheltenham, UK: Stanley-Thornes

Chapter 13

Speech Impairment Secondary to Hearing Loss

Sheila R. Pratt and Nancy Tye-Murray

The study and treatment of speech disorders secondary to hearing loss has a history in the United States dating back to the early 1800s. The literature is large, and this chapter represents a condensation of only portions of that literature. Much has been added to our knowledge of hearing loss and its effects on speech production in recent years because of the research associated with cochlear implants and because of the renewed interest in the role of auditory feedback in the development and control of speech production. Furthermore, technological advancements currently allow for the detection and treatment of hearing loss in early infancy, which has provided additional information about the importance of audition in the early development of speech. However, despite the burgeoning research in the treatment of auditory dysfunction and its impact on speech production, the direct treatment of speech impairment secondary to hearing loss has been limited.

Although speech disorder secondary to hearing loss traditionally is not included within the category of sensorimotor speech disorders, there are numerous reasons for its inclusion. Foremost, audition is a major sensory contributor in the development of speech. It is generally accepted that substantive loss of audition not only interferes with exposure to speech models but also interferes with the internal and external feedback necessary to develop speech normally. The work of Guenther and colleagues (Guenther, 1995; Guenther, Ghosh, & Tourville, 2006) strongly suggests that auditory and somatosensory feedback is fundamental to the development and tuning of the feedforward mechanism that directs speech production in mature speakers. As part of this learning process, speakers develop auditory, somatosensory, and motor representations of speech, and in so doing also develop a mapping of the speech sensorimotor system to the linguistic system. This entire process can be impaired in infants and children with hearing loss. Compounding the problem is that hearing loss occurring in early childhood often results in language delay due to incomplete linguistic models. Therefore, it is often the case with prelingually impaired persons that an impaired motor-speech system interacts with an impaired linguistic system.

The role that audition plays for individuals who have developed normal speech and language has become better understood through the study of postlingually deafened adults whose hearing has been partially restored with a cochlear implant, although the impact of less severe hearing loss on the speech production of mature speakers is less well established. There are three general perspectives. First, in mature speakers, audition contributes to the ability of speakers to make the subtle postural and phonemic adjustments required for intra- and interarticulator coordination, and that without auditory feedback speech intelligibility deteriorates over time (Cowie, Douglas-Cowie, & Kerr, 1982; Zimmermann & Rettaliata, 1981). Others have stated that the adjustments made in ongoing speech are not dependent on an intact auditory system (Goehl & Kaufman, 1984; Sapir & Canter, 1991). A more moderate, intermediate view is held by Lane and Perkell and their associates (Lane & Webster, 1991; Lane, Wozniak, Matthies, Svirsky, & Perkell, 1995; Perkell, Lane, Svirsky, & Webster, 1992; Perkell et al, 1997). These investigators conducted a series of studies with adults who use cochlear implants, and suggested that auditory feedback plays a variable role (Lane et al, 1995). They hypothesized that auditory feedback is used to validate the articulatory and acoustic relations within speakers' internal models of speech. Second, audition is used to monitor environmental conditions, such as background noise and reverberation, and ensures that accommodations are made so that acceptable speech intelligibility is maintained. Accordingly, some speech behaviors and speaking conditions require more or less access to the auditory system. The auditory system is, therefore, a contributor to the integrity of the sensorimotor speech mechanism, although the magnitude of influence is dependent on the maturity of the system, the speech behaviors being produced, and the context within which speech is occurring. Furthermore, some speech production processes may be more susceptible to reduced auditory feedback than others in mature speakers (Lane, Matthies, Perkell, Vick, & Zandipour, 2001; Lane & Perkell, 2005).

◆ Characteristics

Hearing loss sufficient to cause disability is very common in the general population. A recent MarkeTrak survey suggests that over 31.5 million persons in the United States have a hearing loss (Kochkin, 2005). The prevalence of severe-to-profound hearing loss in infants was previously estimated at 1 to 2 in 1000 (Feinmesser, Tell, & Levi, 1982; Martin et al, 1981; Parving, 1985). Estimates of hearing loss emanating from universal screening programs that used screening tools sensitive to less severe hearing loss range from approximately 2.0 to 3.15 per 1000 live births (Finitzo, Albright, & O'Neal, 1998; Prieve et al, 2000; Vohr, Carty, Moore & Letourneau, 1998). According to Blanchfield, Feldman, Dunbar, and Gardner (2001) as many as 738,000 individuals in the U.S. have severe-to-profound hearing loss, of which nearly 8% are under the age of 18. In the 2000–2001 school year, the U.S. Department of Education (2002) reported that 70,767 children between the ages of 6 and 21 received hearing services in the schools, which was 1.2% of the school-aged population with reported disabilities. The inclusion of milder losses elevates the prevalence of permanent hearing loss in children to 14.9% (Niskar et al, 1998).

With age and exposure to such things as noise and ototoxic agents, the prevalence and incidence of hearing impairment and disability increases substantially (Morrell, Gordon-Salant, Pearson, Brant, & Fozard, 1996). With many of the industrialized countries experiencing an overall aging of their populations, the numbers of persons with hearing loss will likely increase (American Speech-Language-Hearing Association, 2006). Approximately 16% of adults in the U.S. reports some difficulty with hearing, and after arthritis and hypertension, hearing impairment is the third most commonly reported chronic condition in persons over 65 (National Center for Health Statistics, 1982; Pleis & Coles, 2003). By age 70 years, approximately 30% of the population perceives themselves as being hearing impaired, and by 80 years, 50% report being hearing impaired (Desai, Pratt, Lentzner, & Robinson, 2001). There also is an indication that the prevalence of hearing impairment in persons 48 to 92 years of age is increasing, especially among men (Wallhagen, Strawbridge, Cohen, & Kaplan, 1997). However, self-reported hearing impairment tends to underestimate the numbers of adults with measurable hearing loss. In a population-based cohort study, Cruickshanks, et al (1998) found that of their 3753 subjects tested (aged 43 to 84) the overall prevalence of hearing loss was 45.9%, and for every 5 years of age the risk of hearing loss increased 90%. Of their subjects under the age of 60 years, 20.6% had a hearing loss in contrast to 90% of those 80 years and older. Similar findings have been found in other studies (Helzner et al, 2005; Lee, Matthews, Dubno, & Mills, 2005).

♦ Speech Characteristics

Although hearing loss is common in the general population, its effects on speech production are most pronounced with individuals whose hearing loss is congenital or acquired in early childhood. Only limited effects, if any, are perceptible with most individuals who acquire their hearing losses later in life (Goehl & Kaufman, 1984). Even in cases of complete or nearly complete adventitious hearing loss, speech remains largely intact for most individuals, although speaking rate may be reduced and articulatory and phonatory precision may be compromised (Kishon-Rabin, Taitelbaum, Tobin, & Hildesheimer, 1999; Lane et al, 1995; Lane & Webster, 1991; Leder et al, 1987; Perkell et al, 1992; Waldstein, 1990). The differences largely are similar in nature but reduced in severity to those observed with prelingually deafened speakers.

In addition to there being a relationship between age of onset and severity of speech impairment, there also is a moderately positive relationship between the severity of hearing loss and the severity of the associated speech difficulties (Levitt, 1987; Smith, 1975; Wake, Hughes, Poulakis, Collins, & Rickards, 2004). For example, speech difficulties in children with mild-to-moderate hearing loss, particularly if well aided, tend to be mild and similar in nature to those of normal-hearing children with developmental articulation disorders (Elfenbein, Hardin-Jones, & Davis, 1994; Oller & Kelly, 1974; West & Weber, 1973). Elfenbein et al observed that these children are characterized by good intelligibility. The speech errors that are present tend to be substitutions of affricates and fricatives. In addition, mild hoarseness and resonance problems may be present in 20 to 30% of this subgroup. Their speech problems are usually evaluated and treated in the same manner as hearing speakers because of the mildness of the problems. Therefore, the following discussion of the effects of hearing loss on speech production largely focuses on speakers with congenital or early childhood hearing loss in the severe-to-profound range.

Individuals with severe-to-profound prelingual hearing loss are diverse relative to speech production skills. Nonetheless, there appears to be a relationship between speech perception and speech production skills (Blamey, Sarant, & Paatsch, 2006; Tye-Murray, Spencer, & Gilbert Bedia, 1995). For instance, Tye-Murray et al found that young cochlear-implant users who were most likely to perceive the place of articulation, nasality, and voicing features were also those implant users who were most likely to produce these features correctly. Children who use hearing aids or cochlear implants and who demonstrate good speech recognition skills generally also speak with relatively good intelligibility (Blamey et al, 2006; Gold, 1980; Osberger, Maso, & Sam, 1993).

Recent data from studies looking at the effectiveness of early intervention, as well as studies looking at the impact of cochlear implants, suggest that these interventions result in greater diversity, with many speakers demonstrating normal to near-normal performance whereas others remain substantively impaired (Peng, Spencer, & Tomblin, 2004; Tobey, Geers, Brenner, Altuna, & Gabbert, 2003). For example, Peng et al evaluated the sentence production skills of 24 children who had an average of 84 months of cochlear implant experience. The percentage of keywords spoken correctly ranged from 6 to 100%, with an average of 71.5%. Previously, many individuals born with profound hearing loss never acquired the speech skills that permitted them to interact easily using spoken language. On average, less than 20% of their words were intelligible to listeners who were not familiar with their speech (Hudgins & Numbers 1942; Markides, 1970; Smith, 1975). Smith evaluated 40 children with varying levels of hearing loss and, on average, only 18.7% (0 to 76%) of their words could be identified by inexperienced listeners. Not surprisingly, there was an inverse relationship between the frequency of segmental and suprasegmental errors, and overall intelligibility. Despite a great deal of idiosyncrasy with individual speakers, common error and difference patterns emerge when groups of speakers with hearing loss are evaluated. The patterns tend to be similar across the severity range except when comparing the extremes of the range (Levitt & Stromberg, 1983).

Furthermore, various parts of the speech production mechanism can be affected. The following subsections are an overview of the common patterns observed in persons with hearing loss by speech production subsystem.

Respiration

The difficulty in controlling respiration for speech has been observed in speakers with severe and profound hearing loss, but rarely in speakers with mild-to-moderate hearing loss. Forner and Hixon (1977) evaluated the respiratory skills of 10 adult speakers with profound prelingual hearing loss and observed that their subjects' vegetative respiratory skills were normal as were their ribcage and abdominal adjustments in anticipation of speech. Nonetheless, respiratory control during speech was faulty. Their subjects often phonated on low lung volumes and spoke within a restricted lung volume range. They also produced fewer syllables per breath unit because of inappropriate pausing due to either inspiration or inefficient air expenditure. Persons with hearing loss can exhibit mean air volume expenditures as high as 100 cc/syllable, with most of the air expended just prior to or during the initial portion of an utterance. In contrast, the normal range is approximately 20 to 40 cc/syllable (Forner & Hixon, 1977; Hardy, 1961; Whitehead & Barefoot, 1983). Whitehead (1982) obtained results similar to Forner and Hixon; however, subjects were grouped according to intelligibility. Whitehead observed that the intelligible speakers with hearing loss had respiratory patterns more similar to normal-hearing speakers and that the less intelligible speakers tended to initiate speech at low lung volumes and continued speaking at levels well below functional residual capacity.

Children with hearing loss also may exhibit difficulty with respiratory control. Those with limited respiratory control tend to produce fewer syllables per breath unit, and exhibit excessive air expenditure per syllable and inappropriate pausing due to this inefficient air expenditure. In studies of children fitted with cochlear implants after 5 years of age Higgins, McCleary, Carney, and Schulte (2003) and Jones, Gao, and Svirsky (2003) found that atypical intraoral air pressure patterns often persisted for several years after implantation. The ability to control the airflow through the glottis is a major contributing factor in the speech breathing difficulties exhibited by some speakers with hearing loss. It has been proposed that the differences are a reflection of abnormal laryngeal postures and reduced control of intrinsic laryngeal muscles. Mixed laryngeal patterns have been observed within and across studies with both hyper- and hypoabduction of the glottis. Speakers with hearing loss are usually able to maintain, although inconsistently, an appropriately open and closed vocal tract, with the less intelligible speakers exhibiting poorer control of laryngeal valving (Hutchinson & Smith, 1976; Whitehead, 1982; Whitehead & Barefoot, 1980). Using transillumination of the glottis, McGarr and Löfqvist (1982) found that some speakers with hearing loss exhibit inappropriate glottal abduction between words. McGarr and Löfqvist suggested that these postures result in inefficient air expenditure, although they did not simultaneously measure airflow in their study.

Others have reported high airflow rates during the production of some consonants and vowels with subjects having difficulty maintaining prolonged continuous phonations (Hutchinson & Smith, 1976; Itoh, Horii, Daniloff, & Binnie, 1982; Whitehead & Barefoot, 1983). In other conditions such as with voiceless fricatives in vowel-consonant-vowel (VCV) syllable contexts, reduced airflow has been observed, suggesting excessive restriction of the airway (Whitehead & Barefoot, 1983). Higgins, Carney, and Schulte (1994) also found evidence of hyperconstriction of the airway. In an aerodynamic and electroglottographic study of phonatory, velopharyngeal, and articulatory function, they found that early deafened adults with intelligible speech exhibited higher than normal subglottal pressures, fundamental frequencies, and laryngeal resistances. Some of their subjects with hearing loss also exhibited low laryngeal abduction quotients, and low phonatory air flows. The indication was that these speakers tended to overdrive and overconstrict their vocal folds during phonation. Higgins et al postulated that the hyperconstriction of the glottis was adopted to increase tactile feedback. They also suggested that intelligible speakers with hearing loss are more likely to use a constricted laryngeal posture whereas less intelligible speakers tend to adopt a hyperabducted posture.

Voice

Given the respiratory and laryngeal valving difficulties that some speakers with hearing loss experience, it is not surprising that vocal abnormalities have been observed in this population. Their instances of hyper- and hypoabduction of the larynx can result in voicing and other phonation errors particularly when poorly timed with upper airway articulation. Differences in vocal quality, pitch, and loudness have been reported as well as associated perturbation of the glottal waveform. The vocal quality of speakers with hearing loss typically is described as breathy, hoarse, or strained (Hudgins & Numbers, 1942; Markides, 1970). As with perceptual judgments of hearing-speakers' voice quality, the interjudge agreement on voice quality is good when using extreme samples but less reliable in the middle ranges. In addition, acoustic glottal measurements of perturbation, such as shimmer and jitter, are much less predictive of perceptual judgments of vocal quality in speakers with hearing loss than for normal-hearing patients with vocal pathologies (Arends, Povel, Van Os, & Speth, 1990). It should be noted that the use of perceptual judgments of vocal quality and glottal acoustic perturbation measures have restricted applicability even with normal-hearing populations (Kreiman & Gerratt, 1998; Kreiman, Gerratt, Precoda, & Berke, 1992; Martin, Fitch, & Wolfe, 1995; Shrivastav, Sapienza, & Nandur, 2005).

Although common, the pitch and loudness characteristics of speakers with hearing loss vary within and across speakers (Higgins et al, 1994). Some speakers with hearing loss use an excessively high habitual fundamental frequency (F0) (Angelocci, Kopp, & Holbrook, 1964; Horii, 1982). Boys may have problems lowering their habitual fundamental frequency to acceptable levels as they progress through puberty, although Osberger (1981) found that adolescent girls with hearing loss produced relatively higher fundamental frequencies than did adolescent boys with comparable hearing losses, indicating that elevated fundamental frequency was not isolated to boys in this age range. Some speakers with hearing loss are monopitch in their speech whereas others exhibit excessive pitch variations. Diplophonia can be present and is likely due to excessive tension of the intrinsic laryngeal muscles. Not surprisingly, difficulty producing contextually appropriate (socially and linguistically) intensity levels is common in speakers with profound hearing loss. Some speak at excessively high intensity levels (Calvert & Silverman, 1975) and others at low levels (Penn, 1955). This difficulty with intensity control may be due, in part, to problems monitoring environmental sounds and the acoustics of a speaker's own voice, but a portion is likely due to inefficient speech breathing and laryngeal control. For several possible pragmatic, linguistic, or speech motor-control reasons, difficulties in modulating intensity and fundamental frequency substantially interfere with intelligibility (Monsen, 1979).

Resonance

There are two resonance characteristics associated with speakers with prelingual severe-to-profound hearing loss: cul-de-sac or pharyngeal resonance, and the presence of improper nasalization resulting in hyper- and hyponasality. Pharyngeal resonance is highly salient perceptually and commonly identified with deaf speech. It is not well understood but appears to be the result of improper lingual and pharyngeal posturing. In a radiographic study of 10 normal-hearing and four deaf women with pharyngeal resonance, Subtelny, Li, Whitehead, and Subtelny (1989) found that the deaf subjects' tongues tended to function from a more neutral position when producing vowels than did those of the hearing subjects. A neutralized tongue position was observed even though the speech of the deaf subjects was intelligible and their vowel productions were considered distinct and correct. While producing high vowels, the deaf subjects also were identified with elevated hyoids, large vertical dimensions of the laryngeal pharynx, retracted tongue roots, and retruded tongue dorsums that were associated with substantive epiglottis deflections toward the pharyngeal walls.

Structural limitations of the velopharyngeal mechanism may account for the nasality problems of some children with hearing loss, but more commonly they are the consequence of improper velopharyngeal timing due to poor auditory feedback. Poor timing may account for the substantial intra- and intersubject variability observed by Higgins et al (2003) when recording nasal airflow from children wearing cochlear implants. Stevens, Nickerson, Boothroyd, and Rollins (1976) evaluated a group of 25 deaf children, and measured nasality as vibration transduced from the lateral surface of the nose with an accelerometer. They found that the children showed substantively more instances of vowel nasalization than did groups of normal-hearing children and adults. They also found that it was not uncommon for nasal consonants to be denasalized and nonnasal consonants to be nasalized by the children with hearing loss. In addition, a relation-ship between the degree of inappropriate nasality and intelligibility was observed, and listener judgments of nasality were consistent with accelerometric findings. Persons wearing cochlear implants may be susceptible to reduced nasalization of nasal sounds given the high frequency emphasis of most implant fittings. Uchanski and Geers (2003) observed that over half of the 181 implanted children in their study produced nasals with abnormally reduced low-frequency energy, which could be a function of the limited low-frequency information provided by most cochlear implant processors. It also should be noted that abnormal nasality has been associated with reduced intelligibility, and often is reflected in abnormal acoustic and accelerometric findings (Goldhor, 1995; Monsen, 1978; Stevens et al, 1976).

Segmental Characteristics

Vowels

Vowels are usually more intact than consonants for speakers with hearing loss. Germane to error pattern, speakers with hearing loss tend to produce low vowels more correctly than high and middle vowels, and back vowels more correctly than front vowels (Nober, 1967; Smith, 1975), although Angelocci et al's (1964) data obtained from early adolescent boys indicated more errors on low vowels than high vowels. Typical vowel errors include substitutions, neutralizations, prolongations, nasalizations, and diphthongizations (Hudgins & Numbers, 1942; Markides, 1970; McGarr, 1987; Smith, 1975; Tye-Murray & Kirk, 1993). Vowel omissions are more rare than are consonant omissions, but substitutions and neutralizations are especially common with substitutions going toward a more central and lax vowel. Angelocci et al's (1964) data showed that vowel place errors occur more frequently than height errors, although McCaffrey and Sussman (1994) found that as the severity of hearing loss increases from severe to profound, the likelihood of vowel height errors increases. There is evidence that the use of a cochlear implant results in dramatically fewer vowel errors. For instance, Markides (1970) studied 46 children between the ages of 7 and 9 years with pure-tone averages (i.e., hearing thresholds averaged for 500, 1000, and 2000 Hz) of 95 dB (presumably the British Standard, although it was not specified). The children misarticulated approximately 56% of all vowels and diphthongs when producing monosyllables elicited with picture cards. In contrast, Tobey et al (2003) reported that on average, 62% of all vowels were produced correctly in a sentence context (which is about a 38% error rate) by children wearing cochlear implants. The children were 8 to 9 years of age and had an average of 5.5 years' experience with their implants.

The neutralization of vowels also affects the suprasegmental aspects of speech by shortening the vowel and reducing stress. Vowel prolongation and diphthongization also are commonly observed and contribute to reduced speaking rate (Uchanski & Geers, 2003). Together, the abnormal temporal patterns of vowels likely result in inappropriate linguistic and coarticulatory cues. In addition to singleton vowels being diphthongized, diphthongs are frequently reduced. For example, the intended word "boy" might be produced as /bi/. Further, diphthong elements can be produced as abutting single vowels. Prolongation and nasalization are common diphthong errors as well (Smith, 1975). In contrast, postlingually deafened adults tend to produce prolonged vowels, although they usually maintain monophthong-diphthong distinctions (Palethorpe, Watson, & Barker, 2003).

The perceptual findings of vowel neutralization have been corroborated with acoustic and movement data. For instance, spectrographic analyses of the speech of deaf speakers indicate a tendency for their first (F1) and second (F2) vowel formants to be centralized when compared with normal-hearing talkers (Monsen, 1976a), although excessively high second formants also have been observed, particularly with high back vowels (Angelocci et al, 1964; Stein, 1980). In a study of 17 adolescent speakers with hearing loss and good vowel intelligibility, McCaffrey and Sussman (1994) found that the F0-F1 and F2-F3 differences of their subjects with severe hearing loss tended to be consistent with those produced by their normal-hearing subjects. The intelligibility of their subjects with profound hearing loss, however, was less than that of the subjects with severe hearing loss, and their formant differences were significantly reduced. If the subjects with severe hearing loss showed a reduction in formant space, it was usually with F2 and F3. McCaffrey and Sussman argued that the F2-F3 difference was more susceptible to reduction because F2 and F3 are less audible than F0 and F1. The reduced space between formants is evident as an overlap in vowel targets, which is consistent with neutralization, perceptual ambiguity, and vowel substitutions. It also suggests abnormal lingual posture or restricted mobility (Monsen, 1978; Osberger, Levitt, & Slosberg, 1979; Subtelny, Whitehead, & Samar, 1992) and may interfere with the development of coarticulation (Guenther, 1995). However, in a study of postlingually deafened adults, Lane et al (2001) found little impact on anticipatory coarticulation despite changes in vowel space, duration, and formant variability.

Along with an overlap in vowel target space, it has been reported that speakers with hearing loss often use an elevated fundamental frequency when producing vowels and that fundamental frequency varies more across vowels produced by speakers with hearing loss than by normal-hearing speakers (Angelocci et al, 1964). They also exhibit reduced variability in their second formants suggesting restricted anterior movement of the tongue (Monsen, 1976a). In addition, it has been hypothesized that changes in F0 and F1 are the primary means with which vowels are differentiated productively by speakers with hearing loss (Angelocci et al, 1964; Monsen, 1976a; Stein, 1980).

Using glossometry, Dagenais and Critz-Crosby (1992) assessed tongue position and shape during vowel production. Ten children with profound hearing loss with unintelligible speech were compared with 10 normal-hearing children. The children with hearing loss tended to assume a flat tongue shape with a high back posture. There was less variability in tongue shape and position across vowels, all of which was consistent with vowel neutralization and reduced formant variability. The normal-hearing children, in contrast, exhibited a greater range of lingual postures and tongue shapes across vowels. They also used more discrete tongue positions and less token-to-token variability.

In a cineographic study of two normal-hearing adults and five deaf adults with varying degrees of intelligibility, Stein (1980) found that the deaf subjects produced reasonable tongue height distinctions between high and middle vowels but that posterior-anterior distinctions were lacking. The movement of the subjects' tongue bodies was limited, and the height distinctions may have been mediated by the mandible. Tye, Zimmermann, and Kelso (1983) observed with cinefluorography that their two prelingually deafened adults had similar tongue positions for /u/ and /æ/ unlike their postlingually impaired and normal-hearing subjects. Zimmermann and Rettaliata (1981) evaluated a deaf adult with a childhood-onset progressive hearing loss. This subject's cinefluorographic results, when referenced to the mandible, indicated reduced distinction in tongue shape between vowels and syllable context. Zimmermann and Rettaliata concluded that the distinctions made in the subject's steady-state vowel postures were established with excessive jaw displacement. Tye-Murray (1991), in a microbeam and cinefluorographic study, observed that her three deaf subjects exhibited somewhat reduced tongue mobility but that their mandibles were not excessively mobile in an absolute sense. They did, however, displace their jaws excessively relative to the mobility of the tongue body. In addition, the deaf subjects moved their tongues in a similar fashion regardless of the vowel being produced, whereas the author's normal subjects showed vowel-distinct movement trajectories.

Consonants

Speakers with severe-to-profound hearing loss typically produce a myriad of consonantal errors. Omissions are very common and have a profound negative impact on intelligibility. Other common errors include voiced-voiceless confusions, substitutions, distortions, and errors in consonant clusters (Hudgins & Numbers, 1942; Smith, 1975; Tye-Murray, Spencer, Gilbert-Bedia, & Woodworth, 1996). Further, consonant errors are somewhat more common in the final than initial syllable position, particularly if they are voiced (Markides, 1970; Osberger, Robbins, Lybolt, Kent, & Peters, 1986; Smith, 1975), although Hudgins and Numbers (1942) observed more errors in the initial position. As is the case with vowel production, use of a cochlear implant appears to greatly enhance consonant production. Markides (1970), in the study noted above, found that children with significant hearing loss erred in articulating nearly 72% of their consonants. In contrast, Tobey et al (2003) reported that their young cochlear implant users produced between 65 and 71% consonants correctly (which is an error rate of approximately 35 to 39%).

One of the most frequent consonant errors is one of voicing. Hudgins and Numbers (1942), in their classic study, found that children with hearing loss tend to de-voice voiced consonants. Markides (1970) observed a similar pattern, and Nober (1967) observed that voiceless sounds are more often correct than are voiced sounds. However, Smith (1975) observed a pattern of voiced productions of voiceless sounds, as did Heider, Heider, and Sykes (1941), and Carr (1953). Pratt (2003) remarked that both types of voicing errors can be observed in some children.

Millin (1971) suggested that the voiced-for-voiceless consonant errors are likely due to a mistiming of the initiation and termination of phonation and can be associated with continuous voicing throughout an utterance. Both voicing and devoicing are likely due to inappropriate temporal coordination of the larynx with the upper airway articulators and not phonologic differences. Further, it has been suggested that listener perceptions of the voicing distinctions may be miscued by the durations of the preceding vowels or durations of segments themselves (Gold, 1980; Osberger & McGarr, 1982; Tobey, Pancamo, Staller, Brimacombe, & Beiter, 1991). For example, stop consonants are perceived as voiceless more frequently when preceded by vowels of shorter duration and voiced when preceded by vowels of longer duration (Raphael, 1972). Also, fricatives prolonged relative to a preceding vowel have an increased likelihood of being perceived as voiceless (Denes, 1955).

The instrumental measurements of voicing are consistent with the perceptions of irregular voicing. In a spectrographic study of voice onset time (VOT), Monsen (1976b) observed a tendency for children with profound hearing loss to reduce the VOTs of their initial voiceless stop consonants, although the more intelligible children produced VOT in a manner consistent with hearing children. The less intelligible children had considerable overlap in their VOTs for the voiced and voiceless sounds, with most of their stops produced within the voiced portion of the VOT continuum. Monsen also failed to show differences in VOT relative to place of articulation. McGarr and Löfqvist (1982) obtained similar results in that they found that some of their adult subjects produced VOTs within the perceptual boundary region for voicing, resulting in increased perceptual confusion. Uchanski and Geers (2003) found that although a majority of their 8- and 9-year-old children with cochlear implants produced VOTs within normal limits, a notable proportion produced excessively long and/or short VOTs. Higgins et al (2003) studied a smaller group of older children who wore cochlear implants and also observed reduced VOTs for voiceless plosives, but contrary to Monsen they observed differences across place. Postlingually deafened adults tend to retain correct voicing distinctions, although the VOTs for voiceless sounds tend to be reduced (Lane, Wozniak, & Perkell, 1994; Waldstein, 1990). It has been suggested that voiced productions are unmarked (default), making them more likely and easier to produce when auditory feedback is reduced or eliminated (Lane & Perkell, 2005). Consonant differences related to place of articulation are evident in the speech of persons with hearing loss. Consonants that are associated with visible facial movements, such as bilabials, are more likely to be spoken accurately than consonants that are less visible, such as /k/ and /g/. Several studies involving small groups of children who had received their cochlear implants prior to 5 years of age also have suggested a developmental pattern with a preference for visible consonants (Chin, Tsai, & Gao, 2003; Serry &

Blamey, 1999, 2001). These findings intimate that deaf and hard-of-hearing children attend to the visual cues in their surrounding language community during speech acquisition. It should be noted, though, that McCaffrey and Sussman (1994) did not find this consistently with vowels. In addition, Osberger et al (1986) argued that the superiority of bilabials may be a function of the lips being more constrained in their movements as compared with other articulators such as the tongue, and that visibility may not be the key or only factor. In support of Osberger et al's argument, consonants made in the middle of the mouth often are in error more than sounds made toward the back of the mouth even though they are more visible (Osberger et al, 1986; Smith, 1975).

Talkers with hearing loss also make manner of articulation errors. Characteristically, deaf and hard-of-hearing individuals are more likely to produce plosive consonants more accurately than nasals, fricatives, glides, or laterals, with affricates being particularly difficult (Nober, 1967; Osberger et al, 1986; Smith, 1975), although Blamey and colleagues (Blamey et al, 2001; Serry & Blamey, 1999, 2001) found that glides and nasals developed prior to stops in a group of children who had received cochlear implants at 5 years of age or younger. In most speakers with prelingual hearing loss manner of articulation also interacts with place of articulation and syllable/word position. For example, the fricatives /z/, /ʃ/, and /s/ are difficult to produce but the fricative /f/ usually is produced correctly nearly as often as the plosives /b/ and /p/. In addition, Osberger et al, (1986) found that although plosives were more often correct than fricatives and nasals in the prevocalic position, these types of sounds have similar error rates in the postvocalic position. It should be noted, however, with the high-frequency emphasis and advanced signal processing applied to most cochlear implants, that many early implanted children acquire affricates and fricatives much more easily than their predecessors and peers who were fitted with hearing aids (Tobey et al, 2003; Uchanski & Geers, 2003).

Finally, a speech error frequently associated with speakers with limited residual hearing is glottalization. It is usually expressed by substituting other sounds with glottal stops, particularly back consonants (Levitt, Smith, & Stromberg, 1976). Glottalization may be used as a mechanism to control the airflow through the glottis and not necessarily as a phonological marker. Further, speakers that use glottalization tend to have relatively poor speech intelligibility (Stevens, Nickerson, & Rollins, 1978).

Suprasegmental

As suggested in the previous discussion, the suprasegmental production of deaf speakers often is aberrant. It clearly is not independent of respiratory and laryngeal function nor is it independent of the segmental aspects of speech. Listeners who hear deaf speech for the first time might describe it as sounding labored, effortful, and lacking in rhythm. Speakers with profound hearing loss tend to speak slowly; they may speak at only half the syllable rate of the normal-hearing population (John & Horwarth, 1965; Voelker, 1935). Even children fitted with cochlear implants who have relatively intact segmental characteristics have been found to produce excessively slow speaking rates when producing sentences (Uchanski & Geers, 2003). The reduced rates may be due to sound prolongations, excessive and inappropriate pauses, and insertion of adventitious sounds between phonemes. Inappropriate pausing can occur either due to poor linguistic awareness of where to insert pauses or poor breath control. Although the slow rate of speakers with hearing loss calls attention to itself, Osberger and Levitt (1979) suggested that not all of the factors that contribute to slow rate significantly interfere with intelligibility. They took samples of speech from speakers with hearing loss and digitally altered the timing by correcting for pauses, relative timing, and absolute syllable duration. They found that only correction for relative timing improved intelligibility, and the improvement was small. Correcting for pauses and syllable duration worsened intelligibility, and when the samples were corrected for both relative timing and pauses, intelligibility was substantially worse than for the uncorrected samples. Although not a direct confirmation, the Osberger and Levitt results are consistent with the assertion of Parkhurst and Levitt (1978) that long pauses, if appropriately placed, may improve intelligibility for speakers with hearing loss by allowing more listener processing time. Maassen (1986) found that when pauses were inserted at word boundaries, the intelligibility of deaf speech improved slightly. He postulated that longer pauses at word boundaries may make the boundaries more salient and ease word recognition. He further postulated that treatment of pauses, other than within word pauses, would not likely result in improved intelligibility. Osberger and Levitt also intimated that targeting syllable duration in therapy may decrease, rather than improve, intelligibility.

Poor fundamental frequency and intensity control contributes to the suprasegmental difficulties of speakers with hearing loss. The fundamental frequency of speakers with hearing loss, aside from being higher than normal, also can sound monotonic or fluctuate inappropriately within words and across utterances (Formby & Monsen, 1982; Monsen, 1979; Parkhurst & Levitt, 1978). They also do not show the increased fundamental frequency variations normally associated with reading (Horii, 1982). That is, their fundamental frequency variations tend to be similar regardless of whether the speech is spontaneous or read. Further, it is not unusual for speakers with hearing loss to produce excessively high fundamental frequencies when they initiate utterances. Then the elevated F0 can suddenly drop within the first few hundred milliseconds of the production as if correcting for overshoot. The lack of laryngeal control across utterances also is illustrated by their differential performance with variations in fundamental frequency contour. For example, declining fundamental frequency contours tend to be easier for speakers with hearing loss to produce than are rising or complex contours (Most & Frank, 1991; Rubin-Spitz & McGarr, 1990).

As indicated previously, the vocal intensity of speakers with hearing loss has been described as both excessively low and excessively high. Like fundamental frequency, it may not vary appropriately with the demands of context or environmental conditions (Hood & Dixon, 1969). Further, the prosody of persons with hearing loss, as reflected in stress and phrasing, often is sufficiently impaired so as to interfere with the conveyance of meaning. When Sussman and Hernandez (1979) asked their subjects to produce stressed and unstressed consonant-vowel (CV) syllables, they found that subjects with hearing loss increased their vocal intensity on stressed syllables but not their fundamental frequency. Some speakers with hearing loss also have difficulty producing contrastive stress consistently (Murphy, McGarr, & Bell-Berti, 1990; Sussman & Hernandez, 1979). When asked to produce contrastive stress, subjects with hearing loss often fail to adjust either fundamental frequency or intensity. Osberger and Levitt (1979) observed that some of their speakers with hearing loss failed to produce durational differences for stressed and unstressed syllables. In contrast, Weiss, Carney, and Leonard (1985) found that intelligible children with hearing loss were able to produce perceptually adequate contrastive stress if allowances are made for expressive language skill. Tye-Murray and Folkins (1990) also observed that deaf adult speakers are able to make the necessary articulatory adjustments to produce known stress patterns, further indicating that difficulties with stress production may be related to linguistic knowledge.

Coarticulation

In normal-hearing speakers, movement tends to proceed continuously from one open posture to the next. In contrast, many speakers with severe-to-profound hearing loss, particularly those with reduced intelligibility, may not move their articulators in a continuous, cyclical fashion but as a series of discrete events. For example, in a cinefluorographic study Tye-Murray (1987) observed that during stop consonant production only two of her five subjects with hearing loss adjusted their tongue and jaw postures appropriately in anticipation of following vowels, and these two subjects had relatively high intelligibility. Tye-Murray argued that a lack of distinctiveness between open postures likely contributed to the other subjects' coarticulatory difficulties. Although Stein (1980) and Zimmermann and Rettaliata (1981) suggested that speakers with profound hearing loss distinguish between open postures by altering jaw height, Tye-Murray's less intelligible subjects exhibited no vowel context effects in either jaw or tongue postures. In addition, Tye-Murray, Zimmermann, and Folkins (1987) found that sometimes deaf speakers do not move their articulators toward the open posture during the closed portions of articulations, as do speakers with normal hearing.

Acoustic studies have tended to support the movement data. Consonant-vowel transitions are more restricted in frequency for speakers with hearing loss than those with normal hearing, which can be attributed to vowel neutralization (Monsen, 1976c; Rothman, 1976). Most speakers with hearing loss reduce the duration of the transitions, although some produce excessively lengthened transitions. The formant transitions also vary little with respect to phonetic context suggesting reduced coarticulatory effects. Further, many speakers with hearing loss inconsistently adjust vowel length to accommodate voicing in the postvocalic position (Monsen, 1974; Whitehead & Jones, 1978) and difficulties adjusting vowel duration in response to changes in syllable number also have been observed (Tye-Murray & Woodworth, 1989). That is, as syllable number increases speakers with hearing loss are inconsistent in their reductions of vowel duration, whereas speakers with normal hearing consistently reduce vowel duration as a function of syllable number (e.g., vowel duration in the word *shade* is longer than in the word *shadiness*). Even intelligible speakers may have some difficulty coordinating their speech movements over time. Waldstein and Baum (1991) and Baum and Waldstein (1991) measured both the anticipatory and perseveratory speech behaviors of a group of intelligible children with profound hearing loss by using temporal and spectral acoustic measures (centroid and F2). The children with hearing loss produced both types of coarticulatory behaviors but to a lesser extent than the normal-hearing subjects. An acoustic analysis performed on consonant-vowel-consonant words spoken in sentence context (Uchanski & Geers, 2003) revealed that, on average, children fitted with cochlear implants produce longer vowel durations relative to total word duration than do children with normal hearing.

Viewing the speech of persons with hearing loss as discrete articulatory events is not supported by an acoustic study by Robb and Pang-Ching (1992). They analyzed the absolute and relative speech timing of 31 young adults with hearing loss who varied with regard to overall intelligibility. Thirteen normal-hearing adults served as controls. Robb and Pang-Ching followed the measurement procedures of Weismer and Fennell (1985) and found that although their subjects with hearing loss were slower and produced greater absolute durations, their relative timing was no different than the normal-hearing subjects. Robb and Pang-Ching also found no relationship between relative timing, and speaker intelligibility or degree of hearing loss. If the speakers with hearing loss produced their speech segments as linearly sequenced independent units, it is unlikely that relative timing would hold across utterances. Similar results have been observed with the speech of other groups associated with temporal disturbances such as people with dysarthria, apraxia, and stuttering (Prosek, Montgomery, & Walden, 1988; Weismer & Fennell, 1985), although McNeil, Liss, Tseng, and Kent (1990) observed irregularities in groups of subjects with apraxia and conduction aphasia. Robb and Pang-Ching argued that the temporal differences observed in speakers with hearing loss were of magnitude and not abnormality. They also suggested that their data were consistent with the temporal properties of speech being biologically constrained and independent, to some extent, of auditory feedback. The data of Tye-Murray (1984) and Tye-Murray and Folkins (1990) support this notion. They observed that when speech tasks require alterations such as changes in rate or stress, deaf speakers are able to make the necessary articulatory adjustments (i.e., jaw and lower lip displacements) online.

◆ Developmental Speech Characteristics

Many infants and young children with hearing loss demonstrate delays and developmental patterns that differ from normal-hearing children, especially if the hearing loss is identified late or after a period of protracted hearing loss. Babbling generally does not appear before 12 months of age (Oller & Eilers, 1988; Oller, Eilers, Bull, & Carney, 1985), and canonical babble (well formed and temporally consistent with adult speech) has been observed as late as 31 months in this population (Lynch, Oller, & Steffens, 1989). Infants also produce fewer instances of canonical babble and include a more limited range of consonants in their babble (Stoel-Gammon, 1988; Stoel-Gammon & Otomo, 1986; Wallace, Menn, & Yoshinaga-Itano, 1998). However, later speech intelligibility is better predicted by the consonant inventory used in emerging spoken language during the second year of life than during babble (Obenchain, Menn, & Yoshinaga-Itano, 1998). The phonetic repertoires of infants with severe-to-profound hearing loss often are restricted when compared with their normal-hearing peers, although there is abundant individual variability (Lach, Ling, Ling, & Ship, 1970; Stoel-Gammon & Otomo, 1986; Wallace et al, 1998; Yoshinaga-Itano & Sedey, 1998). The early speech inventories of infants with severe-to-profound hearing loss consist predominately of motorically easy sounds such as vowels and bilabial consonants. The sounds of their inventories also contain more low-frequency information and are more audible. For example, the babbling of infants with hearing loss often has a high concentration of nasals and glides, which include low-frequency continuant cues (Stoel-Gammon & Otomo, 1986).

Without intensive treatment and appropriate fitting of sensory aids, such as high-quality hearing aids and cochlear implants, the speech sound inventories of many children with hearing loss usually do not attain full maturity. Yoshinaga-Itano and Sedey (1998) found that children with moderate-to-severe hearing losses did not reach a full complement of vowel and consonant sounds until approximately 4 and 5 years of age, respectively, and many children with profound hearing loss had restricted inventories even at 5 years of age. As a result, children with profound hearing loss often reach an early plateau in their speech skill development. For instance, the speech characteristics of many children with severe-to-profound hearing loss demonstrate little improvement in sound inventory and production after 8 years of age even with the initiation of extensive training (Hudgins & Number, 1942, McGarr, 1987; Smith, 1975). Such results making it evident that, like auditory and language interventions, speech production therapy should be an important component of early intervention and that the common practice of delaying speech training in children with hearing loss until they have functional language is developmentally untenable if the goal is for them to be oral communicators.

Several studies have examined the speech characteristics of children aged 8 years and older, and examined performance as a function of age. Hudgins and Numbers (1942) included subjects aged 8 to 20 years in their study. They found little improvement in speech performance as a function of age, as did Smith (1975) in a similar study performed 30 years later. McGarr (1987) studied children longitudinally between the ages of 11 and 14 years. She found little change in the average number and types of vowel and diphthong errors over time. The implication is that intervention (fitting of sensory aids, behavioral) should occur early.

Many factors probably contribute to the development of speech errors that have been reviewed in this section. These factors include a child's home environment, educational placement, and quality and quantity of direct speech intervention received, the child's personality and interest in acquiring spoken language, and other individual characteristics such as developmental delay (Edwards, Frost, & Witham, 2006). However, the most predominant factors are probably the amount and quality of residual hearing, the age of onset and identification, and the age of intervention. There is some indication that age of onset is a critical factor even with speakers with adventitious hearing loss (Lane et al, 1995).

♦ The Role of Audition in Development

Tye-Murray (1992) proposed that auditory information plays five important roles during the acquisition of speech. First, audition allows the child to develop specific principles of articulatory organization. By listening to other members of the language community, a child learns to regulate speech breathing, learns how to flex and extend the tongue body, and learns how to rhythmically alternate between vowels and consonants (i.e., open and closed vocal tract positions). Second, audition enables children to learn how to produce specific speech events. For instance, a child might learn to distinguish /t/ with a rapid downward tongue movement and /l/ with a gesture of slower velocity. Third, children utilize auditory information to develop a system of phonological performance. That is, they learn the phonemes of their language by listening to others use them in speech production. They also learn the rules of acceptability for combining phonemes and syllable structures. Fourth,

auditory information informs a child about the consequences of a particular articulatory gesture, and enables the child to compare those consequences with the speech outputs of other talkers. Fifth, when attending to auditory signals, a child may learn to monitor ongoing speech production, and detect and correct speech errors. Subsequent sections of this chapter discuss teaching methods that may influence a child's acquisition of speech production skills and how the influences of the auditory system in speech production might be augmented or assumed by other mechanisms.

♦ Concomitant Nonspeech Characteristics

Hearing loss may or may not be associated with concomitant deficits. Whether deficits are associated with a hearing loss is largely dependent on the cause of the hearing loss, the site of the lesion, and the developmental status at insult. For example, a noise-induced hearing loss occurring in a young adult has a more limited likelihood of concomitant deficits than a hearing loss in a young child due to bacterial meningitis or a genetic disorder. There are a large number of conditions known to cause or be associated with hearing loss. Approximately 25% of prelingual hearing losses are idiopathic, and 54% of school-aged children with hearing loss report a hearing loss of unknown etiology, making it difficult to clearly associate hearing loss with many co-occurring conditions (Gallaudet Research Institute, 2005; Smith & Van Camp, 2006). This issue becomes more complex with the elderly, in whom hearing loss becomes interrelated with socioeconomic and health care factors as well as cognitive and physical decline (National Center for Health Statistics, 1982).

There are several ways in which causes and associated characteristics have been categorized in the literature. **Table 13–1** is a simple listing of characteristics that have

Table 13–1   Some Nonspeech Deficits Associated with Hearing Loss

A. Cognitive deficits
  1. Mental retardation
  2. Dementia
B. Behavioral disorder
C. Psychiatric disorder
D. Language delay and disorder
E. Learning disability
  1. Reading deficits
  2. Writing deficits
F. Nervous system disease
  1. Motor disturbances
  2. Seizures
  3. Glioma or neuroma
  4. Spina bifida
  5. Impaired taste and smell
  6. Vestibular disturbances

Table 13–1 *(Continued)*   Some Nonspeech Deficits Associated with Hearing Loss

G. Eye disease
  1. Optic degeneration and atrophy
  2. Ocular lens abnormalities
  3. Retinitis pigmentosa
      a. Night blindness
      b. Tunnel vision
      c. Blindness
  4. Oculomotor disturbances
H. Renal disease
I. Musculoskeletal disease
  1. Head and neck abnormalities
      a. Abnormalities of the skull
      b. Malformations of the lip and palate
      c. Eyelid malformations
      d. Abnormal facial features
      e. Malformations of the outer ear
      f. Malformations of the middle ear
      g. Mandible and maxillary malformations
      h. Dental abnormalities
      i. Nasal abnormalities
  2. Digital anomalies
  3. Limb abnormalities
  4. Joint abnormalities
  5. Limb and joint pain
  6. Bone disease
  7. Growth retardation
  8. Vertebral abnormalities
  9. Shoulder abnormalities
  10. Winged scapula
J. Skin disease
  1. Pigmentary disorder
      a. Albinism
      b. White forelock
      c. Vitiligo
      d. Leukonychia
      e. Café-au-lait spots
      f. Axillary freckling
      g. Iris bicolor or heterochromia
      h. Salt-and-pepper retinal pigmentation
  2. Lichenified skin eruptions
  3. Recurrent urticaria
  4. Keratosis
  5. Sun sensitivity
  6. Thick, course hair
  7. Abnormal whorl patterns on hands
  8. Malformed fingernails and toenails
K. Metabolic disease
  1. Diabetes
  2. Goiter
  3. Liver and spleen enlargement
  4. Impaired metabolism of carbohydrates
L. Cardiac and vascular disease
M. Urogenital malformations

been acknowledged to coexist with hearing loss. Some co-occur due to shared causative or predisposing factors, whereas others are a result of the hearing loss. Many of these characteristics occur in constellations or syndromes. It is estimated that approximately 50% of all prelingual hearing losses are genetic in nature and of those approximately 30% are syndromic (Nance, 2003; Smith & Van Camp, 2006). Some of the genetic syndromes commonly associated with hearing loss are listed in **Table 13–2.** As there are well over 400 such identified syndromes associated with hearing loss, readers are encouraged to refer to Toriello, Reardon, and Gorlin (2004) for characteristics specific to particular syndromes.

◆ Evaluation Procedures

Sensory

The first step in the evaluation process is the determination of the speaker's sensory skills. In particular, the determination of aided auditory sensitivity and acuity is important because these measures provide an anchor for predicting what further tests and evaluation procedures would be most appropriate. They also may provide a basis for selecting the most advantageous treatment approach. In addition to auditory testing, visual, tactile, proprioceptive, and kinesthetic perceptual testing may provide useful information relative to treatment, especially if a multisensory treatment approach is used (see Chapter 2). It cannot be assumed that a person with a hearing loss can compensate easily through other modalities such as vision or taction. From what is known about syndromes associated with and causes of hearing loss, a higher likelihood of multimodality impairment should be expected.

Structural

After sensory status has been determined, the integrity of the speech apparatus should be assessed via an age-appropriate oral peripheral examination. The Oral Speech Mechanism Screening Examination-Revised (St. Louis & Ruscello, 1987) is an example of a format that can be used with adults. The protocol described by Robbins and Klee (1987) is an example of a protocol that can be used with children. As with concomitant sensory deficits, people with hearing impairment have a high risk of concomitant oral-facial anomalies such as cleft palate. [When assessing speakers with oral-facial anomalies, the approach described by Dworkin, Marunick, and Krouse (2004) may be useful.] Also, it is generally believed that people with hearing loss have a higher prevalence of dysarthria and apraxia of speech despite there being very little documentation to support this belief. Confirming an apraxia of speech in a person with hearing loss, particularly a child, can be difficult because they often have restricted phonologic and phonetic repertoires, making the distinction between an apraxia effect and a hearing loss effect problematic.

Speech

Speech production can be assessed perceptually as well as instrumentally. The human ear remains the most powerful tool for separating normal from abnormal speech production. It can perceive acoustic nuances associated with abnormalities that are often obscured by noise or complexity in instrumental recordings. However, as with many other sensorimotor speech disorders, some hearing-impaired speakers' errors are so unusual or difficult to explain that the added information provided by instruments may assist in the diagnostic process.

Perceptual

When speakers with hearing loss exhibit mild segmental differences, it is usually acceptable to use assessment protocols developed for hearing individuals. Using articulation and phonology assessment tools that were standardized on hearing individuals is reasonable, particularly if the hearing loss is mild to moderate and the person is well aided. To assess people who are more impaired, there are several assessment protocols that have been developed and standardized to guide the perceptual analysis. Some of the tools are structured to evaluate segmental and suprasegmental aspects of speech whereas others are used to assess overall intelligibility.

An evaluation approach commonly used with young children includes the Phonetic Level and Phonologic Level Speech Evaluation protocols developed by Ling (1976). They are criterion-referenced procedures that accompany Ling's treatment approach, which is discussed later. In the Phonetic Level Speech Evaluation the children's imitative vocal characteristics are judged for presence, pitch, duration, and intensity. Vowels and diphthongs are elicited as single syllables, repeated, alternated, and produced with varying pitch. Simple consonants and blends are evaluated primarily at a structured syllabic-unit level. The syllables are initially elicited as isolated syllables and then repeated, alternated, and produced at varying loudness and pitch levels. Word position effects also are assessed. In contrast, the Phonologic Level Speech Evaluation focuses on the quality and complexity of the children's speech at the discourse level. It is a checklist of the children's vocal control, linguistic structure, phonemic inventory, and intelligibility when speaking voluntarily in a nonstructured situation.

The strength of Ling's two assessment procedures is that they relate directly to his treatment program. They also include tasks that are simple enough so that very young and very involved children can be assessed. Problematic for the procedures is that no normative data accompany the protocols, which are published in the book describing the Ling (1976, 2002) treatment approach. In addition, the reliability and linearity of the protocols has been questioned (Dunn & Newton, 1986; Shaw & Coggins, 1991).

The Central Institute for the Deaf (CID) Phonetic Inventory (Moog, 1989) is similar to the Phonetic Level Speech Evaluation in structure and also is based largely on a syllable unit. It was developed primarily for young children or children with severe speech difficulties. In this test, the

Table 13–2 Some Syndromes Commonly Associated with Hearing Loss According to Major Systems Affected

Syndrome/Disease	Type & Degree of Hearing Loss	Oral	Cognitive/Learning	Psychiatric	Nervous System	Vestibular	Pulmonary	Eye	Renal	Musculo-skeletal	Integu-mentary	Endocrine/Metabolic	Cardio-vascular	Urogenital	Inheritance
					Major System Abnormalities										
Familial streptomycin ototoxicity	S-1 to 4*					X									Mit
Ataxia, hypogonadotrophic hypogonadism, mental retardation, and sensorineural hearing loss (Richards-Rundle)	S-1 to 3-p		X		X*			X		X	X	X		X	AR
Ataxia and sensorineural hearing loss (Lichtenstein-Knorr)	S-4-c p/dp	X			X*			X		X			X		AR
Cockayne	S-1 to 3-dp	X	X		X*			X	X	X	X				AR
Hallgren	S-3-dp		X	X	X*			X	X					X	AR or Mit
Motor and sensory neuropathy, optic atrophy, and sensorineural hearing loss, X-linked (Rosenberg-Chutorian)	S-3-p				X*			X		X				X	XR
Motor and sensory neuropathy with sensorineural hearing loss, autosomal dominant (AD) (Charcot-Marie-Tooth)	S-3-p				X*										AD
Motor and sensory neuropathy with sensorineural hearing loss, autosomal recessive (AR) (Charcot-Marie-Tooth; Bouldin)	S-1 to 4-c/p				X*					X					AR
Motor and sensory neuropathy with sensorineural hearing loss, X-linked (X-L) (Charcot-Marie-Tooth; Cowchock)	S-3-d		X		X*					X					XR

(Continued on page 216)

Table 13–2 (Continued) Some Syndromes Commonly Associated with Hearing Loss According to Major Systems Affected

Syndrome/Disease	Type & Degree of Hearing Loss	Oral	Cognitive/Learning	Psychiatric	Nervous System	Vestibular	Pulmonary	Eye	Renal	Musculo-skeletal	Integu-mentary	Endocrine/Metabolic	Cardio-vascular	Urogenital	Inheritance
Myoclonus epilepsy, ataxia, and sensorineural hearing loss (May-White)	S-2 to 3-dp	X			X*	X		X				X			AD
Myoclonus epilepsy, dementia, and sensorineural hearing loss (Latham-Munro)	S-4-c	X	X	X	X*			X				X	X		AR
Neurofibromatosis, type II (vestibular schwannomas and neural hearing loss)	S-4-dp	X			X*	X		X			X				AD
Infantile Refsum	S-4-c		X		X			X*		X	X	X			AR
Pigmentary retinopathy, diabetes mellitus, hypogonadism, mental retardation, and sensorineural hearing loss (Edwards)	S-2 to 3-dp		X		X			X*		X	X	X	X	X	AR
Pigmentary retinopathy, diabetes mellitus, obesity, and sensorineural hearing loss (Alström)	S-3-dp							X*		X	X	X		X	AR
Norrie (oculoacoustico cerebral dysplasia)	S-1 to 3-dp		X	X	X			X*							XR
Adult Refsum (heredopathia atactica polyneuritiformis)	S-1 to 3-dp				X			X*		X	X	X	X		AR
Usher, types I and II	S-1 to 4-c/p		X	X	X	X		X*							AR
Renal tubular acidosis with progressive hearing loss	S-1 to 4-p				X	X		X	X*	X		X			AR

Major System Abnormalities

216

Table 13–2 *(Continued)* Some Syndromes Commonly Associated with Hearing Loss According to Major Systems Affected

Syndrome	Hearing loss	1	2	3	4	5	6	Inheritance
Alport (nephritis and sensorineural hearing loss)	S-1 to 4-dp	X		X*	X	X	X	XR, AD, or AR
Nonmuscle myosin heavy chain IIA (MYH9A) syndrome	S-2 to 3-dp			X*	X	X		AD
Nephritis, motor and neuropathy with sensorineural hearing loss (Lemieux-Neemeh)	S-1 to 4-dp			X*	X	X		AD
Nephritis, urticaria, amyloidosis, and sensorineural hearing loss (Muckle-Wells)	S-3-dp			X*	X		X	AD
Renal, genital, and middle ear (Winter)	C-1 to 2-c/p	X	X	X*	X		X	AR
Apert (craniosynostosis)	C-1 to 2-c	X	X	X*	X			AD
Branchio-otorenal (BOR); brachio-oto; ear-pit hearing loss	C/S/M-1 to 4-c/d	X	X	Xex	X		X	AD
CHARGE	C/S/M-1 to 4-c	X	X	Xex	X		X	AD or AR
Otofaciocervical	C-1 to 3-c	X	X	Xex	X			AD
Crouzon	C-1 to 2-c	X	X	X*	X			AD
Craniodiaphyseal dysplasia	M-1 to 4-p	X	X	X*	X		X	Unknown
Craniotubular	M-1 to 3-dp	X	X	X*	X			AD or AR
DiGeorge (Pye)	C/M-1 to 4-c	X	X	X	X	X*	X	AD, AR or Ch
Ectodactyly-ectodermal dysplasia clefting (EEC)	C/S/M-1 to 4-c	X	X	X*	X		X	AD
Fibrodysplasia ossificans progressiva (FOP)	C/S-1 to 3-dp	X	X	X*	X			AD
Hyperphosphatasemia (juvenile Paget's)	M-2 to 3-dp	X	X	X*	X	X		AR

(Continued on page 218)

Table 13–2 (*Continued*) Some Syndromes Commonly Associated with Hearing Loss According to Major Systems Affected

Syndrome/Disease	Type & Degree of Hearing Loss	Major System Abnormalities													Inheritance
		Oral	Cognitive/Learning	Psychiatric	Nervous System	Vestibular	Pulmonary	Eye	Renal	Musculo-skeletal	Integu-mentary	Endocrine/Metabolic	Cardio-vascular	Urogenital	
Joint fusion, mitral insufficiency and conductive hearing loss (Forney)	C-1 to 3-c									Xex	X		X		AD
Kniest (metatropic dysplasia, type II)	C/S/M-1 to 3-dp	X						X		X*			X		AD
Lacrimoauriculodento-digital (LADD; Levy-Hollister)	M-1 to 3-C	X						X	X	Xex					AD
Lop ears, micrognathia, and conductive loss	C/M-1 to 3-c	X								Xex					AD
Mandibulofacial dysostosis (Treacher Collins)	C/M-1 to 4-c	X	X			X		X		Xex					AD
Oculoauriculo vertebral (Goldenhar)	C/S-1 to 3-c	X	X		X		X	X	X	X*			X		AD
Osteogenesis imperfecta, types I to IV	C/M-1 to 3-dp	X						X		X*			X		AD
Otopalatodigital, types I and II	C/M-1 to 3-c	X	X		X			X		X*					XR
Severe autosomal recessive osteopetrosis (Albers-Schönberg)	C/M-1 to 2-dp	X	X		X			X	X	X*		X			AR
Stickler (Marshall-Stickler; hereditary arthro-ophthalmopathy)	C/S/M-1 to 3-p	X						X		X*					AD
van Buchem's (generalized cortical hyperostosis)	S/M-1 to 3-dp	X			X			X		X*		X			AR

Table 13–2 *(Continued)* Some Syndromes Commonly Associated with Hearing Loss According to Major Systems Affected

Syndrome	Code											Inheritance
Wildervanck (cervico-oculoacoustic; Klippel-Feil anomaly plus)	C/S/M-1 to 4-c/d	X	X	X	X		X	X		X*			Unknown
Dominant onychodystrophy, coniform teeth, and sensorineural hearing loss (Robinson)	S-1 to 4-c	X		X			X	X*	X				AD
Dominant onychodystrophy, triphalangeal thumbs, and sensorineural hearing loss (Goodman-Moghadam)	S-2 to 3-c						X	X*					AD
Dominant piebald trait and sensorineural hearing loss (Telfer)	S-1 to 4-p	X		X			X	X*					AD
Multiple lentigines (LEOPARD)	S-1 to 3-c/p	X		X	X	X	X	X*	X*			X	AD
Pili torti and sensorineural hearing loss (Björnstad)	S-1 to 4-c						X	X*				X	AR
Waardenburg, types I and II	S-1 to 3-c/p	X		X	X		X	X*	X*		X	X	AD or AR
Diabetes insipidus, diabetes mellitus, optic atrophy, and sensorineural hearing loss (DIDMOAD); Wolfram	S-2 to 3-dp	X	X	X		X	X	X*	X*		X	X	AR
Goiter and profound congenital sensorineural hearing loss (Pendred)	S-1 to 4-c/p			X			X	X	X*		X*		AR
Mucopolysaccharidosis I-H (MPS I-H; Hurler)	C/S/M-1 to 3-p	X	X	X	X		X	X	X*	X*	X	X	AR

(Continued on page 220)

Table 13–2 (Continued) Some Syndromes Commonly Associated with Hearing Loss According to Major Systems Affected

Syndrome/ Disease	Type & Degree of Hearing Loss	Oral	Cognitive/ Learning	Psychiatric	Nervous System	Vestibular	Pulmonary	Eye	Renal	Musculo-skeletal	Integu-mentary	Endocrine/ Metabolic	Cardio-vascular	Urogenital	Inheritance
					Major System Abnormalities										
Mucopolysaccharidosis I-S (MPS I-S; Scheie)	M-1 to 2-p	X			X			X		X	X	X*	X		AR
Mucopolysaccharidosis I-H/S (MPS I-H/S; Hurler-Scheie)	C/S/M-1 to 3-p	X			X		X	X		X	X	X*	X		AR
Mucopolysaccharidosis II (MPS II; Hunter)	S/M-1 to 2-p		X		X	X				X	X	X*	X		XR
Mucopolysaccharidosis III (MPS III; Sanfilipo)	S/M-1 to 2-dp	X	X	X	X					X	X	X*	X		AR
α-D-Mannosidosis	S/3-dp	X	X		X		X	X		X		X*			AR
Electrocardiographic abnormalities, fainting spells, and sudden death with sensorineural hearing loss (Jervell Lange-Nielsen; cardioaudition; surdocardiac; long Q-T)	S-3 to 4-c											X	X*		AR
Sickle cell	C/S/M-1 to 4-p								X	X	X	X	X*		AR
Trisomy 21	C/S/M-1 to 4-c	X	X		X		X	X*		X	X		X	X	Ch*
Turner (Ullrich-Turner)	C/S/M-1 to 2-c	X	X	X	X			X*	X	X	X	X	X	X	Ch*

Note. An X designates each major system that is characteristically affected with each syndrome. Asterisk (*) indicates the major system that is most likely involved and best characterizes the syndrome.

Under the system Musculoskeletal, the superscript ex designates the musculoskeletal malformations are primarily limited to the external ear.

Under type and degree of hearing loss: C, conductive hearing loss; S, sensorineural hearing loss; M, mixed hearing loss. The numbers 1 through 4 refer to the degree of hearing loss with 1 being a mild loss, 2 a moderate loss, 3 a severe loss, and 4 a profound loss. The small letters refer to the time course of the hearing loss: c, congenital hearing loss; d, delayed onset; p, progressive hearing loss with delayed onset.

Under inheritance: AD, autosomal dominant; AR, autosomal recessive; Ch, chromosomal disorder; Mit, mitochondrial.

CHARGE, coloboma, heart disease, atresia choanae, retardation, genital hypoplasia, and ear anomalies; LEOPARD, lentigines, electrocardiographic conduction abnormalities, ocular hypertelorism, pulmonary stenosis, abnormal genitalia, retardation, and deafness.

Source: The information in this table was modified from Gorlin, Toriello, and Cohen (1995) and Toriello, Reardon, and Gorlin (2004).

children are shown a series of printed cards along with spoken models for imitation. The areas tested include suprasegmentals, vowels, diphthongs, and consonants in various syllable configurations. The results are plotted in percent correct per category and are profiled. However, like the Ling assessment procedures, the CID Phonetic Inventory is lacking in normative and validation data. The manual also lacks information for interpreting the profiles and there is no indication that the percentages are equivalent across the categories assessed.

Although out of print, the Fundamental Speech Skills Test (Levitt, Youdelman, & Head, 1990) is a well-constructed tool for assessing speech in persons with substantial speech impairment. It is similar to Ling's two assessment procedures in orientation but is more contained and streamlined. It was developed to test children above 5 years of age and adults who have severe-to-profound hearing loss. It was structured to evaluate phonatory, suprasegmental, and segmental aspects of speech at varying levels of complexity. Speech behaviors are elicited with picture plates containing symbols, syllable strings, words, and pictures. Although not required, patients who can read are at an advantage. The test results are compared with norms based on age and degree of hearing loss, although the derivation of the norms are not made explicit and there is no documentation of reliability or validity.

Unlike the above listed evaluation protocols, the Speech Intelligibility Evaluation (SPINE) (Monsen, 1981) is not an assessment of isolated speech skills but a means to document the overall intelligibility of a speaker's productions at the single-word level. It was developed for individuals with severe-to-profound hearing loss who had at least single-word reading skills. The test is not commercially available, so the materials, consisting of 40 cards with single words printed on them, must be constructed by the examiner. The cards are arranged into 10 phonemically contrastive sets of four cards. The contrasts are primarily of vowel characteristics and voicing. For each set, the cards are individually directed toward the patient and away from the examiner. The patient is asked to produce the word aloud and the examiner records what he/she thinks the patient said. The percentage of words correctly identified by the examiner is the patient's intelligibility score. Although usable normative data have not been reported for the SPINE, validity and reliability results have been published and were acceptably high.

The CID Picture SPINE (Monsen, Moog, & Geers, 1988) was developed to assess speech intelligibility in young children and children who have poor reading skills. It was constructed and administered in the same way as the SPINE except that pictures rather than printed words are used. The materials are commercially available and a standardized format is used. Norms are available and measures of reliability and validity are provided. One limitation of the CID Picture SPINE is that the use of simple pictures reduces the types of contrasts that can be tested. In addition, the vocabulary level of the pictures is uneven and can interact with the results. It is not unusual to have to train young children to recognize some of the pictures.

Subtelny and her associates developed a set of rating scales often referred to as the National Technical Institute for the Deaf (NTID) Speech and Voice Rating Scales (or NTID Rating Scales). Although they are described in several publications, they are published in their most complete form as part of a perceptual training program called the Speech and Voice Characteristics of the Deaf (Subtelny, Orlando, & Whitehead, 1981). The training program includes a series of audiotapes that are used to train judgments of overall intelligibility, pitch, resonance, voice quality, and rate. The rating scales, as part of the training program, include categories for intelligibility, pitch register, pitch control, rate, air expenditure, prosodic features, a breathy-weak voice dimension, a tense-harsh vocal dimension, nasal resonance, and pharyngeal resonance. Each category is assessed on a five-point scale with descriptors applied to each point per category. The speaker reads the rainbow passage (Fairbanks, 1960, p. 127) or the CID Everyday Sentences (Silverman & Hirsh, 1955) and the examiner judges the speech according to all 10 categories. Its use with spontaneous speech also has been described (Subtelny, 1977). Although the training program is an attempt to increase rater reliability, there is some indication that multiple raters should be used when assessing a person's speech with these scales making the scales somewhat impractical.

Of all the NTID Speech and Voice Rating Scales, the intelligibility scale has received the greatest amount of attention partly because intelligibility is an overall characteristic of speech, but also because of the multiple factors that can affect intelligibility ratings. For example, experienced raters tend to score speech as more intelligible than inexperienced listeners (McGarr, 1983; Monsen, 1978, 1983). Context and predictability of speech materials tend to affect all listeners similarly regardless of level of experience, although better speakers benefit from increased context whereas poorer speakers perform less well when context is increased (McGarr, 1983; Sitler, Schiavetti, & Metz, 1983). Further, Schiavetti, Metz, and Sitler (1981) questioned the use of interval scaling procedures when assessing speech intelligibility. Samar and Metz (1988) supported this claim. They found that the validity of the midrange of the NTID intelligibility scale was compromised because of extreme confidence intervals despite acceptable reliability and validity quotients. More recently the Speech Intelligibility Rating scale (Dyar, 1994; Parker & Irlam 1995) has been used to rate the speech intelligibility of children who wear cochlear implants, and although its reliability has been documented when used by experienced listeners, it suffers from many of the inadequacies of the NTID intelligibility rating scale (Allen, Nikolopoulos, Dyar, & O'Donoghue, 2001; Edwards et al, 2006; Peng et al, 2004). Rather than intelligibility rating scales, Samar and Metz recommended using write-down procedures like the SPINE, which tend to be more accurate in the mid-skill range.

Instrumental

As with perceptual tools, the selection of instruments for use in an assessment depends on the characteristics of the patient, the questions needing to be addressed, and the specific purpose of the assessment. For example, if the purpose is to document to a third party that respiratory function for speech is abnormal and needs to be treated, then normative data should be available on the tool selected. The tool also must be sensitive and reliable enough to differentiate normal from abnormal function. For many of the instrumental tools available to clinicians, these types of data are not available, which limits their applicability, particularly with the pediatric population.

Pragmatically, there also is the issue of tool availability, practicality, and ease of use. With the advances in digital signal processing, the increased availability of low-cost computers, and the commercial introduction of user-friendly speech analysis software systems, the options for assessing patients are substantial. Some systems are dedicated to a particular parameter of speech such as fundamental frequency or nasality, but many of the systems are multimodular and include modules that can be used for treatment as well as assessment and are therefore more cost-effective for many clinicians. All of these instrumental measures are addressed in detail in earlier chapters in this volume. Those specific tools and measurement parameters most applicable and most frequently used with deaf and hearing-impaired individuals (acoustic, kinematic, and aerodynamic) are reviewed below.

Acoustic

Acoustic analyses can be done in several ways and can target various speech characteristics (see Chapter 4). Wideband spectrograms have been used to look at the center frequencies of vowel formants, formant transitions, and VOT (McCaffrey & Sussman, 1994; Monsen, 1976a–c; Waldstein, 1990), but wideband spectrograms can be problematic when assessing speakers with hearing loss if the bandwidth of the analysis system is not adjustable, which is particularly true when measuring vowel formants. Speakers with excessively high fundamental frequencies produce spectrograms that represent multiple harmonics rather than formants. In addition to being observed in some speakers with hearing loss, this is commonly observed with hearing infants, young children, and women. This phenomenon is due to the harmonics being excessively spaced relative to the filter bandwidths and can be compensated for by increasing the bandwidth of the analysis filters. Kent and Read (1992) recommended that the bandwidth of the analyzing filter be two to three times as large as the fundamental frequency. Another suggested method for measuring formant frequencies has been to use spectra derived from linear predictive coding because unlike spectra derived with a Fourier analysis, it does not represent the harmonics of the fundamental but rather the formant frequencies and amplitudes. It is therefore less directly dependent on the fundamental frequency and the integrity of the harmonic structure. However, when the reliability of measuring formant frequencies derived with linear predictive coding was compared with analogous measurements from spectrograms, both types of analyses became unstable with samples having fundamental frequencies above 350 Hz (Monsen & Engebretson, 1983). Further, most linear predictive coding algorithms do not account for antiresonances in their models, so the introduction of nasalization and lateralization can be problematic (Kent & Read, 1992).

Fundamental frequency is a common acoustic feature measured with hearing-impaired speakers because of their difficulties with habitual fundamental frequency and F0 control. There are several extractions methods available. They vary from measuring waveforms and narrowband spectrograms by hand to digital computational methods. In addition, many digital acoustic analysis systems provide more than one extraction option. Many of the problems associated with measuring fundamental frequency speakers with hearing loss are the same as those encountered when measuring the fundamental frequency of women and children. Many of the algorithms have difficulty processing high-frequency signals accurately as reflected in frequency doubling, halving, and dropouts. The problem can be compounded by the presence of irregularities in the glottal waveform that are commonly associated with speakers with hearing loss, irregularities that also often preclude the use of fine-grained vocal acoustic analyses such as shimmer and jitter. Electroglottographic, accelerometric, inverse filtering, and other digital signal processing methods can be used to avoid some of these problems and are becoming increasingly more available to clinicians.

Problems associated with nasal resonance can be assessed by viewing palatal movement and by direct measures of inappropriate absence or presence of nasal emission (e.g., nasal mirror, nasal airflow), but acoustically nasal resonance is often measured acoustically with a nasometer. Nasometers compare the relative intensity of sound coming through the nose and the mouth. Normative data are available for standard speech samples but are limited for very young children and speakers who have poor language and reading skills (Dalston & Seaver, 1990; Seaver, Dalston, Leeper, & Adams, 1991). In addition, the headsets are heavy and cumbersome for very young children. Although not a test of resonance per se, Goldhor (1995) developed the Nasal Manner Metric for assessing the distinctiveness of nasal-vowel boundaries. As such, it is considered an acoustic correlate of the phonetic feature of nasality. The metric considers the duration of the nasal segment, the total power of the nasal segment, and the power of the nasal and vowel segments below 750 Hz. This metric has been used successfully with children with normal hearing and children with hearing loss (Uchanski & Geers, 2003). An alternative to acoustic measures is to use an accelerometer attached to the side of the nose. It can be input to many of the analysis systems that read simple voltages. For example, it can be put into the microphone ports of many computer-based speech training systems. Accelerometers have the advantages of being small, noninvasive, and relatively inexpensive. There are data supporting the validity of using them to measure nasality in speakers with hearing loss (Stevens et al, 1976), and some normative data have been collected on normal-hearing adults (Lippmann, 1981). Placement and degree of contact on the nose are major considerations, however, when obtaining accelerometric results (Lippmann, 1981).

Movement

Some data are available on speech movements, but most have been collected on a small number of intelligible adult speakers with concentration on the tongue (Tye et al, 1983; Tye-Murray, 1991; Zimmermann & Rettaliata, 1981). In addition, most of the early data were collected with systems that required exposure to radiation or were not commercially available (i.e., x-ray microbeam, cinefluoroscopy, glossometry). However, methods are readily available with which clinicians can assess laryngeal and palatal movements as well as lingual-palatal contact. Electroglottography and videostroboscopy can be used to provide information about laryngeal movements and postures. Nasal endoscopy and photodetection methods can be used to assess palatal movements (Dalston, 1989; Dalston & Seaver, 1990; Karnell, Seaver, & Dalston, 1988). The use of ultrasound and light emitting diodes tracking systems also shows promise in assessing intraoral movements (Bernhardt, Gick, Bacsfalvi, & Adler-Bock, 2005; Bressmann et al, 2005; Whalen et al, 2005). Although not providing direct information about movement, electropalatometry has been applied to speakers with hearing impairment and can be used to provide information about patterns of lingual-palatal contact. Dagenais and Critz-Crosby (1992) identified five patterns commonly associated with deaf speakers. The patterns included an open configuration with little or no contact, a closed configuration with full lingual-palatal contact, front occlusion with lingual contact around the entire alveolar ridge, back occlusion with contact only toward that back of the palate, and a grooved configuration. Dagenais and Critz-Crosby observed that these patterns often are used idiosyncratically by deaf speakers, particularly those with poor intelligibility. Advances have been made in the construction of electropalatometers and in the quantification of data coming from the devices making them more useful in the diagnosis and treatment of speech disorders (McAuliffe, Ward, & Murdoch, 2006; Scobbie, Wood, & Wrench, 2004).

Airflow

Because many speakers with hearing loss, even intelligible speakers, have difficulty with speech breathing and articulatory control of the airstream, measurement of breathing and airflow may be warranted in many cases. Respiratory and aerodynamic measures are not commonly used clinically with hearing-impaired speakers, although Whitehead (1991) applied oral airflow with hearing-impaired subjects to measure the closure durations of stop consonants, and Higgins et al (1994) reported that airflow measures were easily used even with young children. Nasal and oral airflow can be measured with several commercially available systems, and phonatory airflow, subglottal pressure, and laryngeal resistance can be estimated from these two airflow measures (Smitheran & Hixon, 1981). See Chapter 5 for more on the application of aerodynamic measures.

♦ Treatment Approaches

The treatment approaches for speech impairment secondary to hearing loss have been largely developed according to input and feedback modality rather than process, particularly when it comes to the treatment of children. With adults and older children exhibiting isolated deficits (i.e., elevated pitch) treatments are somewhat more process based. Nonetheless, most treatment approaches remain largely focused on getting sufficient feedback or input to the speaker so normal speech can be acquired or impaired speech modified. Because hearing loss occurring in childhood has a more profound effect on speech than does adventitious hearing loss (Goehl & Kaufman, 1984), most of the treatment approaches described in the literature have been developed for children. However, the speech training of children with hearing loss is often interwoven with language, sensory, and academic training, making it difficult to evaluate the effects of the speech training per se. Compounding the problem is that many of the older, more traditional approaches have been only vaguely described in the literature. The published descriptions for many of the approaches function more as philosophies for treatment and not operationalized treatment guidelines or curricula. How they are implemented may vary widely across clinicians and setting. In addition, there are very little treatment efficacy data available for most of the approaches making statements about their effectiveness limited. Clinicians are therefore encouraged to choose approaches that theoretically best fit a particular client and then collect the needed treatment efficacy data for that and other patients.

Auditory Stimulation Approaches

Auditory approaches have been used extensively and for many years, but they have surprisingly little documentation. Terms such as *acoupedic, auditory-global, auditory-oral, aural-oral,* and *unisensory* have been applied to these approaches with little differentiation between the terms. Davis and Hardick (1981) referred to these approaches generically as auditory stimulation methods.

The auditory stimulation approaches tend to be synthetic and are largely restricted to use with preschool children. The goal of these approaches is to train impaired listeners to glean as much from the auditory signal as possible with the rationale that speech is best learned via the auditory modality. The hallmark of these approaches is extensive auditory stimulation and training used in an effort to get early and consistent use of audition. Critical to the present-day implementation of these approaches is that acoustic signals are optimized through amplification or other auditory prostheses. The reliance on other modalities is minimized because it is argued that they can potentially interfere with audition and therefore interfere with the auditory system developing to its fullest potential. However, some auditory approaches, such as Northcott's (1977) Curriculum Guide, propose that natural communication should be promoted with young children with hearing loss, and natural facial cues and gestures should not be inhibited because they co-occur with oral communication. Common to all of the auditory approaches, speech is not treated directly, but its development is encouraged through auditory stimulation with connected speech produced in context. Naturally occurring strings with natural sounding prosody are promoted, although direct imitation of speech is encouraged and reinforced (Lowell & Pollack, 1974). Training of segmental aspects of speech does not occur in the early years. It is reserved for when the children reach school age. At that time, they continue to receive extensive auditory stimulation but are taught correct speech production with a multisensory approach (Lowell & Pollack, 1974). Other than anecdotal reports and case studies there is little evidence that these approaches are effective or ineffective in promoting speech production.

Analytic Auditory-Oral Approaches

Ling (1976, 2002) and Boothroyd (1982) described in detail two very similar approaches, although Ling's approach is much more detailed and structured than Boothroyd's. In both approaches the auditory modality is the modality of choice for input and sensory feedback when training speech in children with hearing impairment. No attempts are made, however, to restrict the use of naturally occurring nonauditory cues. Auditory training is encouraged but it is not a focus of treatment, and it is acknowledged that many children with hearing loss need supplemental cues such as visual and tactile cues to more easily acquire speech. These modalities are not targeted in therapy unless needed, and their artificial use is extinguished as quickly as possible. Ling is very specific about what speech sounds might need supplementary cues when training. He also is specific about how nonauditory cues may facilitate treatment and establish usable feedback. The Ling and Boothroyd approaches are initially analytic, output-based, and involve extensive use of imitation. They start by training basic skills such as respiration and voicing for speech, and developing skeletal vowel and consonant repertoires. The basic skills are trained simultaneously and interwoven, and once acquired are expanded in developmental and structural complexity with the syllable as the basic unit of training. The order of the segments taught and the syllabic complexity is clearly specified in both approaches.

A deviation from the analytic format is that both approaches encourage the use of newly acquired skills in meaningful, communicative contexts, which Ling refers to as the phonologic level. The phonologic level is in contrast to the initial analytical training level, which Ling refers to as the phonetic level. For all levels, Ling suggests that training occur in short intervals multiple times a day. Ling also provides suggestions for training various skills and includes lists of subskills that should be learned to get systematic approximation of target sounds.

Neither Ling nor Boothroyd have provided direct empirical evidence that their treatment approaches are efficacious. However, Perigoe and Ling (1986) compared two matched groups of children with hearing loss relative to the role of grammatical category in generalization training from phonetic to phonologic level productions. One group received speech training with content words (nouns and verbs), and the other with function words (pronouns and prepositions). The children received 40 sessions of training over a course of 9 months and their performance at both the phonetic and phonologic levels were assessed four different times (once pretreatment, twice during treatment and once at the end of treatment). Although there were no substantive differences between the groups, both groups showed gains but primarily on the final assessment. However, because of inadequate experimental control, and the duration over which treatment occurred, the question remains whether the gains were a product of the training or other factors such as maturation or concurrent educational/therapeutic activities.

In a study designed to assess generalization of voicing (+ and −) to cognates, McReynolds and Jetzke (1986) used an imitative syllabic training procedure similar to those suggested by Ling and Boothroyd. A single-subject, multiple-baseline across behaviors design was employed with counterbalancing and replication. Eight school-age children with severe or profound hearing losses served as subjects and were trained to produce either /t/ or /d/ and /k/ or /g/ in vowel-consonant (VC) nonsense syllables. All eight of the children in the study improved from a baseline of 15% correct production or less to a criterion of 85% correct over two consecutive 20-item trials. Six of the eight children also exhibited significant generalization to the cognates of the sounds with which they were trained. More generalization occurred with voiced target-sound training than with voiceless target-sound training. These data suggest that imitative procedures are effective when correcting speech production in children with hearing impairment and that like normal-hearing children they exhibit generalization within phoneme classes.

Visual Methods

Visual methods are rarely used in isolation to treat the speech of persons with hearing loss. They typically are supplemental to other approaches or they are used as part of the general speech, language, and reading instruction. Visual methods include the use of speech reading, mirrors, cued speech, and graphic symbol systems to teach the proper production of individual speech sounds or prosodic elements. They also include the bulk of the computer-based instructional and feedback systems that are discussed later in this chapter.

The primary goals of speech reading and cued speech are not proper sound production but improved speech reception for oral communication. However, they are frequently used in the initial training of sounds to indicate proper articulatory placements and movements (Jenson, 1971). The use of the hand cues provided in cued speech are particularly useful in providing location information for difficult to view articulations. The hand cues are relatively easy to learn and can be used in speech training even if a child does not use cued speech in his/her daily communications.

The graphic symbols employed in speech instruction vary from pictorial representations of articulatory postures and movements to phonetic symbols and dictionary diacritical marks. These graphic symbol systems are frequently integrated with reading instruction (McGarr, Youdelman, & Head, 1992; Streng, 1955).

Multisensory Approaches

Multisensory Syllabic Unit Approach

Carhart (1947, 1963) advocated a multisensory procedure for teaching speech to children with hearing impairment. He suggested that the performance of the auditory system should be optimized via auditory training and appropriate amplification, particularly with children who have substantial residual hearing. He also suggested visual training in which children are taught to focus on the face, first for gestural cues and then for speech articulator cues. Vibrotactile and kinesthetic information also should be used to train the production of particular sounds as well as train children to monitor their own productions. Therefore, children are taught to monitor their speech not only by how it sounds but also by how it feels. Silverman (1971) expanded Carhart's description of the multisensory approach by including the use of other visual and tactile systems such as orthography, graphic displays, cued speech, finger spelling, visual displays of acoustic signals, and tactile aids. The multisensory syllabic unit approach, often referred to as the traditional approach, is largely analytic. As the name would suggest, the basic unit of treatment is the syllable, although speakers are given feedback about individual phonemes as well as prosody. Phonemes are taught in a predetermined sequence with most therapists beginning with bilabial consonants in conjunction with middle and back vowels (Davis & Hardick, 1981, p. 272). A visual system is usually associated with the sounds taught and other sensory cues are emphasized during the instruction. All phonemes are first taught in isolation or CV and VC syllables. The training then proceeds to CVC, CCVC, and finally CVCCC patterns. In addition, natural voice and prosody is promoted, and children are encouraged to use newly acquired speech skills in context. Especially with children, Carhart (1947) suggested that the social act of speech, not the precise articulation of segments, be the emphasis of speech in context. However, prosody is treated in a very analytic fashion once the children have acquired a sizable phoneme repertoire.

Lexington School for the Deaf Approach

A multisensory approach used at the Lexington School for the Deaf and described by Vorce (1971, 1974) is somewhat more eclectic. The basic philosophy is that speech training should be synthetic and stimulated in naturally occurring contexts whenever possible with emphasis on the whole unit rather than its parts. However, it is acknowledged that many hearing-impaired children, particularly school-age children, benefit from more analytic and structured instruction. Instruction starts with the most natural of environments and stimuli, regardless of age, and becomes more analytic and structured as needed. Magner (1971) suggests that the analytic component should be added when a child indicates an interest in oral expression. The analytic instruction is segmented according to voice/resonance, articulation, and prosody. Somewhat antithetical to the basic philosophy, however, is that artificial feedback and cuing systems are utilized even with infants.

Association Method

The association method is one of the most analytic of the multisensory approaches used with children with hearing loss. It was developed by McGinnis (1963) at the Central Institute for the Deaf for children considered aphasic, but it has been used with children referred to as centrally deaf and children with peripheral hearing loss who appear to have difficulty in more traditional therapeutic and educational settings. These children have been described as having sequencing, memory, perceptual motor, and attention difficulties in addition to their sensory deficits (Davis & Hardick, 1981). The association method starts at the phoneme level where the children learn to produce individual sounds. These individual sounds are then combined into CV syllables and gradually built into words, phrases, and sentences. All the while the sounds are associated with one another and blended, as well as associated with auditory cues, lipreading, objects, pictures, reading, and writing. Speech is not the sole purpose of the treatment approach. It is a core component associated with other elements of the communicative process. The association method has been revised of late and has seen resurgence in its use, but there continues to be little documentation of its effectiveness with children who have hearing loss.

Verbotonal Method

In contrast to the other multisensory approaches, the verbotonal method (developed by Petar Guberina in the 1950s) does not initially stress the use of the auditory system (Craig, Craig, & Burke, 1974). Amplification is introduced gradually and only after the child has associated various prosodic patterns of speech with large body movements. At this early stage, vibratory input rather than auditory input is used, and is introduced by way of vibratory floor panels, vibratory benches, or a personal vibrator placed on the wrist. The stress and rhythmic patterns of speech introduced via vibration are associated with body movements through structured play, role playing, stories, and verbal games. The patterns are ultimately associated with oral speech gestures. Spontaneous speech is encouraged but not demanded, with the primary emphasis on natural sounding prosody. Suprasegmental and segmental aspects of speech are always introduced within the confines of whole body activities, with the utterance being the unit of interest.

Auditory amplification is introduced when the children have developed an awareness of the vibratory patterns and the oral and gestural activities that accompany them. It is usually introduced under earphones with a group or desktop auditory trainer. These auditory trainers (Suvag I and Suvag II, respectively [Polyclinic for the Rehabilitation of Listening and Speech, Zagreb, Croatia]) house filters that are adjusted to match the frequency response of the child's region(s) of usable hearing. For example, a child with residual hearing restricted in the low frequencies is amplified using an extended low-frequency response. After the child has adjusted to amplification and the optimal frequency response has been determined, he/she is transitioned to a wearable device called the Mini Suvag or a hearing aid that can match the desired frequency response. Even after a child has been amplified, vibratory input is often retained.

Craig, Craig, and DiJohnson (1972) assessed the effectiveness of the verbotonal method in training early speech skills by comparing it to what they called the traditional method, although their implementation of the traditional method was not specified. Two groups of preschool children who were hearing impaired served as subjects. The children were randomly assigned to the two different groups, with the group compositions comparable relative to age, intelligence, hearing, lipreading skills, and social skills. One group was trained with the verbotonal method and the other with the traditional method. Using a pretest/posttest design, Craig et al found that both groups of children showed significant improvements in their speech intelligibility, loudness, and pitch. The groups did not differ as a whole, but the higher functioning children in the verbotonal group made substantially greater gains than those in the traditional group. The lower functioning children in both groups made similar gains.

♦ Sensory Aids

As indicated previously, most speech training approaches are dependent on optimizing the use of residual hearing or electrically stimulating the auditory system. Correspondingly, it is generally believed that speech is learned and treated easiest if speakers can monitor their productions via their auditory systems. Therefore, the proper and early fitting and use of auditory sensory aids, as well as auditory and language training, are important components of speech production training. In support of this auditory-based approach to speech treatment is the relationship between the severity of prelingual hearing loss and the extent of speech delay found in children (Levitt, 1987; Smith, 1975; Wake et al, 2004) as well as speech perception skills and any history of previous hearing (Geers, 2004). So also is the relationship between the severity and configuration of hearing loss and the amount of speech deterioration found in older children and adults with prelingual hearing loss. For example, Levitt (1987) and Osberger, Maso, and Sam (1993) found that audiometric configuration had a substantive bearing on speech intelligibility. Furthermore, the growing literature supporting the positive impact of cochlear implants on speech development, as well as the role that auditory-oral-based training programs have played in communication outcomes of children fitted with cochlear implants, strongly supports the maximization of audition for the maximization of speech training (Geers et al, 2002; Tobey et al, 2003; Uchanski & Geers, 2003).

Hearing Aids

Despite the indications of a relationship, the empirical data directly relating speech production to the use of hearing aids, hearing aid fitting procedures, hearing aid configurations, or auditory training are limited at best. For example,

Novelli-Olmstead and Ling (1984) found that children show more improvement when speech and auditory training are combined than when auditory training is used alone. Still, the combined training was not compared with speech training in the absence of auditory training, so it is not known whether speech training was augmented by the auditory training or if the improvement was solely the result of the speech training. Yoshinaga-Itano, Apuzzo, Coulter, and Stredler-Brown (1995) reported that infants who are identified by 3 months, fitted early with auditory prostheses, and placed into an early intervention programs shortly after identification are more advanced in consonant and vowel production when tested at later months than are children identified even as early as 7 or 8 months. However, it is difficult to separate the effects of fitting the prostheses early from other aspects of early intervention. Preliminary data reported by Stelmachowicz, Pittman, Hoover, Lewis, and Moeller (2004) on three infants fitted early with hearing aids suggested delays in sound category acquisition consistent with patterns previously reported in the literature. Sound inventories were impoverished, consonants were more affected than vowels, and sound containing high-frequency cues was particularly limited. In a study with preschool children, Pratt, Grayhack, Palmer, and Sabo (2003) observed that vowel formants produced by children with moderate-to-severe hearing loss were more normal when wearing their hearing aids than when they had them removed. They also observed that hearing aid processors affected the formant structure of the vowels produced by these children. It should be noted, however, that these children had intelligible speech, and the speech tokens measured were considered acceptable productions. Similarly, Higgins et al (1994) tested intelligible prelingually hearing-impaired adults with and without their hearing aids and observed a trend toward increased lip closure, voicing durations, and intraoral pressure, and decreased nasal air flow when the subjects were unaided along with subtle changes in phonation. Although these were not significant differences, Higgins et al argued that the changes may have corresponded to increased tactile feedback used to compensate for the reduced auditory feedback.

Cochlear Implants

In contrast to hearing aids, there is a burgeoning literature associating cochlear implants with improved speech production in persons with adventitious hearing loss and more normal speech development in children fitted early with cochlear implants. The assessment of speech changes of adults with adventitious hearing loss following the insertion of cochlear implants has largely been instrumental in nature because the participants tend to be intelligible and their speech differences are more subtle in nature. Many speakers with adventitious hearing loss exhibit differences in speech timing, respiratory and vocal control, and vowel and consonant precision. All of these differences tend to be subtle in nature but consistent with many of the speech differences common to speakers with prelingual hearing loss. Recovery can occur quickly in some individuals after their implants have been turned on, and can be reversed by turning the implant off and on (Lane et al, 1995; Matthies, Svirsky, Perkell, & Lane, 1996; Perkell et al, 1992). However, some of the problems may persist for some people for several years (Kishon-Rabin et al, 1999). Quite surprising, the severity of decline and recovery is not related to the amount of time a person has been deafened prior to implantation, although it may be related to the age of onset.

The data collected on children are quite different from those collected from adults with adventitious hearing loss. Early work by Osberger, Maso, and Sam (1993) observed that children with profound congenital hearing loss or hearing loss occurring in infancy tend to exhibit only limited improvement in speech intelligibility within the first 2 years after implantation and exhibit slight but notable increases after 2 years. Similarly, Tobey, Angelette, et al (1991) observed relatively small gains in intelligibility within the first year: 18.1% preoperatively to 33.5% at 1 year postoperatively. With improvements in cochlear implant technology and software, along with increasing emphasis on early identification, early implantation, and intensive auditory-oral intervention, more positive outcomes have been observed in children (Geers et al, 2002; Tobey et al, 2003; Uchanski & Geers, 2003). These advancements have resulted in greater numbers of children with profound hearing loss being able to use their auditory systems for speech development. More children are demonstrating intelligible speech and normal sound inventories and speech acoustic characteristics by the time they enter school. However, as indicated previously, cochlear implants also have increased the heterogeneity of speech characteristics and severity observed with children with profound hearing loss. Not all children demonstrate substantive gains from their implants over time. Many children who wear cochlear implants do develop normal or near-normal speech production skills, but many also demonstrate reduced sound inventories and protracted developmental timelines for speech production (Blamey et al, 2001; Serry & Blamey, 1999, 2001).

Children implanted in their teens show pre/postimplantation changes in speech intelligibility and consonant production, but many speech differences persist (Dawson et al, 1995). The data on children implanted prior to 2 years or age and the limited data on those implanted prior to 1 year of age suggest that these children are at a substantive advantage over those implanted later (Nikolopoulos, O'Donoghue, & Archbold, 1999). In addition, children who have intact speech skills prior to the onset of their hearing loss may show deterioration in intelligibility subsequent to their hearing loss but regain much of it following implantation (Osberger et al, 1993). So too, implanted children with some history of normal hearing are at a developmental advantage over children with no normal auditory exposure to speech and language (Geers, 2004).

Computer-Based Visual Aids

As the quantity, complexity, and digital signal processing capabilities have increased in the last decade, so have computer-based speech feedback systems. Correspondingly, their costs have decreased as their accessibility to clinicians has increased. In addition, most of the commercially available systems run on desktop computers, incorporate only a limited number of peripherals, and are multimodular, making them more appealing to clinicians who have limited resources and time, and varied caseloads. The different modules usually respond to various acoustic aspects of speech (e.g., fundamental frequency, voicing, vowel production), although a limited number of systems use lingual-palatal contact or movement as input. The modules of most systems also vary according to the instructional nature of the feedback and the interest level of the speaker (Pratt & Hricisak, 1994). For example, some modules may display characteristics of the acoustic input but provide the speaker with little in the way of information about accuracy or correctness. Other modules may indicate if a target has been reached or they may inform the speaker of the goodness-of-fit between a production and a target. In addition, many of the systems include game-like activities to heighten and maintain the interest of young children. Most of these systems were not developed specifically for speakers with hearing loss, but because they predominately use vision as the modality for feedback they have a great deal of face validity for use with the hearing-impaired population. None of the systems are wearable and are therefore useful primarily in the initial training or correction of productions. Eventually, the speaker must be able to make the target productions without feedback from the computer.

The early treatment applications of computer-based feedback systems with speakers with hearing loss were mixed (Osberger, Moeller, Kroese, & Lippman, 1981). Most early treatment studies were done on prototypes, which restricted their application to current commercially available systems. In addition, many treatment studies have used pretest/posttest designs without adequate controls. For example, Fletcher and Higgins (1980) did not use a control group when assessing the treatment efficacy of TONAR II for improving nasal resonance in children with a profound hearing loss. Fletcher and Hasegawa (1983) treated a young child who had a profound hearing loss with the simultaneous use of electropalatometry and glossometry. They concluded that the child's productions of the /i/, /a/, and /t/ improved with treatment, but they did not establish an adequate pretreatment baseline, and their design was insufficient to document that their system was the sole source of any progress made. Similarly, Bernhardt, Gick, Bacsfalvi, and Ashdown (2003) used electropalatometry in conjunction with ultrasound-based visual feedback with four deaf speakers. Pretest-posttest comparisons of their productions suggested improvement, but the study suffered from inadequate controls, too few subjects, and underspecification of the treatment. Ryalls, Michallet, and Le Dorze (1994) used a group design to compare vowel treatment using the Ling (1976) approach to treatment with the vowel accuracy module of the IBM SpeechViewer (IBM, 1988). They treated two randomly assigned groups of school-aged children with profound hearing loss over a 7-week period. No substantive changes in performance were observed over the course of treatment for either group, but no pretreatment measures were obtained and the groups were too small ($n = 4$) to adequately test for differences between the groups.

In contrast, Dagenais, Critz-Crosby, Fletcher, and McCutcheon (1994) compared Ling's approach to treating consonants with treatment via palatometry. They used a pretest-posttest group design. An adequate number of subjects were used with random assignment to the two treatment groups. Dagenais et al observed gains in both groups on target productions and intelligibility, and they concluded that palatometry was as effective, and possibly more so, than Ling's approach for the treatment of consonant production in school-age children with profound hearing loss. Other studies have also supported the effectiveness of computer-based feedback systems with this population. Using a single subject design, Pratt, Heintzelman, and Deming (1993) found that the vowel accuracy module of the IBM SpeechViewer was effective in the treatment of vowels in young children with hearing loss, although their results were vowel and subject dependent. Pratt (2003) also used a single-subject design and found that the voicing module of the SpeechViewer was effective in training voicing in a child with severe-to-profound hearing loss and largely unintelligible speech. In another study using single-subject design, Ertmer, Stark, and Karlan (1996) found that spectrographic feedback targeting the first and second formants was effective with two 9-year-old deaf children in improving vowel production, although generalization to untreated vowels was limited. Furthermore, clinician support and instruction was an integral component of the treatment protocol. Ertmer and Maki (2000) also compared the efficacy of noninstrumental instruction against noninstrumental instruction plus visual feedback from a spectrographic display. The productions of /m/ and /t/ in monosyllabic words were trained with four deaf teenagers who did not wear hearing aids or cochlear implants. Both treatment approaches resulted in improved performance, but the relative differences between approaches were child and phoneme dependent, making it difficult to determine the influence of the spectrographic display. More recently, Massaro and Light (2004) employed a synthesized speaking head that allowed visual access to the articulators for the treatment of both speech perception and production in a small group of school-age children with hearing loss. These investigators observed positive change from pre- to posttreatment, but with no control group it was difficult to determine if the changes were real and if they were the result of the computer-based treatment program.

The computer-based treatment research suggests that this type of visual feedback can be effectively used with patients with hearing loss, although effectiveness may be dependent on the speech characteristic being treated. Speech features that are particularly susceptible to hearing loss and speech gestures associated with limited visibility and proprioceptive feedback may be particularly responsive to visual feedback. For example, consonant voicing is a speech feature that if not well perceived through audition, may be effectively treated with computer-based visual feedback

because it is not easily viewed, is associated with limited proprioceptive feedback, and requires strict temporal coupling between articulators.

♦ Conclusion

As indicated at the beginning of this chapter, the literature on the effects of hearing loss on speech development and production is vast. Much is known about the consequences of hearing loss on speech production when the hearing loss occurs early in life and is severe to profound in degree. However, the information on persons with mild-to-moderate hearing loss is scant, particularly if the hearing loss occurs in childhood or is progressive in nature. Previously, there was limited information on the effects of adventitious hearing loss on speech production, but with the introduction of cochlear implants this population has received concentrated investigation, and the results suggest a role for audition in speech regulation after the motor speech system has matured. The research has indicated that speech may not be fully mature in early adulthood, that language may influence the role of audition as a sensory feedback mechanism, that speech is affected relatively quickly by auditory deprivation and recovery is equally as quick, and that the duration of the deprivation is not as critical a factor as the age of onset.

In addition to our increased knowledge of the effects of hearing loss on speech production, several assessment tools, both perceptual and instrumental, have become available, although most lack adequate standardization and norms. Further, there are many treatment approaches available, but the efficacy data are limited because few studies have been conducted, and of those that have, adequate experimental control largely has been inadequate. The few well-controlled treatment studies that have been published are promising; however, they tend to indicate that speech treatment is effective with the hearing-impaired population. Finally, the treatment area most notably lacking in efficacy research is the use of hearing aids to promote speech development and preservation. The lack of research in this area is glaring because wearable electroacoustic hearing aids have been available for over 50 years (Lybarger, 1988) and are a fundamental component for many of the direct speech treatment approaches. It is critical that more work be done in this area given the expansion of universal infant hearing screening programs. More infants with hearing loss will be identified shortly after birth, and to effectively treat them, more needs to be known about the effects of hearing aids on developing speech and auditory systems.

References

Allen, C., Nikolopoulos, T.P., Dyar, D., & O'Donoghue, G.M. (2001). Reliability of a rating scale for measuring speech intelligibility after pediatric cochlear implantation. *Otology & Neurotology, 22,* 631–633

American Speech-Language-Hearing Association. (2006). The prevalence and incidence of hearing loss in adults. http://www.asha.org/public/hearing/disorders/prevalence_ adults.htm

Angelocci, A.A., Kopp, G., & Holbrook, A. (1964). The vowel formants of deaf and normal-hearing eleven to fourteen year old boys. *Journal of Speech and Hearing Disorders, 29*, 156–170

Arends, N., Povel, D., Van Os, E., & Speth, L. (1990). Predicting voice quality of deaf speakers on the basis of glottal characteristics. *Journal of Speech and Hearing Research, 33*, 116–122

Baum, S.R. & Waldstein, R.S. (1991). Perseveratory coarticulation in the speech of profoundly hearing-impaired and normally hearing children. *Journal of Speech and Hearing Research, 34*, 1286–1292

Bernhardt, B., Gick, B., Bacsfalvi, P., & Adler-Bock, M., (2005). Ultrasound in speech therapy with adolescents and adults. *Clinical Linguistics and Phonetics, 19*, 605–617

Bernhardt, B., Gick, B., Bacsfalvi, P., & Ashdown, J. (2003). Speech habilitation of hard of hearing adolescents using electropalatography and ultrasound as evaluated by trained listeners. *Clinical Linguistics and Phonetics, 17*, 199–216

Blamey, P.J., Sarant, J.Z., & Paatsch, L.E. (2006). Relationships among speech perception and language measures in hard-of-hearing children. In: P.E. Spencer, M. Marschark (Eds.), *Advances in the Spoken Language Development of Deaf and Hard-of-Hearing Children* (pp. 85–102). London: Oxford University Press

Blamey, P.J., Sarant, J.Z., Paatsch, L.E., Barry, J.G., Bow, C.P., Wales, R.J., Wright, M., Psarros, C., Rattigan, K., & Tooher, R. (2001). Relationships among speech perception, production, language, hearing loss, and age in children with impaired hearing. *Journal of Speech Language & Hearing Research. 44*, 264–285

Blanchfield B.B., Feldman, J.J., Dunbar, J.L., & Gardner, E.N. (2001). The severely to profoundly hearing-impaired population in the United States: prevalence estimates and demographics. *Journal of the American Academy of Audiology, 12*, 183–189

Boothroyd, A. (1982). *Hearing Impairments in Young Children.* Englewood Cliffs, NJ: Prentice-Hall

Bressmann, T., Thind, P., Uy, C., Bollig, C., Gilbert, R.W., & Irish, J.C. (2005). Quantitative three-dimensional ultrasound analysis of tongue protrusion, grooving and symmetry: data from 12 normal speakers and a partial glossectomy. *Clinical Linguistics and Phonetics. 19*, 573–588

Calvert, D. & Silverman, R. (1975). *Speech and Deafness.* Washington, DC: Alexander Graham Bell Association for the Deaf

Carhart, R. (1947). Conservation of speech. In: H. Davis (Ed.), *Hearing and Deafness, a Guide for Laymen* (pp. 300–317). New York: Murray Hill Books

Carhart, R. (1963). Conservation of speech. In: H. Davis & S.R. Silverman (Eds.), *Hearing and Deafness,* revised edition (pp. 387–302). New York: Holt, Rinehart and Winston

Carr, J. (1953). An investigation of the spontaneous speech sounds of five-year-old deaf-born children. *Journal of Speech and Hearing Disorders, 18*, 22–29

Chin, S.B., Tsai, P.L., & Gao, S. (2003). Connected speech intelligibility of children with cochlear implants and children with normal hearing. *American Journal of Speech-Language Pathology, 12*, 440–451

Cowie, R., Douglas-Cowie, E., & Kerr, A. (1982). A study of speech deterioration in post-lingually deafened adults. *Journal of Laryngology and Otology, 96*, 101–112

Craig, W., Craig, H., & Burke, R. (1974). Components of verbotonal instruction for deaf students. *Language Speech & Hearing Services in Schools, 5*, 38–42

Craig, W., Craig, H., & DiJohnson, A. (1972). Preschool verbo-tonal instruction for deaf children. *Volta Review, 74*, 236–246

Cruickshanks, K.J., Wiley, T.L., Tweed, T.S., Klein, B.E., Klein, R., Mares-Perlman, J.A., & Nondahl D.M. (1998). Prevalence of hearing loss in older adults in Beaver Dam, Wisconsin. The Epidemiology of Hearing Loss Study. *American Journal* of Epidemiology, *148*, 879–886

Dagenais, P.A. & Critz-Crosby, P. (1992). Comparing tongue positioning by normal hearing and hearing-impaired children during vowel production. *Journal of Speech and Hearing Research, 35*, 35–44

Dagenais, P.A., Critz-Crosby, P., Fletcher, S., & McCutcheon, M. (1994). Comparing abilities of children with profound hearing impairments to learn consonants using electropalatography or traditional aural-oral techniques. *Journal of Speech and Hearing Research, 37*, 687–699

Dalston, R.M. (1989). Using simultaneous photodetection and nasometry to monitor velopharyngeal behavior during speech. *Journal of Speech and Hearing Research, 32*, 195–202

Dalston, R.M. & Seaver, E. (1990). Nasometric and phototransductive measurements of reaction times among normal adult speakers. *Cleft Palate Journal, 27*, 61–67

Davis, J. & Hardick, E. (1981). *Rehabilitative Audiology for Children and Adults.* New York: John Wiley

Dawson, P.W., Blamey, P., Dettman, S., Rowland, L, Barker, E., Tobey, E., Busby, P., Cowan, R., & Clark, G. (1995). A clinical report on speech production of cochlear implant users. *Ear and Hearing, 16*, 551–561

Denes, P. (1955). Effect of duration on the perception of voicing. *Journal of the Acoustical Society of America, 27*, 761–764

Desai, M., Pratt, L. Lentzner, H., & Robinson, K. (2001). Trends in vision and hearing among older Americans. In: *Aging Trends, No. 2.* Hyattsville, MD: National Center of Health Statistics

Dunn, C. & Newton, L. (1986). A comprehensive model for speech development in hearing-impaired children. *Topics in Language Disorders, 6*, 25–46

Dworkin, J. P., Marunick, M. T., & Krouse, J. H. (2004). Velopharyngeal dysfunction: speech characteristics, variable etiologies, evaluation techniques, and differential treatments. *Language, Speech, and Hearing Services in Schools, 35*, 333–352

Dyar D. (1994). Monitoring progress: the role of a speech and language therapist. In: B. McCormick, S. Archbold, & S. Sheppard (Eds.), *Cochlear Implants for Young Children* (pp. 237–268). London: Whurr

Edwards, L.C., Frost, R., & Witham, F. (2006). Developmental delay and outcomes in paediatric cochlear implantation: implication for candidacy. *International Journal of Pediatric Otolaryngology, 70*, 1593–1600

Elfenbein, J.L., Hardin-Jones, M., & Davis, J. (1994). Oral communication skills of children who are hard of hearing. *Journal of Speech and Hearing Research, 37*, 216–226

Ertmer, D.J. & Maki, J.E. (2000). A comparison of speech training methods with deaf adolescents: spectrographic versus noninstrumental instruction. *Journal of Speech, Language, and Hearing Research, 43*, 1509–1523

Ertmer, D.J., Stark, R.E., & Karlan, G.R. (1996). Eliciting prespeech vocalizations in a young child with profound hearing impairment: usefulness of real-time spectrographic speech displays. *American Journal of Speech-Language Pathology, 4*, 33–38

Fairbanks, G. (1960). *Voice and Articulation Drill Book*, 2nd ed. New York: Harper & Row

Feinmesser, M., Tell, L., & Levi, H. (1982). Follow-up of 40,000 infants screened for hearing defect. *Audiology, 21*, 197–203

Finitzo, T., Albright, K., & O'Neal, J. (1998). The newborn with hearing loss: detection in the nursery. *Pediatrics, 102*, 1452–1460

Fletcher, S.G. & Hasegawa, A. (1983). Speech modification by a deaf child through dynamic orometric modeling and feedback. *Journal of Speech and Hearing Disorders, 48*, 179–185

Fletcher, S.G. & Higgins, J. (1980). Performance of children with severe to profound auditory impairment in instrumentally guided reduction of nasal resonance. *Journal of Speech and Hearing Disorders, 45*, 181–194

Formby, C. & Monsen, R. (1982). Long-term average speech spectra for normal and hearing-impaired adolescents. *Journal of the Acoustical Society of America, 71*, 196–202

Forner, L.L. & Hixon, T.J. (1977). Respiratory kinematics in profoundly hearing-impaired speakers. *Journal of Speech and Hearing Research, 20*, 373–408

Gallaudet Research Institute (2005). *Regional and National Summary Report of Data from the 2004–2005 Survey of Deaf and Hard of Hearing Children and Youth.* Washington, DC: GRI, Gallaudet University

Geers, A.E. (2004). Speech, language, and reading skills after early cochlear implantation. *Archives of Otolaryngology, Head and Neck Surgery, 130*, 634–638

Geers, A., Brenner, C., Nicholas, J., Uchanski, R., Tye-Murray, N., & Tobey, E. (2002). Rehabilitation factors contributing to implant benefit in children. *Annals of Otology, Rhinology, and Laryngology-Supplement, 189,* 127–130

Goehl, H. & Kaufman, D. (1984). Do the effects of adventitious deafness include disordered speech? *Journal of Speech and Hearing Disorders, 49,* 58–64

Gold, T. (1980). Speech production in hearing-impaired children. *Journal of Communication Disorders, 13,* 397–418

Goldhor, R. (1995). The perceptual and acoustic measurement of the speech of hearing-impaired talkers. In: A. Syrdal, R. Bennett, & S. Greenspan (Eds.), *Applied Speech Technology* (pp. 521–545). Boca Raton, FL: CRC Press

Gorlin, R., Toriello, H., & Cohen, M.M. (1995). *Hereditary Hearing Loss and Its Syndromes.* Oxford Monographs on Medical Genetics, 28. New York: Oxford University Press

Guenther, F.H. (1995). Speech sound acquisition, coarticulation, and rate effects in a neural network model of speech production. *Psychological Review. 102,* 594–621

Guenther, F.H., Ghosh, S.S., & Tourville, J.A. (2006). Neural modeling and imaging of the cortical interactions underlying syllable production. *Brain and Language, 96,* 280–301

Hardy, J.C. (1961). Intraoral breath pressure in cerebral palsy. *Journal of Speech and Hearing Disorders, 26,* 309–319

Heider, F., Heider, G., & Sykes, J. (1941). A study of the spontaneous vocalizations of fourteen deaf children. *Volta Review, 43,* 10–14

Helzner, E.P., Cauley, J.A., Pratt, S.R, Wisneiwski, S.R., Zmuda, J.M., Talbott, E.O., de Renkeniere, N., Harris, T.B., Rubin, S.M, Simonsick, E.M, Tylarsky, F.A., & Newman, A.B. (2005). Race and gender differences in hearing loss among older adults: the Health ABC Study. *Journal of the American Geriatrics Society, 53,* 2119–2127

Higgins, M.B., Carney, A., & Schulte, L. (1994). Physiological assessment of speech and voice production of adults with hearing loss. *Journal of Speech and Hearing Research, 37,* 510–521

Higgins, M.B., McCleary, E.A., & Carney, A.E., & Schulte, L (2003). Longitudinal changes in children's speech and voice physiology after cochlear implantation. *Ear and Hearing, 24,* 48–70

Hood, R. & Dixon, R. (1969). Physical characteristics of speech rhythm of deaf and normal-hearing speakers. *Journal of Communication Disorders, 2,* 20–28

Horii, Y. (1982). Some voice fundamental frequency characteristics of oral reading and spontaneous speech by hard-of-hearing young women. *Journal of Speech and Hearing Research, 25,* 608–610

Hudgins, C. & Numbers, F. (1942). An investigation of the intelligibility of speech of the deaf. *Genetic Psychology Monographs, 25,* 289–392

Hutchinson, J. & Smith, L. (1976). Aerodynamic functioning in consonant production by hearing-impaired adults. *Audiology and Hearing Education, 2,* 16–19, 22–25, 34

IBM. (1988). *IBM Personal System/2 Independence Series SpeechViewer Application Software User's Guide.* Boca Raton, FL: Author

Itoh, M., Horii, Y., Daniloff, R., & Binnie, C. (1982). Selected aerodynamic characteristics of deaf individuals' various speech and nonspeech tasks. *Folia Phoniatrica, 34,* 191–209

Jenson, P. (1971). The relationship of speechreading and speech. In: L.E. Connor (Ed.), *Speech for the Deaf Child: Knowledge and Use* (pp. 265–279). Washington, DC: A.G. Bell Association for the Deaf

John, J. & Horwarth, J. (1965). The effect of time distortions on the intelligibility of deaf children's speech. *Language and Speech, 8,* 127–134

Jones, D. L., Gao, S., & Svirsky, M. A. (2003). The effect of short-term auditory deprivation on the control of intraoral pressure in pediatric cochlear implant users. *Journal of Speech, Language, and Hearing Research, 46,* 658–669

Karnell, M.P., Seaver, E., & Dalston, R. (1988). A comparison of photodetector and endoscopic evaluations of velopharyngeal functions. *Journal of Speech and Hearing Research, 31,* 503–510

Kent, R. & Read, C. (1992). *The Acoustic Analysis of Speech.* San Diego: Singular

Kishon-Rabin, L., Taitelbaum, R., Tobin, Y., & Hildesheimer, M. (1999). The effect of partially restored hearing on speech production of postlingually deafened adults with multichannel cochlear implants. *Journal of the Acoustical Society of America, 106,* 2843–2857

Kochkin, S. (2005). MarkeTrak VI: The VA and direct mail sales spark growth in hearing market. *The Hearing Review, 8,* 16–24, 63–65

Kreiman, J. & Gerratt, B.R. (1998). Validity of rating scale measures of voice quality. *Journal of the Acoustical Society of America, 104,* 1598–1608

Kreiman, J., Gerratt, B.R., Precoda, K., & Berke, G.S. (1992). Individual differences in voice quality perception. *Journal of Speech and Hearing Research, 35,* 512–520

Lach, R., Ling, D., Ling, L., & Ship, N. (1970). Early speech development in deaf infants. *American Annals of the Deaf, 115,* 522–526

Lane, H., Matthies, M., Perkell, J., Vick. J., & Zandipour, M. (2001). The effects of changes in hearing status in cochlear implant users on the acoustic vowel space and CV coarticulation. *Journal of Speech, Language, and Hearing Research, 44,* 552–563

Lane, H. & Perkell, J.S., (2005). Control of voice-onset time in the absence of hearing: a review. *Journal of Speech, Language, and Hearing Research, 48,* 1334–1343

Lane, H. & Webster, J.W. (1991). Speech deterioration in postlingually deafened adults. *Journal of the Acoustical Society of America, 89,* 859–866

Lane, H., Wozniak, J., Matthies, M., Svirsky, M., & Perkell, J. (1995). Phonemic resetting versus postural adjustments in the speech of cochlear implant users: an exploration of voice-onset-time. *Journal of the Acoustical Society of America, 98,* 3096–3106

Lane, H., Wozniak, J., & Perkell, J. (1994). Changes in voice-onset time in speakers with cochlear implants. *Journal of the Acoustical Society of America, 96,* 56–64

Leder, S., Spitzer, J., Kirchner, J.C., Flevaris-Phillips, C., Milner, P., & Richardson, F. (1987). Speaking rate of adventitiously deaf male cochlear implant candidates. *Journal of the Acoustical Society of America, 82,* 843–846

Lee, F.S. Matthews. L.J., Dubno, J.R., & Mills, J.H. (2005). Longitudinal study of pure-tone thresholds in older persons. *Ear & Hearing, 26,* 1–11

Levitt, H. (1987). Interrelationships among the speech and language measures. In: H. Levitt, N. McGarr & D. Geffner (Eds.), *Development of Language and Communication Skills of Hearing-Impaired Children. American Speech-Language-Hearing Association Monographs, 26,* 123–139

Levitt, H., Smith, C., & Stromberg, H. (1976). Acoustical, articulatory and perceptual characteristics of the speech of deaf children. In: G. Fant (Ed.), *Proceedings of the Speech Communication Seminar* (pp. 129–139). New York: Wiley

Levitt, H. & Stromberg, H. (1983). Segmental characteristics of the speech of hearing-impaired children: factors affecting intelligibility. In: I. Hochberg, H. Levitt, M.J. Osberger (Eds.), *Speech of the Hearing Impaired: Research, Training and Personnel Preparation* (pp. 53–73). Baltimore: University Park Press

Levitt, H., Youdelman, K., & Head, J. (1990). *Fundamental Speech Skills Test.* Englewood, CO: Resource Point

Ling, D. (1976). *Speech and the Hearing-Impaired Child: Theory and Practice.* Washington, DC: A.G. Bell Association for the Deaf

Ling, D. (2002). *Speech and the Hearing-Impaired Child: Theory and Practice,* 2nd Edition. *Washington, DC: A.G. Bell Association for the Deaf*

Lippmann, R.P. (1981). Detecting nasalization using a low-cost miniature accelerometer. *Journal of Speech and Hearing Research, 24,* 314–317

Lowell, E. & Pollack, D. (1974). Remedial practices with the hearing impaired. In: S. Dickson (Ed.), *Communication Disorders Remedial Principles and Practices* (pp. 440–497). Glenview, IL: Scott, Foresman

Lybarger, S. (1988). A historical overview. In: R. Sandlin (Ed.) *Handbook of Hearing Aid Amplification,* vol. 1 (pp. 1–30). Boston: College-Hill Press

Lynch, M., Oller, K., & Steffens, M. (1989). Development of speech-like vocalizations in a child with congenital absence of cochleas: the case of total deafness. *Applied Psycholinguistics, 10,* 315–333

Maassen, B. (1986). Marking word boundaries to improve the intelligibility of the speech of the deaf. *Journal of Speech and Hearing Research, 29,* 227–230

Magner, M. (1971). Techniques of teaching. In: L.E. Connor (Ed.) *Speech for the Deaf Child: Knowledge and Use* (pp. 245–264). Washington, DC: A.G. Bell Association for the Deaf

Markides, A. (1970). The speech of deaf and partially hearing children with special reference to factors affecting intelligibility. *British Journal of Disorders of Communication, 5,* 126–140

Martin, D., Fitch, J., & Wolfe, V. (1995). Pathologic voice type and the acoustic prediction of severity. *Journal of Speech and Hearing Research, 38,* 765–771

Martin, J.A.M., Bentzen, O., Colley, J., Hennebert, D., Holm, C., Iurato, S., de Jonge, G., McCullen, O., Meyer, M., Moore, W., & Morgon, A. (1981). Childhood deafness in the European community. *Scandinavian Audiology, 10,* 165–174

Massaro, D.W. & Light, J. (2004). Using visual speech to train perception and production of speech for individuals with hearing loss. *Journal of Speech, Language, Hearing Research, 47,* 304–320

Matthies, M.L, Svirsky, M., Perkell, J., & Lane, H. (1996). Acoustic and articulatory measures of sibilant production with and without auditory feedback from a cochlear implant. *Journal of Speech & Hearing Research, 39,* 936–946

McAuliffe, M.J., Ward, E.C., & Murdoch, B.E. (2006). Speech production in Parkinson's disease: I. An electropalatographic investigation of tongue-Palate contact patterns. *Clinical Linguistics and Phonetics, 20,* 1–18

McCaffrey, H.A. & Sussman, H. (1994). An investigation of vowel organization in speakers with severe and profound hearing loss. *Journal of Speech and Hearing Research, 37,* 938–951

McGarr, N. (1983). The intelligibility of deaf speech to experienced and in-experienced listeners. *Journal of Speech and Hearing Research, 26,* 451–458

McGarr, N. (1987). Communication skills of hearing-impaired children in schools for the deaf. In: H. Levitt, N. McGarr & D. Geffner (Eds.), *Development of Language & Communication in Hearing Impaired Children. American Speech-Language-Hearing Association Monographs, 26,* 91–107

McGarr, N. & Löfqvist, A. (1982). Obstruent production in hearing-impaired speakers: interarticulator timing and acoustics. *Journal of the Acoustical Society of America, 72,* 34–42

McGarr, N., Youdelman, K., & Head, J. (1992). *Guidebook of Voice Pitch Remediation in Hearing-Impaired Speakers.* Englewood, CO: Resource Point

McGinnis, M.R. (1963). *Aphasic Children: Identification and Education by the Association Method.* Washington, DC: A.G. Bell Association for the Deaf

McNeil, M.R., Liss, J., Tseng, C., & Kent, R. (1990). Effects of speech rate on the absolute and relative timing of apraxic and conduction aphasic sentence production. *Brain and Language, 38,* 135–158

McReynolds, L.V. & Jetzke, E. (1986). Articulation generalization of voiced-voiceless sounds in hearing-impaired children. *Journal of Speech and Hearing Disorders, 51,* 348–355

Millin, J.P. (1971). Therapy for reduction of continuous phonation in the hard-of-hearing population. *Journal of Speech and Hearing Disorders, 36,* 496–498

Monsen, R.B. (1974). Durational aspects of vowel production in the speech of deaf children. *Journal of Speech and Hearing Research, 17,* 386–398

Monsen, R.B. (1976a). Normal and reduced-phonological space: The production of English vowels by deaf adolescents. *Journal of Phonetics, 4,* 189–198

Monsen, R.B. (1976b). The production of English stop consonants in the speech of deaf children. *Journal of Phonetics, 4,* 29–42

Monsen, R.B. (1976c) Second formant transitions of selected consonant-vowel combinations in the speech of deaf and normal-hearing children. *Journal of Speech and Hearing Research, 19,* 279–290

Monsen, R.B. (1978). Toward measuring how well hearing-impaired children speak. *Journal of Speech and Hearing Research, 21,* 197–219

Monsen, R.B. (1979). Acoustic qualities of phonation in young hearing-impaired children. *Journal of Speech and Hearing Research, 22,* 270–288

Monsen, R.B. (1981). A usable test for the speech intelligibility of deaf talkers. *American Annals of the Deaf, 126,* 845–852

Monsen, R.B. (1983). The oral intelligibility of hearing-impaired talkers. *Journal of Speech and Hearing Disorders, 48,* 286–296

Monsen, R.B. & Engebretson, A. (1983). The accuracy of formant frequency measurements: a comparison of spectrographic analysis and linear prediction. *Journal of Speech and Hearing Research, 26,* 89–97

Monsen, R.B., Moog, J., & Geers, A. (1988). *CID Picture SPINE.* St. Louis: Central Institute for the Deaf

Moog, J. (1989). *CID Phonetic Inventory.* St. Louis: Central Institute for the Deaf

Morrell, CH., Gordon-Salant, S., Pearson, J.D., Brant, L.J., & Fozard, J.L. (1996). Age- and gender-specific reference ranges for hearing level and longitudinal changes in hearing level. *Journal of the Acoustical Society of America, 100,* 1949–1967

Most, T. & Frank, Y (1991). The relationship between the perception and the production of intonation by hearing-impaired children. *Volta Review, 12,* 301–309

Murphy, A., McGarr, N., & Bell-Berti, F. (1990) Acoustic analysis of stress contrasts produced by hearing-impaired children. *Volta Review, 92,* 80–91

Nance, W.E. (2003). The genetics of deafness. *Mental Retardation and Developmental Disabilities Research Review, 9,* 109–119

National Center for Health Statistics & Ries, P.W. (1982). *Hearing Ability of Persons by Sociodemographic and Health Characteristics: United States. Vital and Health Statistics* (Series 10, No. 140, DHHS Publications No. PHS 82–1568. Public Health Service). Washington, DC: U.S. Government Printing Office

Nikolopoulos, T.P., O'Donoghue, G.M., & Archbold, S. (1999). Age at implantation: its importance in pediatric cochlear implantation. *Laryngoscope, 109,* 595–599

Niskar, A.S., Kieszak, S.M., Holmes, A., Esteban, E., Rubin, C., & Brody, D.J. (1998). Prevalence of hearing loss among children 6 to 19 years of age: the Third National Health and Nutrition Examination Survey. *Journal of the American Medical Association, 279,* 1071–1075

Nober, E.H. (1967). Articulation of the deaf. *Exceptional Child, 33,* 611–621

Northcott, W. (1977). *Curriculum Guide, Hearing-Impaired Children (0–3) and Their Parents.* Washington, DC: The A.G. Bell Association for the Deaf

Novelli-Olmstead, T. & Ling, D. (1984). Speech production and speech discrimination by hearing-impaired children. *Volta Review, 76,* 72–80

Obenchain, P., Menn, L., & Yoshinaga-Itano, C. (1998). Can speech development at 36 months in children with hearing loss be predicted from information available in the second year of life? *Volta Review, 100,* 149–180

Oller, D.K. & Eilers, R.E. (1988). The role of audition in infant babbling. *Child Development, 59,* 441–449

Oller, D.K., Eilers, R.E., Bull, D., & Carney, A. (1985). Pre-speech vocalizations of a deaf infant: a comparison with normal metaphonological development. *Journal of Speech and Hearing Research, 28,* 47–63

Oller, D.K. & Kelly, C. (1974). Phonological substitution processes of a hard-of-hearing child. *Journal of Speech and Hearing Disorders, 39,* 65–74

Osberger, M.J. (1981). Fundamental frequency characteristics of the speech of the hearing impaired. *Journal of the Acoustical Society of America, 69,* S68 (A)

Osberger, M.J. & Levitt, H. (1979). The effect of timing errors on the intelligibility of deaf children's speech. *Journal of the Acoustical Society of America, 66,* 1316–1324

Osberger, M.J., Levitt, H., & Slosberg, R. (1979). Acoustic characteristics of correctly produced vowels in deaf children's speech. *Journal of the Acoustical Society of America, 66,* S13 (A)

Osberger, M.J. & McGarr, N. (1982). Speech production characteristics of the hearing impaired. *Speech and Language, 8,* 221–283

Osberger, M.J., Maso, M. & Sam, L. (1993). Speech intelligibility of children with cochlear implants, tactile aids, or hearing aids. *Journal of Speech and Hearing Research, 36,* 186–203

Osberger, M.J., Moeller, M.P., Kroese, J.G., & Lippmann, RR. (1981). Computer-assisted speech training for the hearing impaired. *Journal of the Academy of Rehabilitative Audiology, 14*, 145–158

Osberger, M.J., Robbins, A.M., Lybolt, J., Kent, R., & Peters, J. (1986). Speech evaluation. In: M.J. Osberger (Ed.), *Language and Learning Skills of Hearing-Impaired Students. American Speech-Language-Hearing Association Monographs, 23*, 24–31

Palethorpe, S., Watson, C.I., & Barker, R. (2003). Acoustic analysis of monophthong and diphthong production in acquired sever-to-profound hearing loss. *Journal of the Acoustical Society of America, 114*, 1055–1068

Parker, A. & Irlam, L. (1995). Intelligibility and deafness: the skills of listener and speaker. In: S. Wirz (Ed.), *Perceptual Approaches to Communication Disorders* (pp. 56–83). London: Whurr

Parkhurst, B. & Levitt, H. (1978). The effect of selected prosodic errors o the intelligibility of deaf speech. *Journal of Communication Disorders, 11*, 249–256

Parving, A. (1985). Hearing disorders in childhood; some procedures for detection, identification and diagnostic evaluation. *International Journal of Paediatric Otorhinolaryngology, 9*, 31–57

Peng, S.C., Spencer, L., & Tomblin, J.B. (2004). Speech intelligibility of pediatric cochlear implant recipients with seven years of device experience. *Journal of Speech Language and Hearing Research, 47*, 1227–1235

Penn, J. (1955). Voice and speech patterns of the hard-of-hearing. *Acta Otolaryngologica* (suppl 124)

Perkell, J., Lane, H., Svirsky, M., & Webster, J. (1992). Speech of cochlear implant patients: a longitudinal study of vowel production. *Journal of the Acoustical Society of America, 91*, 2961–2978

Perkell, J.S., Matthies, M.L., Lane, H., Guenther, F.H., Wilhelms-Tricarico, R., Wozniak, J., & Guiod, P. (1997). Speech motor control: acoustic goals, saturation effects, auditory feedback and internal models. *Speech Communication, 22*, 227–250

Perigoe, C. & Ling, D. (1986). Generalization of speech skills in hearing-impaired children. *Volta Review, 88*, 351–366

Pleis, J.R. & Coles, R. (2003). Summary health statistics for U.S. adults: National Health Interview Survey, 1999. *Vital & Health Statistics, Series 10: Data from the National Health Survey, 212*, 1–137

Pratt, S.R. (2003). Reducing voicing inconsistency in a child with severe hearing loss. *Journal of the Academy of Rehabilitative Audiology, 36*, 45–65

Pratt, S.R., Grayhack, J., Palmer, C., & Sabo, D. (2003). Hearing aid influences on vowel production in children. Presented at the American Auditory Society, Scottsdale, AZ, March

Pratt, S.R., Heintzelman, A., & Deming, S. (1993). The efficacy of using the IBM SpeechViewer Vowel Accuracy Module to treat young children with hearing impairment. *Journal of Speech and Hearing Research, 36*, 1063–1074

Pratt, S.R. & Hricisak, I. (1994). Commercially available computer-based speech feedback systems. *Journal of the Academy of Rehabilitative Audiology, 27*, 89–106

Prieve, B., Dalzell, L, Berg, A., Bradley, M., Cacace, A., Campbell, D., De-Cristofaro, J., Gravel, J., Greenberg, E., Gross, S., Orlando, M., Pinheiro, J., Regan, J., Spivak, L., & Stevens, F. (2000). The New York Universal Newborn Hearing Screening Demonstration Project: outpatient outcome measures. *Ear and Hearing, 21*, 104–117

Prosek, R.A., Montgomery, A., & Walden, B. (1988). Constancy of relative timing for stutterers and nonstutterers. *Journal of Speech and Hearing Research, 31*, 654–658

Raphael, L.J. (1972). Preceding vowel duration as a cue to the perception of the voicing characteristic of word-final consonants in American English. *Journal of the Acoustical Society of America, 51*, 1296–1303

Robb, M.P. & Pang-Ching, G. (1992). Relative timing characteristics of hearing-impaired speakers. *Journal of the Acoustical Society of America, 91*, 2954–2960

Robbins, J. & Klee, T. (1987). Clinical assessment of oropharyngeal motor development in young children. *Journal of Speech and Hearing Disorders, 52*, 271–277

Rothman, H.B. (1976). A spectrographic investigation of consonant-vowel transitions in the speech of deaf adults. *Journal of Phonetics, 4*, 129–136

Ryalls, J., Michallet, B., & Le Dorze, G. (1994). A preliminary evaluation of the clinical effectiveness of vowel training for hearing-impaired children on IBM's SpeechViewer. *Volta Review, 96*, 19–30

Rubin-Spitz, J., & McGarr, N. (1990). Perception of terminal fall contours in speech produced by deaf persons. *Journal of Speech and Hearing Research, 33*, 174–180

Samar, V.J. & Metz, D. (1988). Criterion validity of speech intelligibility rating-scale procedures for the hearing-impaired population. *Journal of Speech and Hearing Research, 31*, 307–316

Sapir, S. & Canter, G. (1991). Postlingual deaf speech and the role of audition in speech production: Comments on Waldstein's paper (1990). *Journal of the Acoustical Society of America, 90*, 1672–1673

Schiavetti, N., Metz, D.E., & Sitler, R.W. (1981). Construct validity of direct magnitude estimation and interval scaling: evidence from a study of the hearing impaired. *Journal of Speech & Hearing Research, 241*, 441–445

Scobbie, J.M., Wood, S.E., & Wrench, A.A. (2004). Advances in EPG for treatment and research: an illustrative case study. *Clinical Linguistics and Phonetics, 18*, 373–389

Seaver, E.J., Dalston, R., Leeper, H., & Adams, L. (1991). A study of nasometric values for normal nasal resonance. *Journal of Speech and Hearing Research, 34*, 715–721

Serry, T.A. & Blamey, P.J. (1999). A 4-year investigation into phonetic inventory development in young cochlear implant users. *Journal of Speech, Language, and Hearing Research, 42*, 141–154

Serry, T.A. & Blamey, P.J. (2001). Phonetic inventory development in young cochlear implant users 6 years postoperation. *Journal of Speech, Language, and Hearing Research, 44*, 73–79

Shaw, S. & Coggins, T. (1991). Interobserver reliability using the phonetic level evaluation with severely and profoundly hearing-impaired children. *Journal of Speech and Hearing Research, 34*, 989–999

Shrivastav, R., Sapienza, C.M., & Nandur, V. (2005). Application of psychometric theory to the measurement of voice quality using rating scales. *Journal of Speech, Language, and Hearing Research, 48*, 323–335

Silverman, S.R. (1971). The education of deaf children. In: L.E. Travis (Ed.), *Handbook of Speech and Language Pathology* (pp. 399–430). Englewood Cliffs, NJ: Prentice-Hall

Silverman, S. & Hirsh, I. (1955). Problems related to the use of speech in clinical audiometry. *Annals of Otology, Rhinology and Laryngology, 64*, 1234–1244

Sitler, R.W., Schiavetti, N., & Metz, D. (1983). Contextual effects in the measurement of hearing-impaired speakers' intelligibility. *Journal of Speech and Hearing Research, 26*, 30–34

Smith, C.R. (1975). Residual hearing and speech production in the deaf. *Journal of Speech and Hearing Research, 19*, 795–811

Smith, R.J.H. & Van Camp, G. (2006). Deafness and hereditary hearing loss overview. In: *GeneReviews*. Seattle, WA: University of Washington. http://www.geneclinics.org/profiles/deafness-overview/details.html

Smitheran, J.R. & Hixon, T. (1981). A clinical method for estimating laryngeal airway resistance during vowel production. *Journal of Speech and Hearing Disorders, 46*, 138–146

Stein, D. (1980). A study of articulatory characteristics of deaf talkers. *Dissertation Abstracts International, 41*, 1327B

Stelmachowicz, P.G., Pittman, A.L., Hoover, B.M., Lewis, D.E., & Moeller, M.P. (2004). The importance of high-frequency audibility in the speech and language development of children with hearing loss. *Archives of Otolaryngology, Head and Neck Surgery, 130*, 556–562

Stevens, K.N., Nickerson, R., Boothroyd, A., & Rollins, A. (1976). Assessment of nasalization in the speech of deaf children. *Journal of Speech Hearing Research, 19*, 393–416

Stevens, K., Nickerson, R., & Rollins, A. (1978). On describing the suprasegmental properties of the speech of deaf children. In: D. McPherson & M. Davids (Eds.), *Advances in Prosthetic Devices for the Deaf: A Technical Workshop* (pp. 134–155). Rochester, NY: National Technical Institute for the Deaf

St. Louis, K. & Ruscello, D. (1987). *Oral Speech Mechanism Screening Examination-Revised.* Austin: Pro-Ed

Stoel-Gammon, C. (1988). Prelinguistic vocalizations of hearing-impaired & normally hearing subjects: a comparison of consonantal inventories. *Journal of Speech and Hearing Disorders, 53,* 302–315

Stoel-Gammon, C. & Otomo, K. (1986). Babbling development of hearing-impaired and normally hearing subjects. *Journal of Speech and Hearing Disorders, 51,* 33–41

Streng, A. (1955). *Hearing Therapy for Children.* New York: Grune & Stratton

Subtelny, J. (1977). Assessment of speech with implications for training. In: F. Bess (Ed.), *Childhood Deafness* (pp. 183–194). New York: Grune & Stratton

Subtelny, J., Li, W., Whitehead, R., & Subtelny, J.D. (1989). Cephalometric and cineradiographic study of deviant resonance in hearing-impaired speakers. *Journal of Speech and Hearing Disorders, 54,* 249–263

Subtelny, J., Orlando, N., & Whitehead, R. (1981). *Speech and Voice Characteristics of the Deaf.* Washington, DC: The A.G. Bell Association for the Deaf

Subtelny, J.D., Whitehead, R., & Samar, V. (1992). Spectral study of deviant resonance in the speech of women who are deaf. *Journal of Speech and Hearing Research, 35,* 574–579

Sussman, H. & Hernandez, M. (1979). A spectrographic analysis of the suprasegmental aspects of the speech of hearing-impaired adolescents. *Audiology and Hearing Education, 5,* 12–16

Tobey, E.A., Angelette, S., Murchison, C., Nicosia, J., Sprague, S., Staller, S., Brimacombe, J., & Beiter, A. (1991). Speech production in children receiving a multichannel cochlear implant. *American Journal of Otology, 12* (suppl), 164–172

Tobey, E.A., Geers, A., Brenner, C.A., Altuna, D., & Gabbert, G. (2003). Factors associated with development of speech production skills in children implanted by age five. *Ear and Hearing, 24* (suppl), 36–45

Tobey, E.A., Pancamo, S., Staller, S., Brimacombe, J., & Beiter, A. (1991). Consonant production children receiving a multichannel cochlear implant. *Ear and Hearing, 12,* 23–31

Toriello, H.V., Reardon, W., & Gorlin, R.J. (2004). *Hereditary Hearing Loss and Its Syndromes.* New York: Oxford University Press

Tye, N., Zimmermann, G., & Kelso, J. (1983). "Compensatory articulation" in hearing impaired speakers: a cinefluorographic study. *Journal of Phonetics, 11,* 101–115

Tye-Murray, N. (1984). Articulatory behavior of deaf and hearing speakers over changes in rate and stress: a cinefluorographic study. *Dissertation Abstracts International, 45,* 2128B

Tye-Murray, N. (1987). Effects of vowel context on the articulatory closure postures of deaf speakers. *Journal of Speech and Hearing Research, 30,* 99–104

Tye-Murray, N. (1991). The establishment of open articulatory postures by deaf and hearing talkers. *Journal of Speech and Hearing Research, 34,* 453–459

Tye-Murray, N. (1992). Articulatory organizational strategies and the role of audition. *Volta Review, 94,* 243–260

Tye-Murray, N. & Folkins, J. (1990). Jaw and lip movements of deaf talkers producing utterances with known stress patterns. *Journal of the Acoustical Society of America, 87,* 2675–2683

Tye-Murray, N. & Kirk, K. (1993). Vowel and diphthong production by young cochlear implant users and the relationship between the phonetic level evaluation and spontaneous speech. *Journal of Speech and Hearing Research, 36,* 488–502

Tye-Murray, N., Spencer, L., & Gilbert Bedia, E. (1995). Relationships between speech production and speech perception skills in young cochlear-implant users. *Journal of the Acoustical Society of America, 98,* 2454–2460

Tye-Murray, N., Spencer, L., Gilbert-Bedia, E., & Woodworth, G. (1996). Differences in children's sound production when speaking with a cochlear implant turned on and turned off. *Journal of Speech and Hearing Research, 39,* 604–610

Tye-Murray, N. & Woodworth, G. (1989). The influence of final-syllable position on the vowel and word duration of deaf talkers. *Journal of the Acoustical Society of America, 85,* 313–21

Tye-Murray, N., Zimmermann, G.N., & Folkins, J. (1987). Movement timing in deaf and hearing speakers: Comparison of phonetically heterogeneous syllable strings. *Journal of Speech and Hearing Research, 30,* 411–417

Uchanski, R.M. & Geers, A.E. (2003). Acoustic characteristics of the speech of young cochlear implant users: a comparison with normal-hearing age-mates. *Ear and Hearing, 24* (suppl), 90S-105S

U.S. Department of Education. (2002). To assure the free appropriate public education of all Americans: Twenty-fourth annual report to Congress on the Implementation of Individuals with Disabilities Education Act. http://www.ed.gov/about/reports/annual/osep/2002/index.html

Voelker, C. (1935). An experimental study of the comparative rate of utterance of deaf and normal-hearing speakers. *American Annals of the Deaf, 83,* 274–284

Vohr, B.R., Carty, L., Moore, P.E., & Letourneau, K. (1998). The Rhode Island Hearing Assessment Program: experience with statewide hearing screening (1993–1996). *Journal of Pediatrics, 133,* 353–357

Vorce, E. (1971). Speech curriculum. In: L.E. Connor (Ed.), *Speech for the Deaf Child* (pp. 221–224). Washington, DC: A.G. Bell Association for the Deaf

Vorce, E. (1974). *Teaching Speech to Deaf Children.* Washington, DC: A.G. Bell Association for the Deaf

Wake, M., Hughes, E.K., Poulakis, Z., Collins, C., & Rickards, F.W. (2004). Outcomes of children with mild-profound congenital hearing loss at 7 to 8 years: a population study. *Ear and Hearing, 25,* 1–8

Waldstein, R.S. (1990). Effects of postlingual deafness on speech production: implications for the role of auditory feedback. *Journal of the Acoustical Society of America, 88,* 2099–2114

Waldstein, R.S. & Baum, S. (1991). Anticipatory coarticulation in the speech of profoundly hearing-impaired and normally hearing children. *Journal of Speech and Hearing Research, 34,* 1276–1285

Wallace, V., Menn, L., & Yoshinaga-Itano, C. (1998). Is babble the gateway to speech for all children? A longitudinal study of children who are deaf or hard of hearing. *Volta Review, 100,* 121–148

Wallhagen, M.I., Strawbridge, W.J., Cohen, R.D., & Kaplan, G.A. (1997). An increasing prevalence of hearing impairment and associated risk factors over three decades of the Alameda County Study. *American Journal of Public Health, 87,* 440–442

Weismer, G., & Fennell, A. (1985). Constancy of (acoustic) relative timing measures in phrase-level utterances. *Journal of the Acoustical Society of America, 78,* 49–57

Weiss, A.L., Carney, A., & Leonard, L. (1985). Perceived contrastive stress production in hearing-impaired and normal hearing children. *Journal of Speech and Hearing Research, 28,* 26–35

West, J.J. & Weber, J. (1973). A phonological analysis of the spontaneous language of a four-year-old hard-of-hearing child. *Journal of Speech and Hearing Disorders, 38,* 25–35

Whalen, D. H, Iskarous, K., Tiede, M.K., Ostry, D.J., Lehnert-LeHouillier, H., Vatikiotis-Bateson, E., & Hailey, D.S. (2005). The Haskins Optically Corrected Ultrasound System (HOCUS). *Journal of Speech, Language, and Hearing Research, 48,* 543–553

Whitehead, R.L. (1982). Some respiratory and aerodynamic patterns in the speech of the hearing impaired. In: I. Hochberg, H. Levitt, & M.J. Osberger (Eds.), *Speech of the Hearing Impaired: Research, Training, and Personnel Preparation.* Baltimore: University Park Press

Whitehead, R.L. (1991). Stop consonant closure durations for normal-hearing and hearing-impaired speakers. *Volta Review, 93,* 145–153

Whitehead, R. & Barefoot, S.M. (1980). Some aerodynamic characteristics of plosive consonants produced by hearing-impaired speakers. *American Annals of the Deaf, 125,* 366–373

Whitehead, R.L. & Barefoot, S.M. (1983). Airflow characteristics of fricative consonants produced by normally hearing and hearing-impaired speakers. *Journal of Speech and Hearing Research, 26,* 185–194

Whitehead, R.L. & Jones, K. (1978). The effect of vowel environment on du-ration of consonants produced by normal-hearing, hearing-impaired and deaf adult speakers. *Journal of Phonetics, 6,* 77–81

Yoshinaga-Itano, C, Apuzzo, M., Coulter, D., & Stredler-Brown, A. (1995). The effect of early identification of hearing loss on development. Pre-sented at the Annual Convention of the American Academy of Audiol-ogy, Dallas, TX

Yoshinaga-Itano, C., & Sedey, A. (1998). Early speech development in chil-dren who are deaf or hard of hearing: interrelationships with language and hearing. *Volta Review, 100,* 181–211

Zimmermann, G. & Rettaliata, P. (1981). Articulatory patterns of an adven-titiously deaf speaker: implications for the role of auditory information in speech production. *Journal of Speech and Hearing Research, 24,* 169–178

Chapter 14

Adult-Onset Neurogenic Stuttering

Luc F. De Nil, Elizabeth Rochon, and Regina Jokel

When adults experience a stroke, suffer a head injury, or develop a neurodegenerative disorder or other disorder affecting normal brain functions, they sometimes develop speech disfluencies, which may closely resemble the characteristic speech behaviors typically associated with developmental stuttering. This speech disfluency disorder is most frequently referred to as neurogenic stuttering, although alternative terminology has been proposed over the years, such as acquired stuttering of adult onset (Andy & Bathnagar, 1992), cortical stuttering (Rosenbek, Messert, Collins, & Wertz, 1978), and stuttering associated with acquired neurological disorders (SAAND) (Helm-Estabrooks, 1993), among others. In this chapter, we will primarily use the term *neurogenic stuttering*. One of the earliest references to this disorder can be found in Pick (1899, quoted in Van Borsel, 1997), who wrote that he was "now able to prove that indeed brain disease which may have its localization in different parts of the brain, may lead to speech which on the one hand shows similarities with genuine stuttering and which on the other hand is certainly closely linked to aphasic disturbances of speech" (p. 447).

The incidence of neurogenic stuttering is not known, but it is believed to be relatively rare. However, the recognition of neurogenic stuttering in individuals may be obscured by the presence of other severe communication problems, such as aphasia, apraxia of speech, or dysarthria. Just as for developmental stuttering, neurogenic stuttering is more likely to be seen in men than in women, with gender ratios reported to be as high has 15:1 (Mazzucchi, Moretti, Carpeggiani, Parma, & Paini, 1981). Typically, acquired speech disfluencies develop in individuals who have no prior history of developmental stuttering, although sometimes a developmental stuttering condition may have existed prior to damage to the central nervous system. In the latter case, one can debate whether the condition should be categorized as neurogenic stuttering or be regarded as having triggered a reoccurrence or exacerbation of previously existing developmental stuttering. Given the sometimes questionable reliability of self-reports of recovery from stuttering or of the actual presence or absence of developmental stuttering in childhood, we would argue against excluding such patients from the study of neurogenic stuttering. If reported, their inclusion should be supported by reasonably well-documented evidence that the neurological condition resulted in a significant increase or change in observable stuttering, and by the carefully noted existence of a previous stuttering history.

Neurogenic stuttering needs to be differentiated from psychogenic stuttering, a separate disorder that typically also has its onset in adulthood (Mahr & Leith, 1992). Psychogenic stuttering most likely appears as a consequence of an emotional or psychological trauma and is characterized primarily by a sudden onset related in time to a significant event, with speech disfluencies consisting primarily of repetitions. The frequency of disfluencies in psychogenic stuttering does not appear to respond to typical fluency-enhancing conditions (e.g., singing, masking, choral reading), and initially does not trigger feelings of frustration, avoidance, or coping behaviors (Deal, 1982).

The differentiation between neurogenic and psychogenic stuttering is not always straightforward. Indeed, there have been several reported case studies of individuals in whom neurogenic stuttering was a telltale sign of a slowly developing neurological disorder, but who were initially diagnosed as psychogenic stuttering because of a lack of early evidence of any neurological signs (Lebrun, Retif, & Kaiser, 1983). Conversely, psychological or psychiatric reactions (e.g., depression) to neurological trauma or disease are not rare, and may accompany or possibly trigger the appearance of speech disfluencies. Despite these areas where differential diagnosis between the two adult-onset stuttering disorders may be difficult, this chapter deals exclusively with neurogenic stuttering. Readers interested in psychogenic stuttering are referred to two excellent review articles (Mahr & Leith, 1992; Roth, Aronson, & Davis, 1989).

Most reports of neurogenic stuttering have involved adults. However, if neurological disease or trauma can trigger the onset of stuttering-like symptoms, it should not be assumed a priori that this can occur only in adults. For instance, Nass, Schreter, and Heier (1994) reported on a 2-year-old child who presented with a sudden onset of stuttering, characterized primarily by severe repetitions of initial phonemes, lasting approximately 7 weeks following a second stroke. Increasingly, researchers are recognizing the likely involvement of deficient neurological processes in developmental stuttering (De Nil, 2001; Ingham, 2001), but very little is known about the extent to which early brain damage, such as strokes in children, may trigger stuttering disfluencies and whether or not these disfluencies can be differentiated reliably from developmental stuttering. Because the possible incidence of neurogenic stuttering in young children has received very little attention in the literature, our discussion focuses primarily on neurogenic stuttering in adults.

◆ Subgroups of Neurogenic Stuttering

Over the years, various subgroups of neurogenic stuttering have been proposed. For instance, Canter (1971) and, later, Rosenbek (1984) differentiated between dysarthric stuttering, apraxic stuttering, and dysnomic stuttering. Van Borsel (1997) distinguished between true neurogenic stuttering and stuttering that is drug-induced (pharmacogenic stuttering). More recently, he has suggested further subdivisions based on underlying lesion location, for example, thalamic stuttering (Van Borsel, Van Der Made, & Santens, 2003). Helm-Estabrooks, Yeo, Geschwind, and Freedman (1986) separately described stuttering associated with stroke, head trauma, extrapyramidal disease, tumor, dementia, drug usage, and other causes. Furthermore, she differentiated between transient and persistent neurogenic stuttering, which she believed to be associated with either multifocal unilateral (transient) or bilateral (persistent) lesions (Helm, Butler, & Canter, 1980). Many of these suggested subgroups are based primarily on differences in etiology or primary communication disorder, and may or may not reflect differences in symptomatology of speech disfluencies. In addition, subgroup categorizations are sometimes based on one or very few patients and it may be hard to differentiate between normal intersubject variations and true subgroup characteristics. Nevertheless, the possibility that differences in acquired stuttering may be reflective of loci and nature of the neurological lesions is intriguing and warrants further attention.

This chapter first discusses the important early contributions of Canter, whose descriptions of neurogenic stuttering have significantly influenced research and clinical practice, and then discusses the literature on neurogenic stuttering in persons with stroke, head injury, and neurodegenerative disorders, followed by a brief review of some other conditions that may result in acquired stuttering. We focus primarily on the nature of the speech motor difficulties, as evidenced by the nature of the speech disfluencies, the loci of neurological damage, the occurrence of secondary behaviors, concomitant language or motor disorders, and speech-associated attitudes and emotions. Following this review, we integrate what we know to date about neurogenic stuttering. Finally, a brief overview of diagnostic and treatment approaches that have been used in neurogenic stuttering is offered, along with some final comments on future research directions for this disorder.

◆ Canter's Contributions to Neurogenic Stuttering

In 1971, Gerald Canter published a paper, "Observations on Neurogenic Stuttering: A Contribution to Differential Diagnosis," in which he set out to describe neurogenic stuttering, a behavior that he called a subclass of disfluent speech, to contribute to the differential diagnostic abilities of clinicians working with the stuttering population. Canter described three subclassifications of neurogenic stuttering: (1) dysarthric stuttering in which speech fluency breakdown is a result of "faulty motor execution," and which is observed primarily in patients with Parkinson's disease and cerebellar lesions; (2) apraxic stuttering, seen in patients with apraxia of speech who have lost the ability to translate phonemes into motor speech patterns; and (3) dysnomic stuttering, in which stuttering is associated with word retrieval problems. According to Canter, each of these three subgroups with neurogenic stuttering presented with somewhat distinct types of speech disfluencies. Dysarthric stuttering is more likely to be characterized by tense articulatory blocks, apraxic stuttering consists primarily of "probing repetitions" of a sound as well as silent speech blocks, whereas the features of dysnomic stuttering are word or phrase repetitions prior to word retrieval, in addition to pauses, articulatory gropings, and interjections.

Probably most influential has been Canter's description of seven criteria that in his view could be used for differential diagnosis between developmental and neurogenic stuttering. The criteria he suggested to be associated with neurogenic stuttering are the following:

1. Repetitions and prolongations on final consonants

2. Moments of stuttering occurring primarily on /r/, /l/, and /h/

3. Disfluencies not systematically related to grammatical function (e.g., content versus function words)

4. Disfluencies possibly inversely related to the level of propositionality, with choral speech and repetitions resulting in more disfluencies compared with self-formulated speech

5. Absence of an adaptation effect (i.e., no decrease in disfluency with repeated readings)

6. Absence of marked anxiety about the disfluencies, although annoyance is possible

7. No secondary behaviors (e.g., avoidance or escape behaviors)

Canter's classification of neurogenic stuttering into three subclasses and the subsequent formulation of the diagnostic criteria were based primarily on his clinical observations and experience. Nevertheless, his paper arguably has been one of the most influential papers on the topic of neurogenic stuttering and, directly or indirectly, has guided many published case study reports of patients with neurogenic stuttering. At the same time, however, reviews of the published case studies, as well as several investigations on larger groups of persons with neurogenic stuttering, have cast doubt on the generalizability of Canter's observations. Reviewing the existing literature using Canter's criteria as a guide, Van Borsel (1997) concluded that "clinical symptomatology does not enable one to safely distinguish neurogenic stuttering from developmental stuttering" (p. 21). Ringo and Dietrich (1995) suggested that the clinical usefulness of Canter's criteria could be "increased by elaborating and redefining the details of their characterization" (p. 117). For instance, several reports have documented the presence of reading adaptation (Jokel & De Nil, 2003; McClean & McLean, 1985), secondary behaviors (Ludlow, Rosenberg, Salazar, Grafman, & Smutok, 1987; Van Borsel, Van Lierde, Cauwenberge, Guldermont, & Van Orshoven, 2001), or emotional reactions (Jokel & De Nil, 2003; McClean & McLean, 1985) in patients with neurogenic stuttering. Whether or not neurogenic stuttering tends to be phoneme-specific remains to be investigated, but it almost certainly is not restricted to the phonemes identified by Canter. Although it has become obvious that Canter's criteria are an overgeneralization of his clinical observations, it needs to be pointed out that Canter himself stated that "few of our neurogenic stutterers have shown all of these characteristics; and it should also be emphasized that the presence of one or two of them cannot be considered to be diagnostic of neurogenesis" (Canter 1971, p. 142). Furthermore, he suggested that these criteria should not be used as firm diagnostic measures but rather could lead to forming a hypothesis regarding the presence of neurogenic stuttering, which would need confirmation with further neurological and other diagnostic procedures.

Regardless of the ultimate validity of Canter's criteria, it remains true that his contribution was one of the first papers to address neurogenic stuttering systematically as a disorder in its own right, warranting disorder-specific diagnostic and treatment considerations. There is no question that for clinicians Canter's paper triggered an awareness of the presence of neurogenic stuttering, leading to a significant increase in reported case studies and a greater understanding of the disorder.

Three classes of neurological disorders appear to be most associated with neurogenic stuttering: stroke, head injury, and neurodegenerative diseases. In the following sections we review the characteristics of neurogenic stuttering in each of these as well as in some other conditions.

◆ Neurogenic Stuttering Associated with Stroke

Neurogenic stuttering may occur following a cortical or subcortical stroke in adults. It appears to affect males more than females. Indeed, the male-to-female ratio in the case studies reviewed for this chapter was approximately 5:1.

Case Study 1: Neurogenic Stuttering Associated with Stroke

Z.K., a 55-year-old right-handed man who worked as an asset manager for a large Canadian company, was born in a North-African country but completed his education, including his MBA, in Canada. His past medical history and his family history did not include neurological disease or a history of stuttering. Prior to his stroke he was fluent in English, Arabic, French, and Armenian.

In January 1994 he was admitted to a local hospital with signs of stroke. A computed tomography (CT) scan revealed an infarct in the frontoparietal region of the left hemisphere. Upon admission he presented with some right-sided weakness of his upper limb, Broca's type aphasia, and non-fluent speech, which initially was interpreted as one of the features of his aphasia. Within the first 18 months after the stroke, Z.K. received intensive speech and physical therapy. As his impairments resolved, it became apparent that in addition to the nonfluent speech typical of Broca's aphasia, Z.K. developed disfluencies consistent with stuttering. At the conclusion of his rehabilitation program stuttering was his only speech impediment.

Z.K. was seen again 4 years post-onset. He presented with intact language and cognition (Mini–Mental State Examination score of 30/30). At the time of his assessment, he was repeating single words, sounds, and syllables in initial and medial positions of multisyllabic words. No secondary behaviors were observed on evaluation or reported by the patient. He reported more frequent stuttering while speaking to an unfamiliar person or in public. Formal assessment showed varied frequencies of stuttered moments depending on the speech task. For instance, although monologue and conversational speech yielded disfluency rates of 19.5% each, automatic speech (i.e., naming the days of the week) was completely fluent. Relative to speech, reading was somewhat better with 2% disfluency on single word reading, 13% on sentence reading, and 10% on reading a passage. No adaptation was noted on repeated reading of the passage. His overall score on the Stuttering Severity Instrument-3 was 25, which suggested a moderate severity. Z.K.'s speech fluency improved with pacing and choral speech.

In most cases, the onset of stuttering was a first occurrence, although a few cases have been reported where the stroke triggered a reoccurrence of childhood stuttering (Mazzuchi et al, 1981; Mouradian, Paslawski, & Shuaib, 2000). For instance, Mouradian et al reported on a 68-year-old woman who presented with moderately severe disfluency following a stroke. According to the woman, she had stuttered as a child but had outgrown her stuttering by the age of 12. Although her premorbid normal fluency was confirmed by her daughter who was not aware of the fact that her mother had ever stuttered, it must be noted that the woman's poststroke disfluencies consisted primarily of interjections, part- and whole-word repetitions, phrase repetitions, and revisions. This raises questions regarding the validity of the stuttering diagnosis as only part-word repetitions are typically included in the core behaviors of stuttering (Bloodstein, 1995; Conture, 2001). Because a more comprehensive speech and language evaluation was not possible in this patient, it could not be ascertained to what extent some of the disfluencies may have reflected language deficiencies, such as word retrieval problems due to aphasia.

The brain sites affected by the stroke in patients who develop neurogenic stuttering vary widely and include subcortical regions such as the thalamus and brainstem (Abe, Yokoyama, & Yorifuji, 1993; Van Borsel & Taillieu, 2000), basal ganglia (Nass et al, 1994), and cerebellum (Van Borsel & Taillieu, 2000), as well as cortical regions including temporal and parietal lobe (Ardila & Lopez, 1986; Bijleveld,

Lebrun, & Dongen, 1994; Helm-Estabrooks et al, 1986), supplementary motor area (Van Borsel et al, 2001), and frontal cortex (Van Borsel & Taillieu, 2000). Lesions can occur either unilaterally or bilaterally in the left as well as the right hemisphere. As mentioned before, Helm, Butler, and Benson (1978) have suggested that neurogenic stuttering tends to persist in persons who show bilateral lesions, whereas multifocal unilateral lesions are more likely to be associated with transient stuttering. This may be the result of reduced interhemispheric compensatory mechanisms in bilateral lesions. There is some evidence that compensation for affected functions following stroke is initially accomplished by contralateral compensation in homologous regions immediately following the stroke, whereas long-term recovery of function involves intrahemispheric compensation (Fernandez, Cardebat, Demonet, Joseph, Mazaux, Barat, et al, 2004). Presumably, such interhemispheric compensation would be affected negatively by the presence of bilateral lesions, possibly resulting in more chronic or persistent fluency problems.

Speech disfluencies associated with stroke are likely to be composed of repetitions that involve short segments, such as sounds or syllables, as well as longer words and phrases. In a study of seven individuals with stroke, Rosenbek et al (1978) reported that on average, 72% of all disfluencies consisted of sound and syllable repetitions (including single syllable words), compared with only 14% prolongations. No speech blocks were reported in this study. In some individuals, the occurrence of repetitions appears to be task specific. Abe et al (1993) described a male patient who had suffered a bilateral medial thalamic and brainstem infarct and who showed syllable repetitions but only during spontaneous speech and not during word repetition or reading. Van Borsel et al (2003) also reported on an individual who experienced a thalamic stroke and whose disfluencies consisted primarily of word and part-word repetitions as well as interjections. Similar to the person described by Abe et al, the individual reported on by Van Borsel and colleagues showed a significantly higher frequency of stuttering during propositional speech tasks (e.g., conversation and monologue) as compared with nonpropositional tasks (e.g., counting, word repetition, and reading aloud). This observation raises the possibility that the site of lesion may influence task-specific variability in neurogenic stuttering.

According to Canter's (1971) criteria, repetitions and prolongations in neurogenic stuttering are likely to occur in any position in the word or sentence (initial, medial, or final). However, a review of published case studies of stuttering following stroke reveals that the large majority of disfluencies are observed in word or syllable initial positions. For instance, repetitions in the patient reported by Abe et al (1993) were restricted to initial syllables in words. Similarly, stuttering was restricted to initial parts or sounds of a word in a woman who experienced a right hemisphere stroke at the age of 42 (Fleet & Heilman, 1985). In analyzing the speech disfluencies of seven individuals with stroke, Rosenbek, et al (1978) observed disfluencies primarily in initial word positions, with the most severe patients showing "some instances of medial position repetitions" (p. 87). In our own study of six individuals with stroke, 93% and

95% of disfluencies occurred in word initial position during reading and spontaneous speech, respectively (Jokel & De Nil, 2003; Jokel, De Nil, & Sharpe, 2007). An interesting observation in this study was that individuals with stroke showed a decrease in the frequency of stuttering disfluencies as the reading material became more complex. The ratio of nonstuttering/stuttering disfluency shifted from 0.94 during word reading to 1.48 during paragraph reading. This may indicate that, as the material became more complex, disfluencies resulting from language deficiencies became more prominent compared with the core stuttering disfluencies. As such, in stroke, and possibly other populations as well, the nature of the language and reading material needs to be considered when comparing across studies and across individuals.

Persons with developmental stuttering often show a marked improvement in fluency with repeated readings of the same text, an effect known as adaptation (Bloodstein, 1995). Most likely, adaptation in developmental stuttering is the result of motor practice, and the lack of reading adaptation has been cited to be one of the key differential diagnostic criteria for neurogenic stuttering (Canter, 1971). Helm-Estabrooks and colleagues (1986) listed the lack of adaptation as one of the typical characteristics of stroke-induced stuttering. However, many authors have pointed to the equivocal nature of this criterion, as not all people with developmental stuttering show adaptation (Bloodstein, 1995), and not all individuals with neurogenic stuttering fail to demonstrate adaptation (Mazzuchi et al, 1981; Van Borsel, 1997). It is hard to evaluate the proportion of persons with neurogenic stuttering following stroke who show an adaptation effect because not all case studies indicate whether adaptation was present or not, and if they do, it is not always clear how the effect was assessed, thereby making it difficult to assert the validity or the generalizability of the claim. In our own study of six persons with stroke-induced stuttering, four were able to complete three successive readings of the rainbow passage. Three of these four showed a reduction in the frequency of their disfluencies of more than 30% from the first to the third reading (Jokel & De Nil, 2003; Jokel et al, 2007). This finding casts doubt on whether the presence or absence of reading adaptation indeed is a useful criterion in the differential diagnosis of neurogenic stuttering with an etiology of stroke.

Many studies also do not include information on secondary behaviors or psychological or emotional reactions. Rosenbek et al (1978) reported some accessory features (such as eye blinking and facial grimacing) in three of the seven most severe individuals in their study. However, they observed that "elaborate, florid accessory features of some young adult stutterers were never noted" (p. 88). In our own study, the average score on the S-24, a speech attitude questionnaire commonly used with persons with developmental stuttering, was 18.3. This score is almost identical to that reported for developmental stuttering, suggesting that individuals with stroke-induced stuttering hold the same negative perceptions with regard to their speech competence as do persons with developmental stuttering.

◆ Neurogenic Stuttering Associated with Neurodegenerative Disorders

Neurogenic stuttering has also been observed in persons who develop neurodegenerative diseases. In particular, several case studies have been reported in persons with Parkinson's disease (Hertrich, Ackermann, Ziegler, & Kashel, 1993; Leder, 1996; Louis, Winfield, Fahn, & Ford, 2001), motor neuron diseases (Lebrun et al, 1983), and multiple sclerosis (Mowrer & Younts, 2001).

Case Study 2: Neurogenic Stuttering Associated with Parkinson's Disease

G.N., a right-handed engineer, was diagnosed with idiopathic Parkinson's disease (PD) at the age of 62. He was born in Europe and completed a bachelor's degree in English. He spoke fluent English, Italian, Polish, and German. He had no history of speech or language difficulties, and there was no history of PD in his family.

At the time of his speech fluency assessment, G.N. was 74 years old. His cognitive and language evaluation did not reveal any impairment. Consistent with hypokinetic dysarthria, his speech was characterized by hypophonia and short rushes of poorly articulated speech. In addition he stuttered on single words and sounds in a way that was distinctly different from palilalia. G.N. remarked that the disfluencies appeared gradually approximately 5 years after he was diagnosed with PD. A CT scan revealed moderate age-related brain atrophy.

G.N. appeared mildly disfluent, though by his own appraisal he was "moderate." The most prominent disfluency type was sound repetitions. Other disfluencies took the form of initial syllable and word repetitions and some prolongations. G.N. never stuttered on medial or final sounds/words. No secondary behaviors were observed or reported by the patient.

Formal assessment revealed that the frequency of stuttering was task-dependent. Although G.N. was only 2 to 3% disfluent in reading single words and sentences, reading a passage yielded 12% disfluencies. Because of poor breath support, G.N. could only read the passage twice. There was virtually no difference in the level of fluency between the two readings. Conversational speech was associated with a higher incidence of stuttered moments (19%), whereas automatic speech was 6.7% disfluent. His overall score on the Stuttering Severity Instrument-3 was 23, consistent with a mild stuttering severity. G.N.'s speech fluency was improved with pacing.

Parkinson's disease (PD) tends to affect males more than females and men with PD appear to be much more likely to be affected by neurogenic stuttering, but the small number of reported cases in the literature makes this difficult to judge. PD affects the extrapyramidal brain system and results from the accumulation of fibrous protein deposits in the brain, especially the substantia nigra and locus ceruleus, which may interfere with normal neuronal function (Haass & Kahle, 2000). Because of the selective death of the neurons that normally secrete the neurotransmitter dopamine, the movement characteristics of PD include muscle rigidity (especially of the limbs), resting tremor, festinating gait, lack of facial expression, and general poverty of voluntary movement. Canter (1971) characterized neurogenic stuttering in this population as "dysarthric stuttering," which he described as being characterized by attempts to produce rapid movements, articulatory freezing, and frequent prolongations or silent blocks. It appears that some of the characteristics of neurogenic stuttering in these individuals may be related to their overall movement characteristics. For instance, Louis et al (2001) reported on two patients with PD and neurogenic stuttering, one of whom showed frequent pausing and occasional blocking. The other displayed "pressured speech" and freezing of speech, as well as sound repetitions. Leder (1996) observed a 29-year-old individual with PD whose stuttering was characterized by multiple repetitions, often involving 20 or more repeated units, and blocks. Although the frequent and excessive repetitions could be considered similar to palilalia (Canter, 1971), Van Borsel (1997) views stuttering repetitions in this population as very distinct from palilalic disorders because palilalia tends to produce repetitions primarily affecting speech fragments longer than those typically seen in stuttering. In this light it is interesting to note that Hertrich et al (1993) described a female with PD who showed significant sound, word, and phrase repetitions but only on longer utterances. Few or no stuttering moments were observed on single words and short sentences. Disfluencies occurred on initial as well as final words in phrases, but initial disfluencies tended to involve consonant-vowel segments, whereas final disfluencies were more likely to involve longer syllable-level segments.

The person reported by Leder (1996) represents an interesting case study of how neurogenic stuttering, in the absence of any obvious neurological problems, may be misdiagnosed initially as psychogenic stuttering. Indeed, in this individual, the occurrence of stuttering was the first sign of the onset of PD, which was not diagnosed until approximately 10 months later. Only when she received a diagnosis of PD was the speech diagnosis changed from psychogenic to neurogenic stuttering. Neurogenic stuttering was also one of the first symptoms of a developing motor neuron disease in a 54-year-old man (Lebrun et al, 1983) who gradually developed stuttering-like disfluencies (repetitions of sounds and syllables and occasional prolongations and blocks) that became progressively worse. Following the onset of his stuttering, he developed other neurological symptoms that were initially thought to signal the onset of PD but were ultimately diagnosed as (upper) motor neuron disease. Similarly, Quinn and Andrews (1977) described a 62-year-old businessman for whom gradually developing stuttering may have signaled the early onset of Alzheimer's disease, which was confirmed approximately 7 months later.

Acquired stuttering in a person with multiple sclerosis was reported by Mowrer and Younts (2001). The 36-year-old man in this study showed excessive part- and whole-word repetitions, which occurred primarily in initial position, but also to a lesser extent in medial and final positions. In addition to his excessive disfluencies, his speech was characterized by abnormal prosody, and it was very slow. Multiple sclerosis results from a loss of myelin in the brain, resulting in lesions (plaques or sclerosis). Depending on the localization of this damage, symptoms may include dysarthria, discoordination of articulatory movements, and increased spasticity, which may in part account for the prosodic characteristics and the excessive slow speech of the patient described by Mowrer and Younts (2001).

Very few reports of individuals with neurodegenerative diseases include reports on the presence or absence of secondary behaviors, reading adaptation, or psychological reactions to the stuttering. The case described by Lebrun et al (1983) reported becoming more disfluent when tense or at meetings. The person with PD in the paper by Leder (1996) was reported not to have developed speech fears. No secondary behaviors were observed in the individuals described by Mowrer and Younts (2001) and Leder (1996). According to Helm-Estabrooks (1993), adaptation effects are occasionally seen in these individuals, but very few published reports comment on the presence or absence of this feature. No adaptation effect was observed by Hertrich and colleagues (1993).

◆ Neurogenic Stuttering Associated with Traumatic Brain Injury

Reports of neurogenic stuttering subsequent to a traumatic brain injury (TBI) have often involved victims of motor vehicle accidents (Dworkin, Culatta, Abkarian, & Meleca, 2002; Marshall & Neuburger, 1987; McClean & McLean, 1985), but several papers have also reported cases of penetrating wounds to the head (Lebrun, Bijleveld, & Rousseau, 1990; Lebrun & Leleux, 1985; Ludlow et al, 1987).

Case Study 3: Neurogenic Stuttering Associated with Head Injury

C.W., a 41-year-old predominantly right-handed woman who worked as a teacher, had a history of asthma, epilepsy, and hypoglycemia, all controlled with medications. There was no history of speech or language problems in C.W. or her family, though neither she nor her two siblings were good spellers.

At the age of 32 C.W. was struck in the head by a child on a swing. She lost consciousness and appeared confused upon regaining consciousness. Shortly after the accident she reported the onset of stuttering. She was subsequently diagnosed with head injury and posttraumatic stress disorder. A magnetic resonance imaging (MRI) scan of the head did not reveal any structural abnormalities. A single photon emission computed tomography (SPECT) scan performed at the same time showed bilateral symmetrical hypoperfusion in the frontal lobes.

Although C.W. complained of some comprehension and word finding problems at the time of her fluency assessment, her performance on all language tasks was normal.

On cognitive testing she performed more poorly on the attention subtest of the Mini–Mental State Examination test. C.W. perceived her stuttering as mild, which was inconsistent with her moderate Stuttering Severity Index (SSI)-3 score of 25. She reported particular difficulty with the sounds /s/ and /p/. The sound-specific stuttering was not observed on formal testing; however, C.W. repeated many other initial sounds and initial and medial words in sentences. Sound and syllable repetitions were noted on all tasks, whereas prolongations and a few blocks occurred mostly in reading. No secondary behaviors were noted.

Formal assessment of disfluencies in reading showed that reading single words evoked a much higher severity of disfluency than oral reading of sentences (42% and 28%, respectively). Repeated reading of a passage showed a 50% reduction in disfluencies by the third trial. C.W. was only 12% disfluent in conversational speech, whereas her disfluencies increased to more than 30% on automatic speech tasks. Several therapeutic techniques, such as choral reading, pacing, and reduced speech rate were tried with C.W.; however, none induced any changes. C.W. reported that she found acupuncture, massage therapy, and meditation helpful in alleviating some of the speech problems.

In the case of neurogenic stuttering, analyzing the site of lesion in TBI may provide valuable information about the neural systems involved in speech fluency. However, not all persons with TBI show evidence of neurological lesions upon medical examination, especially those with closed head injury. This may sometimes trigger a diagnosis of psychogenic stuttering. In one of our own studies (Jokel & De Nil, 2003), five of the six patients with medically diagnosed TBI did not show any findings on neuroimaging studies, and four of them were initially diagnosed with psychogenic stuttering. In the absence of an observable neurological lesion, such differential diagnosis can be very difficult to make in the TBI population. Dworkin et al (2002), for instance, described a person who developed stuttering 4 weeks after a motor vehicle accident that resulted in several medical complaints, such as photophobia, nausea, headaches, and cervical tenderness. The diagnosis of psychogenic stuttering was made based on the absence of a neurological lesion, a high frequency of disfluencies without fluent moments, the sudden onset of the stuttering symptoms, and the case history. Marshall and Neuburger (1987) presented three individuals who developed stuttering after sustaining a TBI, two as a result of a motor vehicle accident and one from a fall. Detailed information on the nature and site of the lesion, was not available for all individuals. The person who suffered a fall was diagnosed with a left temporal hematoma that was removed surgically, whereas one of the motor vehicle accident individuals experienced a brainstem concussion.

Other lesion sites noted in persons with neurogenic stuttering are left and right frontal cortex (Helm-Estabrooks et al, 1986; Quinn & Andrews, 1977), bilateral parietal cortex (Lebrun et al, 1990), and unilateral right parietal cortex (Marshall & Neuburger, 1987). Ludlow and colleagues (1987) reported on 10 Vietnam War veterans who had sustained penetrating missile wounds resulting in acquired stuttering as one of the symptoms; five evidenced unilateral right lesions, one had a bilateral lesion, and four had primarily left-lateralized lesions. Interestingly, the localization of the lesions was similar in both hemispheres. These regions included cortical areas (Broca's area, supplementary motor area, primary motor area, supramarginal and angular gyri, and Wernicke's area), subcortical white matter, anterior frontal as well as posterior temporal and the corpus callosum, basal ganglia, and brainstem. In comparison with a control group of traumatically brain injured who did not experience speech disfluencies, the group with neurogenic stuttering was more likely to show lesions in the corpus callosum and the basal ganglia (caudate and lentiform nuclei). Although the site of lesion was somewhat similar between the two groups, Ludlow and colleagues point out that the use of CT scans may have failed to reveal all lesion sites, and individual differences in brain organization for speech may account for differential rates of onset of neurogenic stuttering and recovery from the disorder.

An interesting case study was reported by Helm-Estabrooks et al (1986) of a man who had experienced developmental stuttering since the age of 8 but who no longer stuttered when he emerged from a coma 10 days after a TBI. The authors speculated that the resolution of stuttering might have been a consequence of establishing hemispheric dominance for motor tasks as a result of lesioning one hemisphere. However, because he also displayed slowed dysarthric speech, it is possible that the disfluencies were eliminated or reduced as a result of his other motor speech symptoms. Indeed, based on the published report, improvement of his dysarthria and hemiparesis was associated with a gradual increase in the frequency of his disfluencies, although 1 year later they were still at a level below that seen prior to the accident.

The onset of neurogenic stuttering in TBI individuals tends to be relatively sudden and occurs close to the time of the accident, but sometimes the onset of stuttering is reported a considerable time after the occurrence of the brain injury. For instance, the patient described by Quinn and Andrews (1977) was reported to have started stuttering 2 years post injury, whereas Lebrun and Leleux (1985) reported on an individual whose stuttering symptoms started appearing 32 years after the injury, at the same time as some of his other neurological symptoms gradually worsened. A patient of the first author of this chapter reported the onset of stuttering approximately 1 year after sustaining a fall that resulted in chronic headaches and mild cognitive problems.

Rapid speech rate is one of the main speech characteristics seen in many persons with neurogenic stuttering following TBI. Ludlow et al (1987) described the speech in one person with neurogenic stuttering as "shot from a gun, with intermittent and unpredictable bursts of rapid and unintelligible speech, uncontrolled repetitions or prolongations, and long silences without struggle" (p. 62). All three cases described by Marshall and Neuburger (1987) were characterized as having rapid speech rate, characterized primarily by repetitions of sounds, syllables, words, and phrases. Repetitions were the most frequent disfluency type, followed by less frequently occurring prolongations and occasional blocks, although a case of long blocks, lasting several seconds, at the beginning of words has also been reported

(Lebrun et al, 1990). Lebrun et al's case presented with acquired stuttering following right parietal damage after a missile wound. In addition to the long blocks, the main disfluencies included initial sound and syllable repetitions and prolongations. In our observations of six persons with TBI (Jokel et al, 2007), most disfluencies during reading consisted of repetitions, prolongations, and blocks, although overall they consisted of less than 50% of all disfluencies observed. The proportional frequency of stuttering disfluencies tended to increase during spontaneous speech. Proportionally, the frequency of the disfluencies did not change based on the complexity of the reading material (words, sentences, paragraphs), but in spontaneous speech the frequency of stuttering disfluencies tended to be higher in monologue than in conversation. In most cases described in the literature, disfluencies occur primarily in initial and medial word positions. Again, our observations indicated that individuals with TBI experienced the most disfluencies (82%) in word initial positions, followed by word medial and then word final positions. During spontaneous speech, a higher percentage of word final disfluencies (13%) was present.

As in stroke and neurodegenerative disorders, the presence or absence of a reading adaptation effect in persons with TBI is inconsistent. One individual described by McClean and McLean (1985) showed little adaptation following repeated reading. Of the five persons with TBI who were able to complete the adaptation task in our study, only two showed a decrease in disfluencies of 30% or greater (Jokel et al, 2007). This finding seems in keeping with the observations reported by Helm-Estabrooks et al (1986), who noted that the adaptation effect is rare in patients with head trauma. Although secondary behaviors may be present in some persons with TBI (Lebrun et al, 1990; Ludlow et al, 1987), several reported cases do not seem to show evidence of such coping behavior (Dworkin et al, 2002; Lebrun & Leleux, 1985; McClean & McLean, 1985). Of our six TBI patients, three showed such behaviors and three did not. Secondary behaviors observed in these individuals consisted of more frequent than usual eye blinking, facial grimacing, head bending, foot tapping, and limb or head movements associated with stuttered moments but incongruent with the context.

As noted above, stuttering following a TBI may be more likely to be diagnosed with psychogenic stuttering than with more easily identifiable neurological conditions, especially if no observable neurological lesion can be found. As a result, case studies of acquired stuttering in this population are more likely to include reference to the presence or absence of psychological reactions to the disfluencies. Typically, it is reported that this population is aware of the stuttering but not anxious or overly concerned (Lebrun et al, 1990; Lebrun & Leleux, 1985; McClean & McLean, 1985). Speech-associated attitudes in the six persons with TBI and acquired stuttering in our study were investigated using the S-24 (Andrews & Cutler, 1974), a questionnaire often used in the assessment of adults with developmental stuttering. The range of scores on this test for our cases ranged from 15 to 18 (maximum possible score of 24) with an average score for the group of 16.8. This score placed them in between the average scores typically obtained for nonstuttering (9) and stuttering (19) speakers. However, their uniformly elevated score on the S-24 compared with the fluent speakers attests to a general negative self-perception of speech abilities, which may be an important consideration for diagnosis and intervention.

◆ Neurogenic Stuttering Associated with Other Disorders

Like TBI, several conditions have been reported that are not necessarily correlated with anatomical or functional brain lesions or disorders. Perino, Famularo, and Tarroni (2000) reported on a 26-year-old woman who complained of bilateral frontal and temporal headaches. She developed stuttering 3 hours prior to visiting the hospital. There was no previous stuttering history in this individual or her family. Her medical record was unremarkable except for insulin-dependent diabetes since the age of 6 years. Although her neurological examination, including CT scan and electroencephalogram (EEG), was normal, she experienced severe stuttering. The stuttering consisted of blocks and repetitions (up to 20 repetitions per word) during both reading and conversation. Her headache and stuttering disappeared completely following the administration of analgesic medication (sumatriptan).

Andy and Bhatnagar (1992) described three individuals with chronic pain and who developed stuttering. One had a 20-year history of trigeminal pain and progressively developed stuttering that consisted primarily of prolongations, repetitions, and hesitations. No secondary behaviors or reading adaptation were observed. A second had severe and chronic lower back pain and subsequent development of stuttering. Her disfluencies consisted of hesitations and syllable and word repetitions. No secondary behaviors, anxiety, or reading adaptation were present. A third developed stuttering within 1 year after the onset of chronic pain. Her stuttering consisted primarily of blocks without any secondary behaviors. In each of the three, stuttering had existed for several years. Thalamic brain stimulation for pain alleviation in the left centromedial nucleus of the thalamus resulted in a significant improvement of fluency or elimination of stuttering in all three cases, which was maintained during follow-up ranging from 5 to 8 years.

Several case studies reported on acquired iatrogenic stuttering in adults. Pimental and Gorelick (1985) reported two individuals who developed stuttering following a myelography examination. Myelography is an imaging procedure that checks the integrity of the spinal canal and requires the injection of a dye, in this case metrizamide. Both individuals developed severe aphasia and apraxia of speech together with severe stuttering within hours following the procedure. Stuttering was described as sound, syllable, and word repetitions, prolongations of the initial sound, and blocks accompanied by facial grimaces and struggle. Although the stuttering frequency and struggle spontaneously subsided within the days following its onset, both patients were still

reported to experience mild stuttering disfluencies 3 to 5 months later, and some language difficulties remained. Meghji (1994) described a female who developed stuttering and clumsy speech following administration of fluoxetine for clinical depression, and whose speech difficulties continued after the pharmacological agent was stopped. This person had had a self-reported transient episode of stuttering 2 years prior, and had a brother who reportedly stuttered in elementary school. Her stuttering was characterized by a high frequency of sound and syllable repetitions and easy prolongations during spontaneous speech and reading. There was evidence of lip tremor and eye blinking. Traditional speech therapy resulted in marked improvement of fluency. Several other case studies of drug-induced stuttering have been described in the literature, including stuttering following administration of psychotropic drugs reported by Brewerton, Markowitz, Keller, and Cochrane, (1996), Burd and Kerbeshian (1991), Christensen, Byerly, and McElroy (1996), Ebeling, Compton, and Albright (1997), and epileptic drugs reported by Helm et al (1980), McClean and McLean (1985), and Nissani and Sanchez (1997).

A rather unique case history was reported by Byrne, Byrne, and Zibin (1993) of a 25–year-old man who had been anorexic since the age of 17. Following a 4-month period of severe weight loss, he developed disfluencies that consisted primarily of syllable repetitions with no improvement following task repetition (adaptation). Although he reportedly was slightly annoyed by the disfluencies, there was no evidence of marked anxiety. As his diet improved over the next 2 weeks, stuttering improved and ultimately disappeared altogether. The authors hypothesized that the occurrence of stuttering may have been related to chronic hypoglycemia, which would have resulted in global cerebral disfunction.

◆ Synthesis of Observations

What we know about neurogenic stuttering is based primarily on publications of clinical case studies that report on observations of one or a few individuals seen in clinical practice. Relatively few papers discuss observations on a larger and more homogeneous group, and even fewer reports result from a priori planned systematic group. This is not surprising given the nature and low incidence of the disorder. Indeed, it is probably fair to state that many of these published case studies are based on rather opportunistic clinical encounters.

Although not all clinical reports are equally detailed in their description of the case history and characteristics of the speech, they nevertheless have yielded a rich database that enables us to appreciate the complexity of neurogenic stuttering. However, the heterogeneity of individual speech patterns that are reported makes it challenging to obtain a global picture of the symptomatology of stuttering in this population, if indeed such a picture exists. In this respect, it is potentially problematic that, as the number of reported cases of neurogenic stuttering expands, future published studies may increasingly describe atypical or unusual clinical cases. The danger exists that the idiosyncratic symptomatology of unusual cases may become seen as the norm by which neurogenic stuttering is defined. The obvious solution appears to be the initiation of large-scale prospective studies of speech fluency characteristics in targeted selected populations (e.g., stroke, PD, head injury, etc.), but the resources needed to carry out such studies may be difficult to obtain. Despite these limitations in our current knowledge, some general tentative conclusions regarding neurogenic stuttering can be made.

◆ Site of Lesion

The picture that seems to emerge from the literature on neurogenic stuttering is one in which almost every region of the brain appears to be implicated in the generation or triggering of disfluencies. As discussed before, adult-onset stuttering has been seen in patients with cortical as well as subcortical lesions, and in persons with frontal as well as temporal and parietal lesions. Lesions do not need to be confined to cerebral regions but may involve the cerebellum as well as the brainstem. In addition, lesions may involve both gray and white matter and may be relatively confined to particular areas of the brain, or be diffuse and involving larger areas or even whole hemispheres. Although the study of neurogenic stuttering potentially may help to reveal the neurological basis of speech fluency, the current picture does not appear to be very helpful and has prompted some researchers to state that "neurogenic stuttering ... does not appear to be linked to any specific lesion site" (Van Borsel, 1997, p. 21). Similarly, Mazzucchi et al (1981) concluded "acquired stuttering, like other neurological signs, could be the final dysfunctional result of lesions variously located" (p. 28). The widespread involvement of various cortical and subcortical sites may not come as a surprise given that normal speech and language processes themselves are represented as a highly complex and distributed neural system involving many regions of the brain (Demonet, Thierry, & Cardebat, 2005). Nevertheless, it is possible that some similarities are beginning to emerge. For instance, Ludlow et al (1987) concluded that the data from their 10 individuals with brain injury who showed persistent stuttering are suggestive of involvement of subcortical pyramidal and extrapyramidal systems unilaterally on either the right or the left side. This conclusion, however, appears to be contradictory to the conclusion reached by Helm and colleagues (1978), who stated that transient acquired stuttering is most likely to be associated with unilateral multifocal hemispheric damage, whereas persistent stuttering is more likely to occur with bilateral damage. The fact that Helm and colleagues based their conclusions primarily on observations of stroke and PD, whereas Ludlow and colleagues studied brain injured persons, may suggest that site of lesion leading to acquired stuttering may be affected by the nature of the neurological disorder.

Recent developments in functional imaging research in adults with developmental stuttering has implicated functional overactivation of sensorimotor areas of the brain as one of the brain systems likely to be involved in the cause or maintenance of developmental stuttering (Braun, Varga, Stager, Schulz, Selbie, Maisog, et al, 1997; De Nil, 2001; De Nil, Kroll, Lafaille, & Houle, 2003; Fox, Ingham, Ingham, Hirsch, Downs, & Martin, 1996). Furthermore, Wu and colleagues (1995), using SPECT in persons with developmental stuttering, have observed hypoactivation of the dopamine system in the basal ganglia. Changes in speech fluency appear to be correlated directly with greater normalization of activation in these cortical and subcortical motor areas (De Nil et al, 2003; Fox et al, 1996). Similar functional imaging studies are currently still lacking in neurogenic stuttering, but the findings in developmental stuttering, coupled with observations by Ludlow et al (1987) and others with regard to involvement of pyramidal and extrapyramidal systems in neurogenic stuttering, seem to strongly implicate lesions or deficiencies in the motor system as one of the central neural variables in neurogenic stuttering.

Another argument for the involvement of the motor system in neurogenic stuttering stems from the fact that the disorder often occurs as part of the complex symptomatology of a variety of neurogenic disorders, including but not limited to tumors, dementia, PD, stroke, TBI, and multiple sclerosis, or it may be drug induced. Although several of these disorders, such as stroke, may also affect language faculties, this does not seem to be a prerequisite for the appearance or persistence of neurogenic stuttering. Mazzucchi et al (1981) observed signs of aphasia in 10 of their 16 cases with neurogenic stuttering. However, as they pointed out, the relationship between aphasia and stuttering was not straightforward. For instance, stuttering could precede aphasia, or vice versa. Also, in some individuals, the aphasia was transient but stuttering was persistent, whereas in others the stuttering was transient but the aphasia persisted. Their conclusion that a pathogenically linked association between acquired stuttering and aphasia is unlikely was further supported by the observation that only 6 to 7% of aphasic patients develop neurogenic stuttering. Nevertheless, the co-occurrence of aphasia may aggravate the severity of stuttering. For instance, Farmer (1975) noted a higher frequency of stuttering repetitions among brain-damaged persons with aphasia as compared with those without signs of aphasia. But her definition of stuttering repetitions appears to include word and phrase repetitions, which may not be very appropriate in light of current practices of restricting core stuttering disfluencies largely to within-word disfluencies (Conture, 2001).

◆ Differential Characteristics of Neurogenic Stuttering

In the absence of neurological or physiological markers for neurogenic stuttering, identification of the disorder is based by necessity largely on the presence or absence of behavioral characteristics. As discussed earlier, Canter

(1971) was one of the first to propose a defined set of criteria that could be useful in identifying neurogenic stuttering. Subsequent research and observations have shown clearly that many of these criteria may not be applicable to all or even any individuals with neurogenic stuttering and at the very least need to be qualified (Ringo & Dietrich, 1995). Helm-Estabrooks and colleagues (1986) suggested several speech and other typical behavioral characteristics that could be used to differentiate between various types of neurogenic stuttering. But even a cursory examination of these variables shows the presence of significant overlap of these criteria among the various subgroups identified.

Reviewing the literature, it appears that despite the significant overlap between the various groups discussed here and the considerable interindividual variability, some trends seem to emerge. Neurogenic stuttering associated with stroke is more likely to consist of a higher frequency of syllable and word repetitions, with relatively fewer prolongations and blocks. Aphasia is not always present, but if it is, such individuals may show a higher frequency of disfluencies than persons without aphasia.

In persons with neurodegenerative diseases, such as PD, which progressively and significantly affect the motor system, there is a tendency for the speech disfluencies to mimic the motor problems. For instance, persons with PD tend to show a stuttering pattern characterized by freezing, prolongations, and blocks. Prosodic characteristics, such as rate and stress, are affected more in this population. In some, disfluencies may occur more frequently on longer utterances (e.g., sentences) than on shorter ones, (e.g., words). Often, the stuttering becomes worse as the neurodegenerative disorder progresses.

Acquired stuttering associated with brain injury appears to be characterized by an increased frequency of more tense disfluencies such as repetitions, prolongations, and blocks. Stuttering tends to occur relatively quickly after the traumatic accident, although this does not appear to be a universal characteristic. The speech and disfluencies in these persons are often excessively rapid and "shotgun-like." The rate of disfluencies sometimes appears highly variable, displaying occasional bursts of high energy. Based on our own observations, the frequency of disfluencies in these individuals does not seem to be affected by the complexity of the speech material.

As in developmental stuttering, disfluencies in all individuals with neurogenic stuttering are much more likely to occur on initial positions in the word or the phrase. Disfluencies on medial sounds, to some extent, and definitely final sounds or syllables, although not absent, are relatively rare, with the possible exception of persons with neurodegenerative diseases for whom several case reports seem to suggest a higher likelihood of final disfluencies (Hertrich et al, 1993; Mowrer & Younts, 2001). However, the presence of a significant frequency of medial or final disfluencies, which is extremely rare in developmental stuttering (Wingate, 1979), most certainly suggests a more general problem with speech motor coordination, and should point toward neurogenic stuttering in cases where such a differential diagnosis is in question.

Whether or not the presence of reading adaptation is a marker for neurogenic stuttering is debatable. Many studies do not explicitly report whether or not adaptation was measured and how. However, it is clear that a considerable number of persons with neurogenic stuttering show at least some adaptation effect. At the same time, approximately 50% of people with developmental stuttering do not show a reading adaptation effect (Bloodstein, 1995). Given this inconsistency, it is highly questionable whether testing reading adaptation in individuals has any differential diagnostic value. With regard to secondary behaviors, persons with neurogenic stuttering do not seem to show such behaviors or they occur less frequently, and if they are present, they seem to be less elaborate and more transient than in developmental stuttering. Secondary behaviors in developmental stuttering develop or are learned as a result of struggle, escape, or avoidance reactions (Bloodstein, 1995; Van Riper, 1971). It needs to be kept in mind, however, that many published case studies of neurogenic stuttering have reported on patients who have been experiencing stuttering for a relatively short period of time. Just as in developmental stuttering, it is possible that fully blown secondary behaviors may only appear after they have experienced stuttering for a significant amount of time and in a variety of social and speaking situations. Nevertheless, there is some evidence that even in persons who have experienced acquired stuttering for a longer period of time, secondary behaviors do not appear to be predominant (Ludlow et al, 1987). The same seems to be true of strong negative speech perceptions and emotions. Many people with neurogenic stuttering certainly are aware of their disfluencies and may be somewhat annoyed by them, but often do not show reactions that are as strong as those typically seen in people with developmental stuttering. Again, not all persons with developmental stuttering do show such strong negative reactions, and it remains possible that persons with neurogenic stuttering would develop more such reactions if their disfluencies were to persist. Finally, at least for several individuals with neurogenic stuttering, perceptions around their other significant cognitive, motor, medical, or language problems may be overshadowing any concern they have regarding their stuttering.

◆ Diagnosis and Assessment of Neurogenic Stuttering

It is evident from our review of the neurological and speech characteristics of neurogenic stuttering that the disorder is highly variable between individuals. Although various diagnostic criteria have been proposed in the literature, none of these criteria, either individually or combined, have been proven to be necessary and sufficient for the diagnosis of neurogenic stuttering. Consequently, diagnosis of neurogenic stuttering involves the triangulation of information gathered along different dimensions, including medical history, speech and language history, detailed case history from the patient and family, direct speech fluency observation, and cognitive and language testing, among others.

Several questions need to be addressed during the diagnosis of neurogenic stuttering:

1. *Are the disfluencies reflective of developmental or adult-onset stuttering?* The answer to this question can be very straightforward if it is evident that the individual does not have a history of developmental stuttering and if the acquired stuttering was first noticed following the onset of the neurological condition. If there is a history of recovered or persistent childhood stuttering, the answer may not be easy to obtain. Indeed, the medical problem may have triggered a reoccurrence or aggravation in adulthood of the preexisting developmental fluency problem (Helm-Estabrooks et al, 1986; Marshall & Neuburger, 1987). It is not clear from our current knowledge of neurogenic stuttering whether finding the answer to this question, although possibly of significant theoretical importance, is clinically important to select and plan intervention (see below). However, it is possible that individuals who experience a reoccurrence or aggravation of a preexisting fluency problem may be more likely to develop negative emotional reactions and possibly secondary behaviors, and although this cannot be tested based on currently available information, further research of this aspect seems warranted. If so, this will need to be considered when planning clinical intervention. In any case, a detailed history, if possible, will need to be obtained to provide insight into the presence and nature of any childhood stuttering.

2. *Are the disfluencies the result of neurogenic or psychogenic origin?* This may be a more difficult question to answer for several reasons. First, the absence of a neurological condition, at least at the time of onset of the stuttering, does not preclude that the stuttering may be a precursor to a gradually developing medical condition (Lebrun et al, 1983; Leder, 1996). Second, in several persons, the neurological problem may be present but not necessarily visible during routine examinations, such as may have been the case in some individuals subsequent to motor vehicle accidents discussed earlier. Third, psychogenic stuttering may arise as a psychological reaction to a neurological disease or lesion (Duffy & Baumgartner, 1997; Van Borsel, 1997). According to Mahr and Leith (1992), the defining criteria of psychogenic stuttering include a change in speech pattern suggesting stuttering, a relationship to psychological factors as evidenced by an onset associated with emotional conflict or secondary gain, and the absence of an organic etiology. In addition, they suggest that psychogenic stuttering is often associated with a past history of mental health problems, atypical disfluency features (stereotypical repetitions, no islands of fluency, and no secondary behaviors), and a perception of "la belle indifférence" in which the person shows a lack of emotional responses to the disfluencies. In addition, interactions with persons with psychogenic stuttering not infrequently have a somewhat unusual or bizarre quality (Mahr & Leith, 1992; Van Borsel, 2000) that may be hard to describe in words.

3. *Other issues to be considered*: Although specific diagnostic procedures for assessing neurogenic stuttering are often determined by the nature of the underlying neurological problem, they need to include a detailed case history and speech fluency examination. In addition, the clinician needs to differentiate the stuttering from any other dysarthric or language deficiencies the person may be experiencing. Sometimes, such as in conditions of chronic pain or memory problems, the effect of these problems on the occurrence of stuttering also needs to be evaluated. In addition to the medical and developmental case history questions and medical imaging information relevant to the disease or trauma condition, special attention should be given to probing the possible presence of stuttering or other speech and language problems, and associated coping behaviors, prior to the onset of the disease or brain trauma. Often, patients and their family may not recognize the premorbid presence of disfluencies as stuttering, especially if the current neurogenic stuttering is rather severe. Several textbooks on developmental stuttering include detailed case history forms that may be useful in this respect (Conture, 2001; Guitar, 1998; Manning, 2001).

Speech fluency analysis should include more than an overall estimate of disfluencies. It is necessary to differentiate between disfluencies that occur in normal speech and those associated with stuttering (Conture, 2001; Guitar, 1998; Yaruss, 1998) because an overall higher frequency of typical but not stuttering-related disfluencies may nevertheless give the impression of stuttering in these persons (De Nil, Sasisekaran, Van Lieshout, & Sandor, 2005). Also, although the overall frequency of disfluencies may stay relatively constant in an individual, the proportion of stuttering to normal disfluencies may change significantly across speech tasks differing in complexity (Jokel, 2007). The frequency and type of disfluencies should be determined in a variety of reading and spontaneous speech conditions, including monologue and conversation. Speech material should include simple (e.g., single word) and more complex utterances (sentences and continuous text). Such material can be found in several neurogenic language tests (e.g., Goodglass, Kaplan, & Barresi, 2001). If possible, speech samples should be sufficiently long (at least 200 syllables) to provide a representative sample of current speech fluency and to provide an overall impression of the variability in stuttering across word and phrase loci and grammatical structures. Propositional speech (e.g., story telling or conversation) should be compared with fluency during more automatic speech (e.g., counting or naming the days of the week) because persons with neurogenic stuttering are much more likely than people with developmental stuttering to experience significant disfluencies in the latter speech tasks (Helm-Estabrooks, 1993; Helm-Estabrooks et al, 1986). For the same reason, the affect of fluency-enhancing techniques on the frequency and severity of disfluencies should be evaluated. This may include delayed auditory feedback or masking, choral speech, paced or rhythmic speech, and slow speech. Often, but not always, people with neurogenic stuttering fail to demonstrate significantly improved fluency under these conditions.

In addition to evaluating speech fluency, it is important to test for other deficiencies that may affect or aggravate the presence of disfluencies, or that may be mistaken for stuttering disfluencies. They include aphasia, word-finding problems, oral or verbal apraxia, acquired dyslexias, memory problems, and general sensorimotor problems (Helm-Estabrooks, 1993).

◆ Treatment of Neurogenic Stuttering

Not all persons with neurogenic stuttering require treatment. For some, the stuttering disfluencies are of a transient nature and slowly improve over the course of a few weeks or months. For others, the disorder appears to be more persistent. Reports of successful or unsuccessful treatment of neurogenic stuttering include the use of traditional fluency therapy typically used with developmental stuttering, externally supported fluency using delayed auditory feedback or pacing, medication, and surgery. At present, there is no preferred intervention approach that appears to be useful for all or even a subgroup of persons with neurogenic stuttering.

In many cases, clinicians start with traditional fluency therapy and complement or replace it with other techniques if necessary. Meghji (1994) reported on the successful use of speech therapy techniques on a 27-year-old woman who experienced adult-onset stuttering following administration of an antidepressant drug. Although the nature of the speech techniques was not described, she was reported to speak slowly and fluently after four treatment sessions. Nowack and Stone (1987) reported on the use of speech techniques, including nonrepetitive release of voiceless airflow aimed at producing fluent but slurred speech, and relaxation in two cases. Although they reported improved fluency, at the same time both of these patients were undergoing adjustments to their anticonvulsant medication. This makes it hard to know to what extent the change in disfluency was related to the behavioral rather than pharmacological intervention. Mowrer et al (2001) reported on the use of continuous phonation and vowel prolongation in a case with multiple sclerosis. Significant improvement in frequency of repetitions was observed after two sessions, at which time the focus of therapy shifted to word omissions, morphological errors, and prosody. Therapy was discontinued after 27 weekly sessions. Rubow, Rosenbek, and Schumacher (1986) described the use of stress management consisting of breathing exercises, progressive relaxation, and cognitive reframing in a person with neurogenic stuttering secondary to stroke. Speaking tasks were gradually increased in complexity. After 60 sessions of treatment, the person demonstrated decreased muscle activity in response to stress and improved fluency on single words and during conversation.

Several papers report on the use of delayed auditory feedback (DAF) in neurogenic stuttering. Marshall and Neuburger (1987) describe treatment outcomes for three person with TBI. Each underwent 1 hour of DAF treatment two or three times per week. All three showed reduction in stuttering behaviors on the tasks used in treatment, but there was no generalization to new tasks, or to speaking situations outside the clinic. Upon discontinuation of DAF, one individual was able to maintain a high level of fluency, but two of the three returned to their pretreatment disfluency level within 6 months after termination of treatment. Downie, Low, and Lindsay (1981) used DAF in a patient with PD. Although this person benefited from using the instrument for about a year, adaptation to the delayed feedback gradually occurred and the effectiveness was lost.

Andy and Bhatnagar (1992) described four individuals with adult-onset stuttering, two of whom were treated for chronic pain and one for chronic headaches and seizures, using chronically implanted electrodes for stimulation of the left centromedian nucleus of the thalamus. Thalamic stimulation resulted in elimination of the stuttering in two individuals and significant reduction of stuttering in the other two. Improvement in fluency was maintained at 5 and 8 years postsurgery in these individuals.

Several reports have documented the effectiveness of drug treatment for the alleviation of neurogenic stuttering. Perino and colleagues (2000) described a person with a migraine whose physical symptoms and acquired stuttering were effectively and promptly eliminated following an injection of sumatriptan. The fact that stuttering had occurred suddenly 3 hours prior to the hospital visit and promptly disappeared raises the possibility of psychogenic stuttering. However, the authors felt that they could rule out that possibility given the negative results from an in-depth psychological examination. Baratz and Mesulam (1981) reported the effectiveness of anticonvulsants in controlling stuttering in a person who had developed seizures following a motor vehicle accident. The administration of paroxetine to a person with acquired stuttering following a stroke completely eliminated stuttering within 1 month of starting the treatment (Turgut, Utku, & Balci, 2002). Although not strictly drug related, Byrne and colleagues (1993) reported the development of stuttering in a person with anorexia following a bout of severe weight loss. The stuttering slowly improved in the hospital as he gradually improved his diet and gained weight. They attributed the improvement in fluency to a reestablishment of a more normal body metabolism resulting in a recovery of brain tissue.

◆ Conclusion

Neurogenic stuttering represents a challenging clinical entity as well as a unique research opportunity to delve deeper into the neural mechanisms underlying speech fluency. At the clinical level, neurogenic stuttering typically presents itself as a symptom of a broader and more complex disorder affecting not only one's communication skills, but also one's cognitive, sensorimotor, and even interpersonal abilities. In some individuals, the stuttering may be a minor component of the overall deficit, whereas in others it may represent the major complaint. One of the central themes in the literature has been a focus on differentiating neurogenic stuttering from developmental stuttering. In the clinical setting, however, clinicians often also are faced with differential diagnostic issues relating to word-finding deficits, apraxia of speech, dysarthria, and other neurogenic disorders also affecting speech fluency. Such differentiations are not always easy to make. The question arises as to the therapeutic significance of differential diagnosis. Differentiating stuttering from word-finding deficits would seem to have significant implications for the specific intervention approach that is used clinically. The same may be true for differentiating stuttering from apraxia of speech, although therapeutically there may be more overlap. It is unclear at the present time, however, whether differentiating neurogenic stuttering from developmental stuttering would necessarily result in significant changes in clinical intervention. Indeed, a review of the literature seems to indicate that many clinicians use approaches initially developed for developmental stuttering with a certain degree of success. At this time, it does not seem possible to link various types of clinical intervention with specific subgroups of patients experiencing neurogenic stuttering. Often it appears that clinicians attempt various approaches to find out what works for a given client. A much-needed focus of future research is the systematic investigation of treatment outcomes with larger and more homogeneous groups.

From a research standpoint, neurogenic stuttering offers a unique opportunity to gain a greater understanding of the neural processes underlying speech fluency. Based on the available literature, this form of stuttering likely reflects a basic deficiency in the speech-related sensorimotor neural mechanisms, caused by neurodegenerative conditions or lesions of various types. Language formulation and speech production represents a highly distributed and complex interconnected neural system, which in addition is influenced significantly by other systems involved in attention, emotion, memory, etc. Perhaps not surprisingly, then, neurogenic stuttering has been associated with lesions in many different regions of the brain. It would seem that the current availability of high-resolution structural and functional neuroimaging techniques provides a unique opportunity to try to identify affected regions or systems that are common among many if not all persons with neurogenic stuttering, similar to the work that has been done in apraxia of speech (Dronkers, 1996). Undoubtedly, such investigations will have implications beyond neurogenic stuttering, and will be of interest to researchers in developmental stuttering and other speech fluency disorders. Most likely, this research would necessarily have to involve collaboration among several research centers, given the relatively low incidence of neurogenic stuttering.

References

Abe, K., Yokoyama, R., & Yorifuji, S. (1993). Repetitive speech disorder resulting from infarcts in the paramedian thalami and midbrain. *Journal of Neurology, Neurosurgery & Psychiatry, 56*, 1024–1026

Andrews, G. & Cutler, J. (1974). Stuttering therapy: the relation between changes in symptom level and attitudes. *Journal of Speech and Hearing Disorders, 39*, 312–319

Andy, O.J. & Bhatnagar, S.C. (1992). Stuttering acquired from subcortical pathologies and its alleviation from thalamic perturbation. *Brain and Language, 42*, 385–401

Ardila, A. & Lopez, M.V. (1986). Severe stuttering associated with right hemisphere lesion. *Brain and Language, 27*, 239–246

Baratz, R. & Mesulam, M.M. (1981). Adult-onset stuttering treated with anticonvulsants. *Archives of Neurology, 38*, 132

Bijleveld, H., Lebrun, Y., & Dongen, H.V. (1994). A case of acquired stuttering. *Folia Phoniatrica et Logopaedica, 46*, 250–253

Bloodstein, O. (1995). *A Handbook on Stuttering*, 4th ed. Chicago: National Easter Seal Society

Braun, A.R., Varga, M., Stager, S., Schulz, G., Selbie, S., Maisog, J.M., et al. (1997). Altered patterns of cerebral activity during speech and language production in developmental stuttering: an $H_2^{15}O$ positron emission tomography study. *Brain, 120*, 761–784

Brewerton, T.D., Markowitz, J.S., Keller, S.G., & Cochrane, C.E. (1996). Stuttering with sertraline. *Journal of Clinical Psychiatry, 57*, 90–91

Burd, L. & Kerbeshian, J. (1991). Stuttering and stimulants. *Journal of Clinical Psychopharmacology, 11*, 72–73

Byrne, A., Byrne, M., & Zibin, T. (1993). Transient neurogenic stuttering. *International Journal of Eating Disorders, 14*, 511–514

Canter, G.J. (1971). Observations on neurogenic stuttering: a contribution to differential diagnosis. *British Journal of Disorders of Communication, 6*, 139–143

Christensen, R.C., Byerly, M.J., & McElroy, R.A. (1996). A case of sertraline-induced stuttering. *Journal of Clinical Psychopharmacology, 16*, 92–93

Conture, E.G. (2001). *Stuttering. It's Nature, Diagnosis and Treatment.* Needham Heights, MA: Allyn & Bacon

Deal, J.L. (1982). Sudden onset of stuttering: a case report. *Journal of Speech and Hearing Disorders, 47*, 301–304

Demonet, J.F., Thierry, G., & Cardebat, D. (2005). Renewal of the neurophysiology of language: functional neuroimaging. *Physiological Reviews, 85*, 49–95

De Nil, L.F. (2001). Recent developments in brain imaging research in stuttering. In: B. Maassen, W. Hulstijn, R. Kent, H.F.M. Peters, & P.H.M.M. van Lieshout (Eds.), *Speech Motor Control in Normal and Disordered Speech. Proceedings of the Fourth International Speech Motor Conference* (pp. 150–155). Nijmegen: Uitgeverij Vantilt

De Nil, L.F., Kroll, R.M., Lafaille, S.J., & Houle, S. (2003). A positron emission tomography study of short- and long-term treatment effects on functional brain activation in adults who stutter. *Journal of Fluency Disorders, 28*, 357–380

De Nil, L.F., Sasisekaran, J., Van Lieshout, P.H.H.M., & Sandor, P. (2005). Speech disfluencies in individuals with Tourette syndrome. *Journal of Psychosomatic Research, 58*, 97–102

Downie, A.W., Low, J.M., & Lindsay, D.D. (1981). Speech disorder in parkinsonism—use of delayed auditory-feedback in selected cases. *Journal of Neurology, Neurosurgery, and Psychiatry, 44*, 852

Dronkers, N.F. (1996). A new brain region for coordinating speech articulation. *Nature, 384*, 159–161

Duffy, J.R. & Baumgartner, J. (1997). Psychogenic stuttering in adults with and without neurologic disease. *Journal of Medical Speech-Language Pathology, 5*(2), 75–95

Dworkin, J.P., Culatta, R.A., Abkarian, G.G., & Meleca, R.J. (2002). Laryngeal anesthetization for the treatment of acquired disfluency: a case study. *Journal of Fluency Disorders, 27*, 215–226

Ebeling, T.A., Compton, A.D., & Albright, D.W. (1997). Clozapine-induced stuttering. *American Journal of Psychiatry, 154,* 1473

Farmer, A. (1975). Stuttering repetitions in aphasic and nonaphasic brain damaged adults. *Cortex, 11,* 391–396

Fernandez, B., Cardebat, D., Demonet, J.F., Joseph, P.A., Mazaux, J.M., Barat, M., et al. (2004). Functional MRI follow-up study of language processes in healthy subjects and during recovery in a case of aphasia. *Stroke, 35,* 2171–2176

Fleet, W.S. & Heilman, K.M. (1985). Acquired stuttering from a right hemisphere lesion in a right-hander. *Neurology, 35,* 1343–1346

Fox, P.T., Ingham, R.J., Ingham, J.C., Hirsch, T.B., Downs, J.H., Martin, C., et al. (1996). A PET study of the neural systems of stuttering. *Nature, 382,* 158–162

Goodglass, H., Kaplan, E., & Barresi, B. (2001). *Boston Diagnostic Aphasia Examination.* Baltimore: Lippincott Williams & Wilkins

Guitar, B. (1998). *Stuttering. An Integrated Approach to Its Nature and Treatment,* 2nd ed. Baltimore: Williams & Wilkins

Haass, C. & Kahle, P. J. (2000). Neurodegenerative diseases—Parkinson's pathology in a fly. *Nature, 404,* 341

Helm, N.A., Butler, R.B., & Benson, D.F. (1978). Acquired stuttering. *Neurology, 28,* 1159–1165

Helm, N.A., Butler, R.B., & Canter, G.J. (1980). Neurogenic acquired stuttering. *Journal of Fluency Disorders, 5,* 269–279

Helm-Estabrooks, N. (1993). Stuttering associated with acquired neurological disorders. In: R.F.Curlee (Ed.), *Stuttering and Related Disorders of Fluency* (pp. 205–218). New York: Thieme

Helm-Estabrooks, N., Yeo, R., Geschwind, N., & Freedman, M. (1986). Stuttering: disappearance and reappearance with acquired brain lesions. *Neurology, 36,* 1109–1112

Hertrich, I., Ackermann, H., Ziegler, W., & Kaschel, R. (1993). Speech iterations in parkinsonism—a case-study. *Aphasiology, 7,* 395–406

Ingham, R.J. (2001). Brain imaging studies of developmental stuttering. *Journal of Communication Disorders, 34,* 493–516

Jokel, R. & De Nil, L.F. (2003). A comprehensive study of acquired stuttering in adults. In: K.L. Baker & D.T. Rowley (Eds.), *Proceedings of the Sixth Oxford Dysfluency Conference* (pp. 59–64). Leicester, UK: KLB Publications

Jokel, R., De Nil, L.F., Sharpe, A.K. A comparison of speech disfluencies in adults with acquired stuttering associated with stroke and traumatic brain injury. Submitted to the Journal of Medical Speech-Language Pathology

Lebrun, Y., Bijleveld, H., & Rousseau, J.J. (1990). A case of persistent neurogenic stuttering following a missile wound. *Journal of Fluency Disorders, 15,* 251–258

Lebrun, Y. & Leleux, C. (1985). Acquired stuttering following right brain damage in dextrals. *Journal of Fluency Disorders, 10,* 137–141

Lebrun, Y., Retif, J., & Kaiser, G. (1983). Acquired stuttering as a forerunner of motor-neuron disease. *Journal of Fluency Disorders, 8,* 161–167

Leder, S.B. (1996). Adult onset of stuttering as a presenting sign in a parkinsonian-like syndrome: a case report. *Journal of Communication Disorders, 29,* 471–478

Louis, E.D., Winfield, L., Fahn, S., & Ford, B. (2001). Speech dysfluency exacerbated by levodopa in Parkinson's disease. *Movement Disorders, 16,* 562–565

Ludlow, C.L., Rosenberg, J., Salazar, A., Grafman, J., & Smutok, M. (1987). Site of penetrating brain lesions causing chronic acquired stuttering. *Annals of Neurology, 22,* 60–66

Mahr, G. & Leith, W. (1992). Psychogenic stuttering of adult onset. *Journal of Speech and Hearing Research, 35,* 283–286

Manning, W.H. (2001). *Clinical Decision Making in Fluency Disorders,* 2nd ed. Vancouver, Canada: Singular Thompson Learning

Marshall, R.C. & Neuburger, S.I. (1987). Effects of delayed auditory feedback on acquired stuttering following head injury. *Journal of Fluency Disorders, 12,* 355–365

Mazzucchi, A., Moretti, G., Carpeggiani, P., Parma, M., & Paini, P. (1981). Clinical observations on acquired stuttering. *British Journal of Disorders of Communication, 16,* 19–30

McClean, M.D. & McLean, A. (1985). Case report of stuttering acquired in association with phenytoin use for post-head-injury seizures. *Journal of Fluency Disorders, 10,* 241–255

Meghji, C. (1994). Acquired stuttering. *Journal of Family Practice, 39,* 325–326

Mouradian, M.S., Paslawski, T., & Shuaib, A. (2000). Return of stuttering after stroke. *Brain and Language, 73,* 120–123

Mowrer, D.E. & Younts, J. (2001). Sudden onset of excessive repetitions in the speech of a patient with multiple sclerosis—a case report. *Journal of Fluency Disorders, 26,* 269–309

Nass, R., Schreter, B., & Heier, L. (1994). Acquired stuttering after a 2nd stroke in a 2-year-old. *Developmental Medicine and Child Neurology, 36,* 73–78

Nissani, M. & Sanchez, E.A. (1997). Stuttering caused by gabapentin. *Annals of Internal Medicine, 126,* 410

Nowack, W.J. & Stone, R.E. (1987). Acquired stuttering and bilateral cerebral disease. *Journal of Fluency Disorders, 12,* 141–146

Perino, M., Famularo, G., & Tarroni, P. (2000). Acquired transient stuttering during a migraine attack. *Headache, 40,* 170–172

Pimental, P.A. & Gorelick, P.B. (1985). Aphasia, apraxia and neurogenic stuttering as complications of metrizamide myelography: speech deficits following myelography. *Acta Neurologica Scandinavica, 72,* 481–488

Quinn, P.T. & Andrews, G. (1977). Neurological stuttering—a clinical entity? *Journal of Neurology, Neurosurgery & Psychiatry, 40,* 699–701

Ringo, C. & Dietrich, S. (1995). Neurogenic stuttering: an analysis and critique. *Journal of Medical Speech-Language Pathology, 3,* 111–122

Rosenbek, J., Messert, B., Collins, M., & Wertz, R.T. (1978). Stuttering following brain damage. *Brain and Language, 6,* 82–96

Rosenbek, J.C. (1984). Stuttering secondary to nervous system damage. In: R.F. Curlee & W.H. Perkins (Eds.), *Nature and Treatment of Stuttering: New Directions* (pp. 31–48). San Diego: College-Hill

Roth, C.R., Aronson, A.E., & Davis, L.J. (1989). Clinical studies in psychogenic stuttering of adult onset. *Journal of Speech and Hearing Disorders, 54,* 634–646

Rubow, R.T., Rosenbek, J.C., & Schumacher, J.G. (1986). Stress management in the treatment of neurogenic stuttering. *Biofeedback and Self-Regulation, 11,* 77–78

Turgut, N., Utku, U., & Balci, K. (2002). A case of acquired stuttering resulting from left parietal infarction. *Acta Neurologica Scandinavica, 105,* 408–410

Van Borsel, J. (1997). Neurogenic stuttering: a review. *Journal of Clinical Speech and Language, 7,* 16–33

Van Borsel, J. (2000). Verworven stotteren. In: H.F.M. Peters (Ed.), *Handboek Stem-Spraak-Taalpathologie* (pp. 1–27). Houten: Bohn Stafleu Van Loghum

Van Borsel, J. & Taillieu, C. (2000). Neurogenic stuttering versus developmental stuttering: an observer judgment study. *Journal of Communication Disorders, 34,* 385–395

Van Borsel, J., Van Der Made, S., & Santens, P. (2003). Thalamic stuttering: a distinct clinical entity? *Brain and Language, 85,* 185–189

Van Borsel, J., Van Lierde, K., Cauwenberge, P., Guldermont, I., & Van Orshoven, M. (2001). Severe acquired stuttering following injury of the left supplementary motor region: a case report. *Journal of Fluency Disorders, 23,* 49–58

Van Riper, C. (1971). *The Nature of Stuttering.* Englewood Cliffs, NJ: Prentice-Hall

Wingate, M. E. (1979). The first three words. *Journal of Speech and Hearing Research, 22,* 604–612

Wu, J.C., Maguire, G., Riley, G., Fallon, J., LaCasse, L., Chin, S., et al. (1995). A positron emission tomography [18F]deoxyglucose study of developmental stuttering. *Neuroreport, 6,* 501–505

Yaruss, J.S. (1998). Describing the consequences of disorders: stuttering and the International Classification of Impairments, Disabilities, and Handicaps. [Review]. *Journal of Speech, Language, & Hearing Research, 41,* 249–257

Chapter 15

Apraxia of Speech: Definition and Differential Diagnosis

Malcolm R. McNeil, Donald A. Robin, and Richard A. Schmidt

Darley (1967) is credited with the first reported observation that there was a clinical phenomenon of neurological origin that did not fit into the general categories of the then-accepted neurogenic disorders of speech production (the dysarthrias and aphasia). At the turn of the 20th century (Liepmann, 1900), in the 1960s (Darley, 1967; Jakobson, 1968), and in the more current and commonly accepted framework of speech pathologies (Boone & Plante, 1993; Darley, Aronson, & Brown, 1975a; Hegde, 1991; Palmer & Yantis, 1990), neurogenic speech production disorders have been classified as either linguistic (e.g., phonologic) or motoric. Since Darley's observation and the subsequent accumulation of research into the phenomenon, general introductory and more specialized texts (Duffy, 2005) subdivide motor speech disorders into the dysarthrias and apraxia of speech (AOS).

The movement disorder termed *apraxia* and the original description and elucidation of the general mechanisms of the family of apraxias is usually attributed to Liepmann (1900, 1905, 1913, 1920). Darley's (1969) presentation to the American Speech and Hearing Association on AOS represents the modern emergence of the concept of apraxia applied to speech, although it was not the first time the term was used to describe a phenomenon that fell outside of the accepted clinical classification schema. Like Liepmann, Darley suggested that the term would only be applicable when assurance could be given that the patient had the *intent,* the underlying *linguistic representation,* and the fundamental *motor abilities* to produce speech, but could not do so *volitionally.* Darley further used the term to specify a disorder of the *programming* for speech movements. Thus was set some of the conditions for the identification and psychological specification of AOS. Since the late 1960s, there has been a good deal of research, to a great measure performed by Darley and his students, into the nature and clinical management of AOS. Histories of the term *AOS* (Rosenbek, Kent, & LaPointe, 1984; Square & Martin, 1994; Wertz, LaPointe, & Rosenbek, 1984) and its relationship to oral nonspeech apraxia (Moore, 1975; Roy & Square, 1985; Square-Storer, Roy, & Hogg, 1990), limb apraxias (Duffy & Duffy, 1990; Faglioni & Basso, 1985; Miller, 1986; Rothi & Heilman, 1985; Square-Storer & Roy, 1990), and a variety of other apraxias (e.g., dressing apraxia, writing apraxia, unilateral limb apraxia) have been written elsewhere by limpid-thinking and articulate authors from both the neurology and speech-language pathology disciplines. These histories are not reviewed in this chapter. However, it is important to note that, like all diagnostic categories, the term *AOS* carries with it specific assumptions about its underlying neuroanatomical, neurophysiological, linguistic, and motoric mechanisms. Explicit assumptions about its treatment have emerged (Ballard, Granier, & Robin, 2000; Marquardt & Cannito, 1996; Odell, 2002; Square 1989; Wambaugh & Doyle, 1995). In the context of proposing a definition of AOS, it has been necessary to examine these assumptions and, in doing so, to review a portion of the relevant history.

This chapter reviews the clinical features that differentiate among the general classification of neurogenic, sound-level, speech production disorders, composed of motor speech disorders (apraxia of speech and the dysarthrias) and phonological-level disorders (literal or phonological paraphasia). To do this, it is essential to contrast the phenomenology and the assumptions underlying the labels for these clinical neighbors. These pathologies include (1) the family of dysarthrias, (2) disorders of prosody, and (3) the phonemic paraphasias that cross aphasic classifications but that occur frequently in the individual with so-called conduction aphasia. This chapter also evaluates the current state of defining characteristics of AOS and specifies a tentative inventory of the necessary and sufficient behaviors and conditions used to differentiate it from its nearest clinical neighbors. Although we do not review treatments for AOS in this chapter, we refer the reader to reviews by McNeil, Doyle, and Wambaugh (2000), McNeil, Robin, and Schmidt (1997), Odell (2002), Wambaugh (2002), and Wambaugh, Duffy, McNeil, Robin, and Rogers (2006a,b), and to Chapter 16.

♦ Apraxia of Speech Versus Dysarthria

As discussed in great detail throughout this volume, the dysarthrias are a family of disorders that are in part defined by Darley, Aronson, and Brown (1975a) as "disturbances in muscular control of the speech mechanism resulting from impairment of any of the basic motor processes involved in the execution of speech" (p. 2). As stated, the term is used generically to cover isolated or coexisting motor disorders of respiration, phonation, articulation, resonance, and prosody as well as single or multiple cranial nerve involvement. The term explicitly excludes disorders of speech that have an anatomical structural (e.g., cleft palate), psychological (e.g., hysterical aphonia), learning (e.g., developmental phonological disorders), aprosodia, stuttering, dental, or malocclusal basis. Keys to this definition are the specific set of behaviors and mechanisms implied by the terms *basic motor* and *execution*. One consequence of the basic motor processes part of the definition implies that any movement disorder underlying speech production and dysarthria must be present in the speech apparatus when used to perform *speech* and similar *nonspeech* movements. [See Ballard, Soloman, Robin, Moon, and Folkins (2007) for a detailed discussion of this issue, and Weismer and Liss (1991) for an alternative view.] The restriction of the movement deficits to those involving the "execution" level of movement, encompassed in the definition of dysarthria, are poorly specified by Darley and colleagues as well as by most others who write about sensorimotor speech disorders. However, any one or several of the physiological parameters of tone and reflexes along with the kinematic parameters of strength, speed, range, accuracy, and steadiness are necessarily aberrant in dysarthria. Dysarthria, therefore, can be identified in the absence or presence of any one or a combination of these kinematic/physiological parameters. For example, dysarthria can be identified in the absence of abnormal tone (e.g., hyperkinetic dysarthria), or abnormal reflexes (e.g., ataxic dysarthria). It can be identified in the presence of abnormalities of movement speed (e.g., bradykinesia), strength (e.g., spastic or flaccid dysarthria), range of movement (e.g., hypokinetic or spastic dysarthria), accuracy (ataxic dysarthria), or steadiness (e.g., quick or slow hyperkinetic dysarthria, tremor). In all cases, however, it must be identified in the *speech* of the individual. That is, dysarthria is a disorder of speech production and must be perceived by the listener or felt by the speaker. It cannot be diagnosed only by measuring an abnormal physiological or kinematic variable in the absence of a perceptually evident disorder of speech production unless an acoustic or physiological measure has been shown to predict with certainty that the speech would be perceived as evidencing an abnormality consistent with dysarthria. To date, any such predictions have not been verified.

Tone and reflex abnormalities can be evidenced from pathology of any neural system (e.g., pyramidal, extrapyramidal, cerebellar, vestibular-reticular, lower motor neuron) involved in speech production except the higher conceptual planning and programming levels [see van de Merwe (2007) for a complete discussion of these issues]. Traditionally, planning and programming disorders are not consistent with disorders of tone or reflexes, although disorders at the planning or programming level of motor control could evidence strength, speed, range, accuracy, and steadiness kinematic abnormalities if these discrete movement parameters were involved in the planning or programming deficit. For example, it may be that the motor plan or program assigns a strength parameter to be executed. If this assignment is faulty, then differences in strength might be the result of a programming or planning error. Although the exact parameters of movement that are programmed and that represent the control variables for the motor programmer are not agreed upon, relative timing plays a critical role in the measurement of generalized motor programs (GMPs) as defined by Schmidt and Lee (2005). At the physiological

level, activation of the appropriate motoneurons at the precise times is a reasonable formulation of the neural goal (Grillner, 1982). However, this level of specification does not detail the exact cognitive process that represents motor programming. Schmidt and Lee (2005) discuss the GMP as being operationally measured as the coherence of timing and space of the kinematic landmarks and the absolute assignment of time or amplitude as a parameter. Thus in this sense, motor programming is a process that involves activation of the GMP, parameter specification, and probably concatenation of units of action into a large program (e.g., Klapp, 1995). Within the Klapp (1995, 2003) model, programming advances in stages that involve activation and storage of units of action and subsequent sequencing of these action units into the correct serial order. Using the Schmidt and Lee (2005) definition as applied to AOS, Clark and Robin (1998) have explored GMP error versus parameterization errors using kinematic landmark analyses of nonspeech movements, finding deficits in relative or absolute measures of time and amplitude in AOS but not conduction aphasia. Relative timing of various speech events also plays the primary role in some theories of speech motor control such as coordinative structure theory (Kugler, Kelso, & Turvey; 1980), action theory (Kelso, Tuller, & Harris; 1983), and dynamical systems theory (Kelso, 1995), and replaces the notion of specifically programmed movement in this conceptualization of motor control.

Although Darley, Aronson, and Brown's (1975a) definition of the dysarthrias is inadequate to differentiate AOS from dysarthria, they suggest that with the addition of the aforementioned definitional guidelines, AOS should be separable from the dysarthrias. That is, an absence of tone or reflex abnormalities during speech or nonspeech activities along with a clear differentiation between movement disorders that are manifest only in speech (AOS) and not in comparable nonspeech behaviors (unless a concomitant dysarthria or oral nonspeech apraxia were present) should aid the differential diagnosis. It should also be clear that the differentiation of AOS from dysarthria might be accomplished by perceptual analyses of the speech just as the differentiation of one form of dysarthria is differentiable from another via patterns of finite perceptible speech behaviors. Indeed it has been a major goal of several clinical scientists, spanning the 39 years since Darley's seminal unpublished papers in 1968 and 1969, to describe the pattern of speech behaviors that are characteristic of and isomorphic with AOS.

The first large-scale, comprehensive treatise on AOS was the exhaustive review and analysis of the state of the clinical science by Wertz et al (1984). Based on the aggregate of the published research, a wealth of clinical experience, and a profusion of reason and logic, these authors proposed a definition of AOS that has been the most cited and influential on both research and clinical practice. They defined AOS as "a neurogenic *phonologic* disorder resulting from sensorimotor impairment of the capacity to *select*, program, and/or *execute* in coordinated and normally timed sequences, the positioning of the speech musculature for the *volitional* production of speech sounds" (p. 4, emphasis not in the original). Consistent with, or based on, this definition, the authors proposed that AOS was differentiable from dysarthria on anatomical

Table 15–1   Traditional Differentiating Characteristics of Apraxia of Speech (AOS) and Dysarthria

Feature	AOS	Dysarthria
Lesion Location	Unilateral / anterior	Bilateral if cortical, usually subcortical
Psychophysiological level/mechanism	Motor programming	Movement execution
Observed deviant speech behavior	Speech initiation, selection and sequencing, phoneme substitution, abnormal prosody, infrequent metathetic errors	Sound-level distortions
Speech processes involved	Essentially normal: 1. Resonance 2. Respiration 3. Phonation	Frequent disturbance of 1. Resonance 2. Respiration 3. Phonation
Physiological manifestations	Free from paralysis, paresis, ataxia, involuntary movements	Presence of paralysis, paresis, ataxia, involuntary movements
Influence of non-phonological (phonetic) factors	Effected by word length, error inconsistency	Less effected by word length, errors are more consistent
Oral nonverbal apraxia	Frequently present	Absent

Source: From Wertz, R.T., LaPointe, L.L., & Rosenbek, J.C. (1984). *Apraxia of Speech in Adults: The Disorders and Its Management*. Orlando: Grune & Stratton.

grounds (AOS is unilateral and anterior; dysarthria is bilateral if cortical but usually subcortical), assumed psychophysiological level of impairment (AOS is disturbed motor programming; dysarthria is disturbed movement execution), observed speech behavior (AOS resulting in speech initiation, selection, and sequencing difficulties with a predominance of phoneme substitutions, abnormal prosody, and infrequent metathetic errors; dysarthria is the predominance of sound-level distortions), speech process involvement (AOS entails essentially normal in resonance, respiration, and phonation, and, when affected, the physiological mechanisms are different from dysarthria; dysarthria entails frequent disturbance in resonance, respiration, and phonation), physiological manifestations (AOS patients are free from paralysis or paresis, ataxia, and involuntary movements; dysarthria patients show the presence of paralysis or paresis, ataxia, or involuntary movements), the influence of nonphonological factors (AOS is influenced by such phonetic variables as context, word length, and error inconsistency; dysarthria is less affected by context and word length, and errors are more consistent), and presence of concomitant oral nonverbal apraxia (frequently present in AOS; absent in dysarthria). **Table 15–1** summarizes these contrasts.

◆ Apraxia of Speech Versus Phonemic Paraphasia

It was the dissemination of the dissertation by LaPointe (1969) and the publication by Johns and Darley (1970) that set the stage for the lingering controversy into the description, the mechanisms, and even the existence of AOS. These works followed directly from Darley's (1968) observation that there was a clinical phenomenon that did not fit into the general categories of the then-accepted neurogenic disorders of

speech production, along with his formulation of this clinical entity as something that was consistent with the general notion of apraxia. Immediately following the Johns and Darley publication on the phonemic variability of apraxic speakers, there followed publications by Aten, Johns, and Darley (1971), Deal and Darley (1972), and Rosenbek, Wertz, and Darley (1973) that further described the auditory processing, speech characteristics, and oral sensation of the population, respectively. These publications set the stage for Martin's (1974) influential criticisms of the newly inspired AOS zeitgeist.

In his challenge to the individuals feverishly exploring this newly recognized clinical entity, Martin (1974) objected to the term *AOS* as it was applied to the specific subjects chosen for study by Darley and his students. It is important to note that he did not object, nor did he provide an argument that would support an objection, to the existence of the clinical entity. Martin argued that the speech errors described by this series of studies could be accounted for as easily by linguistic as by motor-programming concepts. This alternative interpretation of the data was designed to inspire a reexamination of the assumptions underlying specific speech errors as evidence for linguistic versus motor attribution. It accomplished this goal and inspired a torrent of studies and critical analysis of the existing data designed to support the motor or the linguistic interpretation. Retrospectively it appears that Martin was right to raise serious questions about the accuracy of the term as applied to the populations being studied experimentally and to the clinical cases presented as prototypical exemplars of the disorder [e.g., "the tornado man" case presented by Darley, Aronson, and Brown (1975b)] and subsequently reported by Square (1996) to have speech symptoms similar to those of patients with parietal lobe lesions and to have had a confirmed left parietal lobe thromboembolic lesion). Numerous studies designed to investigate this alternative explanation, and a sudden interest in the earlier and contemporary descriptions of the speech errors of persons with aphasia followed.

The question for Darley and his colleagues is the question confronted by any clinical pioneer. That is, on what bases does one select subjects for study when trying to identify and characterize a new clinical entity? Without established inclusional and exclusional criteria, derived from careful experimentation, usually accumulated over a long period of time, and without models that specify the levels of breakdown and the potential mechanisms responsible for the phenomena (neither of which were available during Darley's early formulations of AOS), it is difficult or impossible to have confidence that the individuals and groups actually represent the subjects of interest. In other words, it is difficult or impossible to avoid experimental tautologies. Illustrative of this problem is some indirect evidence that Halpern, Keith, and Darley (1976) may have fallen into such a predicament. These authors asked the question whether aphasic patients make errors in the production of phonemes, and if so, is there a discernible pattern to the errors. Being careful researchers, and as the article title implies ("Phonemic Behavior of Aphasic Subjects Without Dysarthria or Apraxia of Speech"), the authors selected subjects who would provide the best test of the hypothesis. That is, they eliminated potential subjects who had concomitant dysarthria or AOS. Twenty-eight of 30 (93%) subjects made *no* phonemic errors. Of those errors produced by the two subjects that did make phonemic errors, 75% were attributable to word-level errors. The authors concluded that aphasic behavior is not characterized by significant breakdown of articulatory performance. This would indeed be an important and surprising finding given the abundant literature describing and quantifying the frequent phonological errors in patients characterized as having aphasia in the absence of motor speech problems. In selecting their subjects for study the authors stated:

Patients were excluded from the study if (1) they made articulation errors referable to significant weakness, slowness, incoordination, or alteration of tone of the speech musculature (dysarthria) or (2) they showed groping, off target, highly inconsistent articulatory errors—primarily substitutions, additions, prolongations, and repetitions—in attempting target words in the context of islands of fluent speech, these errors being especially evident on repetition tasks and increasing in incidence with increase in length of word (apraxia of speech) (p. 366).

The fundamental question is whether the criteria used for eliminating potential participants with AOS actually eliminated participants with aphasia who demonstrate phonological paraphasias. If one examines the typical description of conduction aphasia, the similarities become striking. Goodglass (1992), for example, described the symptomatology of conduction aphasia:

Conversation includes runs of normally articulated words, with generally preserved use of grammatical inflections and syntactic structures. However, speech is marred by more or less frequent errors in the selection and sequencing of phonemes and syllables: these may be omitted, substituted, or transposed, creating literal paraphasias. 2. Auditory comprehension is relatively well preserved and may even be completely normal. 3. The task of repeating words or sentences after the examiner may be particularly deficient, in comparison with the level of fluency observed in conversation (p. 40).

Goodglass goes on to clarify the phonological production difficulties in conduction aphasia:

Because the phonological output difficulties of these patients are linked to the articulatory planning load, the objects or pictures to be named or repeated should include two-, three-, or four-syllable words. Words that involve the proper ordering of two or three consonants (e.g., baseball, elephant, pocketbook) may be insoluble tongue twisters to conduction aphasics, provoking repeated, often unsuccessful, attempts at self-correction (p. 41).

The substitution and omission errors types, islands of fluent, normally articulated speech, and more frequently occurring errors in repetition than in elicited or self-generated speech unmistakably correspond between the descriptions of the two theoretically distinct pathological populations. The addition of the preserved use of grammatical inflections and syntactic structures along with relatively well preserved auditory comprehension in Goodglass's description of conduction aphasia goes even further toward the orthodox description of AOS that is not confounded by aphasia. The increased "planning load" of Goodglass is consistent with the increased word length effect for Darley. Further, the repeated trials and attempts at self-correction of the conduction aphasic may be consistent with the groping, off target, reportedly highly inconsistent articulatory errors of the AOS patient. **Table 15–2** summarizes these and other similarities between AOS and the phonological paraphasias of the person with conduction aphasia.

The precise speech errors that are made by the person with phonological paraphasia (Kohn, 1984; Tuller, 1984) versus people with AOS have also been proposed to differentiate the two populations. Garrett's (1980, 1984) model of language production and its modifications (Buckingham, 1990) have had a major influence on the conceptualization and characterization of the phonological-level errors, especially in conduction and Broca aphasia. The phonetic, and particularly the motoric, levels of speech production are egregiously underspecified in Garrett's and many other such models (Bock, 1982; Dell, 1986, 1988; Levelt, 1989). These levels of speech production have been entirely omitted in some discussions and models designed to explain phonological paraphasias, in spite of the fact that some errors categorized as phonological can be arguably assigned to the subphonemic or motoric levels. Equally notable is at least the attempt to include phonetic and motoric processes in the explanation of aphasic speech production errors by such notable speech researchers as Blumstein (1981), Blumstein and Baum (1987), Buckingham (1979, 1992), and Ryalls (1987).

The descriptions of persons with AOS and phonological paraphasia are perhaps more similar than proponents of their differentiations have demonstrated. Blumstein (1981), for example, summarized the problem and the state of the two pathologies differentiation:

In reality, it would not be surprising to find similar patterns of phonological disintegration whether the errors

Table 15–2   Traditional Characteristics of AOS and Conduction Aphasia

AOS	Conduction Aphasia
Physiology	
Absence of	
1. Muscle weakness	
2. Movement slowness	Intact movement and muscle physiology
3. Movement incoordination	
4. Alterations of muscle tone	
Speech Characteristics	
Groping, off-target, highly inconsistent articulatory errors	Repeated trials, attempts at self-correction
Primarily sound errors of	Sound may be
1. Substitution	1. Substitutions
2. Addition	2. Omissions
3. Prolongation	3. Transpositions
4. Repetition	
Islands of error-free speech	Runs of normally articulated words
Errors especially evident on repetition tasks	More frequently occurring errors on repetition
More errors with increase in word length	Difficulties are linked to the articulatory planning load
Preserved auditory language comprehension	Auditory comprehension is relatively well preserved and may be completely normal
Preserved syntax, semantics and morphology	Generally preserved use of grammatical inflections and syntactic structures
Speech Error Type	
More consonant than vowel	More consonant than vowel
More substitutions than	More substitutions than
1. Distortions	1. Distortions
2. Omissions	2. Omissions
3. Additions	3. Additions
More errors in word initial than final position	More errors in word initial than final position
More error of simplification (e.g., consonant cluster reduction) than complication	More error of simplification (e.g., consonant cluster reduction) than complication
More single feature than multiple feature sound substitutions	More single feature than multiple feature sound substitutions

are articulatory or linguistically based, primarily because theoretical linguistic assumptions are derived from the intrinsic nature or organization. Thus, what is articulatorily simple is phonologically or linguistically simple, and what is articulatorily complex is also linguistically complex (p. 135).

The literature attempting to describe differences between these two populations have, for the most part, selected subjects based on either lesion location (anterior versus posterior) or aphasia syndrome (e.g., Broca, Wernicke, or conduction) or both, with the assumption that persons with Broca aphasia are synonymous with the anterior, and those with Wernicke or conduction aphasia are synonymous with posterior. Broca aphasia is not synonymous with apraxia of speech, although, depending on the exact criteria for its diagnosis, persons with Broca aphasia are likely to have an accompanying motor speech problem along with their agrammatism (Marquardt & Cannito, 1996; McNeil, 1984;

McNeil & Kent, 1990) and typically good (but never "preserved") auditory and reading comprehension. Studies in which lesion location have been correlated with the presence of AOS have not found a relationship using computed axial tomography (Marquardt & Sussman, 1984).

Anterior versus posterior lesions inferred from neurological records and neuropsychological testing by Deutsch (1984) was reported to yield a significant difference between the two lesion groups, with the posterior group producing significantly more polysyllabic sequencing errors than the anterior group. The groups did not differ significantly on monosyllabic or polysyllabic complex errors, fluency errors, phoneme errors (e.g., substitutions, omissions, additions, repetitions, and distortions), or syllable addition errors. The groups were also not different on monosyllabic sequencing errors, or total monosyllabic or polysyllabic errors. Discriminant analysis yielded three measures (percent of polysyllabic sequencing errors, percent of monosyllabic articulation errors, and total number of polysyllabic errors) that correctly classified 89% of the two groups (misclassifying one subject in each group). The premise of the investigation was that there were two forms of apraxia of speech described under various names (e.g., anterior or "efferent kinetic speech apraxia" and posterior or "afferent kinesthetic speech apraxia") by Liepmann (1905, 1913), Luria (1966, 1970), and Canter (1969). The error pattern of the posterior group is most consistent with our description in this chapter of what we have called, and attributed mechanistically to, the phonemic paraphasia. Luria (1966) proposed that Broca's area stored and accessed motor plans or programs for gestures or speech segments and that the parietal lobe (the facial region of the postcentral gyrus) governed the sequencing and transitionalization between speech segments or between nonspeech gestures, a concept endorsed by others (Canter, Trost, & Burns, 1985; Mateer & Kimura, 1977; Ojemann & Mateer, 1979; Poeck & Kerschensteiner, 1975; Riecker, Ackermann, Wildgruber, et al, 2000; Square, Darley, & Sommers, 1982). This assignment is not, however, universal. Liepmann (1905, 1913) for example associated labored articulation of individual speech sounds and distortions of transitionalization to lesions in Broca's areas (frontal lobe) rather than the parietal lobe.

A single and focal cortical or subcortical lesion location underlying either AOS or conduction aphasia has indeed been elusive. In spite of this failure to find differential single and focal lesions between the two populations, Square (1996) has called for a reexamination and a reclassification of AOS based on lesion location within the left hemisphere. This call preceded a renewed interest in specifying the lesion location responsible for AOS. Square-Storer, Roy, and Martin (1997) proposed that AOS can arise from a lesion in parietal or frontal cortex or the frontal subcortex ("frontal quadrilateral space"). They further specified that lesions in any of the following areas can cause AOS: (1) nonprimary motor cortex (Brodmann area 6), including the lateral and mesial premotor (supplementary motor) cortices; (2) frontal pars opercularis (Brodmann area 44); (3) white matter subtending Broca's areas; (4) insula; (5) lenticular nucleus; and (6) midparietal cortex.

Dronkers (1996) reported an overlapping lesion method using computed tomography (CT) and magnetic resonance imaging (MRI) for identifying the lesion site for AOS. She reported that 100% of 25 individuals with the diagnosis of AOS had a left-hemisphere lesion in the precentral gyrus of the insula, whereas 100% of a control group of 19 left-hemisphere lesioned individuals without AOS evidenced no involvement of this area of the insula. The conclusion reached by Dronkers that this area represents a newly identified area for the coordination of speech articulation has received a great deal of attention. This conclusion, subsequently advanced by others (Donnan, Darby, & Saling, 1997), has, however, created as much controversy as it has resolved. The selection of participants for the Dronkers (1996) study, and for the subsequent studies by Ogar, Willock, Baldo, Wilkins, Lundy, and Dronkers (2006), has yielded groups that by the nature of their selection criteria encompass persons with phonological-level deficits or even persons with dysarthria, and who may or may not include persons with

AOS. For example, in the Ogar et al (2006) study, dysarthria was differentiated from AOS by the presence of weakness, predictability, and consistency of errors. However, weakness of the speech musculature is not pathognomonic of dysarthria. *Error consistency* as a differentiating feature between dysarthria and AOS has been challenged. The construct of *error predictability* is also undefined and unsubstantiated as a differential diagnostic feature between AOS and dysarthria. Additionally, it was recognized that the speech production errors in AOS should be differentiated from those generated by an aphasic mechanism. Ogar et al's construct for this differentiation was that "AOS can occur independently of language-related impairments in auditory comprehension, reading comprehension and writing" (p. 344). However, it appears from their summary of the demographic characteristics of their AOS group that only two of the 18 participants were judged to be free from dysarthria, and only one did not have concomitant aphasia. This study, like the Dronkers study, relied on criteria for selection of AOS participants that may include or exclusively involve individuals with concomitant sound-level speech production disorders that are generated from impairments at levels of the system that are not apraxic in origin. The author's reliance on the presence of one or more of the symptoms of "(1) effortful, trial and error groping with attempts at self correction; (2) dysprosody unrelieved by extended periods of normal rhythm, stress and intonation; (3) articulatory inconsistency on repeated productions of the same utterance, and/or (4) obvious difficulty initiating utterances" (p. 344), taken from Wertz et al (1984), is inadequate to diagnose the presence of AOS or to differentiate it from dysarthria or aphasia, its closest clinical neighbors. Consistent with this interpretation of inadequacy, Ogar et al (2006) state: "In future research, it may be fruitful to view AOS as a collection of symptoms that together have traditionally been recognized as a singular motor speech disorders. For example, some of the speech deficits related to AOS are seemingly motoric (e.g., groping) and other more language-like (e.g., transpositions)" (p. 349). It is our contention, as described later in this chapter, that the behavior of "groping" is not unique to AOS. Even more critical is our assertion that sound exchange errors (i.e., "transpositions") are inconsistent with an AOS attribution. Until the criteria for AOS are agreed upon, tested stringently, and used for selection of populations for study, all of the well-intentioned research that continues to populate the literature will remain uninterpretable and impotent to inform a coherent theory of AOS. Likewise, its contribution to the understanding of brain and behavior relationships or its heuristic value in assessing the efficacy of pathology-specific treatments will remain at best unfulfilled or at worst misinformed.

Hillis, Work, Barker, Jacobs, Breese, and Maurer (2004) questioned the findings of Dronkers (1996) based on the overlapping structural lesion methods for identifying the common site of damage responsible for AOS. They examined 40 consecutive individuals with left-hemisphere, middle-cerebral-artery distributional nonlacunar strokes with lesions in the anterior insula, and 40 consecutive individuals without insular damage. They evaluated the participants immediately after onset using diffusion-weighted imaging and perfusion-weighted imaging to identify infracted or hypoperfused (dysfunctional) tissue. They hypothesized that

the association between chronic apraxia of speech and insular damage is an artefact of the coincident associations between (i) insular damage and large MCA [middle cerebral artery strokes; and (ii) chronic apraxia of speech and large left MCA strokes. The basis for this limitation of lesion overlap studies is that such studies typically do not evaluate the probability of the deficit in patients with the identified areas of lesion, but only the probability of the lesion in patients with the deficit. Thus, it is possible that all patients with apraxia of speech have insular damage, but that few patients with insular damage have apraxia of speech (p. 1480).

Behavioral criteria for inclusion in the AOS group included variable off-target articulation, distorted, groping articulation, and impaired prosody, none of which were attributable to weakness, slowness, or reduced range of movement of the muscles for speech. Although each of these behavioral criteria is not uniquely attributable to AOS or any other neurogenic speech production disorder, the pattern of behaviors is consistent with AOS. Additionally, the criteria do not specify behaviors that are inconsistent with the diagnosis (e.g., serial order phonological errors) as was the case for the Dronkers and Ogar et al studies. The results from Hillis et al (2004) revealed no evidence of an association between AOS and left insular damage (structural or hypoperfusional) or between AOS and superior precentral insular gyrus damage. AOS was, however, associated with hypoperfusion and/or infarction (damage) of Broca's area. Indeed, AOS was less likely to be present (12 cases) than absent (19 cases) in persons with left anterior insular damage. AOS was absent in 17 cases with left anterior insular damage and in 32 cases where there was no damage in the anterior insula. The associations were stronger between the presence of AOS and the presence or absence of damage in left Broca's areas, with 26 cases showing AOS and Broca's area lesions and only five cases with AOS and no Broca's area lesion. Likewise, AOS was absent in four cases, with damage to Broca's area and in 45 cases without damage to this area. The authors concluded that the strong association between AOS and damage to Broca's area, either with or without concurrent damage to the insula, more likely reflects a causal relationship than does the relationship between anterior insular damage and AOS. Based on the likelihood that the participants in the Hillis et al study actually displayed AOS, the associations appear more plausible. However, it is interesting that five of the individuals with AOS did not have damage to Broca's area. It is potentially important that each of these individuals had identified damage to the postcentral gyrus, as this lesion site had previously been identified as the only common lesion location in the group of four individuals identified as having AOS without concomitant dysarthria or aphasia by McNeil, Weismer, Adams, and Mulligan (1990).

McNeil et al (1990) reported structural CT lesion data from four very carefully selected persons with AOS but without other accompanying sound-level speech production disorders (dysarthria or aphasia). Each of these individuals met the criteria for AOS later specified by McNeil et al (1997). Two of these "pure" AOS cases had involvement of the insula, as did two of three individuals with phonemic paraphasia (with the diagnosis of conduction aphasia), but without accompanying AOS or dysarthria. Two of the four individuals with AOS, and one of three individuals with conduction aphasia had damage to Broca's area. As with the five individuals from the Hillis et al (2004) study with AOS but without damage to either the insula or Broca's area, these four individuals with "pure" AOS each had damage to the facial region of the post central gyrus.

Robin, Jacks, and Ramage (in press) reported detailed CT scan lesion data from a series of studies by Robin and colleagues from individuals with AOS. The consistent two areas of lesion overlap associated with pure AOS, using the McNeil et al (1997) criteria, were left lateral premotor cortex (Brodmann's area 6) and Broca's area (Brodmann's area 44). Based on these data, and the extant imaging literature in AOS, the authors concluded that there was no evidence to suggest that the insula played a role in AOS. Interestingly, a postcentral gyrus lesion in the persons with pure AOS in this series was not supported, suggesting that perhaps an examination of a motor planning and programming network is critical to understanding the underlying neuropathology in AOS.

From these studies, most with inadequate participant selection criteria, it is clear that identifying a single lesion that predicts the constellation of sign and symptoms that comprise the complex behavioral manifestations of AOS has not been possible. As Hillis et al have speculated, anatomical variability of Broca's area causing the fallacious assignment of lesion location in previous studies, individual variability of cortical organization of the speech production system (termed the "language" by Hillis et al), "or the possibility of a network of brain regions that function in concert to orchestrate speech articulation" (p. 1485) could account for the disparate findings across studies. Given that speech production is such a neurologically complex enterprise, encompassing psychological functions and neurological substrates well beyond those articulated by Dronkers or Hillis and colleagues, it seems without question that there is a broad network of brain regions whose impairment can engineer the complex set of behavioral abnormalities that define AOS.

With the advent of more precise anatomical imaging tools, especially voxel-based symptom lesion mapping (Bates, Wilson, Saygin, Dick, Sereno, Knight, & Dronkers, 2003), more precise prediction of a lesion-to-behavioral-symptom complex may be possible. However, as noted by Robin et al (2007), ultimately the neural mechanisms of action of AOS will be best quantified using functional imaging techniques with hypotheses that are driven by an exacting model of speech production that encompasses the complex process of motor planning and programming.

In summary, it is clear that in addition to the subject selection issues discussed above, brain imaging techniques that allow for quantification of the exact underlying structural and function lesion are needed. These must be combined with the highest level of behavioral measurement to be useful. Ultimately, confusion rendered by the lesion studies discussed above may have arisen because of differential locations involved in motor planning and programming and their connectivity to other brain regions. Thus, understanding the neural circuitry of AOS could potentially aid in the classification of speech motor planning and programming disorders, each with differential speech symptoms.

♦ Speech Sound-Level Characteristics of Apraxia of Speech

The majority of studies attempting to characterize AOS have used the invalid category of Broca aphasia to select subjects. The major findings from these studies, using broad phonetic transcription of the speech, suggest that the anterior (ostensibly apraxic) patients produce (1) more consonant than vowel errors (Darley, 1982; Keller, 1978; LaPointe & Johns, 1975; Lebrun, Buyssens & Henneaux, 1973; Trost & Canter, 1974); (2) more substitution than distortion, omission, or addition errors (Blumstein, 1973; Dunlop and Marquardt, 1977; Johns & Darley, 1970; Klich, Ireland & Weidner, 1979; LaPointe & Johns, 1975; Sasanuma, 1971; Shankweiler, Harris & Taylor, 1968; Trost & Canter, 1974); (3) more errors in the initial than the final position of the word (LaPointe & Johns, 1975); (4) more errors of simplification (e.g., consonant cluster reduction) than complication (Keller, 1984); (5) more single feature than multiple feature sound substitutions (Blumstein, 1973; LaPointe & Johns, 1975; Trost & Canter, 1974); and (6) more place than manner or voicing errors (LaPointe & Johns, 1975; Trost & Canter, 1974). Using participants with "pure" AOS, Odell, McNeil, Rosenbek, and Hunter (1990) found more place errors than other feature errors, more voiceless-sound substitutions for voiced sounds than the converse, and more single feature than multiple feature sound substitutions.

Meuse, Marquardt, and Cannito (1996) reported a phonological process analysis on spontaneous and repeated single-word and narrative productions from 10 participants with Broca aphasia. Ninety-three percent of the total errors exhibited across the three elicitation tasks were accounted for by the 29 processes examined. However, no single process accounted for their criterion of 20% process utilization. The authors concluded that these phonological analyses failed to produce evidence that was consistent with a phonological deficit. This is an interesting conclusion given the unsupported assumption advanced by some (Bowman, Hodson, & Simpson, 1980) and cautiously advanced by others (Kearns, 1980) that errors described by phonological process analysis represent phonological-level deficits. Process analysis has been shown to be a useful way of characterizing speech production errors of children with developmental articulation errors; however, the underlying mechanisms for the so-called phonological processes are unknown and cannot be assigned unambiguously to any level of the speech production system. The cautions offered by Kearns for the utility of characterizing the speech of persons with AOS remains as valid today as it was in 1980. He stated:

It should be noted that the results of process analyses may not represent a patients rules for transforming abstract phonological forms into phonetic realizations. The need to establish minimal qualitative and quantitative criteria for when a process is present has only recently been recognized. There is, in fact, insufficient data available with regards to whether phonological processes are psychologically real (p. 190).

As Blumstein (1981) pointed out, many studies of the posterior patient (both conduction and Wernicke) have found the same pattern of speech errors as with the anterior patients, including more (1) consonant than vowel errors; (2) substitution errors than distortion, omission, or addition errors; (3) errors in the initial than the final position of the word; (4) errors of simplification (e.g., consonant cluster reduction) than complication; and (5) single feature than multiple feature sound substitutions. Blumstein (1981) concluded that anterior (AOS) and posterior aphasic subjects could not be distinguished on the basis of the patterns of phonological errors.

So what speech errors can unambiguously be assigned to the phonological level of speech production? The answer to this question is critical for establishing the differential diagnostic criteria for AOS. As stated earlier, sound substitutions such as voiced for voiceless or voiceless for voiced cognates could result from the selection of the incorrect phoneme or from the mistiming of vocal fold onset with upper airway articulatory timing. Likewise, most other phoneme substitutions cannot be unambiguously attributed to either level of the mechanism. Sound omissions and additions could also be generated from either motor or linguistic mechanisms. Good acoustically and perceptually produced sounds that are mis-sequenced, on the other hand, are very difficult to assign to the motor level of speech production. That is, left-to-right, progressive assimilative or perseverative (e.g., PLAYBACK → PLAYPACK or PLAY-PLACK), right-to-left, regressive, assimilative, or anticipatory (e.g., PLAYBACK → BLAYBACK or BAYBACK), and complete exchange or metathetic (e.g., PLAYBACK → BAYPLACK or BLAY-PACK) errors that are without phonetic or motoric distortions are most consistent with the assignment of an error constructing the phonological buffer or in filling it with mis-selected phonemes from the phonemic lexicon. Although this may seem paradoxical, movement sequencing often described in the motor-programming literature (Square, 1996; Wertz LaPointe, & Rosenbek, 1984) does not equate to the ordering of speech sounds in the speech production process. Nonetheless, as reflected in the title of their manuscript, "Repeated Trials of Words by Patients with Neurogenic Phonological Selection-Sequencing Impairment (Apraxia of Speech)," LaPointe and Horner (1976) appear to have equated phonological selection and sequencing with AOS.

The reason for this interpretation appears to be rooted in the assumption that a phonological selection and sequencing disorder represents one form of apraxia, presumably ideomotor apraxia. Further, the assumption appears to be that these are legitimate behaviors that represent critical characteristics of AOS. Although the validity of this assumption cannot be adequately debated within the confines of this chapter, the relevance of various nonspeech apraxias to AOS has been discussed elsewhere (McNeil et al, 2000). Additionally, the categorization of speech sound-level errors to pre-motoric stages of processing (Dell, 1986; Dell, Burger, & Svec, 1997; Garrett, 1980, 1984; Levelt, 1989, 1999; Levelt & Wheeldon, 1994; Levelt, Roelofs, & Meyer, 1999; Roelofs, 1997; Shattuck-Hufnagel, 1979, 1987) as opposed to ones that are best subsumed under a motor planning or programming impairment have been reviewed elsewhere as well (McNeil, Pratt, & Fossett, 2004). Given the weight of the experimental and theoretical evidence and the dominant paradigm of making a distinction between speech and language at the sound production level, it is our theoretical position that the notion of ideomotor apraxia is not easily or satisfactorily translated to the speech system. Errors proposed to be consistent with this level of impairment are most parsimoniously and validly attributed to the phonological encoding stage of linguistic formulation. Moreover, the notion of substitution errors as the primary differential factor in ideomotor is not well supported in studies that have used kinematic measures and fine-grained perceptual measures of movement and speech. In particular, subjects with ideomotor limb apraxia have marked deficits in relative timing, amplitude, and phase. These deficits disrupt coordination and result in more distorted movements than frank substitutions of movement components (Poizner, Clark, Merians, Macauley, Rothi, & Heilman, 1995). These movement distortions were evidenced during mimicked and actual tool manipulation. Thus, Poizner and colleagues conclude that patients with ideomotor limb apraxia have difficulty translating motor plans into specific kinematic parameters (e.g., relative phase, relative joint angle), and that a model of apraxia must yield the differentiation of persons with aberrant selection of larger conceptual components from those who have impairments in translating those components into kinematic parameters, a definition that is remarkably similar to the definition of apraxia of speech provided later in this chapter.

Finally, the issue of sequencing is explicit in Klapp's model of motor programming and bears comment. This model has two levels. The INT (internal) level represents a stage in motor programming that organizes the internal structure of the unit of action and buffers in working memory each unit that is part of the overall sequence to be produced. INT is where units of action are selected and parameters assigned. The SEQ (sequencing) level is a sequencer that arranges individual units of action into their correct serial order. Maas, Robin, Ballard, Magnuson, and Wright (2006) have reported that subjects with AOS have breakdowns in the INT portion of the model but perform equal to intact participants on the SEQ portion. A similar finding was reported by Deger and Ziegler (2002). Related to the notion of sequencing, it is now known that disorders of sequencing are considered to be critical to the movement disorder found in patients with Parkinson's disease (e.g., Goerendt, Messa, Lawrence, Grasby, Piccini, & Brooks, 2003; Graybiel, 1998). As such, one hypothesis is that AOS represents a fundamental problem with activation or the storage of units of action, and other disorders, such as Parkinson's disease, are driven by movement sequencing difficulties. In essence, there is no evidence in AOS or limb apraxia to support the notion of a sequencing deficit.

◆ Phonetic/Motoric Characteristics of Apraxia of Speech

Although phonological production errors have not differentiated AOS from phonemic paraphasia, perhaps phonetic patterns could. Blumstein (1981), in fact, made this prediction. Based on several studies conducted at that point in time, and later verified by additional research, she concluded that individuals with "anterior" aphasia (presumably AOS) demonstrated impairments of (1) voice onset time (VOT) (Blumstein, Cooper, Goodglass, Statlender, & Gottlieb, 1980; Blumstein, Cooper, Zurif, & Caramazza, 1977; Hoit-Dalgaard, Murry, & Kopp, 1983; Shewan, Leeper, & Booth, 1984) and (2) nasal sounds (Itoh, Sasanuma, Hirose, Yoshioka, & Ushijima, 1980; Itoh, Sasanuma, & Ushijima, 1979) because both dimensions require finite interarticulator timing. Persons with posterior lesions resulting in aphasia have been reported to show no, or only minor, deficits on these phonetic segments (Itoh, Sasanuma, Hirose, Yoshioka, & Sawashima, 1983). Several other phonetic/motoric dimensions have been investigated subsequently.

Durations of vowels and consonants have been investigated in normal speakers, Broca, apraxic, and other aphasic (typically Wernicke) patients. As summarized by McNeil and Kent (1990), between-group differences in vowel durations have generally not been found when the stimuli were monosyllables (Bauman, 1978; Duffy & Gawle, 1984; Gandour & Daradarananda, 1984; Mercaitis, 1983; Ryalls, 1984, 1986). Vowels in multisyllabic words or nonsense utterances have been shown to be significantly longer for apraxic than normal subjects or aphasic subjects (Collins, Rosenbek, & Wertz, 1983; Kent & Rosenbek, 1983; Mercaitis, 1983; Ryalls, 1981, 1987; Strand, 1987; Strand & McNeil, 1996). McNeil and Kent (1990) have speculated that the sensitivity of vowel duration to syllabic or other aspects of utterance complexity may be an important clinical feature of AOS. Consonant durations, though less often studied than vowels, have also generally been found to be lengthened in AOS (Bauman, 1978; Kent & Rosenbek, 1983; Seddoh, Robin, Sim, Hageman, Moon, & Folkins, 1996). These increased segment durations, along with increased intersegment (Mercaitis, 1983) and transition durations (Kent & Rosenbek, 1983), are consistent with the clinical impression that apraxic and Broca aphasic speakers speech rate is reduced (Kent & Rosenbek, 1983; Kent and McNeil, 1987; McNeil, Liss, Tseng, & Kent, 1990). Because these lengthened segments carry no meaning change, it is difficult to attribute them to a phonological or morphological level of dysregulation (McNeil & Kent, 1990). It should also be cautioned that the sheer presence or even number of vowel errors failed to differentiate AOS, conduction aphasic, and ataxic dysarthric groups by Odell, McNeil, Rosenbek, and Hunter (1991b) using perceptual analyses in a single-word task. Further, the number of syllables in a word did not differentially affect the vowel error rate across groups in this study.

◆ Force and Position Control

Movement control and strength of the speech articulators are routinely assessed clinically during speech and non-speech activities in persons with neurological speech production disorders. However, relatively few studies have been conducted to evaluate the parameters of movement, force, or position control with instruments more sensitive and potentially more reliable than the hand and eye typically used in the clinical evaluation. Although the clinical examination of persons suspected of having AOS includes the evaluation of muscle forces produced during nonspeech tasks, if weakness is evidenced during these tasks, the default diagnosis is usually that of dysarthria, not AOS or phonemic paraphasia. If disorders of postural control are evidenced, the diagnosis of either oral-nonverbal apraxia or dysarthria (depending on its precise nature) is likely. In fact, it is usually part of the criteria for the diagnosis of AOS that individual articulator strength (usually measured as maximum muscle force), as well as articulatory positioning (usually measured as accurate articulatory placement and speed of movement), be judged within normal limits.

McNeil et al (1990) investigated the articulatory control of small nonspeech isometric forces and small static positions in normal, pure AOS, conduction aphasic, and ataxic dysarthric individuals. They found that persons identified as having pure AOS without concomitant dysarthria or aphasia tracked, with visual feedback, forces and postures of the articulators that were significantly poorer (off target and more variable) than the nonimpaired persons but not differently from the persons with dysarthria. The aphasic participants' performance fell between the normal and the other two pathological groups, but was not significantly different from either. This latter finding was interpreted as opening the possibility of a fundamental speech motor control deficit accompanying or perhaps accounting for the perceived speech production deficits in conduction aphasia. However, given the very high incidence of oral nonspeech apraxia accompanying the presence of phonemic paraphasia (as well as those displaying AOS; McNeil et al, 2000), this finding might well have an alternative explanation—that this task may have reflected the presence of this nonspeech motor control disorder and not a speech motor control deficit per se.

Hageman, Robin, Moon, and Folkins (1994) compared five apraxic and 23 normal participant's ability to track, with visual feedback, a 0.3-, 0.6-, and 0.9-Hz unpredictable signal with the lower lip, jaw, and voice (f_0). Although the authors did not compare the groups or the conditions statistically, the normal participants achieved a best cross-correlation (disregarding their phase lead or lag) with the predictable targets, and their highest cross-correlations were inversely related to the frequency of the predictable target. Further, the normal participant's poorest cross-correlation occurred with the unpredictable signals for all structures. The apraxic individuals, on the other hand, achieved their highest cross-correlations across all structures for the unpredictable targets, and their correlations were variable across the three frequencies of the predictable

targets. Confounding the interpretation of this finding is the fact that the actual cross-correlational values were similar for the apraxic and normal groups for the unpredictable targets. Interpreting their results, the authors noted that movement control for the nonspeech tasks was impaired in their AOS participants. Also, because the unpredictable target was tracked relatively more accurately than the predictable one for the AOS participants, the authors proposed that the speakers with AOS had problems retrieving or developing an internal model or plan of the intended movement patterns. It must be remembered that as with all of the other studies that have used persons with pure apraxia, the sample sizes are small and the results are difficulty to generalize to other pure apraxic individuals or to individuals with AOS accompanied by other speech production deficits. Nonetheless, given the high confidence in accurate participant selection from these two studies, it remains tenable that the nonspeech movements of individuals with AOS are not normal and that these deficits of static and dynamic force and position-tracking are not related to the clinical detection of oral motor movement or force deficits nor presumably to oral nonspeech apraxia. These data have recently been replicated and expanded using similar tracking tasks by Ballard and Robin (in press) and Robin, Hageman, Clark, and Woodword (2007). Ballard and Robin used participants with AOS and concomitant aphasia, whereas Robin et al compared AOS performance to individuals with conduction aphasia. Importantly, Robin et al found that tracking predictable signals predicted (correlated with) perceptual measures of articulatory accuracy at approximately the 0.85 level. As mentioned above, although it is also clear that oral nonspeech apraxia (buccofacial apraxia; diagnosed by traditional oral motor examinations) and AOS can and do dissociate, it is not so clear whether these differences could be attributed to subtle deficits of oral nonspeech apraxia because the methods of assessment and criteria for judgment are considerably less studied and firmly established than they are for AOS.

◆ Intra- and Interarticulator Kinematics

The measurement of movements within a single articulator has been investigated in several studies using a variety of methods and procedures. Many of the kinematic studies have attempted to account for the slower speech of the apraxic individuals found with both perceptual and acoustic analyses. For example, Itoh et al (1980) reported peak velocities for one apraxic subject that were substantively lower than a normal control subject, and were in the range of those reported for a patient with amyotrophic lateral sclerosis. Using the x-ray microbeam system for simultaneously tracking movements of multiple articulators, Itoh et al (1980) and Itoh and Sasanuma (1984) reported inconsistent interarticulator timing abnormalities between the lip, velum, and tongue dorsum in one person with pure AOS. Using fiberscopic observation of the velum, these authors reported velar timing distortions that were often perceived as sound substitutions in this same individual. They also reported lip and jaw kinematics for ten normal (five young and five aged), five Broca aphasics with AOS, and three Wernicke aphasics without AOS (Itoh & Sasanuma, 1987). Although the Wernicke participants showed no abnormalities in peak velocity or displacement, the AOS participants demonstrated inconsistent articulatory velocity or displacement values that occasionally violated the normal reciprocal relationship between peak velocity and displacement. On these occasions, the apraxic speakers underassigned velocity to a displacement or overassigned both velocity and displacement simultaneously.

Using strain-gauge transducers, McNeil, Caliguiri, and Rosenbek (1989) compared labiomandibular duration, displacements, velocities, and dysmetrias in four pure-AOS and four normal-control participants. The movement durations across the transition from the vowel /a/ in "stop" to the vowel /ae/ in "fast" in the phrase "stop fast" was significantly longer in the AOS participants. Although the average peak velocities were not significantly different between the groups, the AOS participants produced significantly greater lower-lip-plus-jaw displacements than the control participants. Although the finding of a normal peak velocity has been replicated by Robin, Bean, and Folkins (1989) and by McNeil and Adams (1990), the greater displacement in the AOS group has not been replicated in subsequent analyses of these same individuals' productions of other utterances (McNeil & Adams, 1990). In addition to the finding of normal peak velocity, McNeil and Adams also found that these individuals produced abnormally long times to reach peak velocity compared with normal, conduction aphasic, and ataxic dysarthric participants. These authors also reported significantly longer total utterance durations for all three pathological groups compared with the normal participants.

As mentioned above, Robin, Bean, and Folkins (1989) also found normal peak velocities in six carefully selected AOS individuals but failed to find abnormal peak velocity/displacement relationships under conditions of altered speech rate, whether the jaw was blocked or unblocked or whether the utterance was produced correctly or incorrectly. Fromm, Abbs, McNeil, and Rosenbek (1982) reported a descriptive study of three pure apraxic and three normal control participants speech under simultaneous acoustic, kinematic, and electromyographic measurement. Description across structures and analysis levels revealed a variety of intra- and interarticulator temporal and spatial dyscoordinations.

Hardcastle (1987) also described a general dyscoordination of the tongue tip, blade, and body in one apraxic speaker using the electropalatograph. The dyscoordination was described as one of unsmooth transitions between successive lingual gestures with poor anticipatory coarticulation. Consistent with this interpretation of the primary deficit of AOS individuals, Forrest, Adams, McNeil, and Southwood (1991) found, from a kinematic analysis of AOS, conduction aphasia, ataxic dysarthric, and normal controls, phase plane trajectories for closing gestures in the AOS speakers that were decoupled in temporal-spatial relations (i.e., amplitude/velocity relations) relative to the same gestures in the normal participants. These authors noted that these decouplings were strikingly similar to the decomposition of multiarticulate movements evidenced in complex arm trajectories in individuals with limb apraxia (Poizner, Mack, Verfaellie, Rothi, & Heilman, 1990).

Katz, Machetanz, Orth, and Schonle (1990a) reported the labial and velar kinematic results from an investigation into the extent and time course of anticipatory coarticulation in the speech of two normal and two anterior lesioned German aphasic speakers. Using electromagnetic articulography, the aphasic participants with anterior lesions produced on-target productions that were more variable than those of the control participants, and these differences were primarily in the spatial/displacement aspects of the movements. The temporal aspects of the anticipatory coarticulatory movements were judged to be largely intact.

Following Shankweiler and colleagues' (1968) pioneering descriptive electromyographic (EMG) study of two individuals with "phonetic disintegration," or what is most likely consistent with AOS as defined in this chapter, showing a lack of temporal differentiation (i.e., reduced independent movements) among articulators, several EMG studies have been reported. Fromm (1981) and Fromm et al (1982) described antagonistic muscle co-contraction, continuous undifferentiated muscle activity, and EMG shutdown from recording of orbicularis oris superior, orbicularis oris inferior, mentalis, and depressor labi inferior muscles in three AOS participants. To replicate this descriptive study, Forrest et al (1991) compared EMG activity from the same muscles in four individuals in each of the following groups: pure AOS, conduction aphasia, ataxic dysarthria, and normal control. Antagonistic muscle co-contraction, continuous undifferentiated muscle activity, and EMG shutdown did not differentiate any of the groups. In fact, all groups, including the normal control group, demonstrated instances of these patterns. The frequency of their occurrence was not related to the judged severity of the AOS in any group. The authors concluded that it was difficult to conceptualize any group characteristics of AOS on the basis of EMG data because of the heterogeneity of each speaker's patterns of muscle activity.

Hough and Klich (1987) investigated the EMG timing of lip rounding for vowel productions in the context of the vowel shorting that normally accompanies the increase in syllable number (e.g., "short"/"shorten"/"shortening"). These authors concluded that there are measurable linguistic influences on EMG lip-rounding onset activity, and that these influences were preserved, although less consistently applied in their AOS participants compared with the normal controls.

The conclusion reached by McNeil and Kent (1990) relative to the EMG evidence describing AOS remains valid. They suggested that the EMG studies attempting to characterize and differentiate phonemic paraphasia from persons with AOS are meager and in desperate need of replication and careful comparison with equivalent data from normal control and other pathological individuals who share speech symptoms and lesion specificity.

◆ Speech Prosody

Prosodic studies include explorations of intensity, fundamental frequency (F_0), and duration. Relatively few studies have investigated the intensity of AOS speech. Fewer still have investigated these attributes in patients with phonemic paraphasia, as they are rarely identified as having prosodic problems. Kent and Rosenbek (1983) investigated syllable amplitude in persons with AOS, and Lebrun, Buyssens, and Henneaux (1973) reported on syllable amplitude in persons diagnosed with Broca aphasia. Both reported amplitude uniformity, which, along with the temporal regularity, leads to neutralization of stress pattern and dysrhythmia, which is part of the characteristic dysprosody often described in AOS.

F_0 variation (contour) in Broca aphasic individuals have been reported as restricted in range for sentence-level stimuli by Ryalls (1982) and Cooper, Soares, Nicol, Michelow, and Goloskie (1984), but not for within-word level stimuli by (Danly & Shapiro, 1982). Additionally, Broca aphasic individuals have been reported to shorten the obligatory utterance-final lengthening (Danly, de Villiers, & Cooper, 1979).

Odell, McNeil, Rosenbek, and Hunter (1990, 1991a,b) added to the description of the prosodic disturbance in AOS and its differentiation from the prosodic pattern found in persons with phonological paraphasia and the ataxic dysarthria (Odell et al, 1991b). They found that the AOS and ataxic dysarthric subjects had substantially more errors on stressed syllables than the persons with phonemic paraphasia. Further, frequent errors involving sound transitions, as reflected by open juncture, separated the small sample of persons with AOS from those with conduction aphasia who demonstrated virtually no such errors.

Ziegler and von Cramon (1985) investigated lingual-laryngeal, lingual-velar, and lingual-labial coarticulation. They found that in contrast to the normal speakers, the AOS participants failed to provide the necessary coarticulatory acoustic cues for normal listeners to judge the upcoming acoustic event (e.g., vowel) when it was totally or partially removed from the auditory stimulus. McNeil, Hashi, and Southwood (1994) replicated this finding for bilabial gestures for two persons with AOS and also found a similar effect for one of two individuals with conduction aphasia. Using acoustic analyses, Tuller and Story (1987) and Katz (1987) investigated anticipatory coarticulation or the anticipation of an articulatory feature in advance of the production of its parent segment. Although Tuller and Story found that some of their nonfluent aphasic participants did not show evidence of anticipatory coarticulation as early as the fluent aphasic or normal controls, Katz failed to find evidence for a delay of coarticulatory gestures in his aphasic speakers with anterior lesions. Katz, Machetanz, Orth, and Schonle (1990b) performed acoustic analyses on word productions contrasting in postconsonantal vowel rounding produced by two anterior lesioned and two normal German-speaking individuals. Anticipatory labialization was assessed by measuring frequency shift in the F2 peaks and in the transitions. They found anticipatory labial coarticulation in the speakers with aphasia that resembled that

of the two normal speakers. These results are interesting. However, it is not possible to equate findings across these studies with any degree of certainty, as the results derived from individuals categorized as nonfluent or anterior cannot be compared with those selected as having AOS. Indeed, as discussed in a previous section, the relationship of lesion location with the presence of AOS, even the gross localization such as anterior, remains unclear and unassignable.

◆ Variability, Consistency, and Target-Approximation Profile

The consistency of speech errors has been argued as evidence for both a basic motoric (execution level) and a linguistic representational error-assignment level. One argument suggests that because no studies have demonstrated a consistently impaired feature (e.g., place) across all the phonemes in which it appears, it is evidence against a linguistic (representational) mechanism for the speech errors of aphasic or apraxic speakers. Another argument specifies that a consistent error is evidence for a motoric-level error. As stated by McNeil, Odell, Miller, and Hunter (1995), there is no shared set of criteria among clinicians or researchers regarding the direction of prediction or magnitude of effect for the three variables of consistency of error location, variability of error type, or target accuracy on multiple and successive trials. Inconsistency of error location (Wertz et al, 1984), variability of error type (Wertz et al, 1984), and improvement on successive attempts to reach the phonemic/phonetic target (Aten et al, 1971; Darley, 1982; Wertz et al, 1984) are reported to be characteristic of AOS. Likewise, the phonological paraphasic errors of the person with conduction aphasia have been reported to (1) increase in accuracy with successive attempts at the target, (2) be consistent in location of the error in the segment, and (3) be nonvariable in the type of the error (Joanette, Keller, & Lecours, 1980). Though this differential consistency and variability has not been documented, it appears that these are principles used by many clinicians to guide their differential diagnosis of AOS from phonemic paraphasia.

As summarized by McNeil, Odell, Miller, and Hunter (1995), speakers with dysarthria are traditionally described as producing errors that are consistent in error location and nonvariable in type (Darley, Aronson, & Brown, 1975a; Wertz et al, 1984). To test this assumption, McNeil et al carefully selected persons with pure AOS, conduction aphasia, and ataxic dysarthria to assess their consistency of error location, variability of error type, and accuracy of successive approximations on three repeated trials of the same word. They reported that the consistency of error location was higher for the groups with AOS and ataxic dysarthria than for the group with phonemic paraphasia. Conversely, the variability of error type was considerably higher for the persons demonstrating phonemic paraphasia than for those demonstrating AOS and ataxic dysarthria, whose performance was very similar to each other. The individuals with phonemic paraphasia produced more *attempts* (defined as any phonemic or audible nonphonemic utterances occurring prior to the final production that was separated from it by any perceived silence) and *starters* (defined as an audible initial sound, syllable, or word characterized by a smooth transition into the final production, with no perceivable pauses or breaks) with a greater percentage of accurately reached targets for both attempts and starters than the groups with AOS or ataxic dysarthrias. Further, the individuals with phonemic paraphasias produced more attempts and starters at the word level and few at the sound level, whereas the group with AOS produced more attempts and starters at the sound level and none at the word level. The groups produced approximately equal proportions of these trial-and-error gropings at the syllable level. Although the numbers of participants from which these findings are derived are extremely small, the purity of their classification can be used to form the basis from which further studies on larger numbers, and perhaps less isolated impairments, can be conducted. In the interim, data from carefully selected individuals with isolated impairments, using finite systems for analysis such as narrow phonetic transcription, can offer more insight into the nature and phenomenology of the disorder than the sum of data accumulated over the previous 30 years from participants who were poorly defined or with mixed disorders. In addition, data derived from individuals with isolated disorders such as pure AOS or phonemic paraphasia without concomitant AOS or dysarthria provide the basis for productive hypothesis building.

In summary, the individuals with phonemic paraphasia were less consistent in the location of their errors on repeated trials of the same utterance than the subjects with AOS. They were also more variable in the type of errors than those with AOS, and they tended to get closer to the target on successive productions of the target with more starters and attempts along the way. These findings are counter to the current clinical beliefs and may offer insight into both the mechanisms of the error generators in the two populations and into their differential diagnosis. However, until appropriate numbers of carefully selected individuals with pure pathologies can be assessed, using the same stimuli and measurement procedures, along with the appropriate statistical procedures (e.g., discriminant function analysis) for determining their contributions to an overall profile that differentiates the populations, these differential features will remain hypotheses for testing.

Seddoh et al (1996) compared the variability of acoustic durational data between persons with AOS and conduction aphasia. They examined VOT, consonant-vowel transition duration, vowel nucleus duration, and total word duration. Participants were required to repeat 10 times a target word embedded within a phrase. Within-subject variability (standard deviation) served as the dependent measure. The results showed that the absolute duration of these measures did not differentiate AOS from conduction aphasia. Rather, significantly greater within-subject variability for the individuals with AOS resulted in the differences between the groups.

If there has been no *a priori* means of selecting participants for study to describe the phenomenology of the disorder and

to determine the underlying nature of pathology, it must follow that all of the data are suspect relative to their usefulness for setting identification criteria and their validity for assigning underlying mechanisms to the pathological behaviors. If one also examines the performance characteristics of carefully selected AOS and conduction aphasic individuals (described below), the probability is increased that the criteria employed by Halpern et al (1976) and by most other researchers who have contributed to the current database actually did eliminate the persons with aphasia that demonstrated phonological or literal paraphasias. This contamination of the AOS database has been recognized by others. For example, Itoh and Sasanuma (1984) stated, "Those articulatory characteristics of apraxia of speech set forward by Johns and Darley (1970) which have been confirmed by many investigators since then, in fact, might be reflecting an underlying impairment which is not confined to the level of motor programming, . . . but extend into the level of linguistic (phonological) processing . . . as well" (p. 159).

◆ Effort

The notion of excessive effort expended in the production of speech is a frequently appearing characteristic in the sundry descriptions and definitions of AOS. As discussed by Pierce (1991), the notion of effort may be tied, to some degree, to the concepts of consistency, variability, and successive approximations discussed earlier in this chapter. Attempts to self-correct speech errors may give the impression that speech is more effortful to produce, and in fact it may be. However, the notions of consistency, variability, and successive approximations (trial-and-error behavior) toward a correct target cannot unambiguously be assigned to the person with AOS (Hough, 1978; Joanette et al, 1980; Kohn, 1984).

Robin and colleagues (Solomon, Robin, & Luschei, 1994; Solomon, Robin, Mitchinson, VanDaele, & Luschei, 1996; Somodi, Robin, & Luschei, 1995) have investigated the relationships among motor abilities and "sense of effort" in normal and brain-damaged individuals. Robin and colleagues developed reliable measures of "sense of effort" in intact (Somodi et al, 1995; Solomon et al, 1996) and disordered populations such as those with childhood speech disorders (Somodi, Robin, & Luschei, 1995) and Parkinson's disease (Solomon & Robin, 2005). Data from these studies were statistically modeled, and the models predicted "sense of effort" under conditions of fatigue in the intact group but less consistently in the disordered group. Clark and Robin (1998) speculated that brain-damaged individuals may not be sensitive to task demands and may require external feedback to effectively allocate resources to motor or other tasks.

These studies on sense of effort hold as much interest as they do potential clinical promise. However, there is no literature attempting to relate the listener's judgment of the speaker's effort to the actual effort expended by the speaker with AOS. Until this enormously complex set of issues is systematically disentangled, it is very difficult to know what perceptual or linguistic features listeners are attributing to apraxic speech that would make it sound more effortful than the speech of individuals with phonological paraphasia, dysarthria, stuttering, or another speech or language impaired population. Without clarification of these issues with systematic research, it difficult to use the word *effortful* as a necessary or differential feature of AOS.

♦ Apraxia of Speech Defined

Rosenbek and McNeil (1991) proposed that one worthy goal of contemporary clinical scientists interested in speech production and its pathologies is to find *strong neuromotor syndromes* in dysarthria and apraxia of speech. A strong syndrome was defined as one in which neuromuscular abnormalities are identified in predictable distributions across functional components and are related to a pattern of perceptual speech abnormalities with sufficient frequency to

suggest a causal relationship. If the pattern is unique, the syndrome is stronger yet. The authors suggested that the goal of contrasting assumed mechanisms, signs, symptoms, and the presence or absence of concomitant disorders between AOS and dysarthria is eventually to determine the significant characteristics of the groups and find constant differences between them. Having begun, of clinical and experimental necessity, to use the terms *dysarthria* and *apraxia* with their inadequately tested assumptions borrowed from neurology, the search for the defining characteristics and constant differences for AOS has been biased from the onset. The realization of this goal awaits a great deal of clinical experimentation.

Similarly, and more critical to the goals of this chapter, the goal of contrasting assumed mechanisms, signs, and symptoms between AOS and phonemic paraphasia is also eventually to determine the significant characteristics of the groups and find constant differences between them. The review of the phonologic, phonetic, prosodic, and motoric characteristics above provide a foundation for such an enterprise. **Table 15–3** summarizes a tentative (and the

Table 15–3 Tentative List of Characteristics that Differentiate AOS from Phonemic Paraphasia

Apraxia of Speech	Phonemic Paraphasia
Disturbed prosody	
Overall rate	
Slow rate in phonemically on-target or off-target phrases and sentences	Near-normal rate in phonemically on-target phrases and sentences.
Inability to increase rate while maintaining phonemic integrity	Variable ability to increase rate, but within normal ranges, while maintaining phonemic integrity
Microsegmental rate	
Variable, but overall prolonged movement transitions	Variable, but normal movement transition durations
Variable, but prolonged interword intervals in phonemically on-target utterances	Variable, but normal average interword intervals in phonemically on-target utterances
Variable, but abnormally long vowels in multi-syllabic words or words in sentences	Variable, but normal vowel duration in multisyllabic words or words in sentences
Variable, but increased movement durations for individual speech gestures in the production of contextual speech	Variable, but average movement durations within the ranges for normal subjects
Successive self- initiated trials to repair an error leads no closer to the target	Successive self- initiated trials to repair an error leads closer to the target
Stress assignment	
Presence of errors on stressed syllables	No clear relationship between syllabic stress and errors frequency
Phonological characteristics	
With distorted perseverative, anticipatory and exchange phoneme or phoneme cluster errors	With undistorted perseverative, anticipatory and phoneme exchange or phoneme cluster errors
With phoneme distortions	Without phoneme distortions
Presence of distorted sound substitutions, primarily of prolonged phonemes and secondarily devoiced phonemes	Absence of distorted sound substitutions
Other kinematic characteristics	
Difficulty tracking predictable movement patterns with speech articulators	Intact ability to track predictable movement patterns with speech articulators
Intact ability to track unpredictable movement patterns with speech articulators	Intact ability to track unpredictable movement patterns with speech articulators
Other characteristics	
The location of errors in the utterance are consistent from trial to trial	The location of errors in the utterance are not consistent from trial to trial
The types of errors in the utterance are not variable from trial to trial	The types of errors in the utterance are variable from trial to trial

situation has not radically changed since the first edition of this text) list of characteristics that both define AOS and differentiate it from phonemic paraphasia. It remains tentative because although logical and coherent with general clinical observation, it remains substantively untested. That is, it will require systematic verification on relatively large populations who demonstrate characteristics of only one pathological group, or alternatively, on very large groups of carefully described subjects with less pure pathological conditions. Further, when perceptual analyses form the dependent measures, it is essential that narrow phonetic analysis be used to capture the nonphonological as well as the phonological characteristics of the speech errors.

Dabul (1986) proposed a list of 15 speech and nonspeech behaviors that characterize AOS, any five or more of which were sufficient for its diagnose. The list consisted of the exhibition of (1) anticipatory phonemic errors, (2) perseverative phonemic errors, (3) phonemic transposition errors, (4) phonemic voicing substitutions, (5) phonemic vowel substitutions, (6) visible and audible searching behavior, (7) numerous and varied off-target attempts at the word, (8) highly inconsistent errors, (9) increase in errors with increase in phonemic sequence, (10) fewer errors in automatic speech than volitional speech, (11) marked difficulty initiating speech, (12) intrusion of a schwa between syllables or in consonant clusters, (13) abnormal prosodic features, (14) awareness of errors and inability to correct them, and (15) a receptive-expressive gap. Pierce (1991) suggested that only three of these 15 behaviors were unique characteristics of AOS and could be used to differentiate it from phonemic paraphasic speech errors. The three unique behaviors were difficulty initiating speech, intrusion of a schwa, and abnormal prosody. Visible and audible searching, he suggested, might be useful for the differentiation of the two pathologies depending on how searching is defined. He further suggested that the other 11 behaviors are characteristics of both phonemic paraphasia and AOS, or in the case of sound substitutions, are a clear sign of phonemic paraphasia and not apraxic speech.

We respectfully disagree with Pierce's selection of the behaviors listed by Dabul that differentiate the two pathologies. That is, anticipatory, perseverative, and transposition errors are generated at the phonological encoding level of speech production and belong exclusively to the phonemic paraphasic. Errors that are highly inconsistent are also most likely generated by the phonemic paraphasic. From Dabul's list, only the intrusive schwa (when separated from the linguistically derived epenthesis) and abnormal prosody (depending on how it is defined) belong exclusively to the individual with AOS. Errors that increase with increases of phonemic sequences are more frequent with volitional than automatic speech (depending on how the terms *volitional* and *automatic* are operationalized), are uncorrectable with awareness (depending to a great measure on the severity of the disorder), and occur in the context of a receptive-expressive performance gap (depending on the severity of both the speech production deficit and the other aphasic symptoms), belong to both groups. Voicing and vowel substitutions, visible and audible searching, varied off-target attempts at self-correction, and marked difficulty initiating

speech, are more likely to be seen in the phonemic paraphasic; however, they can be seen in both groups.

Following their 40 pages of detailed review of the characteristics of AOS, Wertz et al (1984) condensed their discussion into its four most salient clinical characteristics: (1) effortful, trial and error, groping articulatory movements, and attempts at self-correction; (2) dysprosody unrelieved by extended periods of normal rhythm, stress, and intonation; (3) articulatory inconsistency on repeated productions of the same utterance; and (4) obvious difficulty initiating utterances.

They suggested that those persons revealing these four behaviors in spontaneous and imitative speech are apraxic. Although all of these behaviors are likely to be seen in AOS, only the dysprosody, in the context of the other three (and other) behaviors, is likely to differentiate it from phonemic paraphasia. It will be recalled that the phonemic paraphasic may present with inconsistent trial-and-error behaviors and attempts at self-correction, with a great deal of effort, often at the initiation of an utterance.

It is unlikely that a checklist method of features can be developed that will allow the differential diagnosis of AOS. All of the behaviors that compose the core features of the syndrome can be seen in other neurogenic speech production disorders. It is the behaviors that occur in particular clusters, likely influenced by severity, that allow the differential identification of AOS and other motor speech disorders. It is unfortunate that a large-enough pool of individuals with pure AOS, or an even larger pool of not-so-pure AOS individuals, has not been collected on the same appropriate tasks, using the same methods of measurement, so that cluster analyses, confirmatory factor analyses, or similar statistical procedures could be employed to establish the patterns of behavior that differentiate AOS from its clinical pathological neighbors. Until this is done, the sifting and winnowing of information from diverse populations, using diverse tasks and measurement procedures, along with the continued sharpening of theory, will constitute the grounds for our formal definition of AOS and the criteria by which it is to be identified and eventually managed. It is critical to the clinical theoretician and to the practicing clinician to remember that AOS rarely presents in isolation. Such behaviors as sound substitutions can occur in a person with AOS because they are distortions of the intended sound or because they are phoneme substitutions that occur because of a phonological encoding disruption. In the former case the mechanism might be consistent with the mechanism for AOS. In the latter case it might attributable to a phonological encoding-level error. If it could be established that the mechanism was one attributable to the phonological level of speech processing, it does not mean, and cannot be concluded, that AOS is a phonological disorder. The arguments about whether AOS is a phonological disorders or a motor programming disorder are fatuous. Although the exact manifestations in the speech apparatus are to a large measure yet to be specified, AOS is by definition, a motor planning/ programming disorder. The issue is not one of defining apraxia; that has been done, as clearly delineated in the literature review above. The critical issue is one of specifying to whom the term *AOS* applies. The criteria proposed by

McNeil et al (1997), reiterated here, and used by Wambaugh et al (2006a,b), are, we believe, strong candidates.

Consistent with the proposed mechanisms discussed throughout the chapter, and consistent with the characteristics discussed above and summarized in **Table 15–3** that should eventually differentiate AOS from phonemic paraphasia, the following definition of AOS is proposed:

Apraxia of speech is a phonetic-motoric disorder of speech production. It is caused by inefficiencies in the translation of well-formed and -filled phonological frames into previously learned kinematic information used for carrying out intended movements. These inefficiencies result in intra- and interarticulator temporal and spatial segmental and prosodic distortions. It is characterized by distortions of segment and intersegment transitionalization and coarticulation resulting in extended durations of consonants, vowels, and time between sounds, syllables, and words. These distortions are often perceived as sound substitutions and as the misassignment of stress and other phrasal and sentence-level prosodic abnormalities. Errors are relatively consistent in location within the utterance and invariable in type. It is not attributable to deficits of muscle tone or reflexes, nor to primary deficits in the processing of sensory (auditory, tactile, kinesthetic, proprioceptive), or language information. In its extremely infrequently occurring isolated form, it is not accompanied by the above-listed deficits of basic motor physiology, perception, or language.

♦ Requirements for Additional Research (Persons with "Pure" Apraxia of Speech and Narrow Phonetic Transcription)

There are at least two important experimental methods, in addition to continued theoretical developments, that have clarified the assignment of specific speech errors to specific levels of the linguistic and motoric speech production process. The use of both *narrow phonetic transcription* and the selection of individuals for study who demonstrate *isolated AOS* (i.e., without coexisting aphasia or dysarthria) have enabled the continued specification of linguistic and motoric mechanisms of the speech production process. It must be recognized, however, that isolated AOS and isolated phonemic (literal) paraphasia (phonemic paraphasia in isolation from any convincing signs of dysarthria, AOS, or other signs of aphasia such as evidence of impairments in reading, writing, auditory comprehension, lexical retrieval, etc.) are extremely rare speech-language pathologies. It must also be recognized, however, that "isolated"

pathologies in individuals whose speech is transcribed narrowly may be the only convincing forms of perceptual evidence from which defining characteristics can be formulated. That is, if pathologies frequently or typically coexist, there is little assurance that the data on which the phenomenology of AOS or phonemic paraphasias can be used to set the defining characteristics of either pathological group unless certain error types or certain measurements can unambiguously be assigned to different levels of the speech production system. As so clearly called for by Itoh and Sasanuma (1984), more rigorous criteria for subject selection in research will be mandatory if we are to extract only those articulatory characteristics that are the direct acoustic results of apraxic movements per se and nothing else. Itoh and Sasanuma state, "Our finding[s] ... are clearly in support of the view that faulty programming of speech musculature constitutes the base of the symptom complex called apraxia of speech and that the most natural and reasonable end products of this underlying deficit are (phonetic) distortions" (p. 160). It is only with narrow phonetic transcription that these distortions can be extracted from the phonemic errors that are the natural consequence of categorical speech perception (Lieberman & Studdert-Kennedy, 1978).

Finally, it is imperative that research in speech motor planning and programming be driven by detailed models of speech production. In our view, a close inspection of several speech production models such as those proposed by Guenther, Hampson, and Johnson (1998), Levelt, (1999), Roelofs (1997), and van der Merwe (2007) offer a reasonable start. The combination of detailed models that drive hypothesis testing, along with precise behavioral measures, will yield accurate differential diagnosis and a continued exploration of the neuropsychological mechanisms of AOS. These approaches, combined with temporally and spatially sensitive brain imaging methods, should produce relevant and converging evidence about the neural and cognitive bases of AOS.

♦ Apraxia of Speech Treatment

Although the effective and efficient treatment of AOS is the primary application of differential diagnosis and comprehensive assessment for AOS, its discussion is beyond the scope of this chapter. In addition to Chapter 16, offering principles of treatment relevant for AOS, an ever-increasing literature supports the efficacy of treatment and several limpid reviews of it are available from several sources, including Ballard and Robin (2002), McNeil et al (2000), McNeil et al (1997), Odell (2002), Wambaugh (2002), and Wambaugh et al (2006a,b).

References

Aten, J.L., Johns, D.F., & Darley, F.L. (1971). Auditory perception of sequenced words in apraxia of speech. *Journal of Speech and Hearing Research, 14,* 131–143

Ballard, K.J., Granier, J.P., & Robin, D.A. (2000). Understanding the nature of apraxia of speech: theory, analysis, and treatment. *Aphasiology, 14,* 969–995

Ballard, K.J. & Robin, D.A. (2002). Assessment of AOS for treatment planning. *Seminars in Speech and Language: Apraxia of speech: From Concept to Clinic, 4,* 281–291

Ballard, K.J. & Robin, D.A. (2007). Influence of continual feedback on jaw pursuit-tracking in healthy adults and in adults with apraxia plus aphasia. *Journal of Motor Behavior, 29,* 19–28

Ballard, K.J., Solomon, N.P., Robin, D.A., Moon, J., & Folkins, J. (2007). Non-speech assessment of the speech production system. In: M.R. McNeil (Ed.), *Clinical Management of Sensorimotor Speech Disorders,* 2nd ed. New York: Thieme

Bates, E., Wilson, S.M., Saygin, A.P., Dick, F., Sereno, M.I., Knight, R.T., & Dronkers, N.F. (2003). Voxel-based lesion-symptom mapping. *Nature Neuroscience, 6,* 448–450

Bauman, J.A. (1978). *Sound Duration: A Comparison Between Performances of Subjects with Central Nervous System Disorders and Normal Speakers.* Unpublished doctoral dissertation, University of Colorado

Blumstein, S.E. (1973). *A Phonological Investigation of Aphasic Speech.* Mouton: The Hague

Blumstein, S.E. (1981). Phonological aspects of aphasia. In: M.T. Sarno (Ed.), *Acquired Aphasia* (pp. 129–155). New York: Academic Press

Blumstein, S.E. & Baum, S. (1987). Consonant production deficits in aphasia. In: J.H. Ryalls (Ed.), *Phonetic Approaches to Speech Production in Aphasia and Related Disorders* (pp. 3–22). Boston: College-Hill Press

Blumstein, S.E., Cooper, W.E., Goodglass, H., Statlender, S., & Gottlieb, J. (1980). Production of deficits in aphasia: a voice-onset time analysis. *Brain and Language, 9,* 153–170

Blumstein, S.E, Cooper, W.E., Zurif, E.B., & Caramazza, A. (1977). The perception and production of voice-onset time in aphasia. *Neuropsychologia, 155,* 371–383

Bock, J.K. (1982). Toward a cognitive psychology of syntax: information processing contribution to sentence formulation. *Psychological Review, 89,* 1–47

Boone, D.R. & Plante, E. (1993). *Human Communication and Its Disorders,* 2nd ed. Englewood Cliffs, NJ: Prentice Hall

Bowman, C.A., Hodson, B.W., & Simpson, R.K. (1980. Oral apraxia and aphasic misarticulation. *Clinical Aphasiology, 8,* 89–95

Buckingham, H.W., Jr. (1979). Explanation in apraxia with consequences for the concept of apraxia of speech. *Brain and Language, 8,* 202–226

Buckingham, H.W. (1990). Abstruse neologisms, retrieval deficits and the random generator. *Journal of Neurolinguistics, 5,* 215–235

Buckingham, H.W. (1992). Phonological production deficits in conduction aphasia. In: S.E. Kohn (Ed.), *Conduction Aphasia* (pp. 77–116). Hillsdale, NJ: Lawrence Erlbaum Associates

Canter, G.J. (1969). The influence of primary and secondary verbal apraxia on output disturbances in aphasic syndromes. Paper presented at the Annual Convention of the American Speech and Hearing Association, Chicago

Canter, G.J., Trost, J.E., & Burns, M.S. (1985). Contrasting speech patterns in apraxia of speech and phonemic paraphasia. *Brain and Language, 24,* 204–222

Clark, H. & Robin, D. 1998). Generalized motor programme and parameterization accuracy in apraxia of speech and conduction aphasia. *Aphasiology, 12,* 699–713

Collins, M., Rosenbek, J.C., & Wertz, R.T. (1983). Spectrographic analysis of vowel and word duration in apraxia of speech. *Journal of Speech and Hearing Research, 26,* 224–230

Cooper, W.E., Soares, C., Nicol, J., Michelow, D., & Goloskie, S. (1984). Clausal intonation after unilateral brain damage. *Language and Speech, 27,* 17–24

Dabul, B. (1983). *Apraxia Battery for Adults* (ABA-2). Tigard, OR: C.C. Publications

Danly, M., de Villiers, J.G., & Cooper, W.E. (1979). Control of speech prosody in Broca's aphasia. In: J.J. Wolf, and D.H. Klatt (Eds.), *Speech Communication Papers Presented at the 97th Meeting of the Acoustical Society of America.* New York: Acoustical Society of America

Danly, M. & Shapiro, B. (1982). Speech prosody in Broca's aphasia. *Brain and Language, 16,* 171–190

Darley, F.L. (1967). Lacunae and research approaches to them. IV. In: C. H. Millikan & F. L. Darley (Eds.), *Brain Mechanisms Underlying Speech and Language* (pp. 236–290), New York: Grune & Stratton

Darley, F.L. (1968). Apraxia of speech: 107 years of terminological confusion. Paper presented at the American Speech and Hearing Association, Denver

Darley, F.L. (1969). Aphasia: input and output disturbances in speech and language processing. Paper presented at the American Speech and Hearing Association, Chicago

Darley, F.L. (1982). *Aphasia.* Philadelphia: W.B. Saunders

Darley, F.L., Aronson, A.E., & Brown, J.R. (1975a). *Motor Speech Disorders.* Philadelphia: W.B. Saunders

Darley, F.L., Aronson, A.E., & Brown, J.R. (1975b). *Motor Speech Disorders: Audio Seminars in Speech Pathology.* Philadelphia: W.B. Saunders

Deal, J.L. & Darley, F.L. (1972). The influence of linguistic and situational variables on phonemic accuracy in apraxia of speech. *Journal of Speech and Hearing Research, 15,* 639–653

Deger, K. & Ziegler, W. (2002). Speech motor programming in apraxia of speech. *Journal of Phonetics, 30,* 321–335

Dell, G.S. (1986). A spreading-activation theory of retrieval in sentence production. *Psychological Review, 93,* 283–321

Dell, G.S. (1988). The retrieval of phonological forms in production: tests of prediction from a connectionist model. *Journal of Memory and Language, 27,* 124–142

Dell, G.S., Burger, L.K., & Svec, W.R. (1997). Language production and serial order: a functional analysis and a model. *Psychological Review, 104,* 123–147

Deutsch, S.E. (1984). Prediction of site of lesion from speech apraxic error patterns. In J.C. Rosenbek, M.R. McNeil, & A.E. Aronson (Eds.), *Apraxia of Speech: Physiology, Acoustics, Linguistics, Management* (pp. 113–134). San Diego: College Hill Press

Donnan, G.A., Darby, D.G., & Saling, M.M. (1997). Identification of brain region for coordinating speech articulation. *Lancet, 349,* 221–222

Dronkers, N.F. (1996). A new brain region for coordinating speech articulation. *Nature, 384,* 159–161

Duffy, J.R. (2005). *Motor Speech Disorders: Substrates, Differential Diagnosis and Management,* 2nd ed. St. Louis: Mosby

Duffy, J.R. & Duffy, R.J. (1990). The assessment of limb apraxia: the limb apraxia test. In: E.A. Roy (Ed.), *Neuropsychological Studies of Apraxia and Related Disorders* (pp. 503–531). North Holland: Elsevier Science Publishers

Duffy, J.R. & Gawle, C.A. (1984). Apraxic speakers' vowel duration in consonant-vowel-consonant syllables. In: J.C. Rosenbek, M.R. McNeil, and A.E. Aronson (Eds.), *Apraxia of Speech: Physiology Acoustics, Linguistics, Management* (pp. 167–196). San Diego: College-Hill Press

Dunlop, J.M. & Marquardt, T.P. (1977). Linguistic and articulatory aspects of single word production in apraxia of speech. *Cortex, 13,* 17–29

Faglioni, P. & Basso, A. (1985). Historical perspectives on neuroanatomical correlates of limb apraxia. In: E.A. Roy (Ed.), *Neuropsychological Studies of Apraxia and Related Disorders* (pp. 3–44). North Holland: Elsevier Science Publishers

Forrest, K., Adams, S., McNeil, M.R., & Southwood, H. (1991). Kinematic, electromyographic, and perceptual evaluation of speech apraxia, conduction aphasia, ataxic dysarthria and normal speech production. In: C.A. Moore, K.M. Yorkston, & D.R. Beukelman, (Eds.), *Dysarthria and Apraxia of Speech: Perspectives on Management* (pp. 147–171) Baltimore: Paul H. Brookes

Fromm, D. (1981). *Investigation of Movement/EMG Parameters in Apraxia of Speech.* Unpublished master's thesis, University of Wisconsin-Madison, Madison, Wisconsin

Fromm, D., Abbs, J.H., McNeil, M.R., & Rosenbek, J.C. (1982). Simultaneous perceptual-physiological method for studying apraxia of speech. *Clinical Aphasiology, 10,* 155–171

Gandour, J. & Dardarananda, R. (1984). Prosodic disturbance in aphasia: Vowel length in Thai. *Brain and Language, 23*, 206–224

Garrett, M.F. (1980). Levels of processing in sentence production. In: B. Butterworth (Ed.), *Language Production, Volume 1: Speech and Talk* (pp. 177–220). London: Academic Press

Garrett, M.F. (1984). The organization of processing structure for language production: applications to aphasic speech. In: D. Caplan, A.R. Lecours, & A. Smith, (Eds.), *Biological Perspectives on Language* (pp. 172–193). Cambridge, MA: MIT Press

Goerendt, I.K., Messa, C. Lawrence, A.D., Grasby, P.M., Piccini, P., & Brooks, D.J. (2003). Dopamine release during sequential finger movements in health and Parkinson's disease: a PET study. *Brain, 126*, 312–325

Goodglass, H. (1992). Diagnosis of conduction aphasia. In: S.E. Kohn (Ed.), *Conduction Aphasia* (pp. 3–50). Hillsdale, NJ: Lawrence Erlbaum Associates

Graybiel, A.M. (1998). The basal ganglia and chunking of action repertoires. *Neurobiology of Learning and Memory, 70*, 119–136

Grillner, S. (1982). Possible analogies in the control of innate motor acts and the production of sound speech. In: S. Grillner, B. Lindblom, J. Lubker, A. Persson (Eds.), *Speech Motor Control* (pp. 217–230). Oxford: Pergamon Press

Guenther, F.H., Hampson, M., & Johnson, D. (1998). A theoretical investigation of reference frames for the planning of speech movements. *Psychological Review, 105*, 611–633

Hageman, C.F., Robin, D.A., Moon, J.B., & Folkins, J.W. (1994). Oral motor tracking in normal and apraxic speakers. *Clinical Aphasiology, 22*, 219–229

Halpern, H., Keith, R., & Darley, F.L. (1976). Phonemic behavior of aphasic subjects without dysarthria or apraxia of speech. *Cortex, 12*, 365–372

Hardcastle, W.J. (1987). Electropalatographic study of articulation disorders in verbal dyspraxia. In: J.H. Ryalls (Ed.), *Phonetic Approaches to Speech Production in Aphasia and Related Disorders* (pp. 113–136). Boston: College-Hill Press

Hegde, M.N. (1991). *Introduction to Communicative Disorders.* Austin: Pro-Ed

Hillis, A.E., Work, M., Barker, P.B., Jacobs, M.A., Breese, E.L., & Maurer, K. (2004). Re-examining the brain regions crucial for orchestrating speech articulation. *Brain, 127*, 1479–1487

Hoit-Dalgaard, J., Murry, T., & Kopp, H.G. (1983). Voice onset time production and perception in apraxic subjects. *Brain and Language, 20*, 329–339

Hough, M.S. (1978). *Frequency of Specific Types of Phonological/Motor Errors Produced by Fluent and Nonfluent Aphasic Adults.* Unpublished master's thesis, University of Florida

Hough, M.S. & Klich, R.J. (1987). Effects of word length on lip EMG activity in apraxia of speech. *Clinical Aphasiology, 15*, 271–276

Itoh, M. & Sasanuma, S. (1984). Articulatory movements in apraxia of speech. In: J.C. Rosenbek, M.R. McNeil & A.E. Aronson (Eds.), *Apraxia of Speech: Physiology, Acoustics, Linguistics, Management* (pp. 134–165). San Diego: College Hill Press

Itoh, M. & Sasanuma, S. (1987). Articulatory velocities of aphasic patients. In: J.H. Ryalls (Ed.), *Phonetic Approaches to Speech Production in Aphasia and Related Disorders* (pp. 137–162). Boston: College-Hill Press

Itoh, M., Sasanuma, S., Hirose, H., Yoshioka, H., & Sawashima, M. (1983). Velar movements during speech in two Wernicke aphasic patients. *Brain and Language, 19*, 283–292

Itoh, M., Sasanuma, S., Hirose, H., Yoshioka, H., & Ushijima, T. (1980). Abnormal articulatory dynamics in a patient with apraxia of speech: X-ray microbeam observations. *Brain and Language, 11*, 66–75

Itoh, M., Sasanuma, S., & Ushijima, T. (1979). Velar movements during speech in a patient with apraxia of speech. *Brain and Language, 7*, 227–239

Jakobson, R. (1968). *Child Language Aphasia and Phonological Universals.* The Hague: Mouton

Joanette, Y., Keller, E., & Lecours, A.R. (1980). Sequence of phonemic approximations in aphasia. *Brain and Language, 11*, 30–44

Johns, D.F. & Darley, F.L. (1970). Phonemic variability in apraxia of speech. *Journal of Speech and Hearing Research, 13*, 556–583

Katz, W.F. (1987). Anticipatory labial and lingual coarticulation in aphasia. In: J.H. Ryalls (Ed.), *Phonetic Approaches to Speech Production in Aphasia and Related Disorders* (pp. 221–242). Boston: College-Hill Press

Katz, W., Machetanz, J., Orth, U., & Schonle, P. (1990a). A kinematic analysis of anticipatory coarticulation in the speech of anterior aphasic subjects using electromagnetic articulography. *Brain and Language, 38*, 555–575

Katz, W., Machetanz, J., Orth, U., & Schonle, P. (1990b). Anticipatory labial coarticulation in the speech of German-speaking anterior aphasic subjects: acoustic analyses. *Journal of Neurolinguistics, 5*, 295–320

Kearns, K. (1980). The application of phonological process analysis to the adult neuropathologies. *Clinical Aphasiology, 8*, 187–195

Keller, E. (1978). Parameters for vowel substitutions in Broca's aphasia. *Brain and Language, 5*, 265–285

Keller, E. (1984). Simplification and gesture reduction in phonological disorders of apraxia and aphasia. In: J.C. Rosenbek, M.R. McNeil, and A.E. Aronson (Eds.), *Apraxia of Speech: Physiology, Acoustics, Linguistics and Management* (pp. 221–256). San Diego: College-Hill Press

Kelso, J.A.S. (1995). *Dynamic Patterns: The Self-Organization of Brain and Behavior.* Cambridge, MA: MIT Press

Kelso, J.A.S., Tuller, B., & Harris, K.S. (1983). A dynamic pattern perspective on the control and coordination of movement. In: P.F. MacNeilage (Ed.), *The Production of Speech* (pp. 137–173). New York: Springer-Verlag

Kent, R.D. & McNeil, M.R. (1987). Relative timing of sentence repetition in apraxia of speech and conduction aphasia. In: J.H. Ryalls (Ed.), *Phonetic Approaches to Speech Production in Aphasia and Related Disorders* (pp. 181–220). Boston: College-Hill Press

Kent, R.D. & Rosenbek, J.C. (1983). Acoustic patterns of apraxia of speech. *Journal of Speech and Hearing Research, 26*, 231–249

Klapp, S.T. (1995). Motor response programming during simple and choice reaction time: the role of practice. *Journal of Experimental Psychology: Human Perception and Performance, 21*, 1015–1027

Klapp, S.T. (2003). Reaction time analysis of two types of motor preparation for speech articulation: action as a sequence chunks. *Journal of Motor Behavior, 35*, 135–150

Klich, R.J., Ireland, J.V., & Weidner, W.E. (1979). Articulatory and phonological aspects of consonant substitutions in apraxia of speech. *Cortex, 15*, 451–470

Kohn, S.E. (1984). The nature of the phonological disorder in conduction aphasia. *Brain and Language, 23*, 97–115

Kugler, P.N., Kelso, J.A.S., & Turvey, M.T. (1980). On the concept of coordinative structures as dissipative structures: I. Theoretical lines of convergence. In: G.E. Stelmach (Ed.), *Tutorials in Motor Behavior* (pp. 1–47). Amsterdam: North Holland

La Pointe, L.L. (1969). *An Investigation of Isolated Oral Movements, Oral Motor Sequencing Abilities and Articulation of Brain Injured Adults.* Unpublished doctoral dissertation, University of Colorado

La Pointe, L.L. & Horner, J. (1976). Repeated trials of words by patients with neurogenic phonological selection-sequencing impairment (apraxia of speech). *Clinical Aphasiology, 6*, 261–277

La Pointe, L.L. & Johns, D.F. (1975). Some phonemic characteristics in apraxia of speech. *Journal of Communication Disorders, 8*, 259–269

Lebrun, Y., Buyssens, E., & Henneaux, J. (1973). Phonetic aspects of anarthria. *Cortex, 9*, 126–135.

Levelt, W.J.M. (1989). *Speaking: From Intention to Articulation.* Cambridge, MA: MIT Press

Levelt, W.J.M. (1999). Models of word production. *Trends in Cognitive Sciences, 3*, 223–232

Levelt, W.J.M., Roelofs, A., & Meyer, A.S. (1999). A theory of lexical access in speech production. *Behavioral and Brain Sciences, 22*, 1–75

Levelt, W.J.M. & Wheeldon, L. (1994). Do speakers have access to a mental syllabary? *Cognition, 50,* 239–269

Lieberman, A.M. & Studdert-Kennedy, M. (1978). Phonetic perception. In: R. Held, H. Leibowitz, & H.L. Teuber (Eds.), *Handbook of Sensory Physiology, Volume VII: Perception* (pp. 143–178), Heidelberg: Springer-Verlag

Liepmann, H. (1900). Das Krankheitsbild der apraxia (motorischen asymboli) auf Grund eines Falles von einseitiger apraxie. *Monatschrift fur Psychiatrie and Neurologie, 9,* 15–40

Liepmann, H. (1905). Die linke hemisphaere und das handeln. *Muchener Medizinische Wochenschift, 52,* 2322–2326, 2375–2378

Liepmann, H. (1913). Motor aphasia, anarthria and apraxia. Transactions of the 17th International Congress of Medicine, Section XI, Part II, 97–106

Liepmann, H. (1920). Apraxie. *Ergbenisse Der Ges. Medizin, 1,* 516–543. Reported in: Brown, J.W. (1972). *Aphasia, Apraxia and Agnosia.* Springfield: Charles C. Thomas

Luria, A.R. (1966). *Higher Cortical Functions in Man.* New York: Basic Books

Luria, A.R. (1970). *Traumatic Aphasia: Its Syndromes, Psychology and Treatment.* The Hague: Mouton

Maas, E., Robin, D.A., Ballard, K.J., Magnuson, C.E., & Wright, D.L. (2006). Speech motor programming in apraxia of speech: a reaction time approach. Paper presented at the Conference on Motor Speech, Austin, Texas

Marquardt, T.P. & Cannito, M. (1996). Treatment of verbal apraxia in Broca's aphasia. In: G.L. Wallace (Ed.), *Adult Aphasia Rehabilitation* (pp. 205–228). Boston: Butterworth-Heinemann

Marquardt, T.P. & Sussman, H. (1984). The elusive lesion—apraxia of speech link in Broca's aphasia. In: J.C. Rosenbek, M.R. McNeil, & A.E. Aronson (Eds.), *Apraxia of Speech: Physiology, Acoustics, Linguistics, Management* (pp. 91–112). San Diego: College Hill Press

Martin, A.D. (1974). Some objections to the term apraxia of speech. *Journal of Speech and Hearing Disorders, 39,* 53–64

Mateer, C. & Kimura, D. (1977). Impairment of nonverbal oral movements in aphasia. *Brain and Language, 4,* 262–276

McNeil, M.R. (1984). Current concepts in adult aphasia. *International Rehabilitation Medicine, 6,* 128–134

McNeil, M.R. & Adams, S. (1990). A comparison of speech kinematics among apraxic, conduction aphasic, ataxic dysarthric and normal geriatric speakers. *Clinical Aphasiology, 18,* 279–294

McNeil, M.R., Caliguiri, M., & Rosenbek, J.C. (1989). A comparison of labiomandibular kinematic durations, displacements, velocities and dysmetrias in apraxic and normal adults. *Clinical Aphasiology, 17,* 173–193

McNeil, M.R., Doyle, P.J., & Wambaugh, J. (2000). Apraxia of Speech: a treatable disorder of motor planning & programming. In: S.E. Nadeau, L.J. Gonzales Rothi, & B. Crosson (Eds.), *Aphasia and Language: Theory to Practice* (pp. 221–226). New York: Guilford

McNeil, M.R., Hashi, M., & Southwood, H. (1994). Acoustically derived perceptual evidence for coarticulatory errors in apraxic and conduction aphasic speech production. *Clinical Aphasiology, 22,* 203–218

McNeil, M.R. & Kent, R.D. (1990). Motoric characteristics of adult aphasic and apraxic speakers. In: G.E. Hammond (Ed.), *Cerebral Control of Speech and Limb Movements* (pp. 349–386). North-Holland: Elsevier Science Publishers

McNeil, M.R., Liss, J., Tseng, C.-H., & Kent, R.D. (1990). Effects of speech rate on the absolute and relative timing of apraxic and conduction aphasic sentence production. *Brain and Language, 38,* 135–158

McNeil, M.R., Odell, K.H., Miller, S.B., & Hunter, L. (1995). Consistency, variability, and target approximation for successive speech repetitions among apraxic, conduction aphasic and ataxic dysarthric speakers. *Clinical Aphasiology, 23,* 39–55

McNeil, M.R., Pratt, S.R., & Fossett, T.R.D. (2004). The differential diagnosis of apraxia of speech. In: B. Maassen, R.D. Kent, H.F.M. Peters, P.H.M.M. Van Lieshout, & W. Hulstijn (Eds.), *Speech Motor Control in Normal and Disordered Speech* (pp. 389–413). Oxford, UK: Oxford Medical Publications

McNeil, M.R., Robin, D.A., & Schmidt, R.A. (1997). Apraxia of speech: Definition, differentiation and treatment. In: M.R. McNeil (Ed.), *Clinical*

Management of Sensorimotor Speech Disorders (pp. 311–344). New York: Thieme

McNeil, M.R., Weismer, G., Adams, S., & Mulligan, M. (1990). Oral structure nonspeech motor control in normal, dysarthric, aphasic and apraxic speakers: Isometric force and static position control. *Journal of Speech and Hearing Research, 33,* 255–268

Mercaitis, P.A. (1983). *Some Temporal Characteristics of Imitative Speech in Non-Brain-Injured, Aphasic, and Apraxic Adults.* Unpublished doctoral dissertation, University of Massachusetts-Amherst

Meuse·S., Marquardt, T.P., & Cannito, M. (1996). Phonological analyses of apraxia of speech in individuals with Brocas Aphasia. Paper presented at the Motor Speech Conference, Amelia Island, FL

Miller, N. (1986). *Dyspraxia and Its Management.* Rockville, MD: Aspen

Moore, W.M. (1975). *Assessment of Oral, Nonverbal Gestures in Normal and Selected Brain-Injured Sample Populations.* Unpublished doctoral dissertation, University of Colorado

Odell, K.H. (2002). Considerations in target selection in apraxia of speech treatment. *Seminars in Speech and Language: Apraxia of speech: From Concept to Clinic, 4,* 309–323

Odell, K., McNeil, M.R., Rosenbek, J.C., & Hunter, L. (1990). Perceptual characteristics of consonant productions by apraxic speakers. *Journal of Speech and Hearing Disorders, 55,* 345–359

Odell, K., McNeil, M.R., Rosenbek, J.C., & Hunter, L. (1991a). Perceptual characteristics of vowel and prosody production in apraxic, aphasic, and dysarthric speakers. *Journal of Speech and Hearing Research, 34,* 67–80

Odell, K., McNeil, M.R., Rosenbek, J.C., & Hunter, L. (1991b). A perceptual comparison of prosodic features in apraxia of speech and conduction aphasia. *Clinical Aphasiology, 19,* 295–306

Ogar, J., Willock, S., Baldo, J., Wilkins, D., Ludy, C., & Dronkers, N. (2006). Clinical and anatomical correlates of apraxia of speech. *Brain and Language, 97,* 343–350

Ojemann, G. & Mateer, C. (1979). Human language cortex: Localization of memory, syntax and sequential motor-phoneme identification systems. *Science, 205,* 1401–1403

Palmer, J.M. & Yantis, P.A. (1990). *Survey of Communication Disorders.* Baltimore: Williams & Wilkins

Pierce, R.S. (1991). Apraxia of speech versus phonemic paraphasia: Theoretical, diagnostic, and treatment considerations. In D. Vogel & M.P. Cannito (Eds.), *Treating Disorders Speech Motor Control: For Clinicians by Clinicians* (pp. 185–216). Austin: Pro-Ed

Poeck, K. & Kerschensteiner, M. (1975). Analysis of the sequential motor events in oral apraxia. In: K.J. Zulch, O. Creutzfeldt, & G.C. Galbraith (Eds.), *Cerebral Localization* (pp. 98–109). Berlin: Springer-Verlag

Poizner, H., Clark, M.A., Merians, A.S., Macauley, B., Rothi, L.J., & Heilman, K.M. (1995). Joint coordination deficits in limb apraxia. *Brain, 118,* 227–242

Poizner, H., Mack, L., Verfaellie, M. Rothi, L.J., & Heilman, K.M. (1990). Three dimensional computer graphic analysis of apraxia. *Brain, 113,* 85–101

Riecker, A., Ackermann, H., Wildgruber, D., Meyer, J., Dogil, G., Haider, H., & Grodd, W. (2000). Articulatory/phonetic sequencing at the level of the anterior perisylvian cortex: a functional magnetic resonance imaging (fMRI) study. *Brain and Language, 75,* 259–276

Robin, D.A., Bean, C., & Folkins, J.W. (1989). Lip Movement in Apraxia of Speech. *Journal of Speech and Hearing Research, 32,* 512–523

Robin, D.A., Jacks, A., & Ramage, A.E. (in press). The neural substrates of apraxia of speech as uncovered by brain imaging: a critical review. In: R. Ingham (Ed.), *Neuroimaging in Communication Disorders and Sciences.* San Diego: Plural Publishing

Roelofs, A. (1997). The WEAVER model of word-form encoding in speech production. *Cognition, 64,* 249–284

Rosenbek, J.C. & Jones, H. (2007). Principles of treatment for sensorimotor speech disorders. In: M.R. McNeil (Ed.), *Clinical Management of Sensorimotor Speech Disorders,* 2nd ed. New York: Thieme

Rosenbek, J.C., Kent, R.D., & LaPointe, L.L. (1984). Apraxia of speech: an overview and some perspectives. In: J.C. Rosenbek, M.R. McNeil & A.E.

Aronson (Eds.) *Apraxia of Speech: Physiology, Acoustics, Linguistics, Management* (pp. 1–72). San Diego: College Hill Press

Rosenbek, J.C. & McNeil, M.R. (1991). A discussion of classification in motor speech disorders: dysarthria and apraxia of speech. In: C.A. Moore, K.M. Yorkston, & D.R. Beukelman, (Eds.), *Dysarthria and Apraxia of Speech: Perspectives on Management* (pp. 289–295). Baltimore: Paul H. Brookes

Rosenbek, J.C., Wertz, R.T., & Darley, F.L. (1973). Oral sensation and perception in apraxia of speech and aphasia. *Journal of Speech and Hearing Research, 16,* 22–36

Rothi, L.J. & Heilman, K. (1985). Ideomotor apraxia: gestural discrimination, comprehension and memory. In: E.A. Roy (Ed.), Neuropsychological Studies of Apraxia and Related Disorders (pp. 65–74). North Holland: Elsevier Science Publishers

Roy, E.A. & Square, P.A. (1985). Common considerations in the study of limb, verbal, and oral apraxia. In: E.A. Roy (Ed.), *Neuropsychological Studies of Apraxia and Related Disorders* (pp. 111–162). North Holland: Elsevier Science Publishers

Ryalls, J.H. (1981). Motor aphasia: acoustic correlates of phonetic disintegration in vowels. *Neuropsychologia, 19,* 365–374

Ryalls, J.H. (1982). Intonation in Broca's aphasia. *Neuropsychologia, 20,* 355–360

Ryalls, J.H. (1984). Some acoustic aspects of fundamental frequency of CVC utterances in aphasia. *Phonetica, 41,* 103–111

Ryalls, J.H. (1986). An acoustic study of vowel production in aphasia. *Brain and Language, 29,* 48–67

Ryalls, J.H. (1987). Vowel production in aphasia: towards an account of the consonant-vowel dissociation. In: J.H. Ryalls (Ed.), *Phonetic Approaches to Speech Production in Aphasia and Related Disorders,* (pp. 23–44). Boston: College-Hill Press

Sasanuma, S. (1971). Speech characteristics of a patient with apraxia of speech. *Research in Logopaedics and Phoniatrics, 5,* 85–89

Schmidt, R.A. & Lee, T.D. (2005). *Motor Control and Learning: A Behavioral Emphasis,* 4th ed. Champaign: Human Kinetics

Seddoh, S.A., Robin, D.A., Sim, H-S., Hageman, C., Moon, J.B., & Folkins, J.W. (1996). Speech timing in apraxia of speech versus conduction aphasia. *Journal of Speech and Hearing Research, 39,* 590–603

Shankweiler, D., Harris, K.S., & Taylor, M.L. (1968). Electromyographic studies of articulation in aphasia. *Archives of Physical Medicine and Rehabilitation, 49,* 1–8

Shattuck-Hufnagel, S. (1979). Speech errors as evidence for serial order mechanism in sentence production. In: W.E. Cooper & E.C.T. Walker (Eds.), *Sentence Processing: Psycholinguistic Studies Presented to Merrill Garrett* (pp. 295–242). Hillsdale, NJ: Lawrence Erlbaum Associates

Shattuck-Hufnagel, S. (1987). The role of word onset consonants in speech production planning: new evidence from speech error patterns. In: E. Keller & M. Gopnik (Eds.), *Motor and Sensory Processing in Language* (pp. 17–51). Hillsdale, NJ: Lawrence Erlbaum Associates

Shewan, C.M., Leeper, H.A., & Booth, J.C. (1984). An analysis of voice onset time (VOT) in aphasic and normal subjects. In: J.C. Rosenbek, M.R. McNeil, & A.E. Aronson (Eds.), *Apraxia of Speech: Physiology, Acoustics, Linguistics, Management* (pp. 197–220). San Diego: College-Hill Press

Solomon, N.P. & Robin, D.A. (2005). Perceptions of effort during handgrip and tongue elevation in Parkinson's disease. *Parkinsonism and Related Disorders, 11,* 353–361

Solomon, N.P., Robin, D.A., Luschei, E.S. (1994). Strength, endurance and sense of effort: studies of the tongue and hand in people with Parkinson's disease and accompanying dysarthria. Paper presented at the Motor Speech Conference, Sedona, AZ

Solomon, N.P., Robin, D.A., Mitchinson, S.I., VanDaele, D.J., & Luschei, E.S. (1996). Sense of effort and the effects of fatigue in the tongue and hand. *Journal of Speech and Hearing Research, 39,* 114–125

Somodi, L.B., Robin, D.A., & Luschei, E.S. (1995). A model of sense of effort during maximal and submaximal contractions of the tongue. *Brain and Language, 51,* 371–382

Square, P.A. (1989). *Acquired Apraxia of Speech in Aphasic Adults.* London: Taylor & Francis

Square, P.A. (1996). Apraxia of Speech Reconsidered. In: F. Bell-Berti, & L. J. Raphael (Eds.), *Producing Speech: Contemporary Issues for Katherine Safford Harris* (pp. 375–386). New York: AIP Press

Square, P.A., Darley, F.L., & Sommers, R.I. (1982). An analysis of the productive errors made by pure apractic speakers with differing loci of lesions. *Clinical Aphasiology, 10,* 245–250

Square, P.A. & Martin, R.E. (1994). The nature and treatment of neuromotor speech disorders in aphasia. In: R. Chapey (Ed.), *Language Intervention Strategies in Adult Aphasia,* 3rd ed. (pp. 467–499). Baltimore: Williams & Wilkins

Square-Storer, P.A. & Roy, E.A. (1990). The dissociation of aphasia from apraxia of speech, ideomotor limb, and buccofacial apraxia. In: G.E. Hammond (Ed.), *Cerebral Control of Speech and Limb Movements* (pp. 477–502). North-Holland: Elsevier Science Publishers

Square-Storer, P.A., Roy, E.A., & Hogg, S.C. (1990). The dissociation of aphasia from apraxia of speech, ideomotor limb, and buccofacial apraxia. In: G.E. Hammond (Ed.), *Cerebral Control of Speech and Limb Movements* (pp. 451–476). North-Holland: Elsevier Science Publishers

Square-Storer, P.A., Roy, E.A., & Martin, R.E. (1997). Apraxia of speech: another form of praxis disruption. In: L.J.G. Rothi & K.M. Heilman (Eds.), *Apraxia: The Neuropsychology of Action* (pp. 173–206). Hove, England: Psychology Press

Strand, E.A. (1987). *Acoustic and Response Time Measures in Utterance Production: A Comparison of Apraxic and Normal Speakers.* Unpublished doctoral dissertation, University of Wisconsin-Madison

Strand, E.A. & McNeil, M.R. (1996). Effects of length and linguistic complexity on temporal acoustic measures in apraxia of speech. *Journal of Speech and Hearing Research, 39,* 1018–1033

Trost, J.E. & Canter, G.J. (1974). Apraxia of speech in patients with Broca's aphasia: a study of phoneme production accuracy and error patterns. *Brain and Language, 1,* 65–79

Tuller, B. (1984). On categorizing aphasic speech errors. *Neuropsychologia, 22,* 547–557

Tuller, B. & Story, R.S. (1987). Anticipatory coarticulation in aphasia. In: J.H. Ryalls (Ed.), *Phonetic Approaches to Speech Production in Aphasia and Related Disorders* (pp. 243–260). Boston: College-Hill Press

Van der Merwe, A. (2007). A theoretical framework for the characterization of pathological speech sensorimotor control. In: M.R. McNeil (Ed.), *Clinical Management of Sensorimotor Speech Disorders,* 2nd ed. New York: Thieme Medical Publishers

Wambaugh, J.L. (2002). A summary of treatments for apraxia of speech and review of replicated approaches. *Seminars in Speech and Language: Apraxia of Speech: From Concept to Clinic, 23,* 293–308

Wambaugh, J.L. & Doyle, P.J. (1995). Treatment for acquired apraxia of speech: a review of efficacy reports. *Clinical Aphasiology, 22,* 231–243

Wambaugh, J.L., Duffy, J.R., McNeil, M.R., Robin, D.A., & Rogers, M.A. (2006a). Treatment 2006 guidelines for acquired apraxia of speech: a synthesis and evaluation of the evidence. *Journal of Medical Speech Language Pathology, 14,* 15–32

Wambaugh, J.L., Duffy, J.R., McNeil, M.R., Robin, D.A., & Rogers, M.A. (2006b). Treatment guidelines for acquired apraxia of speech: treatment descriptions and recommendations. *Journal of Medical Speech Language Pathology, 14,* 25–67

Weismer, G. & Liss, J.M. (1991). Reductionism is a dead-end in speech research: perspectives on a new direction. In: C. Moore, K.M. Yorkston, D.R. Beukelman (Eds.), *Dysarthria and Apraxia of Speech: Perspectives on Management* (pp. 15–27). Baltimore: Paul H. Brookes

Wertz, R.T., LaPointe, L.L., & Rosenbek, J.C. (1984). *Apraxia of Speech in Adults: The Disorders and Its Management.* Orlando: Grune & Stratton

Ziegler, W. & von Cramon, D. (1985). Anticipatory coarticulation in a patient with apraxia of speech. *Brain and Language, 26,* 117–130

Chapter 16

Principles of Treatment for Sensorimotor Speech Disorders

John C. Rosenbek and Harrison N. Jones

Ramsey (1970) reminds us "that no man is good enough to cure another without his consent" (p. 7). This then becomes our first principle of treatment of sensorimotor speech disorders. The adult or child with one of these conditions must give permission for treatment. Without permission, nothing, or nothing of value, is possible even from the finest clinician. However, once that permission is granted, other principles come to bear. Fortunately for clinicians relishing ambiguity, unfortunately for those needing uniformity, no single set of principles dominates the treatment landscape. Instead, principles are nearly as numerous as clinicians and their origins as variable. This chapter develops a manageable number of such principles, given the restrictions of a chapter's length and the writers' orientations regarding the overarching goal of treatment. That goal is to achieve the best possible creation or restitution of communication and the communicator's functional performance and quality of life. This goal is addressed by modifying central neural mechanisms, peripheral mechanisms, and performance whenever possible, and by supporting existing mechanisms and performance when change is, or becomes, impossible. That goal is admittedly ambitious; however, nothing less than great ambition will serve either rehabilitationists or their patients.

This chapter also identifies and describes a tendentious list of origins for the treatment principles. The following origins serve as a convenient framework for organizing principles and as a guide to understanding how treatments have evolved over the years:

1. The medical condition(s) causing the sensorimotor speech disorder

2. The signs, functional components, and pathophysiology of the speech deficit

3. Evidence-based practice

4. Models of disablement

5. Knowledge about motor skill learning

6. Knowledge about neuroplasticity

7. Knowledge about muscle plasticity

No claim of superiority of this set of origins over any other is made; rather, this list merely offers the authors a comfortable organization. Nor does the order or length of their discussion suggest relative importance. Successful practice depends on them all, or so it seems to us, and length was determined primarily by their relative newness as influences on treatment.

◆ Medical Condition

Sensorimotor speech disorders most frequently result from disease in adults and from congenital conditions in infants and children. These etiologies and their signs, severity, and medical or surgical managements all generate principles of speech treatment.

Principle: Treatment Decisions Must Take into Account the Full Range of Each Patient's Deficits

The panoply of conditions causing sensorimotor speech disorders typically affects other body systems and functions as well. The resulting signs, such as general weakness or other movement abnormality, fatigue, sensory deficit, cognitive impairment, depression, impaired attention, and the rest must be accommodated in treatment planning. For example, a depressed person may have difficulty practicing between sessions. Cognitive impairment, depending on severity, may require a simpler treatment approach than would be possible with a cognitively intact person. Regardless of the specifics, however, the principle is that expectations, procedures, schedules, and methods must be selected only after considering each patient's total condition.

Principle: Treatment, When Possible, Should Be Interdisciplinary

Interdisciplinary treatment is a legitimate aim for a variety of reasons. Some are prosaic. For example, it is traditional to offer interdisciplinary services to people with multiple handicaps, especially children. The fact of the multiple handicaps and the opportunity for clinicians to reinforce one another's procedures are often cited reasons for this approach. The usual rehabilitation team comprises professionals from physical therapy, occupational therapy, and speech-language pathology. Another reason for interdisciplinary rehabilitation is that the better conditioning and enhanced activity resulting from physical and occupational therapy may well improve cognitive performance. Equally interesting is the possibility that improved cognition can influence motor performance. This last is evidence not so much of the need for interdisciplinary treatment as it is of the need for treatments whose emphasis extends beyond movement. Of course, interdisciplinary care requires the involvement of multiple other disciples, including professionals from medicine and surgery, nursing, neuropsychiatry, rehabilitation counseling, social work, dietetics, and many more. Even administrators and politicians may need to be involved for truly interdisciplinary services. The likelihood of positive patient outcomes will be enhanced with interdisciplinary planning and execution.

Principle: Response to Treatment May Be the Best Predictor of Treatment Outcome

In decades past, physicians were reluctant to refer patients with progressive disease to rehabilitationists because of a bias that nothing could be done. Patients with stroke or other conditions in which spontaneous improvement was expected were often not referred because of the mindset that nothing needed to be done to promote recovery. These attitudes are now pleasantly old-fashioned. Speech signs in degenerative disease can sometimes be eliminated or slowed, or, if severe, can be accommodated by alternative or augmentative communication (Beukelman & Mirenda, 1998). Furthermore, spontaneous recovery is often incomplete and the residual deficits warrant treatment, and even complete recovery can be hastened by intelligent rehabilitation. Regardless of a disease's course or severity, the best determinant of whether any patient can be helped is to measure response to treatment. This requires careful baseline measurement and frequent probing to assess benefit. Some patients, unfortunately, cannot be helped, and clinicians are duty-bound to recognize them and act accordingly. Discharge is disheartening but necessary. However, most patients can be helped and they will demonstrate this potential by their response to appropriate therapy.

♦ Signs, Functional Components, and Pathophysiology

Speech is the product of a complex set of muscle activities and structural movements. Clinicians, to plan treatment, simplify this complexity. One method for doing so is to cluster the muscles and structures into what have come to be known as the functional components of the speech mechanism (Netsell, 1981). The respiratory mechanism, larynx, velopharynx, and orofacial mechanism are the traditional components. Added to the list is prosody in reference to features of intonation, rhythm, and stress resulting from the coordinated activity of all components. There is a certain magic to this list because nearly all dimensions of a dysarthric speech impairment result from the interaction of structures, but the magic can serve clinicians. It allows

them to listen to abnormal speech and create hypotheses about the structure(s) involved. For example, dysphonia implicates the larynx, as does hypernasality the velopharynx. Articulatory imprecision implicates the orofacial mechanism or one or more of its subcomponents (e.g., the lips, jaw, tongue tip, or back of the tongue). Exceptions abound, of course, as when velopharyngeal inadequacy causes consonant imprecision. Nonetheless, clinicians need systems for organizing the often-extensive array of signs in the speech of a speaker with a sensorimotor speech deficit as an early step in treatment planning.

Final selection of a treatment methodology, however, is influenced by other factors, including the underlying pathophysiology. Creating a hypothesis about the pathophysiology underlying the signs also involves a bit of magic. Traditionally, signs were thought to result from weakness, abnormal tone, discoordination, abnormal timing, tremor, or dystonia for the dysarthrias and from programming/planning failure for apraxia of speech (AOS). The primary origins of these hypotheses are the Darley, Aronson, and Brown (1969a,b) publications, and despite the passage of time, most such hypotheses remain untested. Nonetheless, they are useful, when combined with a cataloging of signs and assumptions about contributions of the functional components alone or in combinations, as a framework for some critical treatment principles.

Principle: Catalog the Signs and Relate Them as Closely as Possible to the Functional Components or the Interaction of the Components of the Speech Mechanism

Eliciting the history and careful listening to connected speech and to the results of special procedures, such as speaking with nostrils occluded or with a bite block in place, are the first steps in the evaluation of each patient's impairment. Connected speech is important, of course, because it is the target of treatment. Furthermore, signs, especially of abnormal prosody, appear almost exclusively in connected speech. Special tests are important to clarify the contributions of the functional components to the overall impairment. For example, without special manipulations like providing manual support to the respiratory system, it may be difficult or impossible to know for sure if the respiratory mechanism is making a major contribution to inadequate loudness.

Principle: Establish a Hypothesized Relationship among Signs, Functional Components, and Underlying Pathophysiology

A hypothetical example may serve to illustrate the principle of combining signs, functional components, and underlying pathophysiology. Testing of a patient with traumatic brain injury reveals an inadequately loud voice, reduced range of loudness on both maximum performance testing and in connected speech, and the use of short phrases. Providing manual support to the respiratory system results in increased loudness, a finding in support of the interpretation that a major component of this person's dysarthria is reduced respiratory drive. Performance on the Hixon and Hoit respiratory testing protocol (Hixon & Hoit, 1998, 1999) suggests more specifically that the reduced respiratory drive is caused by abdominal muscle weakness.

This idealized example is admittedly much neater than nature usually provides. However, even when facing one of nature's challenges created by disease, relating the signs to the functional components and to their interactions can be relatively easy for the experienced clinician. On the other hand, confirming or even hypothesizing the underlying pathophysiology is fiendishly difficult. Nonetheless, establishing these relationships, even hypothetically, aids treatment planning, as is suggested in the next principle.

Principle: When Possible, Treatment Should Target the Underlying Pathophysiology

This principle has been advocated over the years (Abbs & Rosenbek, 1985; Murdoch, Thompson, & Theodoros, 1997) and it has a certain heuristic appeal. When weakness is the underlying pathophysiology, muscle strengthening approaches such as inspiratory and expiratory muscle strength training (Sapienza, Brown, Davenport, & Martin, 1999), continuous positive airway pressure (CPAP) training (Kuehn & Wachtel, 1994), and other strengthening programs may be appropriate. Impaired timing and discoordination, such as occurs in the majority of dysarthria types and in AOS, can also be treated, as is evident in the other chapters of this volume. Other targets of speech treatment, spasticity for example, may be more troublesome, although progress is being made.

This principle is easily misinterpreted as supporting the therapeutic use of nonspeech drills. Indeed, respiratory muscle strength training may be one of only a few treatment approaches in which nonspeech activity can be justified, and only then if it is part of a treatment package to transfer improved strength to louder, more prosodic speech. In addition, several conditions such as spasticity, dyskinesia, and even hypokinesia are task specific, and non-speech manipulation of these conditions would seem to make little sense. Equally nonsensical is to treat the discoordination and impaired timing of AOS, ataxic, hyper- and hypokinetic dysarthria with nonspeech drill. This is not to say that nonspeech drills are incapable of altering nervous system states. However, these alterations will be task specific. Practice wagging your tongue and this skill will improve and the brain's circuitry may even be altered, but speech will be uninfluenced.

Given the tortuousness of this principle, why include it? We think there are several reasons. First, Yorkston's (1996) appeal for treatments specific to the various dysarthric types is most likely to be successful if underlying pathophysiology, rather than signs or functional components, are at least one of the therapeutic targets. This is true because the various dysarthric types, with the possible exception of some flaccid dysarthrias, are soft syndromes, which is to say they share multiple signs or features (Rosenbek & McNeil, 1991). Pathophysiology is somewhat more likely to be unique. Second, treatment needs to be efficient. Treating the underlying pathophysiology, especially if it influences several functional components, has time-saving potential.

Third, treatments of pathophysiology, even if they are unsuccessful, can inform scientists about the nature of speech control in normal and abnormal speakers.

Principle: If Treating the Pathophysiology Is Unsuccessful or Impossible, Treatment Can Be Directed Toward One or More Functional Components According to Their Relative Contribution to the Disturbed Speech Signal

The involvement of multiple functional components is the norm in sensorimotor speech disorders, except occasionally in flaccid dysarthria. Nonetheless, their relative contribution to the disturbed speech signal can often be established. For example, if respiratory drive is seriously compromised, speech will be impaired despite the relative integrity of other components. If other functional components are also involved, reduced respiratory drive may further complicate their function. Therefore, the respiratory mechanism is often the proper first target. Similar hierarchies can sometimes occur for all the other functional components as well. The decision is least complicated when a single component is involved. An isolated velopharyngeal inadequacy is an obvious treatment target. In the special case of AOS, it is the orofacial mechanism combined with the articulatory functions of the velopharynx and larynx that are to be targeted. Even in those numerous cases with disrupted timing and coordination of multiple components, attention to one component early on in treatment may be justified. For example, stabilizing the jaw with a bite block may make coordination of the other components easier. More frequently, however, treatments aimed simultaneously at multiple components are most efficient. This may be the explanation for the generalized effects of the Lee Silverman Voice Treatment (LSVT) (Ramig, Countryman, Thompson, & Horii, 1995), delayed auditory feedback (DAF), (Brendel, Lowit, & Howell, 2004), and other systemic treatments.

Principle: Treatment Does Not End and Sometimes Does Not Start with Signs, Functional Components, and Pathophysiology

Thus far we have taken a traditional medical model–oriented approach to principle development. Different, but ultimately complementary, treatment planning decisions arise from a psychosocial approach to sensorimotor speech disorders. Thus, the final principle in this section moves beyond signs, functional components, and pathophysiology. Indeed the next principle may need to be addressed first with some speakers.

Sensorimotor speech disorders are not solely mechanical disorders. At minimum, they are disorders of the person, and, more ambitiously, and with few exceptions, they are disorders of communication among people. Methods to address function in context, including multiple environments, communication partners, and conditions of interference and stress, are required. Nor can the speaker's quality of life be ignored. A later section (see Models of Disablement) extends this principle, but first it is necessary to survey the influence of evidence on the principles of treatment.

◆ Evidence-Based Practice

Sackett and colleagues (1998) define evidence-based practice (EBP) as the "conscientious, explicit and judicious use of current best evidence in making decisions about the care of individual patients" (Sackett, Richardson, Rosenberg, & Hayes, 1998, p. 2). Evidence is important in rehabilitation for several reasons. Medawar (1979) provides the first with his warning about a "conspiracy of goodwill" (p. 50) among clinicians, growing from their need to make things better for the persons they treat. For Medawar, the defense is the randomized clinical trial, the cornerstone of EBP. Dobkin (2003) says EBP has allowed clinicians to become "less defensive about their practices" (p. vii) and has prepared them to contribute to the emerging efforts to "draw upon the data from neuroscience and engineering to harness the physiology of the nervous system and to modulate its function after injury" (p. vii). For us, the evidence has a profound influence on clinician confidence; the better the evidence, the greater the confidence.

Despite these virtues, EBP is sometimes opposed because of concerns that it threatens clinician autonomy. Sackett and colleagues (1998) are careful to stress that EBP "builds on and reinforces, but never replaces, clinical skills, clinical judgment and clinical experience" (p. 5). They recognize that data are no more a blueprint for practice than are stones a house. Data, like stones, must be ordered and placed. In practice, clinicians use their experience as a guide to that critical work. Overlooking experience in the definition of EBP can have negative consequences for practitioners. Indeed, one's experience with particular groups of patients and particular types and severities of sensorimotor speech disorders may sometimes form the best foundation for treatment decisions about a particular patient or patient group.

Despite the intelligent blending of data, experience, and insight, it is important not to reify EBP. Cohen, Stavri, and Hersh (2004) identify missing components in the EBP approach to planning health care. These include their opinion that data, including quantitative data and data from what Berwick (1996) calls real-time science, are often excluded. This chapter's length prohibits a discussion of qualitative research but Damico and Simmons-Mackie (2003) provide an introduction for the speech-language pathologist (SLP). So-called real-time science is easier. This occurs when practitioners form themselves into groups, agree to perform a procedure in generally the same way, systematically exchange personal experiences, and modify the procedure accordingly. Cohen and colleagues (2004) also identify the loss of individual participant response

in group data as another shortcoming of EBP, and argue that evidence of better care because of EBP's emergence is in short supply. Discussion of EBP's limitations is introduced here only as a reminder to clinicians that the principles of treatment derived from EBP, despite the popularity of the notion, are not necessarily what one might predict and are no more important than principles arising elsewhere.

Principle: Clinical Practice Should Be Based on a Synthesis of the Best Available Evidence from Systematic Research and Clinical Expertise

Speech-language pathology has embraced EBP. Reviews of the evidence in dysarthria (Yorkston, 1996; Yorkston, Spencer, & Duffy, 2003) and AOS (Wambaugh, 2002) are good sources of the data. This principle derives from the obvious limits to the strength of evidence in support of most treatments and contains an important distinction: the difference between the best data *possible* and the best data *available*. A fuller appreciation of this distinction requires knowledge of systems for categorizing the available evidence for a given treatment.

Levels of evidence scales allow clinicians to calculate the strength of treatment data for a given approach, and therefore the confidence (when combined with their own experience) they can have in the methods they employ. Multiple systems for establishing evidence exist, including that developed by the American Academy of Neurology (1994). One that works especially well for the literature in sensorimotor speech disorders is derived from Moore, McQuay, and Gray (1995) and appears in **Table 16–1.**

Classifying literature according to this or any other scheme can be daunting to the uninitiated. For example, the notion of trials without randomization may seem a clumsy description. For guidance in learning about such study designs, Shadish, Cook, and Campbell (2002) are an invaluable source. The purpose of the table's inclusion is to reassure clinicians that data come in a variety of forms and that even expert opinion and uncontrolled descriptive studies of a clinician's experience of treating a case contribute to the evidence.

Principle: Treatment Should Be Organized So that Each Patient's Response Contributes to the Next Patient's Care

Clinicians are responsible for organizing each treatment session so they learn as much as or more than the patient does. This requires beginning treatment planning with a hypothesis about what will work for a particular speaker, measuring

Table 16–1   Type and Strength of Evidence Scale

Level	Description
I	Strong evidence from at least one systematic review of multiple well-designed randomized controlled trials
II	Strong evidence from at least one properly designed randomized controlled trial of appropriate size
III	Evidence from well-designed trials without randomization, single group pre-post, cohort, time series, or matched case-controlled studies
IV	Evidence from well-designed nonexperimental studies from more than one center or research group
V	Opinions of respected authorities based on clinical evidence, descriptive studies, or reports of expert committees

Source: Moore, A., McQuay, H., & Gray, J. A. M. (Eds.) (1995). Evidence-based everything. *Bandolier, 12,* 1, with permission.

performance before initiating therapy, treating systematically, measuring performance during and after treatment, and then reassessing one's hypotheses and methods. Such steps, with the possible exception of beginning with a hypothesis, are not incompatible with third-party payer requirements. As a result, every clinician potentially can contribute to the evidence without influencing reimbursement.

◆ Models of Disablement

Jette (1994) defines disability as "the various impact(s) of chronic and acute conditions on the functioning of specific body systems, on basic human performance, and on people's functioning in necessary, usual, expected, and personally desired roles in society" (p. 380). This definition clearly emphasizes the complexity of disability and implies the challenges of its evaluation and treatment. To simplify the complexity and provide guidance, several models of disability have been developed. Nagi (1965) pioneered an early model of disablement that was later refined by numerous other authors, including Verbugge and Jette (1994). The World Health Organization (WHO) also developed a model of disability known most recently as the International Classification of Functioning, Disability, and Health (ICF) (WHO, 2001). Pope and Tarlow introduced the original Institute of Medicine (IOM) model in 1991. The core of all such models is a set of domains. For example, the original IOM model comprised four domains: pathology, impairment, functional limitation, and disability (Pope & Tarlow, 1991). Yorkston, Beukelman, Strand, and Bell (1999) operationally defined these domains for sensorimotor speech disorders, and their discussion deserves to be read in the original. Impairment, for example, is defined by these authors as "slow, weak, imprecise, and/or uncoordinated movements of the speech musculature or inability to plan sequence of speech movements" (p. 16), and is manifested as signs of respiratory, velopharyngeal, laryngeal, or orofacial mechanism involvement. Perceptually, reduced loudness, dysphonia, hypernasality, and consonant imprecision, are all evidence of impairment. The principles included in this section derive from the IOM's revised model of disablement, the IOM-2 (Brandt and Pope, 1997). In our view, this model provides an especially powerful context for management of sensorimotor speech disorders. This model identifies four domains—no disabling condition, pathology, impairment, and functional limitation—as "inherent" to the individual. Disability, however, is seen not as a domain at all, but as the interaction of the disabled person and the environment.

Figure 16–1 is a representation of what Brandt and Pope (1997) call the enabling-disabling process. As can be seen,

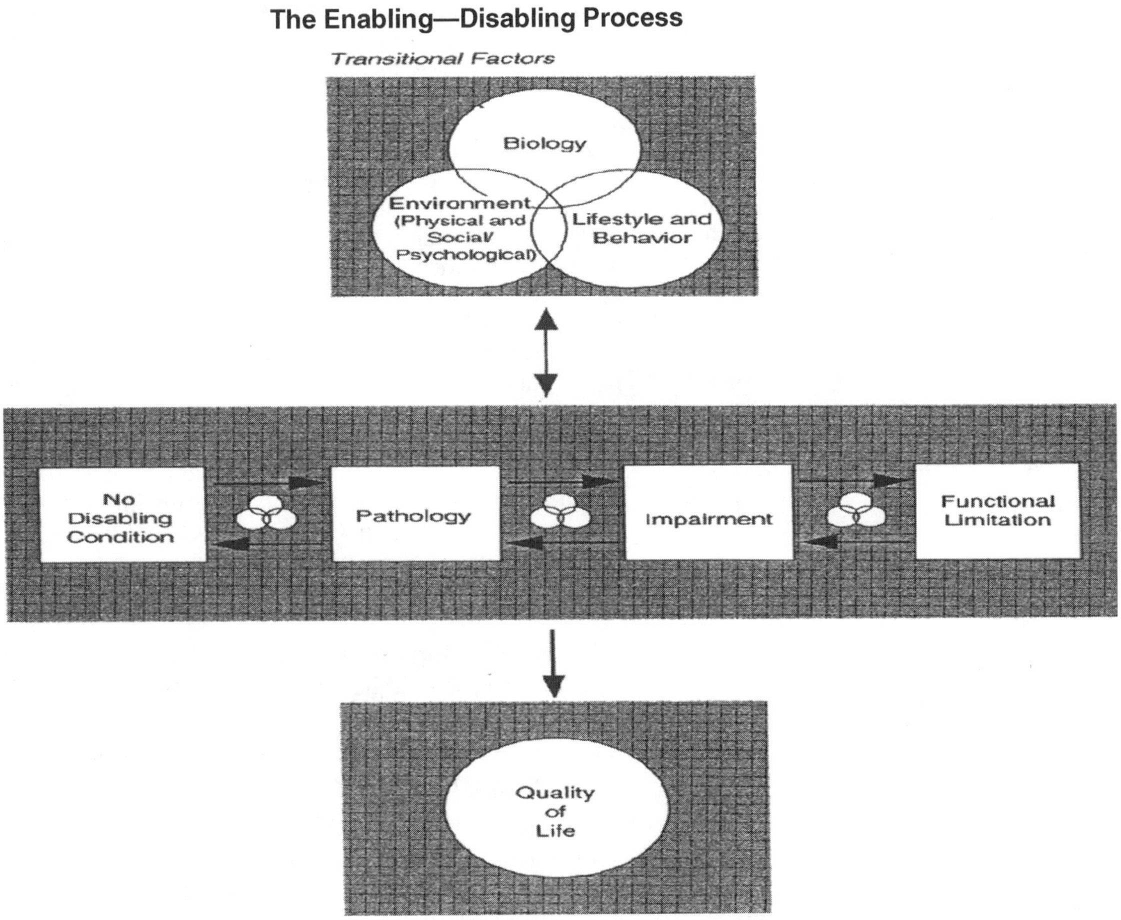

Figure 16–1 Institute of Medicine (IOM-2) model of the enabling-disabling process. [From Brandt, E.N. & Pope, A.M. (Eds.). (1997). *Enabling America: Assessing the Role of Rehabilitation Science and Engineering*. Washington, DC: National Academy Press, with permission.]

boxes represent the domains. The bidirectional arrows between boxes signal the interaction of the domains and the potential influence of disease as portrayed by the left to right arrows, and of rehabilitation by the right to left arrows. Transitional factors that hinder or facilitate movement across the model are also included. Biology (such as age), lifestyle, behavior (such as smoking and overeating), and the environment (again) are the transitional factors. Finally, the concept of quality of life that can be altered by the disabling condition is added. This model serves as a foundation for the following treatment principles.

Principle: Evaluation Requires the Best Possible Assessment of Each Individual's Pre- and Posttreatment Status across the Domains and in Quality of Life

This principle imposes several requirements on the profession and its practitioners. The first is that clinicians have available a repertoire of measurement tools. Speech-language pathology's repertoire for the evaluation of sensorimotor speech disorders has always been relatively long on impairment level measurement approaches. Most grew from Darley, Aronson, and Brown's seminal work (1969a,b). As a result, most approaches are perceptual, requiring the clinician to elicit motor performance, including speech, which the clinician then evaluates. Best possible assessment of impairment also requires acoustic and kinematic measurement (Kent, Weismer, Kent, Vorperian, & Duffy, 1999). Unfortunately, such assessments are in short supply, a condition that must change. Intelligibility, a functional limitation domain measure (Yorkston et al, 1999), is being assessed with increasing sophistication (Kent, 1992). Naturalness, another measure from the functional limitations domain, is more difficult to define and measure, but here, too, progress is occurring (Worrall and Frattali, 2000). Communicative effectiveness, measured by the Communicative Effectiveness Survey (CES) from Donovan and colleagues (2007), is another strategy to assess the domain of functional limitations. Quality of life measurement lags far behind all other measurement. This is unfortunate and must be addressed. As Fleming and DeMets (1996) remind us, the goal of rehabilitation is to change those conditions that are of greatest importance to the person, not those that the clinician thinks are most important or are easiest to measure and treat. Furthermore, speech scientists need to continue providing insights into pathology, especially at the cellular and muscle fiber levels. Speech clinicians, after all, are trainers of cells and fibers, at least in part.

Principle: Collect and Employ the Best Available Data on Each Person's Transitional Factors

Most SLPs take histories more with an eye to understanding what happened to a patient and when, rather than to revealing targets and influences on treatment. Biology, lifestyle and behavior, and the physical, social, and psychological environments have significance beyond history, however. They influence both the disabling (because of disease) and enabling (because of treatment or natural recovery) processes. For example, people with multiple medical diagnoses, because of their genetic inheritance and lifestyle choices, may be more prone to illness, suffer more debilitating and

general effects of that illness, and be less able to respond to treatment. Some of these data, such as age, and other risk factors such as obesity, depression, absence of transportation, and limited financial resources will be easy to obtain from the patient interview and medical record. Others, such as the motivation to participate in treatment, the safety of their environment, and the severity of coexisting illnesses may be more difficult. Nonetheless, time spent tracking down the data is time well spent, as the data influence prognosis and treatment planning and execution.

Principle: Both Persons with the Sensorimotor Speech Disorder and Their Environment Are Potentially Important Therapeutic Targets

None of us, whether well or sick, exists independent of our personal and physical environments. Therefore, treatment planning can profitably consider both. Ideally, clinicians want their therapeutic efforts to be so successful that any patient can exist anywhere. Experience teaches us that expectation's folly. A newer, more powerful idealism is to expect that we can alter human behavior and the environmental influences on that behavior. Foolishly ambitious? Perhaps. Equally foolish, however, is assuming that a clinical treatment focused only on impairment will achieve anything valuable or enduring.

Principle: Treatment Should First Be Targeted at the Domains of Impairment and Functional Limitations If the Clinician Has Reasonable Confidence Improvement Is Possible

This is a reasonably traditional and anodyne principle. SLPs with training in neurogenic communication disorders are skilled in changing speech performance. Increasingly, they know how to enhance functional performance as well. This principle is included, however, as an antidote to the false assumption that improvements in impairment will generalize to functional performance and quality of life. Few notions are further from the truth. Functional performance is most likely to improve if it is specifically targeted in treatment. Improving quality of life is even more problematic. One potential solution is to target treatment at symptoms of greatest significance to the individual. Symptom relief is a powerful influence on quality of life. Even then, however, quality of life may improve slightly or not all, unless the environment can also be changed.

Principle: Altering the Environment, When Appropriate, Should Be as Carefully Done and the Effects as Carefully Measured, as Has Traditionally Characterized the Treatment Planning, Measurement, and Performance Directed at the Impairment

This is a challenging principle despite its relatively long history (Berry & Sanders, 1983). Part of the challenge comes from insecurity about the appropriateness of the SLP's managing the environment. Reimbursement models also contribute to the challenge. How, after all, does one account for time spent trying to arrange transportation? In addition, knowing what specifically is meant by environment is more elusive than knowing what is meant by impairment. Nonetheless, several writers including Brandt and Pope (1997) have identified therapeutically critical components of environment. These are listed in **Table 16–2.** This list summarizes the multiple influences on treatment type, frequency, and duration, on whether treatment can be provided, or accepted if offered, and on prognosis. Primarily, the list serves as a reminder that failure to measure and modify as many of these components as possible means ignoring a major management principle.

♦ Motor Skill Learning

A growing body of literature demonstrating the principles of motor skill learning has emerged. Much of the data in support of these principles derives from experiments in the limbs and animal models, but there is an emerging literature in the bulbar system that can be applied to sensorimotor speech disorders. It has been established that motor skill learning is associated with motor cortex reorganization. These changes in motor cortex are hypothesized to be experience-dependent and driven by skilled movement (Remple, Bruneau, VandenBerg, Goertzen, & Kleim, 2001). Experience-dependent neuroplastic changes have also been observed in other areas of the central nervous system including the somatosensory cortex, auditory cortex (Nadeau, 2002), basal ganglia

(Graybiel, 2004), cerebellum (Boyden, Katoh, & Raymond, 2004), and spinal cord (Wolpaw & Tennissen, 2001). Principles of motor skill learning have been demonstrated in a variety of populations, including healthy young and elderly adults, as well as patients with stroke (Hanlon, 1996; McNeil, Robin, & Schmidt, 1997; Pohl & Winstein, 1999; Winstein, Merians, & Sullivan, 1999), Parkinson's disease (Behrman, Cauraugh, & Light, 2000), and spinal cord injury (Behrman & Harkema, 2000). Winstein and colleagues (1999) state that their findings indicate, "motor learning principles derived from the performance of neurologically healthy participants may be generalizable to individuals with stroke-related unilateral hemisphere brain damage" (p. 983) and presumably to those with other patterns of neurological involvement.

Although activities that are generally thought of as requiring motor skills may include walking or throwing, speech production is also a skilled motor task. Consequently, the literature on skill learning in the limbs may inform the treatment and management of dysarthria and AOS, as has been advocated by other authors (McNeil et al, 1997; Yorkston et al, 1999).

However, principles derived from the motor skill learning literature should be interpreted with caution. For example, Wulf and Shea (2002) have criticized the simple laboratory tasks that are frequently utilized in the motor skills learning literature. These authors emphasize "the need to use more complex skills in motor-learning research" (p. 185). Perhaps more importantly, they state that complex motor skills, like speech, may initially require a facilitative environment for acquisition. This facilitative environment is likely also important to develop trust between a patient and a clinician and establish a motivating environment

Table 16–2   Components of the Psychological, Social, and Physical Environment that May Impact the Delivery and Expectations of Rehabilitation

Psychological and Social Environments	Physical Environments
• Discrimination	• Architecture
• Access to health and medical care	• Transportation
• Appropriate care	• Climate
• Access to technology	• Appropriate technology
• Culture	• Geography
• Employment	• Time
• Family	
• Economy	
• Community organizations	
• Access to social services	
• Traits and personality factors	
• Attitudes and emotional states	
• Access to fitness and health-promoting activities	
• Education	
• Spirituality	
• Independence	

Source: Brandt, E. N. & Pope, A. M. (Eds.). (1997). *Enabling America: Assessing the Role of Rehabilitation Science and Engineering.* Washington, DC: National Academy Press, with permission.

for rehabilitation. A more challenging environment that promotes retention and generalization of motor skills may be implemented following initial success with acquisition level skills.

Principle: Retention and Generalization, Rather than Acquisition, May Be the Best Index of Motor Skill Learning

Acquisition and retention are both terms used to describe different types of learning. Acquisition occurs with skill learning during practice, whereas retention is skill learning in which some permanence across time is demonstrated. Schmidt and Bjork (1996) argue that "the effectiveness of learning is revealed by ... the level of retention shown" (p. 7). However, many of our efforts in the treatment of sensorimotor speech disorders are targeted at the level of acquisition. For example, the ability to complete a consonant-vowel (CV) combination with 90% accuracy may be a short-term goal. Once an individual has accomplished this, the task has been "acquired." Therapy would then likely move to addressing other short-term goals and eventually be discontinued. The third-party payer system also favors acquisition-level measurements of motor skills through, for example, the required use of monthly short-term goals. Retention is often ignored or merely assumed despite its being a critical test of learning. During treatment, it is especially important because rehabilitation does not and cannot continue indefinitely.

Another test of skill learning is generalization, which may be an even more complex form of learning than either acquisition or retention (Poggio & Bizzi, 2004). Generalization occurs when a variation of a skill or behavior can be produced because of learning that occurred during acquisition or retention. For example, the skill may be produced in a new environment (e.g., outside the clinic) or produced under new conditions (e.g., when the individual is under stress or is fatigued) (Schmidt & Bjork, 1992, 1996). In speech treatment, generalization also can include transfer of treatment effects to untreated stimuli and to performance with other listeners. Generalization is as important to treatment success as is retention because time does not permit treatment of all possible speech skills in all the environments where they are required. It is important to acknowledge that conditions that maximize acquisition of motor skills may not promote retention and generalization (Schmidt & Bjork, 1992, 1996). Druckman and Bjork (1991) state, "Learners' performance in the post-training tasks and real-world settings ... are the target of training" (p. 47). In other words, the benefit of a therapy program to improve speech in a patient with a sensorimotor speech disorder should be measured by the retention and generalization of skills.

Principle: Blocked Practice May Promote More Rapid Acquisition of New Skills, Whereas Random Practice May Foster Greater Retention

Blocked practice occurs when movements or tasks are repeated without variation, as may occur during drills. In contrast, during random practice, movements or tasks are mixed during practice sessions (Schmidt & Wrisberg,

2004). The literature on limb movements in healthy individuals demonstrates that the acquisition of new skills occurs more rapidly and with the production of fewer errors under the condition of blocked practice, whereas retention is maximized when practice occurs under random conditions (Knock, Ballard, Robin, & Schmidt, 2000; Schmidt & Wrisberg, 2004; Simon & Bjork, 2001). However, research conducted in healthy adults has indicated that people may prefer blocked practice (Baddeley & Longman, 1978) and their self-assessment of learning may incorrectly predict better learning with this approach (Simon & Bjork, 2001).

Preliminary studies about the effect of blocked versus random practice in the training of motor speech production have been conducted. Adams and Page (2000) found that healthy adult subjects had significantly improved retention of a motor speech task under random practice conditions. Other research in two patients with severe AOS demonstrated that random practice facilitated retention, whereas blocked practice did not (Knock et al, 2000).

Principle: Constant Practice May Promote Acquisition of Motor Skills, Whereas Varied Practice May Foster Retention and Generalization

Constant practice is practice in which learners repeatedly produce a single variation of a skill. In contrast, varied practice is practice in which learners attempt variations of a particular skill. A baseball player throwing a ball different distances to different targets would be participating in varied practice (Schmidt & Wrisberg, 2004). Although the relationship between constant and varied practice appears analogous to the relationship between blocked and random practice, important differences exist. Constant and varied practice schedules are concerned with productions of variations of a particular skill, whereas blocked and random practice schedules emphasize the order of productions. For example, a varied practice schedule may have a baseball player throw a ball 10 feet, 20 feet, and 30 feet, whereas a random practice schedule would ensure that the baseball player did not repeat the same distance throw twice in a row (Schmidt and Wrisberg, 2004). A hypothetical treatment for AOS can demonstrate the concepts of constant and varied practice in speech. The correct production of voiced consonants in the final position of words would be the intended treatment outcome. Constant practice would be the repeated production of the word *bad*. In contrast, varied practice, which is concerned with the production of variations of a skill, could occur with a variety of approaches. Varied practice stimuli could change the vowel preceding the final voiced consonant in the word *bad* to include targets such as *bead, bid,* and *bide.* Another strategy would be to produce different final consonants in the same environment, such as *bad, bag,* and *ban.*

Although varied practice slows acquisition, it is associated with improved retention and generalization of motor and verbal tasks (Schmidt & Bjork, 1996). It has been hypothesized that varied practice leads to the development of sets of rules called schemas that are used to determine the parameter values needed for executing variations of the skill (Schmidt & Wrisberg, 2004). Perhaps most importantly, "varied practice enhances the flexibility or adaptability of movement production, allowing people to apply what they have learned during varied practice to the performance of similar actions they have not specifically attempted before" (Schmidt & Wrisberg, 2004, p. 266). Therefore, varied practice may be particularly beneficial when generalization of motor skills is of primary importance. Although limited data exist regarding the benefit of varied practice in the treatment of sensorimotor speech disorders, varied practice has been advocated by other authors (Duffy, 2005; McNeil et al, 1997).

Principle: Distributed Practice, in Comparison to Massed Practice, May Promote Motor Skill Acquisition and Retention

Although the line between massed and distributed practice is not always clear, massed practice occurs without periods of rest, whereas distributed practice occurs with periods of rest interspersed between trials (Schmidt & Wrisberg, 2004). Distributed practice has long been advocated as a more effective practice schedule for the acquisition and retention of motor skills when compared with massed practice (Baddeley & Longman, 1978; Dail & Christina, 2004; Mackay, Morgan, Datta, Chang, & Darzi, 2002).

Schmidt and Wrisberg (2004) review the effect of massed and distributed practice schedules on motor skill learning and state that, in general, the effect of various practice schedules appears to depend on whether the motor skills are discrete or continuous. An example of a discrete motor task is a basketball player shooting a free throw, whereas running and swimming are continuous motor tasks. When learning discrete motor skills, using a massed practice schedule may not negatively influence learning (and may, in fact, have a positive effect). Contrastingly, when continuous motor skills are being learned, a distributed schedule of practice may be most effective. Additionally, the effects of physical and mental fatigue on learning may especially influence the learning of continuous motor skills, making distributed practice schedules most effective with these activities (Schmidt & Wrisberg, 2004).

Speech appears to fit as a continuous motor skill. Furthermore, the treatment of motor speech disorders often causes physical and mental fatigue for patients with already compromised endurance. Consequently, the most effective practice schedule to be used may be one where practice is distributed. The benefit of distributed practice has been cited by other authors in the motor speech disorders literature (Wertz, LaPointe, & Rosenbek, 1984; Yorkston et al, 1999). Dobkin (2004) also recommends a distributed practice schedule: "Patients are more likely to improve if they practice tasks at home in convenient blocks of 20 min. a few times a day" (p. 532). In summary, the most effective practice schedule for the treatment of sensorimotor speech disorders may be one in which practice occurs for relatively short periods of time interspersed with periods of rest.

Principle: Activities that Occur Prior to Practice May Also Influence Motor Skill Learning

The term *prepractice* has been used by McNeil et al (1997) to describe activities that occur prior to initiating practice trials of a target motor skill. This may be an important time to establish the motivation for learning, often through description of the skills to be learned and of the goals to be achieved. Prepractice is also a time for instructors to provide learners the opportunity to engage in observational learning through the use of modeling and demonstration (Schmidt, 1991).

Although they may not be formally titled, prepractice activities likely occur in the early sessions of most sensorimotor speech disorder treatment. Perhaps the most important lesson here for clinicians working with these patients is that prepractice activities, and in particular instructions, should be clear and simple (Yorkston et al, 1999). McNeil and colleagues (1997) emphasize that "the most important message here is *do not overinstruct*" (p. 333).

Principle: The Type and Amount of Feedback Provided about the Performance of a Motor Skill Can Have a Considerable Impact on Learning

Two different forms of external feedback are usually described in the motor skill learning literature. Knowledge of results (KR) is feedback that indicates the degree of success accomplished with a skill following a trial (Schmidt & Wrisberg, 2004), including verbal feedback such as "You missed that one." Knowledge of performance (KP) provides more specific information about the quality of the movement produced (Schmidt & Wrisberg, 2004). For example, a clinician may be working with patients with hypokinetic dysarthria on decreasing their speech rate and provide feedback such as "Your rate of speech is too fast." Increasing the specificity of feedback with KP is usually associated with improved acquisition (Goodman & Wood, 2004), whereas KR feedback is associated with improved retention. This benefit of KR feedback is particularly valuable during the later stages of training (Knock et al, 2000).

A variety of other factors relative to feedback may affect skill learning, including the frequency with which feedback is provided (Weeks & Kordus, 1998). Research in healthy adults, as well as in adults after stroke, indicates that feedback provided after every trial may be less effective than a reduced frequency feedback schedule (Winstein & Schmidt, 1990; Winstein et al, 1999). It has been hypothesized that excessive feedback may impair motor skill learning due to the suppression of a patient's ability to complete higher-level information processing tasks required to identify target responses (Goodman & Wood, 2004). Furthermore, feedback may most effectively promote skill learning when it is provided following a delay (Knock et al, 2000; Swinnen, Schmidt, Nicholson, & Shapiro, 1990).

Adams and colleagues have been leaders in publishing research on how feedback affects speech sensorimotor learning. Adams and Page (2000) described improved retention of a speech motor skill in healthy subjects when a reduced frequency schedule of feedback was implemented. A similar pattern was identified in a follow-up study of subjects with Parkinson's disease (Adams, Page, & Jog, 2002).

Principle: Implicit and Explicit Learning Systems Appear to Be Disassociated and Neuroanatomically Separate and Thus Provide Opportunities for Strategies in Rehabilitation

Motor skill learning is often discussed in terms of implicit and explicit learning. Implicit learning is defined by Pohl, McDowd, Filion, Richards, and Stiers (2001) as "a broad term used to describe the acquisition of abstract knowledge without awareness of learning" (p. 1781). Boyd and Winstein (2003) more specifically define implicit motor learning as "the capacity to acquire skill through physical practice without conscious recollection of what elements of performance improved" (p. 978). Learning how to swim and learning how to ride a bicycle are examples of motor activities that are largely learned implicitly. In contrast to implicit learning, explicit learning is memory for facts and events (Boyd & Winstein, 2003). Explicit learning occurs consciously and is able to be described by the learner (Dobkin, 2003).

Substantial evidence supporting different neural substrates for implicit and explicit learning exists. Implicit learning is highly distributed throughout multiple neural regions, which include the prefrontal and motor cortices, basal ganglia, and cerebellum (Boyd & Winstein, 2003; Pohl et al, 2001). Explicit learning appears to involve the frontoparietal and temporal cortices, hippocampus, and thalamus (Pohl et al, 2001). Although the neural substrates of implicit and explicit memory are disassociated and neuroanatomically separate, these memory systems "sometimes develop in parallel and can profoundly affect one another" (Boyd & Winstein, 2003, p. 978).

If different neural substrates are indeed involved with implicit and explicit learning, then this clearly has significant implications for rehabilitation, including the treatment of sensorimotor speech disorders. For example, when treating hypokinetic dysarthria associated with Parkinson's disease, implicit learning strategies alone may not be effective due to the importance of the basal ganglia for implicit learning. Conversely, explicit learning networks may be unaffected in Parkinson's disease and thus should possibly play a larger role in rehabilitation for these individuals.

Research by Ho, Bradshaw, Iansek, and Alfredson (1999) supports some of these concepts about implicit and explicit learning and their role in the rehabilitation of sensorimotor speech disorders. Patients with Parkinson's disease and hypophonia demonstrated limited response to implicit learning strategies employed by the researchers to increase vocal intensity (i.e., background noise and instantaneous auditory feedback). Although normal subjects responded by increasing vocal intensity to these conditions, subjects with Parkinson's disease had little response. In contrast, when an explicit learning paradigm was utilized (i.e., explicit instructions regarding volume level), the ability of patients with Parkinson's disease to regulate speech intensity was normalized (Ho et al, 1999). Explicit learning strategies have

also been shown to be beneficial to improve gait in patients with Parkinson's disease (Behrman, Teitelbaum, & Cauraugh, 1998). However, explicit learning strategies may also disrupt implicit motor learning after basal ganglia infarct (Boyd & Winstein, 2004b) and middle cerebral artery stroke (Boyd & Winstein, 2004a). Perhaps the lesson here is that patients may differ in their responses to implicit and explicit learning procedures and giving descriptions and instructions before, during, and after practice may not always be beneficial. Too much information may actually inhibit learning for some patients.

Principle: Learning Experiences Are Most Effective When the Motor Skills and Environmental Conditions of Practice Closely Approximate Conditions of the Target Motor Skill and Environment

This specificity of training principle is well defined in the motor skill learning literature. Schmidt and Wrisberg (2004) define this principle as the idea that "the best practice is that which approximates most closely the movements of the target skill and the environmental conditions of the target context" (p. 194). Task specificity has been shown to be an important factor in the rehabilitation of the upper extremity after stroke (Winstein et al, 2004). Although there are few studies of it in the treatment of sensorimotor speech disorders, the specificity of training principle certainly has a great deal of face validity. For example, this notion can be applied to the treatment of spastic dysarthria. If the target of therapy is for individuals to be able to communicate with their caregiver about their wants and needs using words, therapy will be more effective when using speech skills in words and phrases than in syllables or isolated motor movements. This principle also indicates that the environment in which therapy takes place is critical. If the target environment for the motor skills learned in therapy to take place is a person's home, the treatment may be most effective if provided in the individual's home or in the best approximation of more natural environments.

This principle may explain, at least in part, the challenge of generalization to untreated skills and to other environments. Generalization effects often demonstrate a narrow band of transfer in many aspects of generalization, including generalization to untreated environments. Thus, if a narrow band of transfer to novel environments is expected, the target environment should be included in treatment whenever possible, or the best approximation of that environment should be established during treatment.

Principle: Practice Should Be Intensive and Allow for Multiple Attempts to Complete Targeted Motor Skills

Motor skill training must be intensive in order for motor skill learning to occur. Intensity of practice can refer to the frequency of training sessions, the number of total sessions, the length of training sessions, or the number of trials attempted in a training session. Schmidt and Wrisberg (2004) comment on the importance of intensive practice: "Accomplished performers demonstrate extremely high skill levels because of the enormous amount of time and effort they have devoted to practicing" (p. 248). There is accumulating evidence to support the use of an intensive training schedule in the treatment of sensorimotor speech disorders. For example, performing a high number of trials of targeted motor skills has been reported to be beneficial for persons with AOS (Rosenbek, Lemme, Ahearn, Harris, & Wertz, 1973). Other authors have also advocated that multiple opportunities to practice are beneficial for speech rehabilitation (Duffy, 2005). Although intensive practice schedules may be a challenge for both clinicians and patients, scheduling frequent practice sessions, even two times per day, has been recommended, especially during the early stages of treatment (Rosenbek & LaPointe, 1985). Home therapy activities are an important avenue for patients and clinicians to utilize to increase the intensity of treatment.

Principle: A Traditional Hierarchal Model of Moving from Less to More Complex Tasks May Promote Less Retention and Generalization than Moving from More to Less Complex Tasks

Traditionally, it has been argued that the complexity and/or difficulty of tasks should gradually increase in a hierarchal manner. However, this intuitive approach to arranging tasks may not promote retention and generalization:

> Much evidence speaks against employing the traditional hierarchy of working from less to more complex behaviors. When more complex behaviors are selected, the treatment becomes more difficult, but response generalization is more likely to occur to related behaviors that are of similar or lesser complexity (Ballard, 2001, p. 12).

Wertz and colleagues (1984) also argue that treatment needs to be dynamic and that task complexity should move up and down the continuum of difficulty. Research conducted in the treatment of aphasia also supports these counterintuitive concepts about task complexity. For example, Thompson, Shapiro, Kiran, and Sobecks (2003) have found enhanced generalization when treatment moved from more complex to less complex tasks in patients with aphasia. Another study with similar findings demonstrated that the naming of more difficult atypical items generalized to intermediate and common items, whereas training on typical items did not generalize to intermediate and atypical items (Kiran & Thompson, 2003). It is unknown if this principle is at work in sensorimotor speech disorders, but the small extant database seems to lend support. One way of increasing complexity in a sensorimotor task is to practice multiple, alternating tasks, rather than single tasks. Adams and Page (2000) found that individuals who practiced multiple motor speech tasks had increased retention in comparison to the group that practiced a single task.

Principle: Part Practice May Be Less Effective than Whole Practice for Complex Motor Skills

Whole practice occurs when a motor skill is practiced in its entirety, whereas part practice is practice in which a complex motor skill is broken down into a more simplified form (Schmidt & Wrisberg, 2004). McGuigan and MacCaslin (1954) found that part practice of a complex motor skill such as rifle marksmanship is inferior to whole practice for most participants. Part practice has been found to be beneficial for serial tasks, or tasks in which performance in one part of the task does not affect performance in another part of the task (Schmidt & Wrisberg, 2004). Important for clinicians and researchers interested in sensorimotor speech disorders is the notion that "the least likely candidates for effective part practice are rapid, discrete actions. Research suggests that when such actions are broken down into arbitrary parts, the parts become so changed from the way they operate in the context of the whole that practicing them in isolation contributes little to the whole-task performance" (Schmidt & Wrisberg, 2004, p. 253). The "rapid, discrete actions" noted by these authors are consistent with movements for speech production. This suggests that part practice may not be an effective treatment strategy for motor speech disorders, and a whole practice approach should be used when possible. This principle provides additional support against the use of nonverbal movement training in all but selected cases of sensorimotor speech disorder.

♦ Neuroplasticity

Neuroplasticity can be defined as a relatively persistent change in the nervous system in response to experience. Aging, disease, use (as during therapy), and disuse (as in forced nonuse) are all forms of experience. These changes can be negative, positive, or unrelated to either a specific experience or behavioral change (Nudo, Barbay, & Kleim, 2000). Plasticity is possible for both normal and abnormal brains, regardless of age or gender. The magnitude of positive and negative plastic responses is finite (Schallert et al, 2000) and likely to be more extensive, especially in regard to positive change, in the young than in the old. Both positive or adaptive and negative or maladaptive plasticity are influenced by the type and timing of experience and probably by age and gender, among other influences. An example of the influence of type of experience, reaching for a purpose may be different in effect and performance than merely reaching.

Some plastic changes are immediate, some occur only over time, and the mechanisms for these temporal differences may be unique. Both forms are to be differentiated from the so-called placebo effect or what Moerman and Jonas (2002) call the information effect, which may also be associated with measurable central nervous system change (Benedetti et al, 2004). Furthermore, both an enriched environment and what Dobkin (2003) calls "task-specific behavioral learning" (p. 100) can create positive plastic responses capable of supporting restored or new behaviors. Excellent reviews of the literature in support of these generalities can be found in Kolb (1995), Levin and Grafman (2000), and Dobkin (2003).

Despite this optimism, however, it is important to recognize that what is known most confidently about both positive and negative change in brain mechanisms remains limited. Fortunately, a nascent literature on the bulbar motor system has begun to appear. Typical of this work is a study by Liotti and colleagues (2003) in which the neural correlates of hypokinetic dysarthria pre- and posttreatment were determined using positron emission tomography (PET). The researchers reported that successful treatment was "accompanied by increases in activity in right anterior insula, right basal ganglia, and right dorsolateral prefrontal cortex during phonation, and decreases in activation in cortical motor/premotor regions during phonation and reading" (p. 438). They hypothesized that the distributed neural activity observed before treatment represented abnormal neural function and that treatment induced a more normal and focal pattern of neural activity: "The improvement in speech ... appears to entail a functional brain reorganization suggestive of a shift from an effortful implementation of speech-motor programs caused by the basal ganglia pathology to a more automatic, effortless instantiation of motor actions, and in part possibly relying on improved basal ganglia functioning" (p. 439).

Plasticity studies, whether in animals or humans, are guided by models of the impact of positive or adaptive (use) and negative or maladaptive (injury or disuse) experience on the brain. Nudo and colleagues (2000) propose a simple model **(Fig. 16–2)** of what they call the "interactive effects of use and injury on cortical organization" (p. 169). The model's first message of greatest significance to the creation of principles in sensorimotor speech disorders treatment is that "learning of new motor skills results in predictable changes in the functional organization of motor cortex" (p. 169) specifically to spared neural structures potentially in both hemispheres and at several levels of the neuraxis. The second important message is more implicit but real: disuse can alter neural structures in negative ways.

Despite the potential candidacy of all neural structures for plastic changes, Kolb (1995) observes that "the cortex is the most interesting candidate for neural plasticity" (p. 9). Predictably, therefore, most models and data are derived from experiments involving the cortex. As a result, it is tempting to

conclude that these models and data may have limited application to the rehabilitation of sensorimotor speech disorders because it is commonly assumed that these speech disorders, with the exception of unilateral upper motor neuron dysarthria, spastic dysarthria, and AOS, result from damage to levels of the neuraxis below the cortex. However, this assumption of limited relevance for cortically based models is incorrect for several reasons. The first is that all the dysarthrias, with possible exceptions such as flaccid dysarthria from brainstem or final common pathway lesions, result from disruptions of cortical, subcortical, and cerebellar networks (Van der Merwe, 1997). Second, brainstem structures, including the basal ganglia, appear to be capable of plastic response similar in type to the cortex (Graybiel, 2004; Xu and Wall, 1997, 2000) as is the cerebellum (Boyden et al, 2004) and spinal cord (Wolpaw & Tennissen, 2001). Finally, speech movements require networks extending the length of the neuraxis. Even flaccid dysarthria can be influenced by volitional control unless the lesion has completely destroyed final common pathways. Therefore, it is appropriate to apply principles derived from contemporary, primarily cortically based notions about what can be called use-dependent plasticity to the treatment of the full range of sensorimotor speech disorders.

As mentioned earlier, all plastic changes are not necessarily positive. Two sources of negative influences on nervous system function, in addition to the effects of disease, are important to treatment planning. The first is sensory deprivation or forced nonuse. The second is less well documented but of great concern to clinicians faced with decisions about when and how intensively treatment is to be offered. Intensive experience (treatment) at the wrong time has been shown in rats to cause extension of ischemic lesions in the cortex (Bland et al, 1998; Kozlowski, James, & Schallert, 1996) but not in Parkinson's disease (Sasco, Paffenbarger, Gendre, & Wing, 1992). Potentially neurotoxic effects of intensive treatment at the wrong time, although not yet documented in humans, must be a constant concern for clinicians. Equally speculative, but much more uplifting for practitioners, is the potential neuroprotective effects of certain kinds of treatment. The lesson, therefore, is to stay alert for both the good and bad.

Principle: Nihilism about Neurorehabilitation Is Obsolete and Outdated

Nadeau (2002) states that a paradigm shift has occurred in neurorehabilitation due to the "recent advances in neuroscience and behavioural science [that] have shown that the reconstitution of neural function after injury is plausible" (p. 126). Unfortunately, paradigms shift all the time without some people's noticing. Clinicians in facilities ignorant of what is going on in neurorehabilitation have the obligation to spread the word in scholarly ways. Unfortunately this obligation may sometimes take precedence over the obligation to treat. Fortunately, the database in support of the nervous system's response to appropriate treatment is increasingly robust. Thus, the data can be used to make the point so the clinician does not have to. The clinician is merely required to get those data in the right hands and to remain optimistic about the power of rehabilitation.

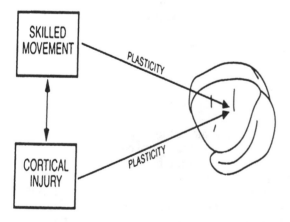

Figure 16–2 The interactive effects of use and injury on cortical organization. [From Nudo, R.J., Barbay, S., & Kleim, J.A. (2000). Rose of neuroplasticity in functional recovery after stroke. In: H.S. Levin & J. Grafman (Eds.), *Cerebral Reorganization of Function After Brain Damage* (pp. 169–197). Oxford: Oxford University Press, with permission.]

Principle: Experience Changes the Brain and Positive Experiences Change It Positively

Kolb (1995) states, "The organization of the brain can be fundamentally altered by experience" (p. 1). The brain's responsiveness to experience is sometimes called use dependent plasticity. Nudo et al (2000) argue that a better term is skill-dependent plasticity because skill training is more powerful than simple use (Karni et al, 1995, 1998; Pascual-Leone et al, 1995). This notion translates directly into sensorimotor speech disorder rehabilitation. Challenging the patient with progressively more demanding targets is likely to be more successful than merely requiring speaking in whatever functional context and with whatever adequacy. Settling for "communication" rather than requiring increased competence of performance may be to deny many speakers the full benefits of treatment. This is not to deny the impact of purpose or functional consequences on skill learning. Increased competence can be achieved with functional drills in functional contexts as long as the treatment goal is improved performance.

Principle: Disuse Has Negative Effects on Brain Organization

Once a function is no longer performed through inability, forced nonuse (such as when a clinician prohibits a behavior), or because of learned nonuse (such as when a speaker quits trying to talk), the nervous system organization on which that function depends shifts in support of activity that is still ongoing. These changes can occur very rapidly. Unknown is whether these conditions make for slower or less complete recovery once rehabilitation is initiated. This principle's lesson for rehabilitationists is that unless otherwise contraindicated, treatment should begin early. However, this principle must be implemented with caution. Recall the earlier mention of the Kozlowski and colleagues (1996) study documenting further damage in the perilesional area of experimentally induced ischemia in rats resulting from intensive early exercise. No human data are available, and this may not be a replicable finding in humans. Regardless, some authors have argued for less intensive therapy in the acute stage of recovery (Bach-Y-Rita, 2002), and clinicians need to be alert for the negative impact of treatment.

Principle: Some Plastic Changes Occur Quickly and Others Occur Later and More Slowly

Evidence exists that plastic change can occur within minutes of beginning training (Karni et al, 1998). Karni and colleagues argue the "quick" learning may reflect "the setting up of a task-specific motor processing routine" (p. 861). "Slow" learning consists of "delayed, incremental gains in performance emerging from continued practice" (p. 862). Similar neural mechanisms may be responsible for both, and both are critical to the retention of learned activity.

This principle impacts treatment in five ways. First, relatively quick changes are not the end of possible improvement, and treatment must be continued over time. Second, retention after treatment ends depends on so-called slow learning in which memories of performance are consolidated. Third, the treatment's first session must be carefully planned to enhance the possibility of setting up an appropriate routine. Fourth, early change may be more than a placebo effect, although it is well known that the placebo effect is accompanied by nervous system as well as behavioral change (Benedetti et al, 2004). Fifth, a period of no or slow change may occur after the quick changes have reached their maximum.

Principle: Neuroplasticity Has Limits

The relatively recent exuberance about plasticity even in older person's brains should not blind us to the fact of its limitations. In some persons, change is impossible because insufficient nervous system remains. In the majority, however, change is possible. Hence, the clinical obligation is, as it has always been, to use the patient's response to treatment as the guide to determine how much is possible. Patients who maintain their gains during no treatment periods have a good prognosis for further improvements. If performance declines or returns to baseline, prognosis for continued improvement is more guarded, assuming treatment has been of sufficient intensity and duration. Failure of generalization to untreated responses similar or identical to treated ones may also be a signal from the nervous system that further plastic responses are unlikely without a different treatment approach. On the other hand, depending on the treatment approach and the target, generalization to dissimilar targets may not be expected, and its absence may have little to do with prognosis. Many of the nervous system's plastic responses are task-specific. This is especially true of the motor skill learning that occurs in dysarthria and AOS treatment. This specificity is yet another reason for avoiding, except perhaps as a last resort, work on skills, such as are involved with oral, nonverbal movements, during speech rehabilitation. Finally, the limits on plasticity in one modality do not predict limits in another. The patient who fails to learn improved speech may well learn alternative communication that depends on different neural substrates for performance.

Principle: Environmental Enrichment and Task-Specific Use Both Have the Potential for Creating Plastic Changes in the Nervous System

Psychologist Donald Hebb took experimental rats home to spend time with the family, and this experience seemed to make them better learners in the laboratory. SLPs need not take patients home, of course. However, inquiring into their environments and influencing those environments to the degree possible can pay dividends when one is doing more focused training. The goals may be as simple as helping an individual keep a diary or increase the number of hours he or she is up and moving around rather than in bed. Homework documented each day may also make a difference. The summary lessons of this principle are that treatment does not begin and end with treatment tasks, and that time spent helping establish the richest possible environment may influence what happens during treatment sessions that may be repetitive, demanding, and relatively sterile.

♦ Muscle Plasticity

Muscles respond with reasonable predictability to use and disuse. In this they resemble the brain. In addition, treatments aimed at changing muscle *structure* such as muscle strengthening exercises, and those aimed at changing muscle *function*, as in motor skill learning, influence the brain. In speech-language pathology, a group of methods posited to influence muscle structure have been grouped together under the rubric of neuromuscular treatment (NMT). The cornerstone of NMT is nonverbal exercise such as pushing against the resistance provided by a tongue blade held by the clinician or moving the tongue in and out of the mouth on command. In addition to the assumption that NMT changes muscle, this approach is driven by two other assumptions. The first is that weakness, and to a lesser degree, abnormal tone and other abnormalities of muscle structure and function, account for the signs of motor speech disorders. The second is that the methods of NMT are the appropriate treatment for these abnormalities. Generations of clinical scientists have voiced their concerns about these assumptions and even more loudly about the methods practiced in their name.

Weakness can serve as an example of these issues. Weakness exists in the bulbar musculature of many dysarthric speakers (Clark, Henson, Barber, Stierwalt, & Sherrill, 2003; Duffy, 2005; Murdoch, Spencer, Theodoros, & Thompson, 1998; Solomon, Lorell, Robin, Rodnitzky, & Luschei, 1995). Proving that weakness is responsible for the speech signs has been devilishly hard, however. Compounding the difficulty is an historic predilection among SLPs for addressing weakness and other muscle abnormalities with nonverbal exercises such as tongue protrusion, massage, and sucking and blowing. Publications by Liss, Kuehn, and Hinkle (1994), Clark (2003), and Weismer and Liss (1991), among others, and an increasing awareness of the general literature on muscle plasticity (Powers & Howley, 2003; Sale, 1988; Sale, McComas, MacDougall, & Upton, 1982; Savage, 1998) seem to be influencing attitudes and, to a degree, even practices. Certainly this literature supports several treatment principles to guide efforts to evaluate traditional NMT and influence muscle plasticity in support of improved speech.

Principle: The Evidence-Based Platform on Which Traditional NMT Rests Is Poorly and Incompletely Built

Clark (2003) reviewed the literature devoted to muscle strengthening and modification of hyper- and hypotonia. Like Hodge (2002), she concludes that the database is inadequate to the confident use of any particular approach. Of strengthening techniques she specifically observes, "Clearly,

the current state of literature is inadequate for establishing that strength training is of benefit for improving speech and/or swallowing function in individuals with neuromuscular impairments" (p. 411). Furthermore, most neuromuscular training programs "do not appear to be based on sound theoretical principles" (p. 411). This is not to say, however, that a sound theoretical basis for a new generation of methods is impossible. Indeed, the literature from a variety of professions outside speech-language pathology provides a robust foundation. Some of these theoretical principles are described below. They are offered so that clinicians can evaluate the theoretical soundness of their favorite treatments and as an impetus for improved methodology.

Principle: Appropriate Neuromuscular Treatment Requires Specificity

Specificity comes in several guises. Clinicians first need to select the target speech behavior and the speech structure(s) responsible for it. Next the clinician has to decide what neuromuscular abnormality is being targeted. Weakness is the nearly reflexive target. Unfortunately, the matter is not so simple. Speech is a submaximum performance task. For example, a significant deficit in strength can occur with no or only minor consequences for speech (Barlow & Abbs, 1983; Kuehn & Moon, 2000; Langmore & Lehman, 1994). The challenge is deciding when weakness is to be targeted. Luschei argues that strengthening may be especially important for the tongue even in relatively minor strength abnormalities because strength is critical for rapid movement. It is unknown if the same is true for other structures. However, weakness accompanying hypertonicity probably should not be a therapeutic target because strengthening may further increase tone. Strength training may also be contraindicated in certain conditions such as amyotrophic lateral sclerosis because muscles so affected may be nearly incapable of recovery after exercise.

If weakness is to be targeted, the next requirement is to select appropriate training tasks because strength training is task specific. In other words, muscles get stronger doing activities for which they are trained but not for other activities. For example, having a patient work to push a tongue blade away from the front of his mouth against increasing resistance may make protrusion stronger but have no impact on tongue movements inside the mouth. Similarly, strength will increase at the rate of movement in which it is trained; the exception is that training strength during fast movements may generalize more to slow than slow does to fast. Train strength during slow movements tongue protrusion and slow but not fast protrusions will be stronger. See Liss and colleagues (1994) for more information on specificity of training.

Clark (2003) states that even appropriate strengthening activities may be inappropriate for some patterns of deficit, and that endurance and power, rather than strength, may sometimes be appropriate therapeutic targets. Endurance can be defined as a relationship of force and time. The greater the endurance, the longer a particular force can be sustained (Robin, Goel, Somodi, & Luschei, 1992). Decreased endurance may be the culprit responsible for speech impairment in some individuals. For these patients, multiple repetitions of submaximum strength exercises may be more appropriate than exercise requiring maximum strength. Fortunately, many strengthening paradigms can improve both strength and endurance. Power, or the rapid production of force, may be another matter. Power may in fact be the critical variable in much speech behavior (Clark, 2003).

Principle: Overload Is Critical

Overload means exercise that demands more than is customary for the performance of a movement or movement sequence. Overload is critical if muscle structure, including hypertrophy in response to strength training, and function are to change. For this reason, the notion that the best treatment for speech is speech is being revised. An alternative notion is that the best treatment for speech is speech and speech-related activity, such as increased respiratory drive under conditions of overload. Overload can be created with varying combinations of frequency, intensity, and duration of activity. Once-a-week practice for 1 month is unlikely to accomplish anything of consequence. Daily practice with systematically more challenging response requirements, and an emphasis on speed of performance (defined humanistically for persons with neurological disease) for 8 to 12 weeks, may improve strength, endurance, and power. An important issue in American health care is money to support such training. One solution for motivated patients is intensive, carefully monitored home practice. Programs for rehabilitation meeting these requirements are CPAP training for velopharyngeal incompetence (Kuehn, 1991; Kuehn et al, 2002), expiratory muscle strength training (Sapienza et al, 1999), and training with the Iowa Oral Performance Instrument (IOPI) (Robin et al, 1992; Stierwalt, Robin, Solomon, Weiss, & Max, 1995). The IOPI, for example, records pressures generated by the tongue against the palate as a surrogate for strength and can be used in a biofeedback paradigm for increasing tongue strength. These programs can serve as guides for clinicians interested in seeing the overload principle in action.

Principle: Early and Later Changes in Response to NMT Are the Responsibility of Different Mechanisms

Early change in response to exercise results from neural adaptation. Mechanisms of adaptation are yet to be determined, but the first response to exercise probably represents the additive effects of involving wider areas of cortical and subcortical neural networks in support of the performance (Powers & Howley, 2003). One effect is to recruit more motor units to the performance. Later changes reflect change in muscle, including muscle hypertrophy, and occur only after weeks of intensive exercise. This principle is worth mentioning for several reasons. One especially important reason has to do with patient motivation. Early change may be followed by a period of dishearteningly slowed improvement. Sagging motivation may be bolstered by patient education about how such exercises work. Another reason is that stopping treatment prematurely robs patients of their full potential for improvement. Premature termination may also hamper the interpretation of the mechanisms of effect for emerging treatments. Finally, an incompletely applied method may appear to be less efficacious than a more traditional treatment and therefore may be dropped inappropriately from the clinical armamentarium.

Principle: Therapeutic Gains Decline When Training Stops

Changes in muscle dissipate unless some level of training continues. This principle is uncomfortable for many clinicians conditioned to thinking of treatment in terms established by third-party payers who set limits on treatment duration and who discourage so-called maintenance therapy. The challenge to the profession, then, is to create maintenance programs and make them the patient's responsibility. Equally as important is providing encouragement to patients so that they continue a maintenance program after therapy is discontinued. By doing so, the neural adaptation portion of change can sometimes be maintained.

♦ Conclusion

Nearly everything clinicians do with those having sensorimotor speech disorders will be helpful. Not all such things will be equally helpful, however. This chapter's list of principles may help clinicians separate the most from the least helpful. That, at least, was the goal of the authors. If these principles simultaneously support the continued transformation of practice, so much the better. Patients deserve the best effort that their clinicians can provide.

References

Abbs, J.H. & Rosenbek, J.C. (1985). Some motor control perspectives on apraxia of speech and dysarthria. In: J. Costello (Ed.), *Speech Disorders in Adults* (pp. 21–58). San Diego: College-Hill Press

Adams, S.G. & Page, A.D. (2000). Effects of selected practice and feedback variables on speech motor learning. *Journal of Medical Speech-Language Pathology, 8,* 215–220

Adams, S.G., Page, A.D., & Jog, M. (2002). Summary feedback schedules and speech motor learning in Parkinson's disease. *Journal of Medical Speech-Language Pathology, 10,* 215–220

American Academy of Neurology. (1994). Assessment: melodic intonation therapy. *Neurology, 44,* 566–568

Bach-Y-Rita, P. (2000). Conceptual issues relevant to present and future neurologic rehabilitation. In: H. S. Levin & J. Grafman (Eds.), *Cerebral Reorganization of Function After Brain Damage* (pp. 357–379). Oxford: Oxford University Press

Baddeley, A.D. & Longman, D.J.A. (1978). Influence of length and frequency of training session on rate of learning to type. *Ergonomics, 21,* 627–635

Ballard, K.J. (2001). Response generalization in apraxia of speech treatments: taking another look. *Journal of Communication Disorders, 34,* 3–20

Barlow, S.M. & Abbs, J.H. (1983). Force transducers for the evaluation of labial, lingual, and mandibular motor impairments. *Journal of Speech and Hearing Research, 26,* 616–621

Behrman, A.L., Cauraugh, J.H., & Light, K.E. (2000). Practice as an intervention to improve speeded motor performance and motor learning in Parkinson's disease. *Journal of the Neurological Sciences, 174,* 127–136

Behrman, A.L. & Harkema, S.J. (2000). Locomotor training after human spinal cord injury: a series of case studies. *Physical Therapy, 80,* 688–700

Behrman, A.L., Teitelbaum, P., & Cauraugh, J.H. (1998). Verbal instructional sets to normalise the temporal and spatial gait variables in Parkinson's disease. *Journal of Neurology Neurosurgery and Psychiatry, 65,* 580–582

Benedetti, F., Colloca, L., Torre, E., Lanotte, M., Melcarne, A., Pesare, M., Bergamasco, B., & Lopiano, L. (2004). Placebo-responsive Parkinson patients show decreased activity in single neurons of subthalamic nucleus. *Nature Neuroscience, 7,* 587–588

Berry, W.R. & Sanders, S.B. (1983). Environmental education: the universal management approach for adults with dysarthria. In: W.R. Berry (Ed.), *Clinical Dysarthria* (pp. 203–216). San Diego: College-Hill Press

Berwick, D.M. (1996). Harvesting knowledge from improvement. *Journal of the American Medical Association, 275,* 877–878

Beukelman, D.R. & Mirenda, P. (1998). *Augmentative and Alternative Communication,* 2nd ed. Baltimore: Paul H. Brookes

Bland, S.T., Humm, J.L., Kozlowski, D.A., Williams, L., Strong, R., Aronowski, J., Grotta, J. & Schallert, T. (1998). Forced overuse of the contralateral forelimb increases infarct volume following a mild, but not a severe, transient cerebral ischemic insult. *Society for Neuroscience Abstracts, 774,* 1955

Boyd, L.A. & Winstein, C.J. (2003). Impact of explicit information on implicit motor-sequence learning following middle cerebral artery stroke. *Physical Therapy, 83,* 976–989

Boyd, L.A. & Winstein, C.J. (2004a). Cerebellar stroke impairs temporal but not spatial accuracy during implicit motor learning. *Neurorehabilitation and Neural Repair, 18,* 134–143

Boyd, L.A. & Winstein, C.J. (2004b). Providing explicit information disrupts implicit motor learning after basal ganglia stroke. *Learning & Memory, 11,* 388–396

Boyden, E.S., Katoh, A., & Raymond, J.L. (2004). Cerebellum-dependent learning: the role of multiple plasticity mechanisms. *Annual Review of Neuroscience, 27,* 581–609

Brandt, E.N. & Pope, A.M. (Eds.). (1997). *Enabling America: Assessing the Role of Rehabilitation Science and Engineering.* Washington, DC: National Academy Press

Brendel, B., Lowit, A., & Howell, P. (2004). The effects of delayed and frequency shifted feedback on speakers with Parkinson disease. *Journal of Medical Speech Language Pathology, 12,* 131–138

Clark, H.M. (2003). Neuromuscular treatments for speech and swallowing: a tutorial. *American Journal of Speech-Language Pathology, 12,* 400–415

Clark, H.M., Henson, P.A., Barber, W.D., Stierwalt, J.A.G., & Sherrill, M. (2003). Relationships among subjective and objective measures of tongue strength and oral phase swallowing impairments. *American Journal of Speech-Language Pathology, 12,* 40–50

Cohen, A.M., Stavri, P.Z., & Hersh, W.R. (2004). A categorization and analysis of the criticisms of evidence-based medicine. *International Journal of Medical Informatics, 73,* 35–43

Dail, T.K. & Christina, R.W. (2004). The spacing effect and metacognition in the learning and long-term retention of a discrete motor task. *Research Quarterly for Exercise and Sport, 75,* 148–155

Damico, J.S. & Simmons-Mackie, N.N. (2003). Qualitative research and speech-language pathology: a tutorial for the clinical realm. *American Journal of Speech-Language Pathology, 12,* 131–143

Darley, F.L., Aronson, A.E., & Brown, J.R. (1969a). Differential diagnostic patterns of dysarthria. *Journal of Speech and Hearing Research, 12,* 249–269

Darely, F.L., Aronson, A.E., & Brown, J.R. (1969b). Cluster of deviant speech dimensions in the dysarthrias. *Journal of Speech and Hearing Research, 12,* 462–496

Dobkin, B.H. (2003). *The Clinical Science of Neurologic Rehabilitation,* 2nd ed. Oxford: Oxford University Press

Dobkin, B.H. (2004). Strategies for stroke rehabilitation. *Lancet Neurology, 3,* 528–536

Donovan, N.J., Velozo, C.A., & Rosenbek, J.C. (2007). The communication effectiveness survey: investigating its item-level psychometric properties. *Journal of Medical Speech – Language Pathology, 15,* 433–447

Druckman, D. & Bjork, R.A. (1991). *In the Mind's Eye: Enhancing Human Performance.* Washington, DC: National Academy Press

Duffy, J.R. (2005). *Motor Speech Disorders: Substrates, Differential Diagnosis, and Management,* 2nd ed. St. Louis: Elsevier Mosby

Fleming, T.R. & DeMets, D.L. (1996). Surrogate endpoints in clinical trials: are we being misled? *Annals of Internal Medicine, 125,* 605–613

Goodman, J.S. & Wood, R.E. (2004). Feedback specificity, learning opportunities, and learning. *Journal of Applied Psychology, 89,* 809–821

Graybiel, A.M. (2004). Network-level neuroplasticity in cortico-basal ganglia pathways. *Parkinsonism & Related Disorders, 10,* 293–296

Hanlon, R.E. (1996). Motor learning following unilateral stroke. *Archives of Physical Medicine and Rehabilitation, 77,* 811–815

Hixon, T.J. & Hoit, J.D. (1998). Physical examination of the diaphragm by the speech-language pathologist. *American Journal of Speech-Language Pathology, 7,* 37–45

Hixon, T.J. & Hoit, J.D. (1999). Physical examination of the abdominal wall by the speech-language pathologist. *American Journal of Speech-Language Pathology, 8,* 335–346

Ho, A.K., Bradshaw, J.L., Iansek, R., & Alfredson, R. (1999). Speech volume regulation in Parkinson's disease: effects of implicit cues and explicit instructions. *Neuropsychologia, 37,* 1453–1460

Hodge, M.M. (2002). Nonspeech oral motor treatment approaches for dysarthria: perspectives on a controversial clinical practice. *Perspectives in Neurophysiological and Neurogenic Speech Disorders, 12,* 22–28

Jette, A.M. (1994). Physical disablement concepts for physical therapy research and practice. *Physical Therapy, 74,* 380–386

Karni, A., Meyer, G., Jezzard, P., Adams, M.M., Turner, R., & Ungerleider, L.G. (1995). Functional MRI evidence for adult motor cortex plasticity during motor skill learning. *Nature, 377,* 155–158

Karni, A., Meyer, G., Rey-Hipolito, C., Jezzard, P., Adams, M.M., Turner, R., & Ungerleider, L.G. (1998). The acquisition of skilled motor performance: Fast and slow experience-driven changes in primary motor cortex. *Proceedings of the National Academy of Sciences of the USA, 95,* 861–868

Kent, R.D. (Ed.). (1992). *Intelligibility in Speech Disorders.* Philadelphia: John Benjamin's Publishing

Kent, R.D., Weismer, G., Kent, J.F., Vorperian, H.K., & Duffy, J.R. (1999). Acoustic studies of dysarthric speech: methods, progress, and potential. *Journal of Communication Disorders, 32,* 141–186

Kiran, S. & Thompson, C.K. (2003). The role of semantic complexity in treatment of naming deficits: training semantic categories in fluent aphasia by controlling exemplar typicality. *Journal of Speech Language and Hearing Research, 46,* 773–787

Knock, T.R., Ballard, K.J., Robin, D.A., & Schmidt, R.A. (2000). Influence of order of stimulus presentation on speech motor learning: a principled approach to treatment for apraxia of speech. *Aphasiology, 14,* 653–668

Kolb, B. (1995). *Brain Plasticity and Behavior.* Mahwah, NJ: Lawrence Erlbaum Associates

Kozlowski, D.A., James, D.C., & Schallert, T. (1996). Use-dependent exaggeration of neuronal injury following unilateral sensorimotor cortex lesions. *Journal of Neuroscience, 16,* 4776–4786

Kuehn, D.P. (1991). New therapy for treating hypernasal speech using continuous positive airway pressure (CPAP). *Plastic and Reconstructive Surgery, 88,* 959–966

Kuehn, D.P., Imrey, P.B., Tomes, L., Jones, D.L., O'Gara, M.M., Seaver, E.J., Smith, B.E., Van Demark, D.R., & Wachtel, J.M. (2002). Efficacy of continuous positive airway pressure for treatment of hypernasality. *Cleft Palate-Craniofacial Journal, 39,* 267–276

Kuehn, D.P. & Moon, J.B. (2000). Induced fatigue effects on velopharyngeal closure force. *Journal of Speech, Language, and Hearing Research, 43,* 486–500

Kuehn, D.P. & Wachtel, J.M. (1994). CPAP therapy for treating hypernasality following closed head injury. In: J.A. Till, K.M. Yorkston, D.R. Beukelman (Eds.), *Motor Speech Disorders: Advances in Assessment and Treatment* (pp. 207–212). Baltimore: Paul H. Brookes

Langmore, S.E. & Lehman, M.E. (1994). Physiologic deficits in the orofacial system underlying dysarthria in amyotrophic lateral sclerosis. *Journal of Speech and Hearing Research. 37,* 28–37

Levin, H.S. & Grafman, J. (Eds.). (2000). *Cerebral Reorganization of Function after Brain Damage.* Oxford: Oxford University Press

Liotti, M., Ramig, L.O., Vogel, D., New, P., Cook, C.I., Ingham, R.J., Ingham, J.C., & Fox, P.T. (2003). Hypophonia in Parkinson's disease: neural correlates of voice treatment revealed by PET. *Neurology, 60,* 432–440

Liss, J.M., Kuehn, D.P., & Hinkle, K.P. (1994). Direct training of velopharyngeal musculature. *Journal of Medical Speech-Language Pathology, 2,* 243–249

Mackay, S., Morgan, P., Datta, V., Chang, A., & Darzi, A. (2002). Practice distribution in procedural skills training: a randomized controlled trial. *Surgical Endoscopy and Other Interventional Techniques, 16,* 957–961

McGuigan, F.J. & MacCaslin, E.F. (1955). Whole and part methods in learning a perceptual motor skill. *American Journal of Psychology, 68,* 658–661

McNeil, M.R., Robin, D.A., & Schmidt, R.A. (1997). Apraxia of speech: definition, differentiation, and treatment. In: M.R. McNeil (Ed.), *Clinical Management of Sensorimotor Speech Disorders.* (pp. 311–344). New York: Thieme

Medawar, P.B. (1979). *Advice to a Young Scientist.* New York: Harper & Row

Moerman, D.E. & Jonas, W.B. (2002). Deconstructing the placebo effect and finding the meaning response. *Annals of Internal Medicine, 136,* 471–476

Moore, A., McQuay, H., & Gray, J.A.M. (Eds.). (1995). Evidence-based everything. *Bandolier, 12,* 1

Murdoch, B.E., Spencer, T.J., Theodoros, D.G., & Thompson, E.C. (1998). Lip and tongue function in multiple sclerosis: a physiological analysis. *Motor Control, 2,* 148–160

Murdoch, B.E., Thompson, E.C., & Theodoros, D.G. (1997). Spastic dysarthria. In: M.R. McNeil (Ed.), *Clinical Management of Sensorimotor Speech Disorders* (pp. 287–310). New York: Thieme

Nadeau, S.E. (2002). A paradigm shift in neurorehabilitation. *Lancet Neurology, 1,* 126–130

Nagi, S. (1965). Some conceptual issues in disability and rehabilitation. In: M. Sussman (Ed.), *Sociology and Rehabilitation* (pp. 100–113). Washington, DC: American Sociological Association

Netsell, R. (1981). The acquisition of speech motor control: a perspective with directions for research. In R. Stark (Ed.), *Language Behavior in Infancy and Early Childhood* (pp. 127–156). New York: Elsevier Science

Nudo, R.J., Barbay, S., & Kleim, J.A. (2000). Rose of neuroplasticity in functional recovery after stroke. In: H.S. Levin & J. Grafman (Eds.), *Cerebral Reorganization of Function After Brain Damage* (pp. 169–197). Oxford: Oxford University Press

Pascual-Leone, A., Nguyet, D., Cohen, L.G., Brasil-Neto, J.P., Cammarota, A., & Hallett, M. (1995). Modulation of muscle responses evoked by transcranial magnetic stimulation during the acquisition of new fine motor skills. *Journal of Neurophysiology, 74,* 1037–1045

Poggio, T. & Bizzi, E. (2004). Generalization in vision and motor control. *Nature, 431,* 768–774

Pohl, P.S., McDowd, J.M., Filion, D.L., Richards, L.G., & Stiers, W. (2001). Implicit learning of a perceptual-motor skill after stroke. *Physical Therapy, 81,* 1780–1789

Pohl, P.S. & Winstein, C.J. (1999). Practice effects on the less-affected upper extremity after stroke. *Archives of Physical Medicine and Rehabilitation, 80,* 668–675

Pope, A.M. & Tarlow, A.R. (1991). *Disability in America: Toward a National Agenda for Prevention.* Washington, DC: National Academy Press

Powers, S.K. & Howley, E.T. (2003). *Exercise Physiology: Theory and Applications to Fitness and Performance,* 5th ed. New York: McGraw-Hill

Ramig, L.O., Countryman, S., Thompson, L.L., & Horii, Y. (1995). Comparison of two forms of intensive speech treatment for Parkinson disease. *Journal of Speech and Hearing Research 38,* 1232–1251

Ramsey, P. (1970). *The Patient as Person.* New Haven: Yale University Press

Remple, M.S., Bruneau, R.M., VandenBerg, P.M., Goertzen, C., & Kleim, J.A. (2001). Sensitivity of cortical movement representations to motor experience: evidence that skill learning but not strength training induces cortical reorganization. *Behavioural Brain Research, 123,* 133–141

Robin, D.A., Goel, A., Somodi, L.B., & Luschei, E.S. (1992). Tongue strength and endurance: relation to highly skilled movements. *Journal of Speech and Hearing Research, 35,* 1239–1245

Rosenbek, J.C. & LaPointe, L.L. (1985). The dysarthrias: description, diagnosis, and treatment. In: D.F. Johns (Ed.), *Clinical Management of Neurogenic Communicative Disorders,* 2nd ed. (pp. 97–152). Boston: Little, Brown

Rosenbek, J.C., Lemme, M.L., Ahern, M.B., Harris, E.H., & Wertz, R.T. (1973). A treatment for apraxia of speech in adults. *Journal of Speech and Hearing Disorders, 38,* 462–472

Rosenbek, J.C. & McNeil, M.R. (1991). A discussion of classification in motor speech disorders. In: C.A. Moore, K.M. Yorkston, & D.R. Beukelman (Eds.), *Dysarthria and Apraxia of Speech: Perspectives in Management* (pp. 289–295). Baltimore: Paul H. Brookes

Sackett, D.L., Richardson, W.S., Rosenberg, W., & Hayes, R.B. (1998). *Evidence-Based Medicine: How to Practice and Teach EBM.* New York: Churchill Livingstone

Sale, D.G. (1988). Neural adaptation to resistance training. *Medicine and Science in Sports and Exercise, 20* (suppl), S135–S145

Sale, D.G., McComas, A.J., MacDougall, J.D., & Upton A.R.M. (1982). Neuromuscular adaptation in human thenar muscles following strength training and immobilization. *Journal of Applied Physiology: Respiration, Environment, Exercise, Physiology, 53,* 419–424

Sapienza, C.M., Brown, J., Davenport, P., & Martin, D. (1999). Inspiratory pressure threshold training for glottal airway limitation in laryngeal papilloma. *Journal of Voice, 13,* 382–388

Sasco, A.J., Paffenbarger, R.S., Gendre, I., & Wing, A.L. (1992). The role of physical exercise in the occurrence of Parkinson's disease. *Archives of Neurology, 49,* 360–365

Savage, J. (1998). *Fundamental Strength Training.* Minneapolis, MN: Learner Publications

Schallert, T., Bland, S.T., Leasure, J.L., Tillerson, J., Gonzales, R., Williams, L., Aronowski, J., & Grotta, J. (2000). Motor rehabilitation, use-related neural events, and reorganization after injury. In: H.S. Levin & J. Grafman (Eds.), *Cerebral Reorganization of Function After Brain Damage* (pp. 145–167). Oxford: Oxford University Press

Schmidt, R.A. (1991). *Motor Learning and Performance: From Principles to Practice.* Champaign, IL: Human Kinetics

Schmidt, R.A. & Bjork, R.A. (1992). New conceptualizations of practice—common principles in three paradigms suggest new concepts for training. *Psychological Science, 3,* 207–217

Schmidt, R.A. & Bjork, R.A. (1996). New conceptualizations of practice: common principles in three paradigms suggest new concepts for training. In: D.A. Robin, K.M. Yorkston, & D.R. Beukelman (Eds.), *Disorders of Motor Speech: Assessment, Treatment, and Clinical Characterization* (pp. 3–23). Baltimore: Paul H. BrookesSchmidt, R.A. & Wrisberg, C.A. (2004). *Motor Learning and Performance,* 3rd ed. Champaign, IL: Human Kinetics

Shadish, W.R, Cook, T.D, Campbell, D.T. (2002). *Experimental and Quasi-Experimental Designs for Generalized Causal Inference.* Boston: Houghton Mifflin

Simon, D.A. & Bjork, R.A. (2001). Metacognition in motor learning. *Journal of Experimental Psychology—Learning Memory and Cognition, 27,* 907–912

Solomon, N.P., Lorell, D.M., Robin, D.A., Rodnitzky, R.L., & Luschei, E.S. (1995). Tongue strength and endurance in mild to moderate Parkinson's disease. *Journal of Medical Speech-Language Pathology, 3,* 15–26

Stierwalt, J.A.G., Robin, D.A, Solomon, N.P., Weiss, A.L., & Max, J.E. (1995). Tongue strength and endurance: relation to the speaking ability of children and adolescents following traumatic brain injury. In: D.A. Robin, K.M. Yorkston, & D.R. Beukelman (Eds.), *Disorders of Motor Speech: Recent Advances in Assessment, Treatment, and Clinical Characterization* (pp. 243–258). Baltimore: Paul H. Brookes

Swinnen, S.P., Nicholson, D.E., Schmidt, R.A., & Shapiro, D.C. (1990). Information feedback for skill acquisition—instantaneous knowledge of results degrades learning. *Journal of Experimental Psychology-Learning Memory and Cognition, 16,* 706–716

Thompson, C.K., Shapiro, L.P., Kiran, S., & Sobecks, J. (2003). The role of syntactic complexity in treatment of sentence deficits in agrammatic aphasia: the complexity account of treatment efficacy (CATE). *Journal of Speech Language and Hearing Research, 46,* 591–607

Van der Merwe, A. (1997). A theoretical framework for the characterization of pathological speech sensorimotor control. In: M.R. McNeil (Ed.), *Clinical Management of Sensorimotor Speech Disorders* (pp. 1–26). New York: Thieme

Verbrugge, L.M. & Jette, A.M. (1994). The disablement process: social science and medicine. *Social Science & Medicine Journal, 38,* 1–14

Wambaugh, J.L. (2002). A summary of treatments for apraxia of speech and review of replicated approaches. *Seminars in Speech and Language, 23,* 293–308

Weeks, D.L. & Kordus, R.N. (1998). Relative frequency of knowledge of performance and motor skill learning. *Research Quarterly for Exercise and Sport, 69,* 224–230

Weismer, G. & Liss, J.M. (1991). Reduction is a dead-end in speech research: perspectives on a new direction. In: C.A. Moore, K.M. Yorkston, & D.R. Beukelman (Eds.), *Dysarthria and Apraxia of Speech: Perspectives on Management* (pp. 15–27). Baltimore: Paul H. Brookes

Wertz, R.T., LaPointe, L.L., & Rosenbek, J.C. (1984). *Apraxia of Speech in Adults.* Needham Heights, MA: Allyn and Bacon

Winstein, C.J., Merians, A.S., & Sullivan, K.J. (1999). Motor learning after unilateral brain damage. *Neuropsychologia, 37,* 975–987

Winstein, C.J., Rose, D.K., Tan, S.M., Lewthwaite, R., Chui, H.C., & Azen, S.P. (2004). A randomized controlled comparison of upper-extremity rehabilitation strategies in acute stroke: a pilot study of immediate and long-term outcomes. *Archives of Physical Medicine and Rehabilitation, 85,* 620–628

Winstein, C.J. & Schmidt, R.A. (1990). Reduced frequency of knowledge of results enhances motor skill learning. *Journal of Experimental Psychology-Learning Memory and Cognition, 16,* 677–691

Wolpaw, J.R. & Tennissen, A.M. (2001). Activity-dependent spinal cord plasticity in health and disease. *Annual Review of Neuroscience, 24,* 807–843

World Health Organization. (2001). *International Classification of Functioning, Disability and Health: ICF.* Geneva: WHO

Worrall, L.E. & Frattali C.M. (Eds.). (2000). *Neurogenic Communication Disorders: A Functional Approach.* New York: Thieme

Wulf, G. & Shea, C.H. (2002). Principles derived from the study of simple skills do not generalize to complex skill learning. *Psychonomic Bulletin & Review, 9,* 185–211

Xu, J. & Wall, J.T. (1997). Rapid changes in brainstem maps of adult primates after peripheral injury. *Brain Research, 774,* 211–215

Xu, J. & Wall, J.T. (2000). Rapid reorganization of subcortical and cortical maps in adult primates. In: H.S. Levin & J. Grafman (Eds.), *Cerebral Reorganization of Function after Brain Damage* (pp. 130–144). Oxford: Oxford University Press

Yorkston, K.M. (1996). Treatment efficacy: dysarthria. *Journal of Speech and Hearing Research. 39,* S46–S57

Yorkston, K.M. & Beukelman, D.R., Strand, E.A., & Bell, K.R. (1999). *Management of Motor Speech Disorders in Children and Adults,* 2nd ed. Austin: Pro-Ed

Yorkston, K.M., Spencer, K.A., & Duffy J.R. (2003). Behavioral management of respiratory/phonatory dysfunction from dysarthria: a systematic review of evidence. *Journal of Medical Speech-Language Pathology, 11,* xiii–xxxviii

Part II

Pathology

Chapter 17

Alport Syndrome

Stacey L. Pavelko, Cynthia A. Eberwein, and Sheila R. Pratt

♦ General Information on Disorder

Alport syndrome is an inherited disorder resulting from changes in the type IV collagen α3/α4/α5 network of the glomerular basement membrane (GBM). It represents the more severe end of the spectrum of hereditary type IV collagen nephropathies, with thin basement membrane nephropathy (TBMN) representing the mild end. Alport syndrome is clinically heterogeneous but is usually associated with hematuria, proteinuria, progressive renal failure, sensorineural hearing loss, and ocular lesions. The juvenile form occurs before 30 years of age and is more severe than the adult form, which has a later onset (Barker et al, 1990).

Diagnostic Signs and Symptoms

The hallmark of Alport syndrome is persistent microscopic hematuria, often associated with proteinuria, progressive renal failure, ocular abnormalities, and high-frequency sensorineural hearing loss (Kashtan, 1998). The presenting sign of Alport syndrome is usually hematuria (Hudson, Tryggvason, Sundaramoorthy, & Neilson, 2003). Differentiating Alport syndrome from TBMN is difficult. Kidney biopsies have been used to confirm suspected Alport syndrome (Kashtan, 1999), although without a clear family history of renal failure it is often difficult to distinguish between the two diseases (Dagher, Wang, Fassett & Savige, 2002). Misdiagnosis of Alport syndrome as TBMN may be quite common, with 10% of families having a biopsy diagnosis of TBMN later being suspected as having Alport syndrome (Buzza, Wilson, & Savige, 2001). More recently, researchers have advocated the use of confocal laser microscopy to examine the epidermal basement membrane of skin biopsies as a less invasive way to diagnose the disease (Muda et al, 2003).

Neuropathology

There have been isolated reports in the literature of seizures, electroencephalogram (EEG) abnormalities, and lesions to the thalami and basal ganglia associated with Alport syndrome (Kawakami et al, 1990; Sener, 1998; Shields, Pataki, & DeList, 1990).

Epidemiology

The gene frequency is estimated to be 1 in 5000 to 1 in 10,000 (Pirson, 1999). Approximately 85% of cases are X-linked dominant, with males being more severely affected than females. In persons with X-linked Alport syndrome, approximately 90% of males and 10% of females develop moderate to severe hearing loss before age 40, and 12% of females and 90% of males reach end-stage renal disease (ESRD) by that same age. Ocular abnormalities are present in 15% of females and 35.2% of males (Jais et al, 2000, 2003). Additionally, esophageal leiomyomatosis, mainly manifested by dysphagia or retrosternal pain has been reported (Antignac & Heidet, 1996).

Autosomal recessive and autosomal dominant cases of Alport syndrome also have been reported. Less than 10% of cases of Alport syndrome are autosomal recessive, with males and females being equally and severely affected (Pirson, 1999). More recently, two cases of autosomal dominant forms of the disease have been reported. In these cases, no patients had signs of ocular abnormalities, 19% had bilateral sensorineural hearing loss and 37.5% had ESRD by age 50 (Pescucci et al, 2004).

Genetics

Alport syndrome is due to defects in type IV collagen, a major component of basement membranes. Six genetically distinct type IV collagen α-chains have been identified, α1 (IV) through α6 (IV). The α3, α4, α5, and α6 chains are expressed selectively in the basement membranes of some tissues, including the eye, kidney, and cochlea, and are believed to be involved in Alport syndrome (Kashtan, Kleppel, & Gubler, 1996). Approximately 85% of patients with Alport syndrome have X-linked inheritance of mutations in the COL4A5 gene (Lemmink, Schröder, Monnens, & Smeets, 1997). In the majority of non–X-linked cases, the transmission appears to be autosomal recessive, with mutations detected in either the COL4A3 or the COL4A4 gene (Lemmink et al, 1997). In cases of autosomal dominant inheritance, mutations have been detected in either the COL4A3 or the COL4A4 gene (Pescucci et al, 2004). No cases of Alport syndrome solely due to mutations in the COL4A6 gene have been reported.

♦ Speech Impairment Associated with Disorder

The speech production skills of persons with Alport syndrome have not been described in the literature. However, the associated hearing loss increases the likelihood of speech production problems, although they are likely to be mild given the onset and magnitude of the hearing losses observed. Sensorineural hearing loss usually begins during the second decade of life as a mild bilateral high-frequency loss (Pirson, 1999). The hearing loss usually progresses to involve middle and lower frequencies, but pure-tone thresholds rarely exceed 60 to 70 dB hearing level (HL). Furthermore, speech recognition skills are usually maintained (Merchant et al, 2004). Depending on the presence and extent of basal ganglion and thalamic involvement, additional motor speech impairment may complicate the clinical presentation.

Diagnostic Signs and Symptoms

With the presence a hearing loss, speech and vocal characteristics consistent with hearing loss may be present (see Chapter 13).

Etiology

Speech and communication deficits may result secondary to hearing loss and the co-occurrence of auditory and visual impairment. Although less common, thalamic and basal ganglia lesions may further compromise speech production.

Neuropathology

Neuropathological manifestations could be due to seizure activity, lesions to the thalami or basal ganglia, or abnormal brain activity.

Associated Cognitive, Linguistic, and Communicative Signs and Symptoms

Individuals with Alport syndrome present with normal intelligence. Speech deficits other than those related to hearing

loss have not been reported in the literature. However, the co-occurrence of hearing loss and visual impairment can substantively impair communication.

Special Diagnostic Considerations

There are no minimal diagnostic criteria for evaluation of speech in Alport syndrome. Diagnosis of Alport syndrome is typically based on hematuria and supported by a positive family history of renal problems as well as renal or skin biopsies. Early evaluation of hearing is recommended to provide a measure of baseline auditory function, as is frequent monitoring of hearing, particularly into the second decade of life (Pirson, 1999). In addition, swallow studies should be considered given the compounded risk of eating and drinking problems due to the possible presence of esophageal leiomyomatosis (Antignac & Heidet, 1996).

Treatment

Onset of progressive sensorineural hearing loss typically does not occur until the second decade of life, and rehabilitation services may be needed at that time. Auditory and visual sensory aids likely will be needed. Esophageal leiomyomatosis may cause dysphagia in some patients, and they should be monitored to ensure safe eating and provided with rehabilitation services as needed.

References

Antignac, H. & Heidet, L. (1996). Mutations in Alport syndrome associated with diffuse esophageal leiomyomatosis. In: K. Tryggvason (Ed.), *Molecular Pathology and Genetics of Alport Syndrome* (pp. 172–182). Basel: Karger

Barker, D.F., Hostikka, S., Zhou, J., Chow, L., Oliphant, A., Gerken, S., et al. (1990). Identification of mutations in the COL4A5 collagen gene in Alport syndrome. *Science, 248,* 1224–1227.

Buzza, M., Wilson, D., & Savige, J. (2001). Segregation of hematuria in thin basement membrane disease with haplotypes at the loci for Alport Syndrome. *Kidney International, 59,* 1670–1676

Dagher, H., Wang, Y.Y., Fassett, R., & Savige, J. (2002). Three novel COL4A4 mutations resulting in stop codons and their clinical effects in autosomal recessive Alport syndrome. *Human Mutation, 20,* 321–322

Hudson, B.G., Tryggvason, K., Sundaramoorthy, M., & Neilson, E. (2003). Alport's syndrome, Goodpasture's syndromes, and type IV collagen. *New England Journal of Medicine, 348,* 2543–2556

Jais, J.P., Knebelmann, B., Giatras, I., De Marchi, M., Rizzoni, G., Renieri, M., et al. (2000). X-linked Alport syndrome: natural history in 195 families and genotype-phenotype correlations in males. *Journal of the American Society of Nephrology, 11,* 649–657

Jais, J.P., Knebelmann, B., Giatras, I., De Marchi, M., Rizzoni, G., Renieri, M., et al. (2003). X-linked Alport syndrome: natural history and genotype-phenotype correlations in girls and women belonging to 195 families: a "European Community Alport Syndrome Concerted Action" study. *Journal of the American Society of Nephrology, 14,* 2603–2610

Kashtan, C.E. (1998). Alport syndrome and thin glomerular basement membrane disease. *Journal of the American Society of Nephrology, 9,* 1736–1750

Kashtan, C.E. (1999). Alport syndrome: is diagnosis only skin deep? *Kidney International, 55,* 1575–1576

Kashtan, C.E., Kleppel, M.M., & Gubler, M.C. (1996). Immunohistologic findings in Alport syndrome. In: K. Tryggvason (Ed.), *Molecular Pathology and Genetics of Alport Syndrome* (pp. 172–182). Basel: Karger

Kawakami H., Murakami T., Murano I., Ushijima T., Taguchi T., Hattori S., et al. (1990). Chronic nephritis, sensorineural deafness, growth and developmental retardation, hyperkinesis, and cleft soft palate in a 5-year-old boy. A new combination? *Nephron, 56,* 214–217

Lemmink, H.H., Schröder, C.H., Monnens, L.A.H., Smeets, H.J.M. (1997). The clinical spectrum of type IV collagen mutations. *Human Mutations, 9,* 477–499

Merchant, S.N., Burgess, B., Adams, J., Kashtan, C., Gregory, M., Santi, P., et al. (2004). Temporal bone histopathology in Alport syndrome. *Laryngoscope, 114,* 1609–1618

Muda, A.O., Massella, L., Giannakakis, K., Renieri, A., Rizzoni, G., & Faraggiana, T. (2003). Confocal microscopy of the skin in the diagnosis of X-linked Alport syndrome. *Journal of Investigative Dermatology, 121,* 208–211

Pescucci, C., Mari, F., Longo, I., Vogiatzi, P., Caselli, R., Scala, E., et al. (2004). Autosomal-dominant Alport syndrome: natural history of a disease due to COL4A3 or COL4A5 gene. *Kidney International, 65,* 1598–1603

Pirson, Y. (1999). Making the diagnosis of Alport's syndrome. *Kidney International, 56,* 760–775

Senner, R.N. (1998). Hereditary nephritis (Alport Syndrome): MR imaging findings in the brain. *Computerized Medical Imaging & Graphics, 22,* 71–72

Shields, G.W., Pataki, C. & DeList, L.E. (1990). A family with Alport syndrome and psychosis. *Schizophrenia Research, 3,* 235–239

Chapter 18

Amyotrophic Lateral Sclerosis

William D. Hula and Saša A. Živković

◆ General Information on Disorder

The terms *amyotrophic lateral sclerosis* (ALS) and *motor neuron disease* (MND) are often used interchangeably. However, although MND includes different clinical syndromes that may affect lower or upper motor neurons, or both, ALS is the most common adult motor neuron disease causing degeneration of both upper and lower motor neurons (Brooks, Miller, Swash, & Munsat, 2000). It is a neurodegenerative disorder resulting in progressive weakness and death, usually from respiratory failure. Diagnosis is based on clinical and electrodiagnostic findings, together with the absence of neuroimaging or laboratory evidence of another disorder that may mimic ALS. Initially, patients usually present with bulbar or asymmetric limb weakness, followed by progression locally, before involving other regions. Rarely, patients report pain or paresthesias. Weakness affects skeletal and bulbar muscles, and ocular weakness is apparent only in end-stage patients receiving prolonged ventilatory support (Borasio & Miller, 2001). Bulbar symptoms are the initial presenting signs in 20 to 30% of cases overall, and >50% in older women (Li, Alberman, & Swash, 1990). Differential diagnosis includes delayed postpolio syndrome, tandem cervical myelopathy and lumbosacral radiculopathies, multifocal motor neuropathy, lead intoxication, and polymyositis.

◆ Diagnostic Signs and Symptoms

Early signs and symptoms are variable, but the clinical findings that emerge over time are characterized by a combination of upper motor neuron (UMN) (spasticity, hyperreflexia, pathological reflexes, pseudobulbar affect) and lower motor neuron (LMN) (weakness, hypotonia, hyporeflexia, fasciculations, muscle atrophy) signs in a widespread distribution. Diagnosis of clinically definite ALS requires the presence of UMN and LMN signs in at least three body regions (e.g., lumbosacral, thoracic, cervical, bulbar) (Brooks et al, 2000). Sialorrhea is frequently present, and is related to dysphagia, rather than excessive production of saliva. Fasciculations are seen in nearly all patients, and when they occur in conjunction with weakness and upper motor neuron signs, are highly suggestive of ALS. Benign fasciculations can occur in normal individuals, and are not associated with other neurological signs.

Neuropathology

The neuropathological findings in ALS are distinct, with loss and degeneration of the large anterior horn cells of the spinal cord and lower cranial motor nuclei of the brainstem. Upper motor neurons in the motor cortex are affected as well. Histopathological studies of the central nervous system demonstrate neuronal atrophy with relative increase in lipofuscin and loss of Nissl substance, with accumulation of phosphorylated neurofilaments and ubiquitin-positive inclusions (Brooks et al, 2000; Hirano, 1996). These findings can be seen in other neurodegenerative disorders as well. Additionally, small eosinophilic granular inclusions, known as Bunina bodies, can be identified in anterior horn cells (Hirano, 1996).

Epidemiology

The annual incidence of ALS has been estimated as 0.3 to 2 per 100,000 population, with a prevalence of up to 9 per 100,000. Mean age of onset is 57 years, with a median survival of 4.0 years (Ringel et al, 1993). In 5% of patients the onset of symptoms occurs before the age of 30. Traditionally, ALS has been considered more common in men, but newer studies show identical incidence in men and women (Sorenson, Stalker, Kurland, & Windebank, 2002).

Genetics

The etiology of nonfamilial ALS remains unknown, and 5 to 10% of cases are familial. In most of these families there is evidence of autosomal dominant inheritance, whereas autosomal recessive inheritance is rare (Figlewicz & Orrell, 2003). In 20% of familial cases, a mutation in the enzyme *superoxide dismutase* has been demonstrated, but the relevance of this finding for other cases of ALS is unclear. These patients present at a slightly earlier age, but their presentation and course are almost indistinguishable from nonfamilial ALS. A second gene associated with juvenile ALS has been identified as *alsin* (Figlewicz & Orrell, 2003).

◆ Speech Impairment Associated with Disorder

ALS is associated with progressive mixed spastic-flaccid dysarthria and dysphagia. Although both spastic and flaccid signs are typically present, either may predominate and the pattern may evolve over time (Darley, Aronson, & Brown, 1969). The majority of patients develops dysarthria and become anarthric by the time of death (Saunders, Walsh, & Smith, 1981).

Diagnostic Signs and Symptoms

The most prominent perceptual characteristics of the dysarthria associated with ALS include imprecise consonants, hypernasality, harsh voice, slowed rate, monopitch, short phrases, and distorted vowels (Darley et al, 1969). Nonspeech oral motor findings include hyperreflexia, increased tone, and slow movements in systems with UMN involvement, and hyporeflexia, low tone, fasciculations, and muscle atrophy in systems with LMN involvement.

Etiology and Neuropathology

The speech impairments observed in ALS are due to the loss and degeneration of neurons in the motor cortex, the corticobulbar and (to a lesser extent) corticospinal tracts, and the motor neurons of brainstem, and spinal cord.

Associated Cognitive, Linguistic, and Communicative Signs and Symptoms

Pseudobulbar affect is common in ALS (Borasio & Miller, 2001). Contrary to traditional views of ALS as a disorder only of motor function, it has been associated in some cases with frontal lobe dysfunction, and studies have shown mild declines in cognitive or language performance in up to one third of cases (Massman et al, 1996).

Special Diagnostic Considerations

Given that bulbar presentation is not uncommon, the observation of progressive UMN and LMN signs on motor speech and oral-motor nonspeech exam, absent other compelling explanation, should provoke the appropriate medical referrals to rule out a diagnosis of ALS. Marked declines in speech intelligibility in ALS are preceded by slowing of speech rate, with precipitous drops in intelligibility occurring when speech rate falls below 100 to 120 words per minute (WPM) (Ball, Willis, Beukelman, & Pattee, 2001). Reduced intelligibility in ALS has been most strongly linked to impaired velopharyngeal and phonatory function, with lingual articulatory function also implicated (Kent et al, 1992).

Treatment

Palatal prostheses have been reported to increase intelligibility in ALS patients (Esposito, Mitsumoto, & Shanks, 2000), and a range of alternative and augmentative communication (AAC) options are available. AAC interventions should anticipate the progression of patients' symptoms, taking into account factors including individual needs, hand function, and mobility (Yorkston, Strand, Miller, Hillel, & Smith, 1993). Interventions focusing on speaker, listener, and situation-oriented communication strategies may also be useful (Duffy, 1995).

References

Ball, L.J., Willis, A., Beukelman, D.R., & Pattee, G.L. (2001). A protocol for identification of early bulbar signs in amyotrophic lateral sclerosis. *Journal of the Neurological Sciences, 191,* 43–53

Borasio, G.D. & Miller, R.G. (2001). Clinical characteristics and management of ALS. *Seminars in Neurology, 21,* 155–166

Brooks, B.R., Miller, R.G., Swash, M., & Munsat, T.L. (2000). El Escorial revisited: revised criteria for the diagnosis of amyotrophic lateral sclerosis. *Amyotrophic Lateral Sclerosis and Other Motor Neuron Disorders, 1,* 293–299

Darley, F.L., Aronson, A.E., & Brown, J.R. (1969). Differential diagnostic patterns of dysarthria. *Journal of Speech and Hearing Research, 12,* 246–269

Duffy, J. (1995). *Motor Speech Disorders: Substrates, Differential Diagnosis, and Management.* St. Louis: Mosby

Esposito, S.J., Mitsumoto, H., & Shanks, M. (2000). Use of palatal lift and palatal augmentation prostheses to improve dysarthria in patients with amyotrophic lateral sclerosis: a case series. *Journal of Prosthetic Dentistry, 83,* 90–98

Figlewicz, D.A. & Orrell, R.W. (2003). The genetics of motor neuron diseases. *Amyotrophic Lateral Sclerosis and Other Motor Neuron Disorders, 4,* 225–231

Hirano, A. (1996). Neuropathology of ALS: an overview. *Neurology, 47,* S63–S66

Kent, J.F., Kent, R.D., Rosenbek, J.C., Weismer, G., Martin, R., Sufit, R., et al. (1992). Quantitative description of the dysarthria in women with amyotrophic lateral sclerosis. *Journal of Speech and Hearing Research, 35,* 723–733

Li, T.M., Alberman, E., & Swash, M. (1990). Clinical features and associations of 560 cases of motor neuron disease. *Journal of Neurology, Neurosurgery, and Psychiatry, 53,* 1043–1045

Massman, P.J., Sims, J., Cooke, N., Haverkamp, L.J., Appel, V., & Appel, S.H. (1996). Prevalence and correlates of neuropsychological deficits in amyotrophic lateral sclerosis. *Journal of Neurology, Neurosurgery, and Psychiatry, 61,* 450–455

Ringel, S.P., Murphy, J.R., Alderson, M.K., Bryan, W., England, J.D., Miller, R.G., et al. (1993). The natural history of amyotrophic lateral sclerosis. *Neurology, 43,* 1316–1322

Saunders, C., Walsh, T., & Smith, M. (1981). Hospice care in the motor neuron diseases. In: C. Saunders & J. Teller (Eds.), *Hospice: The Living Idea* (pp. 223–235). London: Edward Arnold

Sorenson, E.J., Stalker, A.P., Kurland, L.T., & Windebank, A.J. (2002). Amyotrophic lateral sclerosis in Olmsted County, Minnesota, 1925 to 1998. *Neurology, 59,* 280–282

Yorkston, K. M., Strand, E., Miller, R., Hillel, A., & Smith, K. (1993). Speech deterioration in amyotrophic lateral sclerosis: implications for the timing of intervention. *Journal of Medical Speech-Language Pathology, 1,* 35–46

Additional Reading

Dangond, F. (2006). Amyotrophic lateral sclerosis. http://www.emedicine.com/neuro/topic14.htm

Mitsumoto, H. & Munsat, T.L. (2001). *Amyotrophic Lateral Sclerosis. A Guide for Patients and Families.* New York: Demos

Shaw, P.J. & Strong, M.J. (2003). *Motor Neuron Disorders (Blue Books of Practical Neurology,* vol. 28). Boston: Butterworth-Heinemann

Yorkston, K.M., Miller, R.M., & Strand, E.A. (1995). *Management of Speech and Swallowing Disorders in Degenerative Disease.* Tucson, AZ: Communication Skill Builders

Chapter 19

Angelman Syndrome

Robin L. Alvares

♦ General Information on Disorder

Angelman (1965) described three "puppet" children with distinctive appearance, seizures, motor delays, frequent and inappropriate laughing, and lack of speech. Reports of individuals with these characteristics resurfaced in the mid-1980s, and larger-scale studies of individuals with Angelman syndrome (AS) emerged (Clayton-Smith, 1992, 1993; Williams & Frias, 1982; Williams et al, 1995a; Zori et al, 1992).

Diagnostic Signs and Symptoms

Diagnostic criteria have been developed such that all individuals with AS exhibit the following characteristics: severe developmental delay, lack of or minimal speech production, ataxia or tremulous limbs, and frequent laughing, smiling, and hand-flapping (Williams et al, 1995a). Additional anatomical, neurological, motor, and behavioral characteristics occur with varying frequency. Physical characteristics may include hypopigmentation, prognathia, widely spaced teeth, microcephaly, and scoliosis (Clayton-Smith & Laan, 2003). Motor signs include distal lower limb spasticity and ataxic-like gait (Beckung, Steffenberg, & Kyllerman, 2004) and a motor speech disorder. Individuals often exhibit abnormal electroencephalogram (EEG) and seizures, hyperactivity, fascination with water, socially inappropriate laughter, and sleep disturbances.

Neuropathology

There have been few cases available for postmortem study; however, some abnormalities that have been reported include cerebellar hyperplasia (Williams & Frias, 1982), unilateral temporal hypoplasia (Van-Lierde, Atza, Giardino, & Viani, 1990), decreased myelinization and thinning of the corpus callosum (Zori et al, 1992).

The majority of individuals with AS experience seizures (90%), and seizures typically occur before age 3 (Zori et al, 1992) and are often of the "absence" or "myoclonic" variety (Guerrini, Carrozzo, Rinaldi, & Bonanni, 2003). Although there is no definitive characteristic EEG pattern associated with AS, most individuals exhibit delta, theta, and posterior discharge patterns suggestive of seizure activity (Valente, Andrade, Grossman, Kok, Fridman, Koiffmann, & Marques-Dias, 2003).

Epidemiology

Williams (2003) suggested 1 in 15,000 children and young adults have AS. Most patients identified in North America have been Caucasian; however, the syndrome has been observed in all racial groups and shows no apparent gender predilection (Williams et al, 1995b).

Genetics

Several genetic sequelae may result in AS. All interfere with the expression of the *UB3EA* gene. At present, there are four known genetic phenotypes of AS.

The most common genetic cause of AS is deletion of the 15q11–13 region of the maternally derived chromosome. Approximately 70% of individuals with AS are considered deletion positive. Paternal uniparental disomy (UPD) accounts for approximately 7% of cases of AS. UPD occurs when both 15th chromosomes are inherited from the father. Individuals with UPD tend to exhibit less severe developmental delays (Clayton-Smith & Laan, 2003). Three percent of individuals with AS have an identifiable imprinting center defect. In this phenotype, a portion of the 15th chromosome responsible for replicating the 15q11–13 region is defective. Approximately 10% of individuals with AS have a mutation of the *UBE3A* gene in the 15q11–13 region. The remaining 10% of individuals have no identifiable genetic anomaly.

In many cases, AS appears to be a spontaneous mutation. Several recent studies have suggested a link between some cases of AS and in vitro fertilization (Green, 2004; Ludwig, Katalinic, Gross, Varon, & Horsthemke, 2004).

♦ Speech Impairment Associated with Disorder

One clinical diagnostic criterion for Angelman syndrome is a marked lack of speech. Individuals with Angelman syndrome either use no speech or only a limited number of words, though nonspeech vocalizations and the meaningful use of intonation are observed (Alvares & Downing, 1998; Angelman, 1965; Clayton-Smith, 1992, 1993; Williams et al, 1995a; Williams & Frias, 1982).

Diagnostic Signs and Symptoms

Craniofacial characteristics associated with the syndrome include prognathia, which entails protruding and wide mouth with widely spaced teeth.

Etiology

Anatomical and motor differences do not appear to account entirely for the diminished speech production in individuals with AS. It has been argued that there is a gap between expressive and receptive communication that may be explained by a severe oral motor problem that resembles apraxia of speech (Alvares & Downing, 1998; Jolleff & Ryan, 1993).

Neuropathology

At present, no specific neuropathology has been associated with the clinical, oral, and motor picture observed in AS.

Associated Cognitive, Linguistic, and Communicative Signs and Symptoms

Individuals with AS tend to exhibit severe to profound mental retardation; however, due to diminished speech production and motor and attention deficits in these individuals, it may be difficult to assess. Some researchers have reported a phenotypic overlap between AS and autism in a subgroup with AS (Peters, Beaudet, Madduri, & Bacino, 2004).

Special Diagnostic Considerations

Feeding and swallowing problems have not been widely reported in the literature; however, several cases of dysphagia have been reported anecdotally. Several individuals with AS have gastrostomy tubes.

Treatment

Developmental delays may limit the potential for effective treatment of speech and feeding problems for most individuals with AS. Clinicians and families have reported difficulty with behavioral interventions to discourage mouthing and instead have sought appropriate objects to provide oral input. Some clinicians have anecdotally reported success with oral brushing or vibration prior to feeding to increase oral input and improve feeding; however, no documented efficacy evidence has accompanied these observations. Likewise, successful therapeutic strategies for the development of usable speech, such as intensive oral motor therapy, have not been documented in the literature and have only been described anecdotally. Many individuals with AS demonstrate adequate oral motor control in the ability to use some meaningful speech, and others are able to combine limb gestures with meaningful intonation. It is suggested that a combination of speech and nonspeech modalities be used to provide communication systems that maximize opportunities for meaningful communication (Alvares & Downing, 1998). Gestures (Calculator, 2002), sign language, picture systems, and voice output augmentative/alternative communication systems have been used with varying rates of success.

References

Alvares, R.L. & Downing, S. F. (1998). A survey of expressive communication skills in children with Angelman syndrome. *American Journal of Speech-Language Pathology, 7,* 14–24

Angelman, H. (1965). "Puppet" children, a report on three cases. *Developmental Medicine and Child Neurology, 7,* 681–688

Beckung, E., Steffenburg, S., & Kyllerman, M. (2004). Motor impairments, neurological signs, and developmental level in individuals with Angelman syndrome. *Developmental Medicine and Child Neurology, 46,* 239–243

Calculator, S.N. (2002). Use of enhanced natural gestures to foster interactions between children with Angelman syndrome and their parents. *American Journal of Speech-Language Pathology, 11,* 340–355

Clayton-Smith, J. (1992) Angelman's syndrome. *Archives of Disease in Childhood, 67,* 889–891

Clayton-Smith, J. (1993). Clinical research on Angelman Syndrome in the United Kingdom: observations on 82 affected individuals. *American Journal of Medical Genetics, 46,* 12–15

Clayton-Smith, J., & Laan, L. (2003). Angelman syndrome: a review of the clinical and genetic aspects. *Journal of Medical Genetics, 40,* 87–95

Green, N.S. (2004). Risks of birth defects and other adverse outcomes associated with assisted reproductive technology. *Pediatrics, 114,* 256–259

Guerrini, R., Carozzo, R., Rinaldi, R., & Bonanni, P. (2003). Argelman Syndrome: etiology, clinical features, diagnosis, and management of symptoms. *Pediatric Drugs, 5*(10), 646–661

Jolleff, N. & Ryan, M.M. (1993). Communication development in Angelman's syndrome. *Archives of Disease in Childhood, 69,* 148–150

Ludwig, M., Katalinic, A., Gross, S., Varon, R. & Horsthemke, B. (2004). *Fertility and Sterility, 82,* S49

Peters, S.U., Beaudet, A.L., Madduri, N. & Bacino, C.A. (2004). Autism in Angelman syndrome: implications for autism research. *Clinical Genetics, 66,* 530–536

Valente, K.D., Andrade, J.Q., Grossmann, R.M., Kok, F., Fridman, C., Koiffmann, C.P., & Marques-Dias, M.J. (2003). Angelman syndrome: difficulties in EEG pattern recognition and possible misinterpretations. *Epilepsia, 44,* 1051–1063

Van-Lierde, A., Atza, M.G., Giardino, D., & Viani, F. (1990). Angelman's syndrome in the first year of life. *Developmental Medicine and Child Neurology, 32,* 1011–1016

Williams, C.A. (2003). *Incidence Statistics. How Common Is Angelman Syndrome?* Aurora, IL: Angelman Syndrome Foundation

Williams, C.A., Angelman, H., Clayton-Smith, J., Driscoll, D.J., Hendrickson, J.E., Knoll, J.H.M., Magenis, R.E., Schnizel, A., Wagstaff, J., Whidden, E.M., & Zori, R.T. (1995a). Angelman syndrome: consensus for diagnostic criteria. *American Journal of Medical Genetics, 56,* 237–238

Williams, C.A. & Frias, J.L. (1982). The Angelman ("happy puppet") syndrome. *American Journal of Medical Genetics, 11,* 453–460

Williams, C.A., Zori, R.T., Hendrickson, J., Stalker, H., Marum, T., Whidden, E.Y., Driscol, D.J. (1995b). Angelman syndrome. *Current Problems in Pediatrics, 25,* 216–231

Zori, R.T., Hendrickson, J., Woolven, S., Whidden, E.M., Gray, B., & Williams, C.A. (1992). Angelman syndrome: clinical profile. *Journal of Child Neurology, 7*(3), 270–280

Chapter 20

Apraxia of Speech in Childhood

Thomas Campbell and Sharon A. Gretz

◆ General Information on Disorder

Consistent with the definition and identifying characteristics of adult acquired apraxia of speech (McNeil, Robin, & Schmidt, 1997), childhood apraxia of speech (CAS) is a phonetic-motor disorder of speech production characterized by a disruption in the planning and programming of voluntary, complex motor activity for speech production. The core clinical features of CAS that have been hypothesized to distinguish it from other childhood disorders of speech-sound production include abnormal articulatory transitions, resulting in increased durations between speech sounds and syllables, and increased speech-sound durations; and abnormal lexical and sentence stress patterns. These children also display difficulty in establishing and maintaining appropriate articulatory postures, resulting in reduced articulatory precision especially when producing longer and more complex syllable structures. The basic underlying cause of the disorder has been hypothesized to be a deficit in the translation of an abstract phonological code into a motor command (Maassen, 2004; McNeil et al, 1997).

Diagnostic Signs and Symptoms

Children with CAS often display several speech characteristics and clinical outcomes that may be important features of the child's overall clinical profile, but they have not been proven to differentiate CAS from other childhood speech-sound disorders. Severely reduced speech intelligibility, inconsistent omissions and substitutions of consonant phonemes and vowel distortions have been reported to be important speech characteristics of young children with apraxia of speech. For very young children suspected of having CAS, few verbal attempts or a complete paucity of consonant and vowel productions have been reported as potential diagnostic markers. In addition, it has been posited that children with CAS display reduced speech-sound normalization rates and often require lengthy treatment programs to achieve intervention goals. Finally, the expressive language skills of these children have been described as significantly lower than their receptive language abilities. However, these clinical characteristics have also been reported for children with various other developmental and acquired speech-sound production disorders. To date, no studies have appropriately examined the sensitivity and specificity of these clinical characteristics for classifying

children with apraxia of speech. This has primarily been due to the lack of an agreed upon definition of CAS among clinicians and researchers.

Neuropathology

Childhood apraxia of speech can result from stroke, tumor, and seizure disorder, or from diffuse cortical damage associated with traumatic brain injury. However, the neuropathology of CAS is unknown for the vast majority of children. The reported neurological findings and profiles of these children vary considerably, with no consistent anatomical localization accounting for the severe motor-speech deficit. Emerging data suggest that the key to uncovering the neural mechanisms that are associated with CAS are dependent on understanding the neurogenetic expression of specific genes and proteins that are associated with normal and abnormal brain development (Vargha-Khadem, Gadian, Copp, & Mishkin, 2005).

Epidemiology

Prevalence estimates for CAS range from 1 to 2 children per 1000 to 10 to 12 children per 1000 (Shriberg, Aram, & Kwiatkowski, 1997). The ratio of affected males to females has been estimated to be 2:1 (Lewis et al, 2004b). The prevalence rate of CAS may be higher in children with other comorbid diagnoses (Maassen, 2004). It is important to note that previously reported prevalence estimates have not been verified with appropriately designed epidemiological investigations.

Genetics

Familial aggregation studies suggest that CAS is a highly heritable speech disorder. Lewis et al (2004b) reported that in a group of 22 children diagnosed with CAS, 86% had at least one nuclear family member with a history of speech and language disorders, and 59% of the children with CAS had at least one affected parent. These percentages of affected nuclear family members are higher than those reported for children with speech delay of unknown origin (Campbell et al, 2003).

Familial aggregation alone does not provide ample evidence for a genetic cause of CAS, given that such findings could be linked to various cultural transmission variables including environmental factors. However, results from recent molecular genetic studies suggest that a mutation of one or more genes may underlie apraxia of speech in some individuals, although it should be noted that the majority of these studies have not employed a consistent and well-defined definition of CAS. Lai, Fisher, Hurst, Vargha-Khadem, and Monaco (2001) reported that a mutation of the *FOXP2* gene, located on the chromosomal band 7q31, was associated with severe apraxia of speech in the three generational KE family. Recently, MacDermot et al (2005) detected genetic variants that alter FOXP2 protein sequences in a separate group of children with an unsubstantiated diagnosis of apraxia of speech. As the control mechanisms of the *FOXP2* gene and associated proteins are further specified, important information will likely emerge concerning the neuronal processes involved in childhood apraxia of speech and other speech and language disorders.

◆ Speech Impairment Associated with Disorder

The general speech characteristics of children suspected of having apraxia of speech were described earlier (see General Information on Disorder). As noted, many of these speech characteristics are not be specific to CAS and overlap with other types of pediatric speech disorders. Data reported by Shriberg, Campbell, Karlsson, Brown, McSweeny, and Nadler (2003) are consistent with the core-identifying speech characteristics, which include abnormal intersegment transitions, reduced speaking rate, and abnormal lexical and sentence stress patterns. In addition, the maintenance of articulatory precision when producing longer and more complex syllable structures has been shown to be compromised, even after speech intelligibility has normalized.

Diagnostic Signs and Symptoms

The diagnostic signs and symptoms associated with the speech deficit of CAS were outlined earlier (see Diagnostic Signs and Symptoms under the heading General Information on Disorder).

Neuropathology and Etiology

As mention previously, the neuropathology and etiology of CAS are unknown for the majority of affected children.

Associated Cognitive, Linguistic, and Communicative Signs and Symptoms

A variety of linguistic deficits have been reported to occur frequently in CAS. Both receptive and expressive language deficits have been reported, with receptive skills often being superior to expressive skills (Lewis, Freebairn, Hansen, Iyengar, & Taylor, 2004a). Academic difficulties also have been noted including reading (decoding and comprehension) and spelling.

Special Diagnostic Considerations

There are two special diagnostic considerations for the assessment of children with apraxia of speech. First, there are likely to be specific differences in the clinical presentation of apraxia of speech in children and adults because children are in the process of speech and language development. Difficulty in the motor planning and programming of speech-sound production during the primary period of speech and language development predictably has important effects on other cognitive-linguistic functions. This may result in quite different clinical profiles for younger and older children with apraxia of speech. These differences between the child and adult versions of the disorder notwithstanding, our view is that many of the core speech characteristics described previously are the same for children and adults. Second, and most important, without a clear and agreed-upon definition of the disorder, both clinicians and researchers will find it difficult to differentiate with acceptable sensitivity and specificity children with apraxia of speech from other childhood speech-sound production disorders.

Treatment

Intervention programs for children with apraxia of speech consist of a variety of approaches including integral stimulation methods, motor-articulatory placement approaches, tactile-kinesthetic techniques, as well as various rhythmic and gestural approaches (Square, 1999; Strand & Skinder, 1999). Treatment efficacy and effectiveness data for children with apraxia of speech have not been reported for any specific treatment method. However, positive treatment outcomes have been reported for children who have clinical profiles consistent with the diagnosis of apraxia of speech using a hybrid integral stimulation approach (Campbell, 1999). Some children with the most severe or resistant CAS may require augmentative or alternative communication to assist in communication interactions (Cumley & Swanson, 1999).

References

Campbell, T.F. (1999). Functional treatment outcomes in young children with motor speech disorders. In: A.J. Caruso & E.A. Strand (Eds.), *Clinical Management of Motor Speech Disorders in Children* (pp. 385–396). New York: Thieme

Campbell, T.F., Dollaghan, C.A., Rockette, H.E., Paradise, J.L., Feldman, H.M., Shriberg, L.D., Sabo, D., & Kurs-Lasky, M. (2003). Risk factors for speech delay in three-year-old children. *Child Development, 74,* 346–357

Cumley, G.D., & Swanson, S. (1999). Augmentative and alternative communication options for children with developmental apraxia of speech: three case studies. *Augmentative & Alternative Communication, 15,* 110–125

Lai, C.S.L, Fisher, S.E., Hurst, J.A., Vargha-Khadem, F., & Monaco, A.P. (2001). A novel forkhead-domain gene is mutated in a severe speech and language disorder. *Nature, 413,* 519–523

Lewis, B.A., Freebairn, L.A., Hansen, A., Iyengar S., & Taylor, H.G. (2004a). School-age follow up of children with childhood apraxia of speech. *Language Speech and Hearing Services in the Schools, 35,* 122–140

Lewis, B.A., Freebairn, L.A., Hansen, A., Taylor, H.G., Iyengar, S., & Shriberg, L.D. (2004b). Family pedigrees of children with suspected childhood apraxia of speech. *Journal of Communication Disorders, 37,* 157–175

Maassen, B. (2004) Speech output disorders. In: L. Verhoeven & H. van Balkom (Eds.), *Classification of Developmental Language Disorders* (pp. 175–190). Mahway, NJ: Lawrence Erlbaum Associates.

MacDermot, K.D., Bonora, E., Sykes, N., Coupe, A.M., Cecilia, S.L., Lai, C.S.L. Vernes, S.C., Vargha-Khadem, F., McKenzie, F., Smith, R.L., Monaco, A.P. & Fisher, S.E. (2004). Identification of FOXP2 truncation as a novel cause of developmental speech & language deficits. *American Journal of Human Genetics, 76,* 1074–1080

McNeil, M.R., Robin, D.A., & Schmidt, R.A. (1997). Apraxia of speech: definition, differentiation and treatment. In: M.R. McNeil (Ed.), *Clinical Management of Sensorimotor Speech Disorders* (pp. 311–344). New York: Thieme

Shriberg, L.D., Aram, D.M., & Kwiatkowski, J. (1997) Developmental apraxia of speech: I. descriptive and theoretical perspectives. *Journal of Speech, Language, and Hearing Research, 40,* 273–285

Shriberg, L.D., Campbell, T.F., Karlsson, H.B., Brown, R.L., McSweeny, J.L., & Nadler, C.J. (2003). A diagnostic marker for childhood apraxia of speech: the lexical stress ratio. *Clinical Linguistics and Phonetics, 17,* 549–574

Square, P.A. (1999). Treatment of developmental apraxia of speech: tactile-kinesthetic, rhythmic, and gestural approaches. In: A.J. Caruso & E.A. Strand (Eds.), *Clinical Management of Motor Speech Disorders in Children* (pp. 149–185). New York: Thieme

Strand, E.A. & Skinder, A. (1999). Treatment of developmental apraxia of speech: integral stimulation methods. In: A.J. Caruso & E.A. Strand (Eds.), *Clinical Management of Motor Speech Disorders in Children* (pp. 109–148). New York: Thieme

Vargha-Khadem, F., Gadian, D.G., Copp, A., & Mishkin, M. (2005). FOXP2 and the neuroanatomy of speech and language. *Nature Review Neuroscience, 6,* 131–138

Chapter 21

Athetoid Cerebral Palsy

Debra M. Suiter and Michael P. Cannito

◆ General Information on Disorder

Athetoid cerebral palsy is the second most common form of cerebral palsy (Taft, 1995). Athetosis is characterized by fluctuations in muscle tone and is sometimes associated with uncontrolled, involuntary movements (Molnar, 1973). Children with athetoid cerebral palsy present with impaired postural stability, oromotor dysfunction, and, possibly, cognitive deficits (Yokochi, Shimabukuro, Kodama, Kodama, & Hosoe, 1993). Generally, all four limbs are affected. There may also be a history of dysphagia, drooling, and dysarthria. In addition, hearing loss is frequently associated with athetoid cerebral palsy.

Diagnostic Signs and Symptoms

The hallmark of athetosis is unbalanced and fluctuating muscle tone (Molnar, 1973). Athetosis can vary in severity from that detectible only with a maximum performance test and restricted to a single body part, such as a single speech articulator, to very severe and present throughout the body. Infants with athetoid cerebral palsy typically present with a specific set of motor symptoms, including difficulty maintaining a symmetric supine posture, decreased upper extremity forward extension, limited neck and trunk stability, and either asymmetric or excessive opening of the mouth (Molnar, 1973). Signs and symptoms that may be present in infancy include generalized hypotonia, poor spontaneous movements, difficulty feeding, continuous head-turning to one side, and occasional extensor spasms (Yokochi et al., 1993). Children fail to achieve sitting balance at the expected developmental age, and there is a delay in the disappearance of several primitive reflexes including the asymmetric tonic neck, Moro, and Galant reflexes (Yokochi et al., 1993). Children with athetoid cerebral palsy present with involuntary writhing movements of the hands, feet, and face. These movements may not become evident until 18 months of age and may appear as late as 3 years (Molnar, 1973). Movements are frequently exacerbated by times of emotional stress and during adolescence. Athetosis may coexist with other motor deficits, including dystonia, chorea, and other forms of dyskinesia (Molnar, 1973).

Neuropathology

Athetosis results from basal ganglia damage. Specific lesion site is dependent on the etiology of the disorder. Individuals with kernicterus (bilirubin encephalopathy) usually present with lesions in the globus pallidus, subthalamic nucleus, and hippocampus, whereas individuals with perinatal anoxia usually present with lesions involving the putamen, basal ganglia, and thalamus (Hayashi, Satoh, Sakamoto, & Morimatsu, 1991). Clinical presentation differs depending on the lesion site. Individuals with athetosis resulting from kernicterus present with rigidospasticity and fluctuating athetoid movements, whereas individuals with athetosis resulting from perinatal anoxia exhibit a variety of muscle tone abnormalities, including hypotonia, mild spasticity, and rigidospasticity (Hayashi et al, 1991).

Epidemiology

The overall incidence of cerebral palsy is 2 to 4 cases per 1000 live births. Despite recent advances in perinatal care, the prevalence of cerebral palsy, approximately 2%, has remained unchanged over the past 30 years (Taft, 1995). Athetoid cerebral palsy accounts for approximately 10 to 20% of all cases of cerebral palsy (Taft, 1995).

Genetics

Most cases of athetoid cerebral palsy are attributable to perinatal complications. However, genetic factors may contribute to the development of athetoid cerebral palsy. Reports indicate a frequency of familial recurrence of athetoid cerebral palsy of 1.6% (Amor, Craig, Delatycki, & Reddihough, 2001). This incidence is roughly equivalent to the recurrence risk for cerebral palsy in general. Several conditions, including parental consanguinity, male gender, advanced paternal age, and microcephaly, have been associated with an increased risk of recurrence of athetoid cerebral palsy (Amor et al, 2001). It has also been suggested that some cases of athetoid cerebral palsy are due to autosomal-recessive inheritance, whereas others are due to X-linked recessive inheritance (Amor et al, 2001).

◆ Speech Impairment Associated with Disorder

Individuals with athetoid cerebral palsy present with hyperkinetic or athetoid dysarthria (Darley, Aronson, & Brown, 1975). Speech intelligibility is usually reduced significantly. Articulation is characterized by abnormally large jaw range of motion, lingua-mandibular dependence, slow and variable rate of production, prolonged transition times for articulatory movements, and retrusion of the lower lip (Kent & Netsell, 1978). Respiration is characterized by persistence of belly breathing, that is, contraction of the diaphragm with little or no thoracic expansion, beyond 6 months of age, and paradoxical breathing (depression of the upper chest during inhalation) (Love, 2000). Phonation is characterized by monopitch, low pitch, and forced vocal quality. Resonance is characterized by difficulty in achieving and maintaining velopharyngeal closure (Love, 2000).

Diagnostic Signs and Symptoms

Athetosis is characterized by irregular, variable involuntary movements. Individuals with athetoid cerebral palsy may exhibit several involuntary motor responses of the orofacial mechanism, including facial grimacing, spasms, blocking, tongue thrusting, and gagging (Neilson & O'Dwyer, 1984). The dysarthria that occurs in athetoid cerebral palsy is thought to be a result of these involuntary movements. However, research indicates that some aspects of speech production, including syllable production, are affected by irregular voluntary rather than involuntary movements. Neilson and O'Dwyer studied speech articulation using electromyography in a group of individuals with athetoid cerebral palsy and noted that abnormal involuntary movements typically occurred between, rather than during, production of syllables. Movement patterns during syllable production were consistent and reproducible. The authors concluded that irregular voluntary movements were the primary cause of speech production errors evidenced in athetoid dysarthria. However, respiratory and phonatory function and their effects on speech production were not examined in this study. In addition, abnormal involuntary movements that were noted between syllable productions may affect other aspects of speech production such as syllable timing and prosody, both of which are disordered in athetoid dysarthria. Thus, both involuntary and voluntary irregular movements likely contribute to speech patterns evidenced in athetoid dysarthria.

Etiology

Two etiologies have been linked to athetoid cerebral palsy: (1) kernicterus, and (2) perinatal anoxia or perinatal hypoxic-ischemic encephalopathy (Molnar, 1973). Kernicterus can occur due to Rh incompatibility between the mother and fetus, an infection causing destruction of infant red blood cells, or a genetic factor preventing adequate bilirubin clearance from the blood. Routine testing for Rh incompatibility and improvements in prevention of bilirubin

accumulation led to a significant decline in reported cases of kernicterus in the 1970s and 1980s. However, the 1990s saw a reemergence of kernicterus. This was attributed to early discharge of term infants, which typically occurs before their bilirubin levels peak (MMWR, 2001). Currently, perinatal asphyxia is the most common cause of athetoid cerebral palsy.

Neuropathology

Athetoid dysarthria may result in part from a motor learning deficit (Kent & Netsell, 1978). Motor learning principles suggest that motor commands are developed by forming correlations between previously learned motor activities and the sensory consequences of those activities. The periventricular lesions commonly found in cerebral palsy may interrupt the flow of neural activity from the basal ganglia and lateral areas of the cerebellum to the motor and premotor cortex, thus impairing sensorimotor integration in the premotor cortex (Neilson & O'Dwyer, 1984). This would impede motor learning.

Cerebral damage in the periaqueduct area may delay or interrupt the development of neural centers involved in the control of respiration and phonation (Love, 2000). Such damage may account for the persistence of immature breathing patterns, such as belly breathing and abnormal breathing patterns such as paradoxical breathing, both frequently observed in children with athetosis.

Associated Cognitive, Linguistic, and Communicative Signs and Symptoms

Children with athetoid cerebral palsy present with various degrees of cognitive ability, ranging from significant cognitive deficits to normal cognitive abilities (Love, 2000). Individuals with lesions in the thalamoputaminal region typically exhibit lower intelligence quotients than those with lesions of the globus pallidus and subthalamic nucleus (Hayashi et al, 1991). Language abilities vary and may parallel the degree of cognitive deficit.

Special Diagnostic Considerations

The hallmark of athetoid cerebral palsy is fluctuating and unbalanced tone. There is a broad range of intelligibility deficit (mild to significant) that is similar to that seen in other forms of cerebral palsy.

Treatment

Treatment typically focuses on improving overall speech intelligibility through behavioral intervention or providing augmentative alternative communication.

References

Amor, D.J., Craig, J., Delatycki, M., & Reddihough, D. (2001). Genetic factors in athetoid cerebral palsy. *Journal of Child Neurology, 16*, 793–797

Darley, F.L. Aronson, A.E., & Brown J.R. (1975). *Motor Speech Disorders.* Philadelphia: W.B. Saunders.

Hayashi, M., Satoh, J., Sakamoto, K., & Morimatsu, Y. (1991). Clinical and neuropathological findings in severe athetoid cerebral palsy: a comparative study of globo-Luysian and thalamo-putaminal groups. *Brain and Development, 13*, 47–51

Kent, R. & Netsell, R. (1978). Articulatory abnormalities in athetoid cerebral palsy. *Journal of Speech and Hearing Disorders, 43*, 353–373

MMWR. Kernicterus in full-term infants—United States 1994–1998 (2001, June 15). *Morbidity Mortality Weekly Report*, 491–494

Love, R. (2000). *Childhood Motor Speech Disability,* 2nd ed. Needham Heights, MA: Allyn & Bacon

Molnar, G.E. (1973). Clinical aspects of cerebral palsy. *Pediatrics Annals, 2,* 10–27

Neilson, P.D. & O'Dwyer, N. (1984). Reproducibility and variability of speech muscle activity in athetoid dysarthria and cerebral palsy. *Journal of Speech and Hearing Research, 27*, 502–517

Taft, L.T. (1995). Cerebral palsy. *Pediatric Review, 16*, 411–418

Yokochi, K., Shimabukuro, S., Kodama, M., Kodama, K., & Hosoe, A. (1993). Motor function of infants with athetoid cerebral palsy. *Developmental and Medical Child Neurology, 35*, 909–916

Chapter 22

Cerebellar Mutism

Geoffrey V. Fredericks and Joseph R. Duffy

◆ General Information on Disorder

Cerebellar mutism (CM) is a form of mutism that may develop following surgical resection of posterior fossa (PF) tumors, predominately in children (Retake, Grubb, Aram, Hahn, & Ratcheson, 1985). Other terms used to describe it include *cerebellar mutism and subsequent dysarthria* (van Dongen, Catsman-Berrevoets, & van Mourik, 1994), *posterior fossa syndrome* (Doxey, Bruce, Sklar, Swift, & Shapiro, 1999), and *cerebellar mutism syndrome* (JanBen et al, 1998).

Although CM is typically associated with PF tumors in children, it occasionally has been reported in adults (Turgut, 1998). Tumor types include astrocytomas, ependymomas, and primitive neuroectodermal tumors (PNET). Associated tumor locations most often include the fourth ventricle, cerebellar vermis or paravermal areas, the left or right cerebellar hemisphere, and the pons (Doxey et al, 1998; Turgut, 1998).

The postoperative latency to onset of mutism may range from 0 to 7 days (Turgut, 1998). The period of mutism generally lasts for 4 to 8 weeks, but may range from a few days up to 12 months (Doxey et al, 1999). Following resolution of the mutism, a period of dysarthria is usually evident.

Diagnostic Signs and Symptoms

The diagnostic signs of cerebellar mutism are discussed in detail later.

Neuropathology

The underlying mechanism(s) that leads to CM is uncertain. Both multifactorial (e.g., organic and psychogenic causes) and specific organic etiologies have been postulated (Ferrante, Mastronardi, Acqui, & Fortuna, 1990), but psychogenic causes are unlikely in the vast majority of cases (Duffy, 2005). Other specific organic hypotheses include ischemia secondary to transient vasospasm of the blood supply to the cerebellum (Al-Anazi, Hassounah, Sheikh, & Barayan, 2001), cerebro-cerebellar diaschisis (Germano et al, 1998), damage to the dentatothalamocortical tracts (Crutchfield, Sawaya, Meyers, & Moore, 1994), splitting the vermis (Dailey, McKhann, & Berger, 1995), and postoperative meningitis and hydrocephalus (Ferrante et al, 1990).

Epidemiology

The incidence of CM ranges from 1.6% (Koh, Beckwitt Turkel, & Baram, 1997) to approximately 9% of all PF tumor resections in children (Dailey et al, 1995; Doxey et al, 1999).

Genetics

Because CM develops postoperatively, it does not have a primary genetic basis.

◆ Speech Impairment Associated with Disorder

The speech characteristics following the resolution of CM have been poorly described. Typically, speech is described as "dysarthric" and has been characterized by audible respirations, monotonous or a "high-pitched whiny" vocal quality, reduced or alternating loudness, a hoarse phonatory quality, slowed rate, and imprecise articulation (Pollack, Polinko, Albright, Towbin, & Fitz, 1995; van Dongen et al, 1994). In the authors' experience, following the resolution of the mutism, an ataxic dysarthria characterized by audible inspiration, slow rate, irregular articulatory breakdowns, vowel distortions, reduced pitch and loudness variation, and a scanning or "syllable-by-syllable" prosodic pattern of production is present.

Diagnostic Signs and Symptoms

Mutism may manifest itself immediately after surgery or may be delayed in onset from hours to days postoperatively during which speech is typically normal or, occasionally, dysarthric (Dailey et al, 1995; JanBen et al, 1998). The onset of mutism may co-occur with other cognitive and behavioral changes. Among these, the most typical are the presence of whining and social withdrawal (Pollack et al, 1995). During the period of mutism, attempts at speech production may be characterized by grunting or "whining" (Retake et al, 1985). An oropharyngeal apraxia has been frequently reported and its resolution may occur before or at the time of speech return (Dailey et al, 1995; Pollack et al, 1995). The return of speech is often heralded by the emergence of audible laughter or crying, followed by the production of phonemes or single words, progressing to the production of phrases and sentences (Retake et al, 1985; van Dongen et al, 1994). Full recovery of speech may occur over a period of 1 to 12 months postoperatively

(Cochrane, Gustavsson, Poskitt, Steinbok, & Kestle, 1994) but residual dysarthria has been reported as long as 2.5 years postoperatively (Retake et al, 1985), and may be permanent.

Etiology

Cerebellar mutism is typically associated with the resection of PF tumors, but it has also been reported in cases of cerebellitis (Cakir, Karakisi, & Kocanaogullari, 1994), rupture of cerebellar arteriovenous malformations (Al-Anazi et al, 2000), midbrain cavernous malformation and hematoma resection (Wang, Winston, & Breeze, 2002), and pontine lesions (Frim & Ogilvy, 1995).

Neuropathology

The underlying mechanism(s) that cause CM were discussed earlier.

Associated Cognitive, Linguistic, and Communicative Signs and Symptoms

Various cognitive, linguistic, behavioral, and neurological deficits may emerge following cerebellar tumor resection, including in people with CM. Language deficits (e.g., difficulty with syntax comprehension, reduced mean length of utterance), difficulty with problem solving, visuospatial deficits, apathy, abulia, whining, inattention, irritability, emotional lability, transient eyelid apraxia, cranial nerve (CN) palsies (e.g., CN VI, VII), and dysphagia have been reported. (Dailey et al, 1995; Levisohn, Cronin-Golomb, & Schmahmann, 2000; Pollack et al, 1995; Siffert et al, 2000).

Special Diagnostic Considerations

Because of the relatively high incidence of CM (and the possibility of associated cognitive, linguistic, or behavioral deficits that may follow PF tumor resection), both children and adults undergoing PF tumor resection should have their speech and language screened postoperatively, and, ideally, preoperatively. Nonspeech oromotor functions, including praxis, also should be assessed, especially if mutism develops.

Treatment

Management of CM, with or without additional language, cognitive, and behavioral deficits, is appropriate early post-onset. Counseling of parents, the patient, and staff unfamiliar with CM about the probable basis of the mutism, its potential duration, and the probability of ongoing speech deficits after the mutism resolves is essential. During the mute period, the implementation of augmentative communication devices may be beneficial, depending on the presence or absence of other confounding variables (e.g., changes in behavior or cognition). Oromotor and respiratory control exercises emphasizing speech or speech-like movements may be appropriate. Following the resolution of the mutism, a dysarthria is typically present. Therapy to improve physiological functioning, as well as compensatory strategies to improve intelligibility and speech naturalness, should be considered, as necessary. Intervention targeting language and cognitive deficits should also be considered, if appropriate.

References

Al-Anazi, A., Hassounah, M., Sheikh, B. & Barayan, S. (2001). Cerebellar mutism caused by arteriovenous malformation of the vermis. *British Journal of Neurosurgery, 15,* 47–50

Cakir, Y., Karakisi, D., & Kocanaogullari, O. (1994). Cerebellar mutism in an adult: case report. *Surgical Neurology, 41,* 342–344

Cochrane, D.D., Gustavsson, B., Poskitt, K.P., Steinbok, P., & Kestle, J.R.W. (1994). The surgical and natural morbidity of aggressive resection for posterior fossa tumors in childhood. *Pediatric Neurosurgery, 20,* 19–29

Crutchfield, J. S., Sawaya, R., Meyers, C. A., & Moore III, B. D. (1994). Postoperative mutism in neurosurgery: report of two cases. *Journal of Neurosurgery, 81,* 115–121

Dailey, A.T., McKhann G.M. II, & Berger, M.S. (1995). The pathophysiology of oral pharyngeal apraxia and mutism following posterior fossa tumor resection in children. *Journal of Neurosurgery, 83,* 467–475

Doxey, D., Bruce, D., Sklar, F., Swift, D., & Shapiro, K. (1999). Posterior fossa syndrome: identifiable risk factors and irreversible complications. *Pediatric Neurosurgery, 31,* 131–136

Duffy, J.R. (2005). *Motor Speech Disorders: Substrates, Differential Diagnosis, and Management,* 2nd ed.) St. Louis: Elsevier Mosby

Ferrante, L., Mastronardi, L., Acqui, M., & Fortuna, A. (1990). Mutism after posterior fossa surgery in children: report of three cases. *Journal of Neurosurgery, 72,* 959–963

Frim, D.M. & Ogilvy, C.S. (1995). Mutism and cerebellar dysarthria after brain stem surgery: case report. *Neurosurgery, 36,* 854–857

Germano, A., Baldari, S., Caruso, G., Caffo, M., Montemagno, G., Cardia, E., et al. (1998). Reversible cerebral perfusion alterations in children with transient mutism after posterior fossa surgery. *Child's Nervous System, 14,* 114–119

JanBen, G., Messing-Junger, A.M., Engelbrecht, V., Gobel, U., Bock, W.J., & Lenard, H.G. (1998). Cerebellar mutism syndrome. *Klinische Padiatrie, 210,* 243–247

Koh, S., Beckwitt Turkel, S., & Baram, T.Z. (1997). Cerebellar mutism in children: report of six cases and potential mechanisms. *Pediatric Neurology, 16,* 218–219

Levisohn, L., Cronin-Golomb, A., & Schmahmann, J.D. (2000). Neuropsychological consequences of cerebellar tumour resection in children: cerebellar cognitive affective syndrome in a paediatric population. *Brain, 123,* 1041–1050

Pollack, I.F., Polinko, P., Albright, A.L., Towbin, R., & Fitz, C. (1995). Mutism and pseudobulbar symptoms after resection of posterior fossa tumors in children: incidence and pathophysiology. *Neurosurgery, 37,* 885–893

Rekate, H.L., Grubb, R.L., Aram, D.M., Hahn, J.F., & Ratcheson, R.A. (1985). Muteness of cerebellar origin. *Archives of Neurology, 42,* 697–698

Siffert, J., Young Poussaint, T., Goumnerova, L.C., Scott, R.M., LaValley, B., Tarbell, N.J., et al. (2000). Neurological dysfunction associated with postoperative cerebellar mutism. *Journal of Neuro-Oncology, 48,* 75–81

Turgut, M. (1998). Transient "cerebellar" mutism. *Child's Nervous System, 14,* 161–166

van Dongen, H.R., Catsman-Berrevoets, C.E., & van Mourik, M. (1994). The syndrome of "cerebellar" mutism and subsequent dysarthria. *Neurology, 44,* 2040–2046

Wang, M.C., Winston, K.R., & Breeze, R. (2002). Cerebellar mutism associated with a midbrain cavernous malformation. Case report and review of the literature. *Journal of Neurosurgery, 96,* 607–610

Chapter 23

Corticobasal Degeneration

Neila J. Donovan

◆ General Information on Disorder

Corticobasal degeneration (CBD) is one of the levadopa-non-responsive degenerative neurological movement disorders that fall under the classification of Parkinson-plus syndromes (Lang, 2003). It was first reported by Rebeiz, Kolodny, and Richardson (1968). Once considered rare, it now accounts for approximately 3% of cases seen by movement disorder specialists in the United States (Dickson et al, 2002). The onset of CBD typically occurs between the 6th and 7th decades of life and progresses to death in a median of 10 years, with reported ranges from 2.5 to 12.5 years (Wenning et al, 1998). CBD has no known cause or cure. Because there is significant overlap of clinical symptomatology among CBD, progressive supranuclear palsy, and frontotemporal dementia (Dickson et al, 2002; Kertesz, Martinez-Lange, Davidson, & Munoz, 2000; Lang, 2003), definitive diagnosis of CBD can only be made at autopsy. In fact, the emerging literature reserves the term *corticobasal degeneration* for cases that have histopathological evidence to support the label and applies the term *corticobasal syndrome* (CBS) to the clinical diagnosis (Lang, 2003).

Diagnostic Signs and Symptoms

The clinical diagnosis of CBD is typically made in the presence of a triad of core clinical features: (1) progressive asymmetrical rigidity and apraxia (typically of an upper extremity), (2) accompanied by additional cortical involvement (i.e., alien limb phenomenon, cortical sensory loss, myoclonus, aphasia) (Kertesz, 2003), and (3) basal ganglionic dysfunction (i.e., bradykinesia, dystonia, tremor) (Lang, 2003).

Computed tomography (CT) and magnetic resonance imaging (MRI) scans of individuals diagnosed with CBD reveal progressive cortical atrophy that may occur in the anterior cerebral cortex, the frontoparietal region, or the superior temporal cortex, accompanied by atrophy in the caudate or the substantia nigra (Armstrong, Cairns, & Lantos, 2000). Others have reported bilateral but asymmetrical atrophy of the lateral ventricles, and middle or posterior segments of the corpus callosum (Josephs, Tang-Wai, & Boeve, 2002).

Neuropathology

Microscopically, the neuropathology of CBD includes prominent intracellular accumulations of abnormal filaments formed by the microtubule-associated protein tau (Piboolnurak & Waters, 2003). These lead to neuronal and glial pathology, as well as neuronal loss in the anterior cerebral cortex, the frontoparietal region, the superior temporal cortex, substantia nigra, thalamus, lentiform, subthalamus, red nuclei, midbrain tegmentum, and locus ceruleus (Gibb, Luthert, & Marsden, 1989).

Epidemiology

The incidence and prevalence of CBD in the United States is unknown. However, in Europe the incidence of new cases in CBD is 0.6 to 0.9 case per 100,000 people per year. The prevalence is 4.0 to 7.3 per 100,000 persons (Delacourte, 2004).

Genetics

The Office of Rare Diseases criteria for CBD reported no definite familial cases of CBD (Dickson et al, 2002). CBD and frontotemporal dementia and parkinsonism linked to chromosome 17 (FTDP-17) have significant histological overlap; therefore, it is imperative to obtain an accurate family history of neurodegenerative disease.

◆ Speech Impairment Associated with Disorder

The motor speech disorders of CBD have not been studied; however, the presence of dysarthria (Wenning et al, 1998) and apraxia of speech have been reported (Duffy, 1995; Frattali, Grafman, Patronas, Makhlouf, & Litvan, 2000; Kertesz, 2003). The progression of the motor speech disorder may eventually render the individual unable to speak, requiring the use of an augmentative or alternative communication system.

Diagnostic Signs and Symptoms

The literature contains reports of cases in which apraxia of speech was the earliest symptoms of CBD (Duffy, 1995; Gibb et al, 1989; Graham, Bak, & Hodges, 2003a; Graham, Bak, Patterson, & Hodges, 2003b; Rosenfield, Bogatka, Viswanath, Lang, & Jankovic, 1991). Duffy proposed that an individual with CBD might present with hypokinetic or hyperkinetic dysarthria due to basal ganglia degeneration, spastic dysarthria due to upper motor neuron degeneration, and ataxic dysarthria due to cerebellar atrophy.

Etiology

Cortical and subcortical atrophy associated with CBD have the potential to affect the components of the motor speech system including motor planning (prefrontal, parietal, and temporal lobes), motor programming (putamen loop of the basal ganglia, and cerebellum), and execution of speech (Van der Merwe, 1997).

Magnetic resonance imaging results for individuals with CBD who have participated in speech and language studies included asymmetric cortical atrophy with widening of the sylvian fissures; interhemispheric fissures and dilation of cortical sulci in the frontal, parietal, or temporal lobes; periventricular white matter abnormalities with hyperintensities in frontal, temporal, occipital, or parietal lobes (Graham et al, 2003a,b; Kertesz, 2003; Kertesz et al, 2000); and atrophy of the corpus callosum (Frattali et al, 2000).

Neuropathology

As previously stated, the neuropathology of CBD includes prominent intracellular accumulations of abnormal filaments formed by the microtubule-associated protein tau (Piboolnurak & Waters, 2003). These lead to neuronal and glial pathology, and neuronal loss in cortical and subcortical areas of the brain.

Associated Cognitive, Linguistic, and Communicative Signs and Symptoms

In addition to the motor speech problems reported, CBD also causes significant cognitive and linguistic deficits (Frattali et al, 2000; Graham et al, 2003a; Kertesz et al, 2000). Language disorders reported in the literature have included mild to severe primary progressive aphasia (at times the presenting symptom of CBD) (Frattali et al, 2000; Kertesz et al, 2000). The presence of phonological, writing, and spelling deficits associated with CBD in the absence of measurable aphasia have been reported (Graham, Bak, Patterson, et al, 2003). In addition to language disorders, various cognitive disorders including memory deficits, dementia, constructional apraxia, visuospatial impairment, and frontal dysfunction have been reported (Graham et al, 2003a).

Special Diagnostic Considerations

If dysarthria or apraxia of speech are among the earliest signs of CBD, then the speech-language pathologist who deals with motor speech disorders must have an assessment battery that will allow for the differential diagnosis of the dysarthrias—one from another, and from apraxia of speech. Perceptual categorization of the dysarthrias is an accepted method for the differential diagnosis of the dysarthrias and apraxia of speech (Duffy, 1995).

Treatment

Treatment should focus on maintenance or improvement of communication behaviors that the individual can utilize to maintain independent functioning as long as possible. At this time there is no evidence for or against the treatment of motor speech disorders associated with CBD. However, there is evidence of positive treatment effects from other degenerative neurological diseases to use as a foundation for planning appropriate treatments for the motor speech disorders associated with CBD (Yorkston, 1996). For instance, when intelligibility is moderately impaired, treatment may focus on training the individual and communication partners to use strategies to achieve meaningful communicative exchanges. Advance planning for the acquisition and use of an assistive/augmentative communication devise is also very important (Yorkston, Beukelman, Strand, & Bell, 1999).

References

Armstrong, R.A., Cairns, N.J., & Lantos, P.L. (2000). A quantitative study of the pathological lesions in the neocortex and hippocampus of twelve patients with corticobasal degeneration. *Experimental Neurology, 163,* 348–356

Delacourte, A. (2004). *Cerebral aging and neurodegeneration.* http://perso.wanadoo.fr/adna

Dickson, D.W., Bergeron, C., Chin, S.S., Duyckaerts, C., Horoupian, D., Ikeda, K., et al. (2002). Office of rare diseases neuropathologic criteria for corticobasal degeneration. *Journal of Neuropathology and Experimental Neurology, 61,* 935–946

Duffy, J.R. (1995). *Motor Speech Disorders: Substrates, Differential Diagnosis, and Management.* St. Louis: Mosby

Frattali, C. M., Grafman, J., Patronas, N., Makhlouf, F., & Litvan, I. (2000). Language disturbances in corticobasal degeneration. *Neurology, 54,* 990–995

Gibb, W.R.G., Luthert, P.J., & Marsden, C.D. (1989). Corticobasal degeneration. *Brain, 112,* 117

Graham, N.L., Bak, T.H., & Hodges, J.R. (2003a). Corticobasal degeneration as a cognitive disorder. *Movement Disorders, 18,* 1224–1232

Graham, N.L., Bak, T.H., Patterson, K., & Hodges, J.R. (2003b). Language function and dysfunction in corticobasal degeneration. *Neurology, 61,* 493–499

Josephs, K., Tang-Wai, D., & Boeve, B.F. (2002). Clinicopathologic and imaging correlates in corticobasal degeneration. *Neurology, 58,* A132

Kertesz, A. (2003). Pick complex: an integrative approach to frontotemporal dementia: primary progressive aphasia, corticobasal degeneration, and progressive supranuclear palsy. *Neurology, 9,* 311–317

Kertesz, A., Martinez-Lange, P., Davidson, B.A., & Munoz, D.G. (2000). The corticobasal degeneration syndrome overlaps progressive aphasia and frontotemporal dementia. *Neurology, 55,* 1368–1375

Lang, A.E. (2003). Corticobasal degeneration: selected developments. *Movement Disorders, 18,* S51–S56

Piboolnurak, P., & Waters, C.H. (2003). Corticobasal degeneration. *Current Treatment Options in Neurology, 5,* 161–168

Rebeiz, J.J., Kolodny, E.H., & Richardson, E.P., Jr. (1968). Corticodentatonigral degeneration with neuronal acromasia. *Archives of Neurology, 18*, 20–33

Rosenfield, D.B., Bogatka, N.S., Viswanath, A.E., Lang, A.E., & Jankovic, J. (1991). Speech apraxia in cortical-basal ganglionic degeneration [abstract]. *Annals of Neurology, 30*, 296–297

Van der Merwe, A. (1997). A theoretical framework for the characterization of pathological speech sensorimotor control. In: M.R. McNeil (Ed.), *Clinical Management of Sensorimotor Speech Disorders* (pp. 1–26). New York: Thieme

Wenning, G.K., Litvan, I., Jankovic, J., Granata, R., Mangone, C.A., McKee, A.S., et al. (1998). Natural history and survival of 14 patients with corticobasal degeneration confirmed at postmortem examination. *Journal of Neurology, Neurosurgery and Psychiatry, 64*, 184–189

Yorkston, K.M. (1996). Treatment efficacy: dysarthria. *Journal of Speech and Hearing Research, 39*, S46–S57

Yorkston, K.M., Beukelman, D.R., Strand, E.A., & Bell, K.R. (1999). *Management of Motor Speech Disorders in Children and Adults,* 2nd ed. Austin, TX: Pro-Ed

Chapter 24

Creutzfeldt-Jakob Disease

Tepanta R.D. Fossett and Damirez T. Fossett

◆ General Information on Disorder

Creutzfeldt-Jakob disease (CJD) is a rare, medically untreatable, and rapidly progressive neurodegenerative disease that affects the central nervous system (CNS). It is one of a family of prion diseases or transmissible spongiform encephalopathies that include human and nonhuman types. It is transmitted by prion proteins and may be familial, iatrogenic [e.g., contamination from dura mater and corneal grafts, human growth hormone, or neurosurgical instrumentation (Brown et al, 2000)], or sporadic in nature. Subtypes of this disease have been identified, such as Gerstmann-Sträussler-Scheinker (GSS), variant Creutzfeldt-Jakob (vCJD), fatal familial insomnias (FFI), and sporadic fatal insomnia (SFI), but these forms of CJD are not addressed in this chapter. Although there is a large range (Niewiadomska et al, 2002), the mean age of onset of CJD has been reported to be around 60 years of age with a decrease in incidence after age 70 (Collins, Lawson, & Masters, 2004). The typical time course of CJD from onset of signs and symptoms to death ranges from a few months to 2 years. The median duration of the disease is 4 to 5 months (Collins et al, 2004), with approximately 90% of affected individuals surviving about 1 year. Although sudden onset of symptoms may occur, usually there is a gradual onset of nonspecific symptoms (Collins et al, 2004).

Diagnostic Signs and Symptoms

Clinical features of CJD include the gradual onset of a progressive dementia, pyramidal tract signs such as weakness, hyperreflexic, and hypertonicity of the extremities, and extrapyramidal signs such as tremor, rigidity, and slowness of movement. Other features can include myoclonus, amyotrophy, cortical blindness, seizures, and signs of cerebellar dysfunction. Some investigations have suggested that peripheral nervous system impairment may frequently occur with CJD as well (Niewiadomska et al, 2002). Additional signs and symptoms that may occur include depression, insomnia, lethargy, agitation, emotional lability, personality changes, and visual disturbances.

Common diagnostic measures include radiographic analyses, electroencephalography, and examination of cerebral spinal fluid. Although any of these measures may yield unremarkable findings and demonstrate varying sensitivity and specificity, some characteristic diagnostic results are suggestive of CJD. Computed tomography (CT) imaging is most often normal in patients with CJD. Initial CT scans that are normal may progress to show atrophy later in the course of the disease. Perhaps the most beneficial effect of CT imaging is to rule out other focal lesions as the cause of the patient's symptoms. Magnetic resonance imaging (MRI) findings suggestive of CJD include cerebral atrophy, and T2-weighted images may show increased, symmetrical signals in the caudate nucleus and putamen (Collins et al, 2004), as well as other subcortical structures. There are no enhancing lesions and there is no mass effect. Electroencephalography typically shows a pattern of periodic synchronous sharp wave complexes, which is rather pathognomonic of CJD. The detection of the 14-3-3 protein in the cerebrospinal fluid is also a common finding. Postmortem diagnostic procedures include histopathological assessment and immunodiagnostic evaluation of brain tissue.

Neuropathology

Microscopically, CJD is characterized by spongiform vacuolar (vesicles in the cell) changes in the nerve cells of the cortical and subcortical gray matter. In later stages of the disease, there is typically a loss of neurons and replacement of these neurons by fibrillary gliosis. The white matter tracts are typically spared. Atrophy can be either diffuse or localized to particular anatomical regions of the brain, such as the cerebellum, thalamus, basal ganglia, or cortex. There are generally none of the characteristic findings of inflammation. All of the changes are believed to be caused by a proteinaceous infectious particle—smaller than a virus—called a prion. CJD is identified neuropathologically in postmortem examination by spongiform changes that may occur in localized or diffuse brain regions, neuronal degeneration, and gliosis (Niewandowski et al, 2002).

Epidemiology

The incidence of CJD is reported to be approximately 1 case per million, with sporadic CJD accounting for 85% of those cases (Hannah et al, 2001). From 5 to 15% of CJD cases are familial or genetic in nature (Niewiadomska et al, 2002), whereas iatrogenic cases compose a negligible portion of

CJD cases (Brown et al, 2000). Changes in screening criteria for donor material and the increased availability of synthetic materials should further decrease the incidence of iatrogenic cases of CJD (Brown et al, 2000; Hannah et al, 2001). A retrospective study of the incidence of CJD using histologically confirmed cases of CJD, however, suggests that the true incidence may be higher, as the disease may be clinically misdiagnosed in older persons (Bruton, Bruton, Gentleman, & Roberts, 1995).

Genetics

In CJD the normal prion protein takes on an abnormal structure and physiochemical changes occur (Prusiner, 1998; Prusiner & Scott, 1997). This process facilitates the conversion of surround prion proteins to infectious proteins. How and why abnormal prion protein conversion occurs is unclear at this time.

◆ Speech Impairment Associated with Disorder

The speech production skills of persons with CJD have not been well described. Reports in the literature frequently do not mention the presence of speech signs or symptoms, or alternatively, provide diagnostically uninformative descriptions (i.e., slurred speech, hesitant, slow). There is one report that identified pseudobulbar speech in the initial or middle stages of CJD in five patients (Otto et al, 1998). Muteness is common during the middle and later stages of the disease, and average disease duration preceding muteness has been reported to be about 4 months (Otto et al, 1998).

Diagnostic Signs and Symptoms

No specific diagnostic signs or symptoms for speech in CJD have been identified. The neuropathology of this disorder, however, suggests that they are likely and that several different types of dysarthria may be demonstrated. As brain damage in CJD may occur in cortical and subcortical structures affecting the pyramidal and extrapyramidal systems as well as the cerebellum, and as brain damage is progressive and may be localized to a particular lobe or occur diffusely, either a focal or mixed dysarthria is hypothesized as the primary presenting dysarthria in CJD. These dysarthrias would include signs of spastic, ataxic, or hyperkinetic dysarthria. Spastic dysarthria is likely to be the most prominent dysarthria in CJD, as it results from bilateral damage to the direct and indirect activation pathways and is commonly associated with diffuse or multifocal CNS disease and cognitive disturbance (Duffy, 1995). Clinical signs might include pathological oral reflexes, drooling, slow movements, and reduced range of movement (Duffy, 1995). The

speech characteristics for each of these dysarthria types are available in Duffy (1995). The clinical speech picture for the dysarthrias presented in CJD is likely to change over time, as the disease is progressive in nature.

Etiology

The etiology of the speech behaviors noted in CJD is brain damage that affects the pyramidal and extrapyramidal activation systems and cortical and subcortical structures, specifically the basal ganglia, as well as the cerebellum.

Neuropathology

Based on various analytic techniques, both pre- and postmortem, neuropathological changes in CJD include diffuse damage that primarily affects the cerebral cortex, basal ganglia, and cerebellar circuits, whereas individual cranial nerves are often intact. Damage to these areas produces changes in strength, tone, reflexes, range of movement, and overall motor control.

Associated Cognitive, Linguistic, and Communicative Signs and Symptoms

Although the most obvious symptom patients with CJD present with is a rapidly progressive dementia, other signs and symptoms include the presence of aphasia, deficits in verbal fluency, the presence of phonemic and semantic paraphasias, perseverations, and progressively less initiation of communicative attempts.

Special Diagnostic Considerations

There are no special diagnostic considerations for evaluation of speech in CJD. Akinetic mutism has been used as one criterion for CJD (Otto et al, 1998); however, it typically does not occur until the middle to late stages of the disease, thus not aiding in initial differential diagnosis. It is possible, but unlikely, that a suspicion of CJD will be based on speech signs or symptoms, as the neuropathology of the disease is not consistent among persons and as the etiology of the most frequently occurring type of CJD, sporadic, is unknown. Additionally, changes in other cognitive behaviors (i.e., memory) are more dramatic and tend to have a more profound impact on daily functioning early in the disease.

Treatment

Although CJD is rapidly progressive and fatal, an array of direct treatments (Yorkston, Beukelman, & Bell, 1999) with a special attention to alternative and augmentative communication (AAC) during early intervention and training might be considered. Additionally, because of the patient's increasingly limited communicative abilities, it is suggested that treatment goals emphasize counseling the caregiver on communicative strategies that can prolong and facilitate any communicative interaction.

References

Brown, P., Preece, M., Brandel, J.-P., Sato, T., McShane, L., Zerr, I., et al. (2000). Iatrogenic Creutzfeldt-Jakob disease at the millennium. *Neurology, 55,* 1075–1081

Bruton, C.J., Bruton, R.K., Gentleman, S.M., & Roberts, G.W. (1995). Diagnosis and incidence of prion (Creutzfeldt-Jakob) disease: a retrospective archival survey with implications for future research. *Neurodegeneration, 4,* 357–368

Collins, S.J., Lawson, V.A., & Masters, C.L. (2004). Transmissible spongiform encephalopathies. *Lancet, 363,* 51–61

Duffy, J.R. (1995). *Motor Speech Disorders.* St. Louis: Mosby Yearbook

Hannah, E.L., Belay, E.D., Gambetti, P., Krause, G., Parchi, P. Capellari, S., et al. (2001). Creutzfeldt-Jakob disease after receipt of a previously unimplicated brand of dura mater graft. *Neurology, 56,* 1080–1083

Niewiadomska, M., Kulczycki, J., Wochnik-Dyjas, D., Szpak, G. M., Rakowicz, M., Lojkowska, W., et al. (2002). Impairment of the peripheral nervous system in Creutzfeldt-Jakob disease. *Archives of Neurology, 59,* 1430–1436

Otto, A., Zerr, I., Lantsch, M., Weidehass, K., Riedemann, C., & Poser, S. (1998). Akinetic mutism as a classification criterion for the diagnosis of Creutzfeldt-Jakob disease. *Journal of Neurology, Neurosurgery, & Psychiatry, 64,* 524–528

Prusiner, S.B. (1998). Prions. *Proceedings of the National Academy of Science, 95,* 13363–13383

Prusiner, S.B. & Scott, M.R. (1997). Genetics of prions. *Annual Review of Genetics, 31,* 139–175

Yorkston, K.M., Beukelman, D.R., & Bell, K.R. (1999). *Clinical Management of Dysarthric Speakers.* Boston: College-Hill Press

Additional Reading

Kretzschmar, H.A., Ironside, J.W., DeArmond, S.J., & Tateishi, J. (1996). Diagnostic criteria for sporadic Creutzfeldt-Jakob disease. *Archives of Neurology, 53,* 913–920

Chapter 25

Deletion Syndrome

Ilias Papathanasiou and Vaia Varsami

◆ General Information on Disorder

Deletion of 22q11 has been associated with velocardiofacial syndrome (VCFS), Shprintzen syndrome, DiGeorge sequence (DGS), conotruncal anomaly face (CTAF), Caylor cardiofacial syndrome, and autosomal dominant Opitz-G/BBB syndrome (McDonald-McGinn, Kirschner, Goldmuntz, et al, 2003). According to McDonald-McGinn et al, individuals with the 22q11 deletion syndrome have a range of findings and symptoms, including congenital heart disease (74% of individuals), particularly conotruncal malformations; palatal abnormalities (69%), particularly velopharyngeal incompetence (VPI); cleft plate (sometimes submucosal); learning disabilities (70–90%); and characteristic facial features. These facial features include a long face with a prominent nose and a squared-off nasal tip, narrow palpebral fissures, hooded eyelids, and a small mouth. The ears are often small with attached ear lobs. Fingers are long and hyperextensible. Additional findings are feeding difficulties (30%), hypocalcemia (50–70%), immune deficiency (77%), renal anomalies, laryngotracheoesophageal anomalies, hearing loss (both conductive and sensorineural), and skeletal abnormalities. Finally, growth hormone deficiency, autoimmune disorders, and seizures have also been reported. Furthermore, Shprintzen, Goldberg, Golding-Kushner, et al (1992) have reported that these individuals develop psychosis as a frequent clinical feature, usually in late adolescence or early adulthood.

Diagnostic Sign and Symptoms

Clinical features present in individuals with suspected 22q11.2 deletion may include congenital heart disease, palatal abnormalities (especially VPI), hypocalcemia, immune deficiency, learning disabilities, and at times characteristic facial features. When an individual is suspected to have 22q11.2 deletion syndrome, the diagnosis takes place following a fluorescence in-situ hybridization (FISH) test using probes from the DiGeorge chromosomal region (DGCR), where a submicroscopic deletion of the chromosome 22 is detected. McDonald-McGinn et al (2003) reported that fewer than 5% of individuals with clinical symptoms of the 22q11.2 deletion syndrome have normal routine cytogenetic studies and negative FISH testing. The clinical symptoms in such cases are due to chromosomal rearrangements involving the DGCR such as translocation between chromosome 22 and other chromosomes.

Neuropathology

Although the majority of individuals with the deletion 22q11.2 syndrome have a hypotonia and learning disabilities, specific neurological findings are rare. Seizures have been reported in some individuals but are most often associated with hypocalcemia. Rarely, ataxia and atrophy of the cerebellum have been reported.

Epidemiology

The incidence 22q11.2 deletion syndrome is estimated as high as 1 in 2000 live births (Lees, 2001). This includes the velocardiofacial syndrome, whose incidence has been estimated at 1 in 5000 (Pike & Super, 1997).

Genetics

The 22q11.2 deletion syndrome results from a microdeletion on the chromosome 22q11. About 5 to 10% of affected individuals have a parent who also carries the deletion and it has been inherited in an autosomal dominant manner. About 90 to 95% of cases have a de novo deletion of the 22q11.2. A very small percentage (<1%) of individuals with clinical findings of 22q11.2 deletion syndrome have chromosomal rearrangements instead of deletions involving 22q11.2, such as translocation between chromosome 22 and another chromosome.

◆ Speech Impairment Associated with Disorder

The presence of severe hypernasality due to velopharyngeal dysfunction is the most common speech disturbance that is associated with 22q11.2 deletion syndrome. This velopharyngeal dysfunction in some cases is associated with submucous cleft palate. The speech characteristics as described by Shprintzen (1997) are mainly articulatory, delayed onset of speech, global glottal stop substitutions for essentially all consonants except for the nasal consonants, and high pitch voice.

Diagnostic Signs and Symptoms

The 22q11.2 deletion syndrome is diagnosed from the specific pattern of the communicative impairments associated with the other characteristics of the syndrome, such as the facial appearance, cardiac anomalies, cleft palate, and learning disabilities. When children are developing speech, the global glottal stop substitution is one major characteristic of the articulatory impairment. Although glottal stop substitutions are common in children with cleft plate or cleft lip and palate, they are not typically substitutions for all consonants, and often there are other compensatory substitutions in response to both velopharyngeal dysfunction and oral anomalies (Shprintzen, 1997). Unlike other children with clefts, children with 22q11.2 deletion syndrome do not develop pharyngeal fricatives, pharyngeal stops, mid-dorsal stops, and other abnormal substitutions (Shprintzen, 1997).

Etiology

The etiology of the speech behavior noted in this syndrome is the result of the changes in the genes, which affects the function of the oropharyngeal tract.

Neuropathology

Early studies have attributed the velopharyngeal dysfunction observed in the 222q11.2 deletion syndrome to cranial nerve VII involvement (Mercer & Pigott, 2001). This is expressed by the hypodynamic faces associated with the hypodynamic palate and pharynx observed in these patients. Similarly, Shprintzen, Goldberg, Young, et al (1981) reported that pharyngeal hypotonia is present in 90% of the cases, which is correlated with general hypotonia. Arvedson and Brodsky (2002) report that findings on videofluoroscopy swallow studies suggest that the underlying problems of the swallowing and feeding difficulties present are due to dysmobility in the pharyngoesophageal area.

Associative Cognitive, Linguistic, and Communicative Signs and Symptoms

Shprintzen (1997) reports that in addition to distorted speech characteristics, individuals with 22q11.2 deletion syndrome present with delayed and impaired specific aspects in auditory memory and processing. He also reports the presence of conductive hearing loss caused by chronic middle ear disease secondary to both immune deficiency

and clefting. Furthermore, in 15% of the cases sensorineural hearing loss is found and may be unilateral or bilateral; it is usually mild, although moderate to severe cases do occur.

Another important clinical characteristic observed in early adulthood in cases with 22q11.2 deletion syndrome is bipolar affective disorder, with many patients developing psychotic episodes (Shprintzen et al, 1992). In young children the behavioral disorders noted include learning disabilities with their associated typical affect and temperament, which results in poor social interaction and pragmatic-type communication difficulties. The early manifestation of behavioral problems is highly predictive of the development of adult psychiatric disorders.

Special Diagnostic Considerations

There are no special diagnostic considerations for evaluation of speech in patients with 22q11.2 deletion syndrome. The velopharyngeal dysfunction needs to be evaluated with nasopharyngoscopy and multiview radiology while simultaneously recording or videotaping the speech. In addition videofluoroscopic swallow studies can be used for the investigation of feeding and swallowing difficulties. Perceptual assessment of speech and aerodynamic and acoustic measures of speech is necessary to evaluate the effect of the velopharyngeal dysfunction in speech. Finally, articulatory tests and intelligibility ratings are important to evaluate the articulatory patterns observed.

Treatment

As children with 22q11.2 deletion present difficulties from the first days of life, speech and language pathology intervention may be essential for most of their life. Initial evaluation and advice for the feeding difficulties, followed by intervention for speech production (especially consonants) and therapy for hypernasality, are the main streams of the intervention. In addition, prosthetic or surgical management of the hypernasality is indicated in many cases; however, detailed evaluation of the velopharyngeal dysfunction as well as the cooperation of the child are necessary for these techniques to succeed. The presence of behavioral problems can be an obstacle in the treatment and management of cases with 22q11.2 deletion and always need to be addressed.

References

Arvedson, J.C. & Brodsky, L. (2002). *Pediatric Swallowing and Feeding: Assessment and Management,* 2nd ed. Albany NY: Singular Thompson Learning

Lees, M. (2001). Genetics of cleft lip and palate. In: A.C.H. Watson, D.A. Sell, & P. Grunwell (Eds.), *Management of Cleft Lip and Palate.* London: Whurr

McDonald-McGinn, D.M., Kirschner, R., Goldmuntz, E., et al. (2003). 22q11.2 deletion syndrome. Genereviews. www.genetests.org

Mercer, N.S.G. & Pigott, R.W. (2001). Assessment and surgical management of velopharyngeal dysfunction. In: A.C.H. Watson, D.A. Sell, & P. Grunwell (Eds.), *Management of Cleft Lip and Palate.* London: Whurr

Pike, A.C. & Super, M. (1997). Velocardiofacial syndrome. *Postgraduate Medical Journal, 73,* 771–775

Shprintzen, R.J. (1997). *Genetics, Syndromes and Communication Disorders.* San Diego: Singular

Shprintzen, R.J., Goldberg, R.B., Young, D., et al. (1981). The velo-cardio-facial syndrome: a clinical and genetic analysis. *Pediatrics, 67,* 167–172

Shprintzen, R.J., Goldberg, R.B., Golding-Kushner, K.J., et al. (1992). Late onset psychosis in the velo-cardio-facial syndrome. *American Journal of Medical Genetics, 42,* 141–142

Chapter 26

Duchenne Muscular Dystrophy

Kimberley M. Docking and Bruce E. Murdoch

◆ General Information on Disorder

Duchenne muscular dystrophy (DMD) is a genetic X-linked disease primarily affecting males. It is characterized by a progressive weakness and degeneration of the skeletal muscles that control movement. DMD is caused by genetic mutational deficiencies or absence of dystrophin in muscles (Jay & Vajsar, 2001; Kiliaridis & Katsaros, 1998).

Diagnostic Signs and Symptoms

DMD commonly presents in early childhood with a rapid and progressive course (Anderson, Head, Rae, & Morley, 2002; Jay & Vajsar, 2001). Most boys with DMD begin to walk at a later developmental age than their normally developing peers, and are noted to stand or walk on the forward part of their foot later in development. Excessively large and well-developed calf muscles (pseudohypertrophy) are also a common finding associated with this disease as well as orthopedic abnormalities (Jay & Vajsar, 2001). By age 12, most individuals with DMD are unable to walk, and by the age of 20 they often require the use of a respirator (Anderson et al, 2002).

Generalized muscular weakness and wasting affecting the muscles of the hips, pelvic area, thighs, and shoulders, and eventually involving all striated musculature, is a common progression in individuals with DMD and includes the tongue, facial, masticatory, and respiratory muscles (Anderson et al, 2002; Jay & Vajsar, 2001). Cardiac involvement is also a frequent finding in this population due to weakness of the heart muscles, and often underpins the mortality of individuals with DMD.

Neuropathology

Evidence of disordered central nervous system (CNS) architecture has been noted in individuals with DMD, as well as anomalies and absences associated with neurons that normally express dystrophin (Anderson et al, 2002). At the biochemical level, indications of CNS pathology are represented by the abnormal bioenergetics of the CNS and an increase in the levels of choline-containing compounds. Functionally, EEG abnormalities are associated with DMD, with evidence indicating that synaptic function is affected adversely by the absence of dystrophin (Anderson et al, 2002; Kiliaridis & Katsaros, 1998).

Epidemiology

Duchenne muscular dystrophy is a fatal hereditary disease and the most frequent of the muscular dystrophies. It is the second most commonly occurring genetically inherited disease in humans, and affects approximately 1 in 3300 to 1 in 3500 live male births (Anderson et al, 2002; Kiliaridis & Katsaros, 1998; Kim, Wu, & Black, 1995). Onset is often between 2 and 5 years of age, with survival rare beyond the early 30s (Jay & Vajsar, 2001).

Genetics

An X-linked recessive disease, DMD is the result of mutations in the gene that regulates dystrophin. When the Xp21 gene on the X-chromosome fails to make the protein dystrophin, DMD occurs (Kiliaridis & Katsaros, 1998). DMD is inherited by males through their mothers, who are carriers of DMD but exhibit no symptoms.

◆ Speech Impairment Associated with Disorder

Both speech and language delay are common features of DMD, in addition to poor concentration, learning difficulties, or problem behaviors (Mohamed, Appleton, & Nicolaides, 2000). Significant speech and articulation deficits are reported in as many as one third of individuals with DMD (Mohamed et al, 2000; Smith, Sibert, & Harper, 1990). Deficits in the motor speech domain are primarily due to skeletal muscle weakness, and hence dysarthric features are more likely to predominantly represent the flaccid type.

Weaknesses in the muscle groups of most speech subsystems are demonstrated by individuals with DMD, particularly the respiratory, laryngeal, tongue, and lip muscles. DMD is also responsible for weakness of masticatory muscles and difficulties in the preoral phase of swallowing (Willig, Paulus, Lacau Saint Guily, Beon, & Navarro, 1994). As a result of weaknesses in these muscle groups, individuals with DMD may demonstrate features such as poor maximal oral breath pressure, sustained phonation, and maximum vocal intensity, as well as a disruption to the prolongation of vocalized tone (Sanders & Perlstein, 1965). Reduced strength associated with protrusion and lateralization of the tongue may also result, as well as a high incidence of articulatory errors on sounds that require tongue tip elevation and protrusion (Eckardt & Harzer, 1996; Sanders & Perlstein, 1965). Lack of consistency in strength, range of motion, and rate of lateralization of the tongue has also been reported (Sanders & Perlstein, 1965).

A weakness of all the facial muscles, including the lips, is commonly demonstrated by a characteristic round face devoid of tone and flat affect (Sanders & Perlstein, 1965). Poor maximum pressure of lip approximation (indicating weakness of the orbicularis oris) and difficulty pursing (weakness of orbicularis oris) and spreading lips (weakness of lip retractors, zygomaticus, and risorius) are also considered characteristic. A high prevalence of malocclusions has also been noted in DMD populations, which is strongly related to the involvement of orofacial muscle weakness associated with DMD (Eckardt & Harzer, 1996; Kiliaridis & Katsaros, 1998).

Etiology

The motor speech difficulties experienced by individuals with DMD are largely due to the skeletal muscle pathology. However, a disruption of normal motor control function may also have an impact on the ability of these children to learn and carry out movement, and to compensate for weaknesses and structural abnormalities in skeletal muscle.

Neuropathology

Dystrophin has been demonstrated to be deficient in DMD cortical synapses, indicating a role in cognitive impairment (Anderson et al, 2002; Kim et al, 1995). Evidence suggests that dystrophin deficiency may affect not only normal muscle function but also normal synaptic CNS function (Kim et al, 1995). In the brain, dystrophin is found in the neurons where it is associated with the postsynaptic membrane, particularly in cortical and hippocampal neurons and in cerebellar Purkinje cells (Blake & Kroger, 2000). It is generally accepted that the primary cause of cognitive impairment, and therefore likely linguistic deficits, in DMD is the lack of functional dystrophin in regard to the dystrophin-deficient cortical synapses, rather than a secondary consequence of the muscle disease (Blake & Kroger, 2000; Kim et al, 1995).

Associated Cognitive, Linguistic, and Communicative Signs and Symptoms

Nonprogressive cognitive deficits commonly present in as many as one third of individuals with DMD, with evidence suggesting that deficits in verbal intelligence, language, and reading ability predominate (Billard, Gillet, Barthez, Hommet, & Bertrand, 1998; Blake & Kroger, 2000; Kim et al, 1995). A specific cognitive profile of overall poor working memory and difficulty on measures requiring attention to complex verbal information has been consistently reported (Hinton, De Vivo, Nereo, Goldstein, & Stern, 2000; Wicksell, Kihlgren, Melin, & Eeg-Olofsson, 2004). Selective impairment of verbal working memory in boys with DMD is therefore likely to contribute to limited academic achievement, commonly reported across all areas (writing, reading, math).

Special Diagnostic Considerations

Together with the progressive nature of this condition, it is important to consider the developmental impact of age when assessing and managing motor speech function in individuals with DMD.

Treatment

Strategies that utilize the individual's remaining strengths and potential are essential for the successful management of motor speech symptoms associated with DMD. Maximizing communication within the context of daily life situations may involve the use of traditional behavioral therapy approaches combined with alternative and augmentative communication (AAC) in the early intervention phase.

Treatment targeting respiratory support is a particularly important consideration for the individual with DMD, with a focus on postural control and appropriate positioning to counteract muscle weakness interfering with respiration and phonation. Articulation should adopt a functional approach, with compensatory strategies playing an important role. As diagnosis often occurs in early childhood, formulation of treatment goals targeting articulation should consider developmental acquisition, with developmental stimulation programs an effective addition to the treatment program (Smith et al, 1990).

References

Anderson, J.L., Head, S.I., Rae, C., & Morley, J.W. (2002). Brain function in Duchenne muscular dystrophy. *Brain, 125,* 4–13

Billard, C., Gillet, P., Barthez, M., Hommet, C., & Bertrand, P. (1998). Reading ability and processing in Duchenne muscular dystrophy and spinal muscular atrophy. *Developmental Medicine and Child Neurology, 40,* 12–20

Blake, D.J. & Kroger, S. (2000). The neurobiology of Duchenne muscular dystrophy: learning lessons from muscle? *Trends in Neuroscience, 23,* 92–99

Eckardt, L. & Harzer, H. (1996). Facial structure and functional findings in patients with progressive muscular dystrophy (Duchenne). *American Journal of Orthodontics and Dentofacial Orthopaedics, 110,* 185–190

Hinton, V.J., De Vivo, D.C., Nereo, N.E., Goldstein, E., & Stern, Y. (2000). Poor verbal working memory across intellectual level in boys with Duchenne dystrophy. *Neurology, 54,* 2127–2132

Jay, V., & Vajsar, J. (2001). The dystrophy of Duchenne. *Lancet, 357,* 550–552

Kiliaridis, S., & Katsaros, C. (1998). The effects of myotonic dystrophy and Duchenne muscular dystrophy on orofacial muscles and dentofacial morphology. *Acta Odontologica Scandinavica, 56,* 369–374

Kim, T.-W., Wu, K., & Black, I.B. (1995). Deficiency of brain synaptic dystrophin in human Duchenne muscular dystrophy. *Annals of Neurology, 38,* 446–449

Mohamed, K., Appleton, R., & Nicolaides, P. (2000). Delayed diagnosis of Duchenne muscular dystrophy. *European Journal of Paediatric Neurology, 4*, 219–223

Sanders, L.J., & Perlstein, M.A. (1965). Speech mechanism in pseudohypertrophic muscular dystrophy. *American Journal of Disorders in Childhood, 109*, 538–543

Smith, R.A., Sibert, J.R., & Harper, P.S. (1990). Early development of boys with Duchenne muscular dystrophy. *Developmental Medicine and Child Neurology, 32*, 519–527

Wicksell, R.K., Kihlgren, M., Melin, L., & Eeg-Olofsson, O. (2004). Specific cognitive deficits are common in children with Duchenne muscular dystrophy. *Developmental Medicine and Child Neurology, 46*, 154–159

Willig, T.N., Paulus, J., Lacau Saint Guily, J., Beon, C., & Navarro, J. (1994). Swallowing problems in neuromuscular disorders. *Archives of Physical Medicine and Rehabilitation, 75*, 1175–1181

Additional Reading

Cotton, S., Voudouris, N.J., & Greenwood, K.M. (2001). Intelligence and Duchenne muscular dystrophy: full-scale, verbal and performance intelligence quotients. *Developmental Medicine and Child Neurology, 43*, 497–501

Hinton, V.J., De Vivo, D.C., Nereo, N.E., Goldstein, E., & Stern, Y. (2001). Selective deficits in verbal working memory associated with a known genetic etiology: The neuropsychological profile of Duchenne muscular dystrophy. *Journal of the International Neuropsychological Society, 7*, 45–54

Chapter 27

Ehlers-Danlos Syndrome

Joan C. Arvedson and Bonnie Heintskill

♦ General Information on Disorder

Ehlers-Danlos syndrome (EDS) is a heterogeneous group of inheritable generalized connective tissue disorders characterized by joint hypermobility, skin hyperextensibility, and tissue fragility. Connective tissue supports skin, bones, tendons, ligaments, blood vessels, and other organs. This defect is a result of faulty collagen, a protein that serves as "glue" by giving strength and elasticity to the connective tissue. Weak connective tissues create problems with movements and attachments of joints and the endurance of tissues in the body. Six major types of EDS are classified according to distinct features (**Table 27–1**).

Diagnostic Signs and Symptoms

Signs and symptoms differ by type and degree, although basic common signs include, but are not limited to, (1) skin problems—soft velvet-like texture, fragility that causes easy bruising or tears, and severe scarring; (2) joint problems—loose/unstable and prone to dislocations, pain, early onset of osteoarthritis, and hyperextensibilty; (3) miscellaneous problems—musculoskeletal pain, hypotonia, gum disease, arterial/intestinal/uterine fragility, and hearing loss (Hawthorn, 2000). Diagnostic signs include dystrophic "cigarette paper" scarring, tongue hypermobility (Gorlin's sign) (Gorlin, Cohen, & Levin, 1990), and eyelid extensibility (Metenier's sign).

Diagnosis of the more common EDS types (classic [CEDS] and hypermobility [HEDS]) is by family history and clinical evaluation. Fine motor deficits may be early signs of EDS as well as a marker for later-appearing speech motor deficits. EDS individuals have a high proportion of oral problems that include hard tissue defects of the teeth, high cusps and fissures on crowns, high incidence of tooth fractures, periodontal diseases, and fragile/sensitive mucous membranes (e.g., Norton & Assael, 1997).

Neuropathology

Neurological signs are variable among and within EDS types and can often be explained on the basis of the inherent connective tissue defects (Beighton, De Paepe, Steinmann, Tsipouras, & Wenstrup, 1998). A defect in collagen or in another extracellular matrix (ECM) protein such as tenascin during fetal development has been described in association with epilepsy and cerebral cortical dysplasia (e.g., Thomas,

Bossan, Lacour, et al, 1996), and bilateral focal polymicrogyria (Echaniz-Laguna, de Saint-Martin, Lafontaine, et al, 2000). Neuromyopathy is characterized by weak hypotonic muscles and hypoactive deep reflexes. Intracranial vascular abnormalities, although uncommon, are the most serious neurological hazards and have caused death in some EDS individuals (Beighton et al, 1998).

Epidemiology

The overall incidence of EDS may be about 1 in 5000 births worldwide with significant differences among types (**Table 27–1**). Incidence figures will likely be higher as the various types of EDS are recognized more readily.

Genetics

Transmission of the common types of EDS is autosomal dominant. Defective synthesis of type V collagen, a minor type of fibrillar collagen combining two (1(V) chains and one (2(V) chain has been found in approximately 15%. Mutations in the COL5A1 and COL5A2 gene that code for both chains were identified (e.g., Nicholls, Oliver, McCarron, et al, 1996). Intensive studies are under way to identify the genes when COL5A1 and COL5A2 genes are unaffected.

♦ Speech Impairment Associated with Disorder

Speech characteristics are consistent, with flaccid dysarthria related to hypermobility, hypotonia, and a poor sense of proprioception. The result is imprecise articulation, deletion of final consonants, fading at ends of phrases that appears related to fatigue, and dysfluency because of incoordination of articulators, laryngeal and oral movements, and reduced proprioceptive feedback of oral movements. Developmental delays result in speech becoming increasingly difficult over time. Weak neck muscles make it difficult to maintain adequate upright posture, with a negative impact on swallowing. Many EDS individuals experience daily pain in masticatory muscles and demonstrate temporomandibular joint problems, noted in reduced mouth opening and a clicking sound (Hagberg, Korpe, & Berglund, 2004). Fragile oral mucosa and dentition problems are also seen.

Table 27–1 Types of Ehlers-Danlos Syndrome (EDS)

Type of EDS	Classic Type (CEDS) (Types I & II)	Hypermobility (HEDS) (Type III)	Vascular (Type IV)	Kyphoscoliosis (Type VI: ocular-scoliotic)	Arthrochalasia (Type VIIB)	Dermatospraxis (Type VIIC)
Inheritance	Autosomal dominant	Autosomal dominant; not clear how mutations lead to clinical features; recessive inheritance possible	Autosomal dominant; sporadic new mutations	Autosomal recessive	Autosomal dominant; most cases sporadic, caused by new mutations in COL1A1 or COL1A2 gene	Autosomal recessive
Collagen affected	Mutations in COL1A1, COL1A2, COL5A1, COL5A2, & TNXB (not clear; lead to clinical features)	No distinctive biochemical collagen finding yet	Mutations in COL3A1 gene; Proa1 (III) chain of collagen type III encoded by COL3A1	Mutations in PLOD gene; enzyme lysyl hydroxylase is essential for stable cross-links	Alters structure and processing of type I collagen, weakens connective tissue in skin, bones, and other tissues	Mutations in ADAMTS2 gene completely inactivate gene, Connective tissue is weakened
Major diagnostic characteristics	Skin hyperextensibility; widened atrophic scars; joint hypermobility; pes planus	Generalized joint hypermobility; early onset chronic joint pain; variable skin symptoms; mitral valve prolapse common	Thin translucent fragile skin; soft, but not overly stretchy; extensive easy bruising; joint hypermobility; atrial/intestinal/uterine fragility or rupture	Generalized joint laxity; severe muscle hypotonia; scoliosis at birth (progressive); scleral fragility and rupture of ocular globe	Very loose skin; severe generalized joint hypermobility with recurrent subluxations; bilateral congenital hip dislocation; kyphoscoliosis	Soft, doughy skin: fragile and bruises easily; sagging, redundant skin; loose joints; congenital umbilical hernia
Minor diagnostic characteristics	Smooth velvety skin; muscle hypotonia; delayed gross motor development; easy bruising; surgical complications; hernias; positive family history	Recurring joint dislocations in large or small joints; chronic joint/limb pain may be debilitating; bruising; positive family history	Tendon and muscle ruptures; talipes equinovarus (clubfoot) frequent at birth	Stretchy, soft skin, prone to bruising and scarring; Marfan-like appearance; osteoporosis is common; unpredictable tearing of arteries	Delayed motor skills; soft velvety skin, moderately stretchy, fragile, and prone to bruising; not usually to scar abnormally; early onset arthritis	Small chin; blue tinge to sclera (part of eyeball); mild overgrowth of body hair
Prevalence per type: (all types: 1 in 5000)	One of most common; 1 in 20,000 to 40,000	Most common; as many as 1 in 5000–20,000	1 in 250,000	Fewer than 60 cases reported worldwide	Very rare; ~30 cases reported worldwide	Fewer than 10 cases reported worldwide

Source: Types of Ehlers Danlos, The Canadian Ehlers Danlos Association, Bolton, Ontario, & Lavallee, Mark, M.D., Report at EDNF National Conference, Buffalo, NY, July 2004; http://www.ghr.nlm.nih.gov/ghr/disease/ehlersdanlossyndrome.

Diagnostic Signs and Symptoms

Speech and hearing problems related to EDS include, but are not limited to, imprecise articulation related to loose joints and a poor sense of proprioception. Hoarseness/weak voice is likely related to tissue fragility, laryngeal hypotonia, and limited lung capacity. Limited mouth opening due to temporomandibular joint problems underlie difficulties in biting into thick pieces of food and chewing (Hagberg et al, 2004). Speech-language pathologists noting hyperextensibility of the tongue should consider EDS a possible diagnosis. Hearing impairment appears related to hypermobility of joints of the bones in the middle ear. Dizziness may be noted.

Etiology

Speech behaviors appear directly related to faulty collagen and weak joints and secondarily to the resulting hypotonicity. These poor attachments to muscles and cartilage interfere with actions needed to move the articulators to produce speech, to chew and swallow, and to transmit sound.

Neuropathology

Neuropathological changes in EDS vary among types. These changes may relate to central nervous system deficits and are noted at the muscle level.

Associated Cognitive, Linguistic, and Communicative Signs and Symptoms

Cognitive or linguistic deficits (reported in approximately 18%) may occur, but are not necessary for the diagnosis. Hearing loss is noted in type VI (Toriello, Reardon, & Gorlin, 2004).

Special Diagnostic Considerations

There are no specific diagnostic considerations for evaluation of speech motor skills in EDS. Signs of hyperextensibility of the tongue and hypotonia should be explored. Physical examination may reveal a small mandible and a high, arched palate (Shprintzen, 1997).

Treatment

Treatment for speech problems should be planned individually, given the variability in symptoms, signs, and severity. Articulation intervention goals may include increased strength of weak articulators, increased breath support to assist airflow, and slowed rate of speech with shorter utterances (Hunter, Morgan, & Bird, 1998). Voice disorders may require focus on vocal hygiene to maintain healthy vocal folds and to facilitate diaphragmatic breathing. Fluency focus may include slowed rate of speech and respiratory support/timing. Audiological workup should be completed before initiating speech-language intervention. Assistive devices (e.g., hearing aids) should be fitted as early as possible when indicated. Evidence of treatment outcomes is needed.

References

Beighton, P., De Paepe, A., Steinmann, B., Tsipouras, P., & Wenstrup, R. (1998). Ehlers-Danlos syndrome: revised nosology, Villefranche, 1997. *American Journal of Medical Genetics, 77*, 31–37

Echaniz-Laguna, A., deSaint-Martin, A., Lafontaine, A.L., Tasch, E., Thomas, P., Hirsh, E., Marescaux, C., & Andermann, F. (2000). Bilateral focal polymicrogyria in Ehlers-Danlos syndrome. *Archives of Neurology, 57*, 123–127

Gorlin, R.J., Cohen, M.M., Hennekam, R.C.M. (2001). *Syndromes of the head and neck*. 4th ed. (p. 515). New York: Oxford University Press

Hagberg, C., Korpe, L., Berglund, B. (2004). Temporomandibular joint problems and self-registration of mandibular opening capacity among adults with Ehlers-Danlos syndrome. A questionnaire study. *Orthodontic Craniofacial Research, 7*, 40–46

Hawthorn, M. (2000). *Hearing impairment and Ehlers-Danlos syndrome.* The Ehlers-Danlos UK Support Group Web site: www.atv.ndirect.co.uk

Hunter, A., Morgan, A.W., & Bird, H.A. (1998). A survey of Ehlers-Danlos syndrome: hearing, voice, speech and swallowing difficulties—is there an underlying relationship? *British Journal of Rheumatology, 37*, 803–804

Nicholls, A.C., Oliver, J.E., McCarron, S., Harrison, J.B., Greenspan, D.S., & Pope, F.M. (1996). An exon skipping mutation of a type V collagen gene (COL5A1) in Ehlers-Danlos syndrome. *Journal of Medical Genetics, 33*, 940–946

Norton, L.A. & Assael, L.A. (1997). Orthodontic and temporomandibular joint considerations in treatment of patients with Ehlers-Danlos syndrome. *American Journal of Orthodontics and Dentofacial Orthoptics, 111*, 75–84

Shprintzen, R. (1997). *Genetics, Syndromes, and Communication Disorders* (p. 191). San Diego: Singular

Thomas, P., Bossan, A., Lacour, J.P., Chanalet, S., Ortonne, J.P., & Chatel, M. (1996). Ehlers-Danlos syndrome with subependymal periventricular heterotopias. *Neurology, 46*, 1165–1167

Toriello, H.V., Reardon, W., & Gorlin, R.J. (Eds.). (2004). *Hereditary Hearing Loss and Its Syndromes* (p. 146). New York: Oxford University Press

Chapter 28

Encephalitis

Justine V. Goozée and Bruce E. Murdoch

◆ General Information on Disorder

Encephalitis refers to an inflammation of the brain, which can be caused by a range of microorganisms including bacteria (e.g., *Mycobacterium tuberculosis,* leptospirosis), amoeba (e.g., *Balamuthia mandrillaris*), rickettsiae (e.g., Rocky Mountain spotted fever, endemic typhus), fungi (e.g., cryptococcus), and parasites (e.g., cerebral malaria, *Toxoplasma gondii;* Kennedy, 2004). The most typical central nervous system (CNS) invaders, however, are viruses including herpes viruses, arboviruses, enteroviruses, and childhood viruses (Bonthius & Karacay, 2002). The herpes viruses include herpes simplex virus type 1 and 2, human herpesvirus-6 (HHV-6), cytomegalovirus, varicella zoster (chicken pox and shingles), and the Epstein-Barr virus. The arboviruses are viruses that are transmitted from animals to humans by mosquitoes (e.g., Eastern and Western equine, West Nile, and Japanese encephalitis) and ticks. Enteroviruses (e.g., Coxsackie virus) enter the body through, and multiply in, the gastrointestinal tract, and then invade the CNS.

A secondary form of encephalitis, termed postinfectious encephalitis, can result when a virus infects the brain secondarily after infecting other parts of the body (e.g., measles, rubella, and varicella), rather than by direct, primary invasion. Encephalitis may also manifest as part of a reaction to vaccinations (Brodsky & Stanievich, 1985; Kennedy, 2004).

Diagnostic Signs and Symptoms

The presenting signs and symptoms of encephalitis may include fever, chills, malaise, headache, stiff neck, nausea, vomiting, altered mental state, behavioral changes, confusion, impaired consciousness, speech disturbances, motor weakness, cranial nerve dysfunction, and focal or generalized seizures (Bonthius & Karacay, 2002; Marshall, 1982). The pattern of signs and symptoms may differ, however, depending on the type of microorganism contracted, and the site and extent of the inflammation.

The onset of encephalitis is typically acute, but it can also develop more gradually (Robinson & Gilbert, 1986). The duration of the illness is typically a few weeks (Marshall, 1982), but resultant neurological sequelae can persist. The outcomes of encephalitis vary between individuals, from no neurological effects through to persistent effects of varying severity in approximately 25 to 40% of individuals (Brodsky & Stanievich, 1985; Robinson & Gilbert, 1986). In others, the disease is fatal.

Neuropathology

The damage sustained to the CNS following infection can be focal or multifocal, but typically diffuse. Some viruses appear to demonstrate a preference for affecting certain prescribed, localized regions. For example, the typical sites of damage caused by the herpes simplex virus are the temporal and frontal lobes; for the Coxsackie virus it is the basal ganglia; the encephalitis symptoms expressed by the West Nile virus and the varicella virus suggest that the brainstem and cerebellum, respectively, may form target regions (Bonthius & Karacay, 2002; Peatfield, 1987).

The nature of the damage sustained to the CNS in encephalitis can comprise acute inflammation with neuronal necrosis or damage, cerebral edema, demyelination and lesioning of the white matter, and circulatory disturbances including hemorrhages, hypoperfusion, and diminished cerebrovascular reserves (Okamoto, Ashida, & Imaizumi, 2001; Robinson & Gilbert, 1986).

Epidemiology

In regard to the incidence of encephalitis, two forms are recognized: sporadic (i.e., can occur at any time of the year) and epidemic (i.e., part of an outbreak). The various types of encephalitis are reported to be relatively rare (Bonthius & Karacay, 2002; Brodsky & Stanievich, 1985). Herpes simplex virus type 1 is considered to be the most common sporadic encephalitis type. Epidemic outbreaks of encephalitis have occurred in different geographical regions and are typically caused by arboviruses (Robinson & Gilbert, 1986).

Genetics

Not applicable, given that encephalitis results from microbial infection.

◆ Speech Impairment Associated with Disorder

The literature on speech disturbances resulting from encephalitis appears to be composed almost exclusively of viral encephalitis cases. Dysarthria with articulatory, laryngeal, and respiratory subsystem involvement through to mutism have been observed following viral encephalitis. A review of 15 patients with influenza B–associated encephalitis indicated that shortly after onset one patient presented with dysarthria and bulbar paralysis, whereas another three patients demonstrated mutism (Newland et al, 2003). Of the three patients who were initially mute, only one demonstrated complete resolution of neurological and speech disturbances. Outcomes for the other two patients included ataxia in one patient, and oromotor apraxia, difficulty with rhythmic speech, and difficulty coordinating phonation and respiration, with resolution of other motor disturbances, in the other patient. A child presenting with bulbar paralysis had a concurrent respiratory viral infection and died.

A more detailed case study described the articulatory deficits exhibited by a 5-year-old boy who had viral encephalitis at around 6 months to 1 year of age. Observations revealed poor motor coordination, limited range and control of tongue movements, and retraction of lips with no ability to protrude lips. The child expressed his needs through grunting and a small vocabulary set, with poor articulation (Kastein, 1952).

A reportedly rare syndrome, known as operculum or Foix-Chavany-Marie syndrome, can result from bilateral focal cortical damage of the anterior opercular region following encephalitis (Prats, Garaizar, Uterga, & Urroz, 1992). A clinical feature of the syndrome is pseudobulbar palsy, with anarthria or mutism in severe cases. Impairments of mastication and swallowing (van der Poel, Haenggeli, & Overweg-Plandsoen, 1995) and focal facial seizures have also been observed (van der Poel et al, 1995). Persistent speech deficits (i.e., mutism) have been noted at follow-up, in the company of normal language comprehension (Prats et al, 1992).

A vocal tremor was noted during the acute stage of encephalitis in a man (Marshall, 1982). The long-term follow-up of a female who had contracted Japanese encephalitis revealed that, as part of a resulting complex of severe intellectual and motor disabilities including generalized dystonia, she exhibited laryngeal dystonia, an attenuated pharyngeal reflex, and dysphagia (Hamano et al, 2004). Paroxysmal attacks of respiratory disturbance and inspiratory stridor due to abduction restriction of the vocal cords (a feature of her laryngeal dystonia) were also observed. Consistent with her symptoms, magnetic resonance imaging (MRI) revealed basal ganglia lesions (Hamano et al, 2004).

Diagnostic Signs and Symptoms

No specific diagnostic signs or symptoms for speech following encephalitis are recognized. Any speech disturbances that are exhibited are dependent on the nature, site(s), and extent of neurological damage. Given the potential for focal, multifocal, or diffuse damage to the CNS, a range of speech deficits may present following encephalitis.

Neuropathology

Neuronal necrosis and white matter lesioning can occur at any site in the CNS following encephalitis, including the cerebral cortex, basal ganglia, brainstem, cerebellum, and their connections. Damage to these sites in turn can result in disturbances in the strength, tone, coordination, or range of movement of the speech musculature.

Associated Cognitive, Linguistic, and Communicative Signs and Symptoms

A range of cognitive-linguistic impairments has been reported following encephalitis. Case reports have included diagnoses of motor aphasia, anomic aphasia, and fluent aphasia, but with exceptional features not consistent with the classic aphasia syndrome of Wernicke's aphasia. Subcortical dementia has also been reported subsequent to basal ganglia damage caused by Coxsackie virus encephalitis. The sequelae of herpes virus encephalitis have included anterograde and retrograde memory dysfunction, auditory agnosia, and semantic impairments. Long-term behavioral changes in the form of emotionalism, irritability, anxiety, and depression have also been observed.

Special Diagnostic Considerations

Speech disturbances may present as one of a myriad of other signs and symptoms (e.g., fever, headache, altered mental state) at the onset of encephalitis. There are no special diagnostic considerations for the evaluation of speech following encephalitis.

Treatment

The paucity of studies reporting speech disturbances following encephalitis may be indicative of a relatively small incidence of occurrence or, as Marshall (1982) proposed, may be related to the nature and typical management of encephalitis. With encephalitis being a life-endangering disease, of typically brief duration (i.e., a few weeks), referral to a speech pathologist is often not made (Marshall, 1982). Medical treatment of encephalitis is largely symptomatic and supportive. Antiviral medication and antibiotics may be prescribed.

References

Bonthius, D.J. & Karacay, B. (2002). Meningitis and encephalitis in children. An update. *Neurology Clinics, 20*, 1013–1038

Brodsky, L. & Stanievich, J. (1985). Sensorineural hearing loss following live measles virus vaccination. *International Journal of Pediatric Otorhinolaryngology, 10*, 159–163

Hamano, K., Kumada, S., Hayashi, M., Naito, R., Hayashida, T., Uchiyama, A., & Kurata, K. (2004). Laryngeal dystonia in a case of severe motor and intellectual disabilities due to Japanese encephalitis sequelae. *Brain and Development, 26*, 335–338

Kastein, S. (1952). Speech and language habilitation in a post-encephalitic child. *American Journal of Mental Deficiency, 56*, 570–577

Kennedy, P.G.E. (2004). Viral encephalitis: causes, differential diagnosis, and management. *Journal of Neurology, Neurosurgery, and Psychiatry, 75*(suppl 1), i10–i15

Marshall, R.C. (1982). Language and speech recovery in a case of viral encephalitis. *Brain and Language, 17,* 316–326

Newland, J.G., Romero, J.R., Varman, M., Drake, C., Holst, A., Safranek, T., & Subbarao, K. (2003). Encephalitis associated with influenza B virus infection in 2 children and a review of the literature. *Clinical and Infectious Diseases, 36,* 87–95

Okamoto, M., Ashida, K.I., & Imaizumi, M. (2001). Hypoperfusion following encephalitis: SPECT with acetazolamide. *European Journal of Neurology, 8,* 471–474

Peatfield, R.C. (1987). Basal ganglia damage and subcortical dementia after possible insidious Coxsackie virus encephalitis. *Acta Neurologica Scandinavica, 76,* 340–345

Prats, J.M., Garaizar, C., Uterga, J.M., & Urroz, M.J. (1992). Operculum syndrome in childhood: a rare cause of persistent speech disturbance. *Developmental Medicine and Child Neurology, 34,* 359–364

Robinson, M.J. & Gilbert, G.L. (1986). Meningitis and encephalitis in infancy and childhood. In: M.J. Robinson (Ed.), *Practical Paediatrics* (pp. 235–243). Melbourne: Churchill Livingstone

van der Poel, J.C., Haenggeli, C.A., & Overweg-Plandsoen, W.C. (1995). Operculum syndrome: unusual feature of herpes simplex encephalitis. *Pediatric Neurology, 12,* 246–249

Additional Reading

Smyth, V., Ozanne, A.E., & Woodhouse, L.M. (1990). Communicative disorders in childhood infectious diseases. In: B.E. Murdoch (Ed.), *Acquired Neurological Speech/Language Disorders in Childhood* (pp. 148–176). London: Taylor & Francis

Chapter 29

Fragile X Syndrome

Vaia Varsami and Ilias Papathanasiou

◆ General Information on Disorder

Fragile X syndrome (FXS) is a genetic disorder and one of the most common inherited forms of learning disabilities and mental retardation. FXS is reported in the literature under different names, such as Escalante syndrome, Martin-Bell syndrome (MBS), Renpenning syndrome 2, autism–fragile X (AFRAX) syndrome, fra(X)(q27) syndrome, marker X syndrome, and X-linked mental deficiency–megalotestes syndrome, to name a few. The clinical picture of FXS is dominated by mental retardation, poor sensory perception and integration of information, characteristic physical features, delayed speech and language development, and behavioral problems. FXS gets its name from the appearance of the section of the X chromosome, at Xq27.3, which microscopically looks "fragile." More precisely, FXS is caused by a mutation in the *FMR-1* (fragile X mental retardation) gene, located on the X chromosome (Verkerk et al, 1991). This gene is responsible for instructing the cell to produce FMRP, a protein assumed to be essential for proper mental functioning. The X-linkage indicates that the frequency of the syndrome is greater in males, who are usually more severely affected, than in females. Unlike other X-linked conditions, FXS exhibits an unusual inheritance pattern. For instance, males can have the *FMR-1* gene but show no effects of the syndrome. At least 20% of males who are carriers of the fragile X gene are unaffected. The clinical signs of fragile X appear gradually during childhood. The syndrome does not seem to affect life expectancy, and no particular cause of death is reported for affected individuals (Blancquaert & Caron 2002)

Diagnostic Signs and Symptoms

The clinical diagnosis is not easy to make. Individuals with FXS syndrome present with a cluster of *physical* (e.g., elongated face with prominent jaw, large ears, high arched palate, macro-orchidism, recurrent ear infections, joint laxity, congenital hip dislocation, scoliosis, poor muscle tone, mitral valve prolapse, seizure disorders, strabismus), *developmental* (e.g., intellectual and learning disabilities, fine and gross motor delays, coordination difficulties, speech and language delays), and *behavioral* characteristics (e.g., attention-deficit disorder, autistic-like behaviors, hyperarousal, sensory defensiveness, mood instability with aggression or depression). Neurological examination is usually normal, but tremor, apraxia, and a broad-based gait are occasionally recorded (Murray, 1997). Clinical diagnostic testing is based on the detection of an alteration in the *FMR-1* gene. More than 99% of affected individuals have a full mutation in the *FMR-1* gene caused by an increased number of cytosine, guanine, guanine (CGG) trinucleotide repeats (>200 typically) accompanied by aberrant methylation of the *FMR-1* gene. Both increased trinucleotide repeats and methylation changes in *FMR-1* can be detected by molecular genetic testing. Clinically, molecular genetic testing is performed by using two techniques, Southern blot and polymerase chain reaction (PCR), which are performed sequentially (Warren & Nelson, 1994). The Southern blot method is used to identify large expansions and determine the gene's methylation status, followed, if need be, by PCR to accurately determine the size of the normal and premutated alleles. Prenatal tests (amniocentesis, chronic villus sampling, and percutaneous umbilical blood sampling [PUBS]) give evidence of a fetus presenting with FXS. All three tests carry the risk of miscarriage. However, a couple with a family history of fragile X syndrome or mental retardation should consult a medical geneticist or a genetic counselor to learn more about the risks of this disorder in their offspring.

Neuropathology

Recent studies have reported that FMRP is most abundant in neurons and appears to play a role in structural and functional maturation of synapses (Weiler & Greenough 1999). FMRP is found in both nucleus and cytoplasm, where it binds with messenger RNAs (mRNAs) associated with ribonucleoproteins (RNPs) specifically associated with polyribosomes. FMRP-associated RNPs are located in the cell body, as well as in the dendrites, at the base of dendritic spines. Thus, FMRP may play a role in synaptic function and plasticity and may be partially responsible for the reduction of neuronal connections that normally occurs during early development. Lower levels of FMRP are believed to be related to less neuronal pruning, and therefore to atypical brain development (Irwin, Galvez, & Greenough, 2000). However, the role of FMRP has still not been completely elucidated, and the neuropathological or pathophysiological bases of the syndrome are still unknown. More studies are needed to identify how FMRP modulates translation of interacting messages, and whether the messages modulated differ in cell body and dendrite. However, studies have revealed that premutation carriers later in life exhibit neurological features such as tremor and ataxia (Berry-Kravis et al, 2003). Neuroimaging studies have shown that males and females with FXS often have a smaller cerebellar vermis and larger caudate, thalamus, and hippocampus (Roberts, Hennon, & Anderson, 2003).

Epidemiology

Evidence is lacking about the true incidence of FXS. Recent studies have estimated a prevalence of affected FXS carriers of 16 to 25 in 100,000 males (Turner, Webb, Wake, & Robinson, 1996). The prevalence of females is assumed to be approximately one-half the male prevalence. The prevalence of females who are unaffected FXS carriers has been found to be quite high.

Genetics

The genetics of FXS syndrome are quite complicated. On a normal X chromosome, the *FMR-1* gene includes a DNA sequence of CGG, which contains less than 50 copies of the CGG repeat. Individuals with between 50 and 200 repeats are often "premutation" (PM) carriers of fragile X who have mild symptoms or no symptoms at all. When the number of repeats increases, the chemical modification process called DNA methylation (the *FMR-1* gene becomes methylated—shuts down—and, as a consequence, production of FMRP is inhibited) is more likely to occur. It is this chemical modification that appears to inactivate the *FMR-1* gene responsible for FMRP production, which leads to deficits in cognitive processing. Why methylation of this region of DNA leads to the symptoms of FXS is not understood. Mental impairment in FXS appears to correlate with DNA containing more than 200 repeats. In that case, individuals have a full mutation, and most males are impaired and 50% of females show some learning disabilities. However, there are exceptions, including individuals with enormous numbers of repeats who have no apparent impairment.

◆ Speech Impairment Associated with Disorder

Speech problems are characterized by echolalia, rapid and fluctuating rate, and dysfluency. Generalized oral motor difficulties and oral and verbal dyspraxia are reported, with difficulty repeating multisyllabic sequences, low muscle tone, and motor planning problems.

Diagnostic Signs and Symptoms

Diagnostic signs or symptoms for speech in FXS are variable and not consistent among affected individuals with FXS. However, recent studies on speech problems associated with FXS reveal the presence of developmental oral and verbal dyspraxia, which could be related to the general motor coordination and planning difficulties reported in FXS.

In addition, hypotonicity is almost always mentioned in the syndrome's physical characteristics, but no link between poor muscle tone and possible dysarthric speech has been reported.

Etiology

The etiology of speech problems in children with FXS has not been fully explained.

Neuropathology

The neuropathology of the syndrome does not account for the oral or verbal dyspraxia a child with FXS may present. In addition, hypotonicity, tremor, and a broad-based gait are occasionally recorded but are not fully explained on a neuropathological basis. Further neuroimaging research needs to be conducted to verify the underlying neuropathology of FXS.

Associated Cognitive, Linguistic, and Communicative Signs and Symptoms

Most affected males are moderately to profoundly mentally impaired, with an IQ of less than 50, whereas females have an IQ of between 70 and 85 (Murray et al, 1997). Cognitive impairment includes difficulties with reasoning and making inferences, memory, processing, and integration of information. Language is characterized by phonological difficulties as well as perseveration, syntactic, and word retrieval difficulties. Pragmatic difficulties are also present, including poor topic maintenance in conversation, difficulty answering direct questions, gaze aversion, and autistic-like behaviors.

Special Diagnostic Considerations

There are no special diagnostic considerations for evaluation of speech in FXS. Oral and verbal dyspraxia alone cannot be used as criterion for diagnosis. Speech delay problems are often one of the earliest diagnostic signs.

Treatment

Although there is currently no cure for FXS, a multidisciplinary team approach, consisting of speech-language pathologists, pediatricians, special educators, physical and occupational therapists, and psychologists, is suggested to alleviate the symptoms. Intervention and treatment plans should be personalized by considering each individual's developmental level, strengths, weaknesses, and needs while considering the characteristics common among individuals with FXS.

References

Berry-Kravis, E., Lewin, F., & Wuu, J., et al. (2003). Tremor and ataxia in fragile X premutation carriers: blinded videotape study. *Annals of Neurology, 53,* 616–623

Blancquaert, I. & Caron, L. (2001). *Fragile X Syndrome: The Role of Molecular Diagnosis and Screening in An Integrated Approach to Services. Report Prepared by (AÉTMIS 01–1 RE).* Montreal: AÉTMIS

Irwin, S.A., Galvez, R., & Greenough, W.T. (2000). Dendritic spine structural anomalies in fragile-X mental retardation syndrome. *Cerebral Cortex, 10,* 1038–1044

Murray, J., Cuckle, H., Taylor, G., & Hewison, J. (1997). Screening for fragile X syndrome: information needs for health planners. *Journal of Medical Screening, 4,* 6–94

Roberts, J., Hennon, E.A., & Anderson, K. (2003). Fragile X syndrome and speech and language. *The ASHA Leader, 8,* 726–727

Turner, G., Webb, T., Wake, S., & Robinson, H. (1996). Prevalence of fragile X syndrome. *American Journal of Medical Genetics, 64,* 196–197

Verkerk, A.J.M.H., Pieretti, M., Sutcliffe, J.S., et al. (1991). Identification of a gene (FMR-1) containing a CGG repeat coincident with a breakpoint cluster region exhibiting length variation in fragile X syndrome. *Cell, 65,* 905–914

Warren, S.T. & Nelson, D.L. (1994). Advances in molecular analysis of fragile X syndrome. *Journal of the American Medical Association, 271,* 536–542

Weiler, I.J. & Greenough, W.T. (1999). Synaptic synthesis of the fragile X protein: possible involvement in synapse maturation and elimination. *American Journal of Medical Genetics, 83,* 248–252

Additional Reading

Hagerman, R.J. & Silverman. A.C. (1991). *Fragile X Syndrome: Diagnosis, Treatment, and Research.* Baltimore: Johns Hopkins University Press

Chapter 30

Goldenhar Syndrome and Hemifacial Microsomia: The Oculo-Auriculo-Vertebral Spectrum

Cynthia A. Eberwein, Stacey L. Pavelko, and Sheila R. Pratt

◆ General Information on Disorder

Oculo-auriculo-vertebral spectrum (OAVS) refers to a complex of congenital anomalies that involve structures arising from the first and second brachial arches. It is heterogeneous in expression and severity, and one of the most common syndromes with asymmetric manifestations. Variants of the spectrum are referred to as Goldenhar syndrome, Goldenhar-Gorlin syndrome, oculo-auriculo-vertebral dysplasia, hemifacial microsomia, lateral facial dysplasia, and first and second branchial arch syndrome.

Diagnostic Signs and Symptoms

Oculo-auriculo-vertebral spectrum typically is characterized by craniofacial anomalies that are either unilateral in nature or bilateral, with one side worse than the other. A unilateral external ear abnormality often is viewed as a required feature for diagnosis (Gorlin, Cohen, & Hennekam, 2001). A range of pinna and external ear canal differences may be evident, including preauricular skin tags or sinuses, and are frequently seen in combination with macrostomia, aplasia of the parotid gland, and epibulbar dermoids (Allanson, 2004). Facial asymmetry is present in 65% of cases, with marked asymmetry occurring in approximately 20% of cases (Soltan & Holmes, 1986), and approximately 10 to 30% of cases have bilateral involvement (Rollnick, Kaye, Nagatoshi, Hauck, & Martin, 1987). Unilateral or bilateral cleft lip or palate occurs in approximately 7 to 15% of patients (Rollnick et al, 1987). Submucosal clefts, high vaulted palates, and asymmetries of the palate and faucial pillars are frequently observed. Malocclusion is very common. Cranial base and cervical vertebral anomalies are consistent with OAVS. Anomalies are commonly observed in multiple organ systems (Allanson, 2004).

Neuropathology

Cranial defects can contribute to brain malformations (Allanson, 2004). Across reported cases, nearly all of the cranial nerves have been implicated but most commonly the lower portion of the facial nerve due to bony involvement of the facial canal (Aleksic et al, 1984; Bassila & Goldberg, 1989). Although most hearing loss is conductive due to malformations of the external and middle ear structures, in a substantive number of cases inner ear malformations contribute to sensorineural hearing loss that can be unilateral or bilateral (Carvalho, Song, Vargervik, & Lalwani, 1999).

Epidemiology

The incidence of OAVS is estimated at approximately 1 in 5600 births, with a male-to-female ratio of at least 3:2 and a right side to left side involvement ratio of 3:2 (Grabb, 1965). The pathogenesis of OAV spectrum is somewhat unclear, with various explanations proposed (Araneta et al, 1997; Gorlin et al, 2001; Lam, 2000; Soltan & Holmes, 1986). However, it is generally believed that sometime between 3 and 45 days gestation, the sequence is initiated by disturbances in neural crest cells that impede development of craniofacial structures.

Genetics

Most cases of OAVS are sporadic; however, familial cases of autosomal dominant and autosomal recessive inheritance have been reported. Discordance in monozygotic twins, as well as rarer cases of concordance in monozygotic twins and triplets, has been reported (Ferrari, Silengo, Ponzone, & Perugini, 1999). In addition, some chromosomal anomalies have been associated with OAVS, which further suggests a possible genetic link, although a clear basis for OAVS has not been established (Josifova, Patton, & Marks, 2004).

◆ Speech Impairment Associated with Disorder

Although it is reasonable to expect speech disorders given the multisystem anomalies associated with this spectrum, the literature provides only limited data regarding the presence of speech signs and symptoms associated with OAVS. Cleft lip or palate, cranial nerve and central nervous system dysfunction, tongue dysfunction, pharyngeal and laryngeal abnormalities, and hearing loss are associated with this disorder, any of which can contribute to speech production problems.

Diagnostic Signs and Symptoms

Problems with articulation can be observed due to structural and neural abnormalities throughout the head and neck, and contribute to reduced intelligibility. Although dysarthria with OAVS has not been addressed specifically in the literature, it should be expected given the likelihood of peripheral and central neural involvement. Velopharyngeal inadequacy and unilateral hypoplasia of the pharyngeal constrictors and other pharyngeal muscles can contribute to abnormal resonance, hypernasality and nasal emission even in the absence of a cleft palate (D'Antonio, Rice, & Fink, 1998). Abnormal voice quality is common (e.g., harsh/breathy voice and high pitch voice) due to laryngeal or pharyngeal abnormalities, including vocal fold abnormalities and supraglottic dysmorphology (D'Antonio et al, 1998). Upper airway obstructions and pulmonary dysfunction can interfere with respiratory support for vocalization. Depending on the presence, configuration, and severity of a hearing loss, speech and vocal characteristics consistent with hearing loss also may be present (see Chapter 13).

Little research has been conducted to evaluate the phonological processes associated with OAVS, although a recent study of four Dutch children diagnosed with OAVS reported speech errors consistent with dentalization, final consonant and unstressed syllable deletion, and cluster reduction, as well as voice and resonance problems (Van Lierde, Van Cauwenberge, Stevens, & Dhooge, 2004).

Etiology

Speech and language deficits can result directly from the musculoskeletal and neural abnormalities of the head and neck region, as described earlier. They also can arise secondary to hearing loss, pulmonary dysfunction, and cognitive impairment.

Neuropathology

Neuropathological manifestations can be due to abnormalities of one or more cranial nerves as well as the brain malformations mentioned previously. These anomalies may be further associated with damage to the ventricles, cerebellum, or pons, and result in additional changes in tone, reflexes, strength, range of movement, and overall motor control.

Associated Cognitive, Linguistic, and Communicative Signs and Symptoms

Most individuals with OAVS present normal intelligence with only 5 to 15% demonstrating some sort of mental retardation, and approximately 10% showing some learning disability. Delays in expressive and receptive language have been reported despite normal cognitive functioning (Van Lierde et al, 2004).

Special Diagnostic Considerations

The diagnosis of OAVS is typically based on craniofacial signs/symptoms that are asymmetric in nature and supported by computed tomography (CT) or magnetic resonance imaging (MRI) results. Early evaluation of oral-motor integrity, hearing, vision, lip and palate, as well as laryngeal and pharyngeal integrity should be made, as failure to diagnose anomalies in these structures could result in protracted speech and language problems. In cases of severe laryngeal/pharyngeal dysmorphology, assessments of obstructive sleep apnea and intubation risk should be conducted. Also, swallow studies should be considered given the compounded risk of eating and drinking problems with the inclusion of facial nerve dysfunction (de Swart, Verheij, & Beurskens, 2003).

Treatment

As OAVS begins early in fetal development and can impact numerous systems, patients might require early intervention services from a range of health care providers. Reports in the literature suggest that speech and language services are likely to be successful in patients without mental retardation (Belenchia & McCardle, 1985). Treatment goals depend on the structures affected and the severity of the involvement, with initial efforts focused on identifying anomalies and their potential impact on the development of speech, hearing, language, and eating.

References

Aleksic S., Budzilovich, G., Greco, M., McCarthy, J., Reuben, R., Margolis, S., et al. (1984). Intracranial lipmas, hydrocephalus and other CNS anomalies inoculoauriculo-vertebral dysplasia (Goldenhar-Gorlin syndrome). *Child's Brain*, 11, 285-297

Allanson, J. (2004). Genetic hearing loss associated with external ear abnormalities. In: H.V. Toriello, W. Reardon, & R.J. Gorlin (Eds.), *Hereditary Hearing Loss and Its Syndromes*, 2nd ed. (pp 83-125). New York: Oxford University Press

Araneta, M.R., Moore, C., Olney, R., Edmonds, L., Karcher, J., McDonough, C., et al. (1997). Goldenhar syndrome among infants born in military hospitals to Gulf War veterans. *Teratology*, 56, 244-251

Bassila, M.K. & Goldberg, R. (1989). The association of facial palsy and/or sensorineural hearing loss in patients with hemifacial microsomia. *Cleft Palate Journal*, 26, 289-291

Belenchia P. & McCardle, P. (1985). Goldenhar's syndrome: a case study. *Journal of Communication Disorders*, 18, 383-392

Carvalho, G.J., Song, C., Vargervik, K., & Lalwani, A. (1999). Auditory and facial nerve dysfunction in patients with hemifacial microsomia. *Archives of Otolaryngology-Head and Neck Surgery*, 125, 209-212

D'Antonio, L.L., Rice, R., & Fink, S. (1998). Evaluation of pharyngeal and laryngeal structure and function in patients with oculo-auriculo-vertebral spectrum. *Cleft Palate and Craniofacial Journal*, 35, 333-341

de Swart, B.J., Verheij, J.C., & Beurskens, C.H. (2003). Problems with eating and drinking in patients with unilateral peripheral facial paralysis. *Dysphagia*, 18, 267-273

Ferraris, S., Silengo, M., Ponzone, A., & Perugini, L. (1999). Goldenhar anomaly in one of triplets derived from in vitro fertilization. *American Journal of Medical Genetics*, 84, 167-168

Gorlin, R., Cohen, M., & Hennekam, R. (2001). *Syndromes of the Head and Neck*, 4th ed. New York: Oxford University Press

Grabb, W.C. (1965). The first and second branchial arch syndrome. *Plastic and Reconstructive Surgery*, 36, 485-508

Josifova, D.J., Patton, M., & Marks, K. (2004). Oculoauriculovertebral spectrum phenotype caused by an unbalanced t(5;8)(p15.31;p23.1) rearrangement. *Clinical Dysmorphology*, 13, 151-153

Lam, C.H. (2000). A theory on the embryogenesis of oculoauriculo-vertebral (Goldenhar) syndrome. *Journal of Craniofacial Surgery, 11*, 547–552

Rollnick, B.R., Kaye, C.I., Nagatoshi, K., Hauck, W., & Martin, A.O. (1987). Oculoauriculovertebral dysplasia and variants: phenotypic characteristics of 294 patients. *American Journal of Medical Genetics*, 26, 361-375

Soltan, H.C. & Holmes, L.B. (1986). Familial occurrence of malformations possibly attributable to vascular abnormalities. *Journal of Pediatrics*, 108, 112-114

Van Lierde, K.M., Van Cauwenberge, P., Stevens, I., Dhooge, I. (2004). Language, articulation, voice and resonance characteristics in 4 children with Goldenhar syndrome: a pilot study. *Folia Phoniatrica et Logopaedica*, 56, 131-143

Chapter 31

Guillain-Barré Syndrome

Ilias Papathanasiou and John Ellul

◆ General Information on Disorder

Guillain-Barré syndrome (GBS) defines a recognizable clinical entity that is characterized by rapidly evolving symmetric ascending limp weakness, areflexia, and a variable degree of autonomic dysfunction. Diagnosis is made on the basis of clinical presentation and examination, and confirmed with cerebrospinal fluid (CSF) examination and serial electrophysiologic studies. The condition occurs worldwide, affecting patients of all ages and both sexes (Alter, 1990). Two thirds of cases of GBS are preceded by an acute infectious process that triggers a self-limited autoimmune response. GBS, however, embraces a heterogeneous group of pathological entities, including acute inflammatory demyelinating polyneuropathy (AIDP), acute motor axonal neuropathy (AMAN), acute motor sensory axonal neuropathy (AMSAN), and Miller Fisher syndrome (MFS), which have distinctive clinical features and pathogenesis.

The prognosis is generally favorable, although it is a serious disease with mortality up to 10% and residual functional disability in approximately 25% of the cases. Treatment involves supportive care, and cardiac and respiratory monitoring. Intravenous immunoglobulin is the treatment of choice and is safer and more convenient to administer than plasma exchange (Hahn, 1998). It seems, however, that treatment reduces the time to recovery, without significantly altering the proportion of patients with persistent deficit. The use of corticosteroids alone or combined with intravenous immunoglobulin has not been found to be effective, but this subject is still controversial (van Koningsveld et al, 2004).

Diagnostic Signs and Symptoms

The initial symptoms are usually painful peripheral paresthesias, but no definite sensory findings are found on examination. The limb weakness is generally symmetric and often most marked in the proximal muscles. The paralysis is typically ascending and evolves over hours to a few days, or at the most up to 4 weeks. The legs are usually more affected than the arms. Symptoms may progress to affect the facial muscles (bilateral facial palsy in 50% of the cases), as well as oropharyngeal and respiratory muscles. Atypical presentations may include initial bilateral facial weakness often followed by a descending version of the disorder. Autonomic dysfunctions, such as fluctuation in blood pressure, postural hypotension, and cardiac dysrhythmias,

occur in most patients. Transient bladder dysfunction may occur in severe cases, but it is not a prominent feature. Areflexia or hyporeflexia occurs during the early stages of the disease, and is an invariable feature that strongly supports the diagnosis. The Miller Fisher syndrome (MFS) has distinct clinical features and is characterized by ophthalmoparesis, ataxia, and tendon areflexia. The term MFS should be used in cases that conform to this description, and by common usage cases with facial and bulbar palsy are accepted within the definition (Hughes, Hadden, Gregson, & Smith, 1999). The typical CSF pattern consists of an elevated protein level (100 to 1000 mg/dL) without accompanying elevation of cell count. CSF protein may not rise until the end of the first week. Similarly, early neurophysiological studies reveal normal conduction velocities in many patients.

Neuropathology

Two thirds of patients report an antecedent acute infectious illness (1 to 3 weeks prior to neuropathic symptoms), usually respiratory or gastrointestinal. The most frequently encountered pathogen is *Campylobacter jejuni*. Cytomegalovirus and Epstein-Barr virus, varicella-zoster virus, and *Mycoplasma pneumoniae* are also encountered. The popular hypothesis to explain the association between acute infection and GBS is that there is cross-reactivity between lipopolysaccharide components of the pathogen and peripheral nerve gangliosides (molecular mimicry) (Yuki et al, 2004). The early lymphocytic and subsequent macrophage infiltrates in the spinal roots and peripheral nerves cause segmental stripping of myelin, which leads to the characteristic electrophysiological findings of slowing nerve-conduction velocities, delay in F waves, and conduction block. This autoimmune reaction is self-limited, and remyelination sets in promptly, which correlates with a quick and complete recovery. In those with severe disease, demyelination is accompanied by loss of nerve axons. The degree of axonal loss is correlated with a slower speed of recovery and worse functional outcome. In some GBS subtypes, however, the primary insult is believed to be the loss of sensory or motor axons.

Epidemiology

Current epidemiological studies suggest an incidence of 1 to 2 in 100,000 annually, with a slight male preponderance (Alter, 1990; Cheng et al, 2000; Chroni et al, 2004). The incidence rises with age, with a slight peak in late adolescence and young adulthood, coinciding with an increased risk of infections with *C. jejuni* and cytomegalovirus. A second peak is observed in the elderly.

◆ Speech Impairment Associated with Disorder

Dysarthria is the commonest speech disturbance that is associated with GBS. However, the clinical presentation is variable and related to the site of lesion. For instance, in MFS, bilateral facial paralysis resulting in dysarthria is among the primary observed clinical symptoms, whereas in other GBS subtypes dysarthria could be a mild and secondary feature. Furthermore, the detailed speech production skills of patients with GBS have not been well studied.

Diagnostic Signs and Symptoms

Sudden onset of facial weakness with associated sensory loss is usually evident during the early stages of the disease in half of the patients with GBS. Facial, oropharyngeal, and ocular muscles are first affected only in MFS; as in other subtypes, weakness starts from the proximal muscles. Symptoms are usually bilateral and symmetrical, with muscular tone reduced and tendon reflexes diminished or absent. Subsequently, dysarthria, which is described as flaccid, could be observed (Freed, 2000; Murdoch, Ward, & Theodoros, 2000). The physical parameters of the movements affected are range, strength, and tone. Within the first few weeks recovery is very good, and muscle wasting and atrophy are not common. Examination of the speech subsystems shows that the respiratory-phonatory and the articulation are affected due to associated respiratory failure and muscle weakness, resulting in breathiness, harsh voice, audible inspiration, monopitch, monoloudness, and distortion of the consonants (Murdoch et al, 2000). Other speech characteristics may include hypernasality with nasal emission due to the disruption of the palatopharyngeal valve. Similar symptoms sometimes may occur in chronic demyelinating neuropathies, but these conditions are characterized by gradual onset of symptoms, slow recovery, and less favorable prognosis (Duffy, 1995).

Etiology

The etiology of the speech behavior noted in GBS is the widespread inflammatory segmental demyelination, which affects the cranial and spinal respiratory nerves.

Neuropathology

Demyelination and sometimes axonal loss, which characterize GBS, lead to physical weakness, reduced tone, and areflexia or hyporeflexia of the facial, oropharyngeal, and ocular muscles, and occasional sensory loss of the speech mechanisms.

The MFS has distinct immunological and pathological features. The current hypothesis is that certain *C. jejuni* strains give rise to a characteristic pattern of antibodies that recognize epitopes expressed specifically in the nodal regions of oculomotor nerves as well as in dorsal-root ganglion cells and cerebellar neurons (Kornberg et al, 1996), which results in the features of ophthalmoplegia, ataxia, and areflexia.

Associative Cognitive, Linguistic, and Communicative Signs and Symptoms

No associated cognitive, linguistic, or communicative signs or symptoms have been reported in patients with GBS.

Special Diagnostic Considerations

There are no special diagnostic considerations for evaluations of speech in patients with GBS. Due to sudden onset of symptoms, speech evaluation should take place immediately, as in some cases it could contribute to the differential diagnosis of the condition, such as in cases of MFS, where the facial weakness is a prominent feature. In severe cases of GBS, evaluation of speech at the early stages could be impossible as patients are often ventilated within hours from the onset of symptoms. Additionally, the impact of the condition on the ability to swallow is more profound and dramatic and might require more urgent care.

Treatment

Prognosis in patients affected by GBS is generally very good, as only a small percentage have long-term problems. In severe cases, patients might be unable to produce any speech, and therefore alternative and augmentative communication (AAC) might be considered as an option. Neuromuscular treatment for speech and swallowing, such a strength training exercises, endurance exercises, and power training, are the basis for intervention to promote the quickest recovery and should be done at any stage of the disease (Clark, 2003). Finally, counseling of the individual and the caregiver on communicative abilities and strategies can be also offered based on the patient's needs.

References

Alter, M. (1990). The epidemiology of Guillain-Barre syndrome. *Annals of Neurology, 27* (suppl), S7–12

Cheng, Q., Jiang, G.X., Press, R., Andersson, M., Ekstedt, B., Vrethem, M., Liedholm, L.J., Lindsten, H., Brattstrom, L., Fredrikson, S., Link, H., & de Pedro-Cuesta, J. (2000). Clinical epidemiology of Guillain-Barre syndrome in adults in Sweden 1996–97: a prospective study. *European Journal of Neurology, 7,* 685–692

Chroni, E., Papapetropoulos, S., Gioldasis, G., Ellul, J., Diamadopoulos, N., & Papapetropoulos, T. (2004). Guillain-Barre syndrome in Greece: seasonality and other clinico-epidemiological features. *European Journal of Neurology, 11,* 383–388

Clark, H.M. (2003). Neuromuscular treatments for speech and swallowing: a tutorial. *American Journal of Speech, Language, and Pathology, 12,* 400–415

Duffy, J. (1995). *Motor Speech Disorders: Substrates, Differential Diagnosis and Management.* St Louis: Mosby

Freed, D. (2000). *Motor Speech Disorders: Diagnosis and Treatment.* San Diego: Singular Thomson Learning

Hahn, A.F. (1998). Guillain-Barre syndrome. *Lancet, 352,* 635–641

Hughes, R.A., Hadden, R.D., Gregson, N.A., & Smith, K.J. (1999). Pathogenesis of Guillain-Barre syndrome. *Journal of Neuroimmunology, 100,* 74–97

Kornberg, A.J., Pestronk, A., Blume, G.M., Lopate, G., Yue, J., & Hahn, A. (1996). Selective staining of the cerebellar molecular layer by serum IgG in Miller-Fisher and related syndromes. *Neurology, 47,* 1317–1320

Murdoch, B., Ward, L., & Theodoros, D. (2000). Dysarthria: clinical features, neuroanatomical framework and assessment. In: I. Papathanasiou (Ed.), *Acquired Neurogenic Communication Disorders: A Clinical Perspective.* London: Whurr

van Koningsveld, R., Schmitz, P.I., Meche, F.G., Visser, L.H., Meulstee, J., & van Doorn, P.A. (2004). Effect of methylprednisolone when added to standard treatment with intravenous immunoglobulin for Guillain-Barre syndrome: randomised trial. *Lancet, 363,* 192–196

Yuki, N., Susuki, K., Koga, M., Nishimoto, Y., Odaka, M., Hirata, K., Taguchi, K., Miyatake, T., Furukawa, K., Kobata, T., & Yamada, M. (2004). Carbohydrate mimicry between human ganglioside GM1 and Campylobacter jejuni lipooligosaccharide causes Guillain-Barre syndrome. *Proceedings of the National Academy of Science of the United States of America, 101,* 11404–11409

Chapter 32

Hashimoto's Encephalopathy

Joseph R. Duffy

◆ General Information on Disorder

Hashimoto's encephalopathy (HE) is a rare, potentially life-threatening, and incompletely understood autoimmune, thyroid-related neurological disease. It may represent a complication of Hashimoto's disease, or Hashimoto's thyroiditis, a form of chronic autoimmune thyroiditis (Ferracci, Bertiato, & Moretto, 2004). More descriptive terms for HE have been recommended, including *corticosteroid-responsive encephalopathy associated with autoimmune thyroiditis* (Sawka, Fatourechi, Boeve, & Mokri, 2002), *encephalopathy associated to autoimmune thyroid disease* (Canton, de Fabregas, Tintore, Mesa, Codina, & Simo, 2000), and *recurrent acute disseminated encephalomyelitis* (Chaudhuri & Behan, 2003).

Diagnostic Signs and Symptoms

HE develops acutely or subacutely. Its most frequent signs include seizures, rapidly progressive dementia, psychosis, personality change, myoclonus, ataxia, rigidity, movement disorders, pyramidal tract signs, occasional stroke-like episodes, and hallucinations (Seipelt, Zerr, Nau, Mollenhauer, Kropp, Steinhoff, Wilhelm-Gossling, Bamberg, Janzen, Berlit, Manz, Felgenhauer, & Poser, 1999). Stupor, coma, and amnesia have also been reported (Chaudhuri & Behan, 2003; Kalita, Misra, Rathore, Pradhan, & Das, 2003). The clinical presentation of HE can be similar to that associated with Creutzfeldt-Jacob disease (Kalita et al, 2003; Seiplet et al, 1999).

The presence of high titers of antithyroid antibodies in serum is considered diagnostic of HE in patients with acute or subacute encephalopathy (Kalita et al, 2003). Of interest, HE can be present in the absence of known thyroid disease. That is, many patients have biochemically normal thyroid function.

There are no pathognomonic electroencephalogram (EEG) or neuroimaging findings in HE. A variety of EEG abnormalities can be present (Henchey, Cibula, & Helveston, 1995). Magnetic resonance imaging (MRI) sometimes identifies generalized atrophy or diffuse or focal white matter abnormalities (McCabe, Burke, Connolly, & Hutchinson, 2000). Single photon emission computed tomography (SPECT) may show widespread or lateralized cortical hypoperfusion that may normalize with clinical recovery (Forchetti, Katsamakis, & Garron, 1997; Garrard, Hodges, De Vries, Hunt, Crawford, Hodges, & Balan, 2000; Kalita et al, 2003).

Hashimoto's encephalopathy usually responds to steroid treatment with remission of clinical signs and symptoms in approximately 80% of cases. Relapses can occur and some patients have lasting deficits (Garrard et al, 2000; McCabe et al, 2000).

Neuropathology

An autoimmune basis for HE is suggested by high titers of antithyroid antibodies, its fluctuating course, and its responsiveness to immunosuppressive (steroid) therapy (Kalita et al, 2003). Neuropathological data are limited, but hypotheses about its specific pathogenesis include autoimmune reactions to antigens shared by the thyroid gland and the CNS, autoimmune cerebral vasculitis, immune complex deposition, cerebral hypoperfusion, edema-induced cerebral dysfunction, and toxic effects of thyroid-releasing hormone (Ferracci, Mretto, Candeago, Cimini, Conte, Gentile, Papa, & Carnevale, 2003). The role of antithyroid antibodies is unclear. They may not be a direct cause of HE but instead may be a marker for other undetermined antibodies that cross the blood–brain barrier and initiate an autoimmune encephalopathy (Boers & Colebatch, 2001).

Epidemiology

The incidence of HE is not established. Prevalence has been estimated at 2.1 in 100,000 (Ferracci, Bertiato, & Moretto, 2004). Average age at onset is 47 years (Seipelt et al, 1999), but HE can occur in the young and old. It affects more women than men (Seipelt et al, 1999).

Genetics

Specific genetic mechanisms have not been established.

◆ Speech Impairment Associated with Disorder

Although the speech production deficits associated with HE have not been described, the expectation would be that those signs frequently appearing in hyperkinetic dysarthria would be present, especially those associated with tremor and myoclonus.

Diagnostic Signs and Symptoms

Sensorimotor speech disorders are uncommon. One review found dysarthria (type unspecified) in only 7% of cases (Seiplet et al, 1999). Palatal tremor and myorhythmic or myoclonic facial movements have been reported in some cases (Erickson, Carrasco, Grimes, Jabbari, & Cannard, 2002,). Apraxia of speech has not been reported.

Because the medical literature often ignores speech abnormalities unless they are handicapping, it is possible that speech disorders are underreported. The frequent presence of ataxia, tremor, myoclonus, extrapyramidal signs, and stroke-like episodes suggests that any central nervous system (CNS)-based dysarthria, at least theoretically, can occur.

Etiology

The effects of the encephalopathic process on the sensorimotor speech system are the presumed cause of any speech deficits. It seems that multiple loci are possible, including the upper motor neuron pathways and the basal ganglia and cerebellar control circuits.

Neuropathology

As is the case for the general signs and symptoms of HE, the precise neuropathology underlying any associated speech disorders is unclear and, probably, variable.

Associated Cognitive, Linguistic, and Communicative Signs and Symptoms

Cognitive deficits that can impact on communication are noted frequently and they sometimes persist following steroid therapy. Case studies implicate memory and attention deficits (e.g., amnestic syndrome, impaired delayed recall of verbal materials, impaired concentration) and impaired executive functions (Garrard et al, 2000; McCabe et al, 2000). Confusion, limb apraxia, and visuospatial deficits have also been described (Garrard et al, 2000; Seo, Lee, Park, Kim, & Yun, 2003).

Aphasia without nonaphasic cognitive-communication deficits has not been described, but language difficulties (e.g., word finding problems, circumlocution, semantic errors, reduced word fluency) are occasionally noteworthy, although usually only vaguely described (Garrard et al, 2000; McCabe et al, 2000; Seo et al, 2003).

Treatment

Therapy for HE is primarily medical (e.g., steroids), and subsequent recovery is good in many patients. Impairment-directed or compensation-directed behavioral management for associated communication disorders has not been described. Such treatments are not appropriate when consciousness is reduced, and they may not be appropriate if psychosis is present or if the desire or drive to communicate is limited. Memory deficits may require modification of therapy goals and methods. Compensatory strategies seem most appropriate prior to or during medical treatment. Following medical treatment, both impairment-directed and compensation-directed treatments could be considered for residual deficits.

References

Boers, P.M. & Colebatch, J.G. (2001). Hashimoto's encephalopathy responding to plasmapheresis. *Journal of Neurology, Neurosurgery & Psychiatry, 70*, 132

Canton, A., de Fabregas, O., Tintore, M., Mesa, J., Codina, A., & Simo, R. (2000). Encephalopathy associated to autoimmune thyroid disease: a more appropriate term for an underestimated condition. *Journal of Neurological Sciences, 176*, 65–69

Chaudhuri, A. & Behan, P. O. (2003). The clinical spectrum, diagnosis, pathogenesis and treatment of Hashimoto's encephalopathy (recurrent acute disseminated encephalomyelitis). *Current Medicinal Chemistry, 10*, 1945–1953

Erickson, J.C., Carrasco, H., Grimes J.B., Jabbari, B., & Cannard, K.R. (2002). Palatal tremor and myorhythmia in Hashimoto's encephalopathy. *Neurology, 58*, 504–505

Ferracci, F., Bertiato, G., & Moretto, G. (2004). Hashimoto's encephalopathy: epidemiologic data and pathogenetic considerations. *Journal of Neurological Sciences, 217*, 165–168

Ferracci, F., Mretto, G., Candeago, R. M., Cimini, N., Conte, F., Gentile, M., Papa, N., & Carnevale, A. (2003). Antithyroid antibodies in the CSF: their role in the pathogenesis of Hashimoto's encephalopathy. *Neurology, 60*, 712–714

Forchetti, C.M., Katsamakis, G., & Garron, D.C. (1997). Autoimmune thyroiditis and a rapidly progressive dementia: global hypoperfusion on SPECT scanning suggests a possible mechanism. *Neurology, 49*, 623–626

Garrard, P., Hodges, J.R., De Vries, P.J., Hunt, N., Crawford, A., Hodges, J.R., & Balan, K. (2000). Hashimoto's encephalopathy presenting as "myxoedematous madness." *Journal of Neurology, Neurosurgery & Psychiatry, 68*, 102–103

Henchey, R., Cibula, J., & Helveston, W. (1995). Electroencephalographic findings in Hashimoto's encephalopathy. *Neurology, 45*, 977–981

Kalita, J., Misra, U. K., Rathore, C., Pradhan. P. K., & Das, B. K. (2003). Hashimoto's encephalopathy: clinical, SPECT and neurophysiological data. *Quarterly Journal of Medicine, 96*, 455–457

McCabe, D.J.H., Burke, T., Connolly, S., & Hutchinson, M. (2000). Amnesic syndrome with bilateral mesial temporal lobe involvement in Hashimoto's encephalopathy. *Neurology, 54*, 737–739

Sawka, A.M., Fatourechi, V., Boeve, B.F., & Mokri, B. (2002). Rarity of encephalopathy associated with autoimmune thyroiditis: a case series from Mayo Clinic from 1950 to 1996. *Thyroid, 12*, 393–398

Seipelt, M., Zerr, I., Nau, R., Mollenhauer, B., Kropp, S., Steinhoff, B.J., Wilhelm-Gossling, C., Bamberg C., Janzen, R.W., Berlit, P., Manz, F., Felgenhauer, K., & Poser, S. (1999). Hashimoto's encephalitis as a differential diagnosis of Creutzfeldt-Jakob disease. *Journal of Neurology, Neurosurgery & Psychiatry, 66*, 172–176

Seo, S.W., Lee, J.D., Park, S.A., Kim, K.S., & Yun, M.J. (2003). Thyrotoxic autoimmune encephalopathy: a repeat positron emission tomography study. *Journal of Neurology, Neurosurgery & Psychiatry, 74*, 504–506

Chapter 33

Huntington's Disease

Pam Enderby

◆ General Information on Disorder

Huntington's disease (HD) is a neurodegenerative disorder of the nervous system that causes progressive deterioration of physical and cognitive abilities and emotional control. It leads to severe incapacitation and eventually death, generally 15 to 25 years after the onset of symptoms. HD is a genetic disorder, but the symptoms do not usually appear until the ages of 30 years and above. However, it can affect children as young as 2, and these children do not usually live into adulthood. Involvement of the basal ganglia is one of the earliest signs, causing physical decline with involuntary movements called chorea, leading to abnormal gait, imprecise speech, and difficulty with swallowing as early symptoms. Chorea (Greek for "dance") refers to irregular, flowing, and random involuntary movements that often possess a writhing quality. Early onset may give the appearance of general restlessness, and it is often worsened by stress and anxiety and subsides during sleep. As the involuntary movements become worse, they not only affect daily activity but also may be present at rest and when inactive. With the progression of HD, cognitive impairments become more noticeable, commonly starting with short-term memory loss and leading to difficulty with planning and problem solving and eventually a general dementia. A concomitant symptom of HD is emotional changes, which include personality change, such as increases in impulsiveness, disinhibition, mood swings, and aggression. Some of these are difficult to identify as being primary symptoms, as it is possible that some may be secondary, caused by frustration, anxiety, and depression linked to insight into the inevitable decline associated with the condition (Higgins, 2001; Pflanz, Besson, Ebmeier, & Simpson, 1991; Ward and Dennis, 2003).

Diagnostic Signs and Symptoms

Onset is insidious, and it has been noted that onset may be later when the gene has been inherited from the mother rather than the father. Some of the early symptoms may be subtle, and thus diagnosis would depend on the sensitivity of the assessment techniques. The genetic mutation causes brain cells to die, and initially the cells in the basal ganglia seem to be susceptible, causing problems with involuntary movements and parkinsonian-like symptoms. Further deterioration leads to cerebral atrophy, particularly in the frontal parts of the brain, which are associated with behavioral change and dementia. Dysarthria is present in the majority of patients (Podoll, Caspary, Lange, & Noth, 1998; Young, Shoulson, & Penney, 1986). Psychiatric disorders are evident in all cases to some extent. Buxton (1976) identified different clusters of symptoms, which included amnesia and confusion, dementia, and schizophrenia-like manifestations. Although apathy has been noted as a prominent feature in some cases, others note the common pattern of irritability culminating in outbursts of verbal and physical aggression (Jason et al, 1997).

Neuropathology

Huntington's disease is a degenerative disorder in which neuronal loss occurs, particularly in the caudate nucleus and putamen. The pathogenesis of this condition is probably related to the accumulation of polyglutamine-containing protein fragments that are resistant to degradation within the nuclei of neurons and leads to cell death and atrophy (Becher et al, 1998).

Epidemiology

The estimates of the prevalence of HD in persons of European descent are between 2 and 10 per 100,000. The condition appears to be far more common in those of European origins than in other ethnic groups. Genetic counseling and advice is having an affect on incidence and thus prevalence.

Genetics

Huntington's disease is an autosomal dominant condition with virtually full penetrance, so that each offspring of an affected parent has a 1 in 2 risk of inheriting the mutant gene and being affected if he or she survives until the age of onset. Sensitivity and specificity of the genetic test for HD is high, and the mutation rate is low, with most new cases of HD having a parent with the HD gene.

◆ Speech Impairment Associated with Disorder

Huntington's disease results in hyperkinetic dysarthria. It generally has less impact on language ability and structure as compared with those with dementia of Alzheimer's type (Aminoff, Marshall, Smith, & Wyke, 1975). However, spontaneous speech is often halting, with reduced fluency, some stuttering-like behaviors, and word finding and naming difficulties. Podoll et al (1988) attributes deficits to a variety of nonlinguistic factors associated with attention deficits and conversational apathy, among others. As the disease advances, functional communication decreases and many patients become mute in the late stages, making it even more difficult to gauge the degree of cognitive impairment.

Etiology

The etiology of speech behaviors associated with HD is comparable to that of the disease overall as described above.

Neuropathology

It has been noted in patients with HD that the frontal lobes atrophy more markedly and at an earlier stage than the other cortical lobes, indicating the underlying cause of early psychiatric symptoms. The hyperkinetic dysarthria is related to an increase in movement or lack of control of movements associated with damage to the extrapyramidal system and cerebral atrophy. The speech symptoms reflect this decline.

Associated Cognitive, Linguistic, and Communicative Signs and Symptoms

Patients, even at a relative presymptomatic stage, have reported having difficulty in planning and programming cognitive and motor tasks, in shifting mental set, and in other tests of mental flexibility (Brandt & Butters, 1986). These authors suggest that this finding, along with the absence of the aphasia and agnosic problems, may suggest early onset of subcortical dementia. Reading is frequently relatively preserved until later, whereas writing is impaired, but this may be due to physical and other contributory factors rather than specific dysgraphia.

Special Diagnostic Considerations

Hyperkinetic dysarthria is less commonly seen than hypokinetic dysarthria. It is characterized by involuntary movements of the oral musculature leading to uncoordinated breathing and speech, and choreic movements of the face and tongue, which often protrudes. Patients have difficulty in maintaining oral positions, for example if they are asked to stick their tongue out in a static position. The voice is often harsh, with a strained, strangled sound, and it is frequently overloud. The pitch is frequently low, and there is imprecision in consonant production. Whereas patients with spastic dysarthria or hypokinetic dysarthria tend to undershoot their targets for articulation, patients with hyperkinetic dysarthria tend to overshoot. The fluctuation of vocal range, pitch,

and volume is excessive with this patient group as compared with others.

Treatment

Dal Bello-Haas (2002) describes a useful framework for the rehabilitation of people with neurodegenerative diseases that is proposed to assist with planning care and maximizing the quality of life. In this approach the author suggests a system for selecting interventions along with continuum of care by staging neurodegenerative diseases into early, middle, and late stages and relating them to the individual's impairments, functional limitations, and disabilities. This approach would assist greatly with the speech-language pathologist's intervention in patients with HD. Therapeutic management at an early stage would emphasize prevention and compensatory and restorative interventions. For example, providing information and support to the patient and family can in itself be rehabilitative. Working with the family in identifying methods of improving the communication environment may be helpful; for example, developing memory books with pictures of names and places that relate to relevant or favored activities or situations not only may be a mechanism for ensuring that different caregivers become familiar with the patient's history, but also can be used at a later stage to prompt communication or for problem solving. As it is likely that the patients will have swallowing problems, nutrition is one aspect of preventive care that should be addressed as soon as possible. Patients with chorea use a high number of calories, and introducing methods to maintain body weight is desirable.

Compensatory techniques for the person with HD can sometimes be useful. These frequently use memory prompts of a simple nature, such as pointing boards. Other measures to improve functional communication can be discussed with caregivers. These include the usual approaches to assisting communication with those who have dementia, for example ensuring that concrete nouns rather than pronouns be used to facilitate comprehension and communication. Increasing nonverbal communication, such as facial expression and pointing to accompany ordinary communication, can assist in maintaining engagement.

There have been some reports of the successful use of communication aids by persons with HD, but these approaches must be introduced at the right time and it is important to monitor usage with the patient's decline in abilities. The Huntington's Disease Association (in the United States, United Kingdom, and Australia) provides leaflets on strategies to enhance communication in HD patients. They emphasize that, for communication to be more effective, the listener has to consciously accept responsibility for the conversation exchange and change their behaviors, as it is difficult for the person with HD to retain or adapt strategies that may help. The speech-language pathologist can provide invaluable support to the main caregivers in analyzing methods of enhancing patients' communication and swallowing skills.

References

Aminoff, M.J., Marshall, J., Smith, E.M., & Wyke, M.A. (1975). Pattern of intellectual impairment in Huntington's chorea. *Psychological Medicine, 5*, 169–172

Becher, M.W., Kotzuk, J.A., Sharp, A.H., Davies, S.W., Bates, G.P., Price, D.L., & Ross, C.A. (1998). Intranuclear neuronal inclusions in Huntington's disease. *Neurobiology of Disease, 4*, 387–397

Brandt, J. & Butters, N. (1986). The neuropsychology of Huntington's disease. *Trends in Neurosciences, 93*, 118–120

Buxton, M. (1976). Diagnostic problems in Huntington's chorea and tardive dyskinesia. *Comprehensive Psychiatry, 17*, 325–333

Dal Bello-Haas, V.A. (2002). Framework for rehabilitation of neurodegenerative diseases: planning care and maximizing quality of life. *Neurology Report, 26*, 115–129

Higgins, D.S. (2001). Chorea and its disorders. *Neurology Clinic, 19*, 707–722

Jason, G.W., Suchowersky, O., Pajurkova, E.M., Graham, L., Klimek, M.L., Garber, A.T., & Poirier-Heine, D. (1997). Cognitive manifestation of Huntington's disease in relation to genetic structure and clinical onset. *Archives of Neurology, 54*, 1081–1088

Pflanz, S., Besson, J., Ebmeier, K.P., & Simpson, S. (1991). The clinical manifestation of mental disorder in Huntington's disease: a retrospective record study of disease progression. *Acta Psychiatrica Scandinavica, 83*, 53–60

Podoll, K., Caspary, P., Lange, H.W., Noth, J. (1988). Language functions in Huntington's disease. *Brain, 111*, 1475–1503

Ward, C.D. & Dennis, N.R. (2003). Huntington's disease. In: R. Greenwood, M.P. Barnes, T.M. McMillan, & C.D. Ward (Eds.), *Handbook of Neurological Rehabilitation*, 2nd ed. (pp. 553–567). East Sussex: Psychology Press, 553–567

Young, A.B., Shoulson, I., & Penney, J.B. (1986). Huntington's disease in Venezuela: neurological features. *Neurology, 36*, 244–249

Chapter 34

Kennedy Disease/Syndrome

Edythe A. Strand

♦ General Information on Disorder

Kennedy syndrome is a spinobulbar muscular neuropathy that occurs in midlife in men, and is characterized by progressive weakness of bulbar and spinal muscles and gynomastia. It is one of several diseases caused by degeneration of motor neurons. Motor neuron diseases are broadly divided into categories depending on the anatomy of motor neuron loss, familial inheritance, and age of onset (Windebank, 2003). *Amyotrophic lateral sclerosis* (ALS) is the term used when both upper and lower motor neurons are involved, and it usually involves both spinal and bulbar musculature. Upper motor neuron degeneration of the spinal musculature is typically referred to as primary lateral sclerosis, whereas pseudobulbar palsy refers to progressive degeneration of upper motor neurons in the brainstem. There are a group of lower motor neuron disorders, typically referred to as spinal muscular atrophy (SMA), that are genetic diseases seen in childhood or adolescence, and less commonly in adulthood (see related chapters).

Kennedy disease (KD) is an adult form of SMA. It is often called spinal bulbar muscular atrophy (SBMA) as it affects both spinal and bulbar motor neurons. Kennedy, Alter, and Sung (1968) first described this disease, reporting 11 male members of two families who all exhibited slowly progressive spinal and bulbar muscular atrophy. He noted that although this form of the disease was pathologically similar to other forms of degeneration of lower motor neurons, there were specific differences, including (1) relatively late onset, (2) consistent early involvement of bulbar and proximal muscle groups, (3) sex-linked recessive inheritance, and (4) normal life expectancy. The disease is very slowly progressive. It affects only men. Onset is typically between 30 and 50 years, although some patients report mild symptoms much earlier. Life span is usually not greatly reduced.

Diagnostic Signs and Symptoms

The primary characteristics of KD are progressive spinal and bulbar muscular weakness and gynomastia. Muscle cramping and fasciculations may occur early, followed by proximal greater than distal weakness, and atrophy of the muscles in the face and limbs. Reflexes become diminished or absent. Progressive difficulty with speech and swallowing occurs due to weakness in the bulbar musculature. Individuals may experience aspiration, and aspiration-related pneumonia becomes a greater risk as the disease progresses. Signs of androgen insensitivity are also common in men with KD. These include gynecomastia, low sperm count, testicular atrophy, and impotence. Cognition is usually unimpaired.

Diagnosis of KD is usually made through the combination of clinical presentation and specific tests. Electromyography (EMG) is used to determine the presence and distribution of motor neuron loss. A blood test is used to check for elevated serum creatine phosphokinase (CPK) levels (which can result from reduced muscle mass accompanying muscle wasting). Finally, genetic tests using a blood sample can determine if the KD gene is present. Because KD is often confused with ALS, a few differentiating factors are important to note. Although KD affects only men, ALS occurs in both men and women. Onset is typically younger in KD than in ALS. Progression is slower in KD, and weakness is more proximal than in ALS. Only lower motor neurons are affected in KD, but both upper and lower motor neurons degenerate in ALS. KD is always inherited, whereas only approximately 10% of ALS is familial. Cervical spondylosis with narrowing of the spinal canal can be seen in KD, but is not associated with ALS (Fischer, Wullner, Klockgether, Schroder, & Wilhelm, 2001), and thus should be considered when presented with a patient with motor neuron deficits.

Neuropathology

The neuropathology in the spinal muscular atrophy syndromes involves the selective degeneration of the anterior horn cells of the spinal cord or brainstem. The mechanisms involved in the degeneration of motor neurons are still not clear. The degeneration of the motor neurons results in progressive weakness as well as atrophy of the muscles and loss of tendon reflexes. In KD the bulbar and proximal musculature is preferentially involved.

Epidemiology

The prevalence of KD is estimated at 1 in 40,000 (Greenland and Zajac, 2004). The number may actually be larger, as it is considered to be an underdiagnosed disorder and can often be misdiagnosed. The incidence and prevalence in other countries is unknown, but it is thought to be similar to that seen in the United States. Age of onset is typically 40 to 60 years, but may begin as early as the mid-30s. The disease typically runs a course of two to three decades and does not significantly compromise life expectancy. There is no racial predilection reported. Because KD is X-linked, only males express the full phenotype. Women who are carriers have occasionally been reported to develop mild symptoms. Daughters of individuals with KD carry a 50% risk of being carriers, which in turn carries a 50% risk of their sons having the disease gene and a 50% risk of their daughters being carriers. Individuals with KD with no family history have been reported, but the spontaneous mutation rate is not known.

Genetics

The genetic basis of KD was discovered by La Spada, Wilson, Lubahn, Harding, and Fischbeck (1991) when they mapped the gene to the long arm of the X chromosome. This region encodes the androgen receptor *(AR)* gene. KD was therefore determined to be caused by a genetic mutation of the *AR* gene on the X chromosome. It is an X-linked recessive disease.

The *AR* gene provides instructions for making a protein called the androgen receptor. (Proteins are constructed from information that is contained in DNA, which is composed of long chains of molecules that are abbreviated as C, A, G, and T). Androgen receptors allow the body to respond to hormones that are important for normal male sexual development. In one region of the *AR* gene, a segment of DNA that is known as CAG is repeated several times and is called a trinucleotide repeat. The *AR* gene has been mapped to chromosome X;q;11–12, where the gene defect has been localized. In the normal population, CAG repeats vary from 10 to 36, but in KD the number of repeats varies from 40 to 62 (LaSpoda et al, 1991). The expanded CAG region changes the structure of the androgen receptor protein, which leads to loss of motor neurons in the brainstem and spinal cord. The number of repeats correlates with disease severity. This is the only known mutation of the androgen receptor gene associated with motor neuron degeneration.

◆ Speech Impairment Associated with Disorder

Kennedy disease is associated with flaccid dysarthria, which is characterized by weakness, hypotonia, reduced reflexes, atrophy, and fasciculations. There may be progressive weakness with use. There is typically no cognitive or language dysfunction, and no apraxia of speech.

Diagnostic Signs and Symptoms

The flaccid dysarthria of KD is characterized primarily by weakness of the lips, tongue, velum, and laryngeal musculature. Initial symptoms are often tongue weakness, with fasciculations of the face and tongue, and tongue atrophy.

Speech is imprecise, due to a decreased range of motion and strength of articulatory contacts. Hypernasality and a weak voice are typical. The etiology of the flaccid dysarthria is the degeneration of lower motor neurons in the brainstem.

Neuropathology

The degeneration of lower motor neurons causes the progressive weakness and therefore the progressively more severe flaccid dysarthria.

Associated Cognitive, Linguistic, and Communicative Signs and Symptoms

Typically there are no cognitive or linguistic deficits. It might be predicted that the polyglutamine repeats that occur in the disease could lead to cognitive trouble because that is what causes Huntington's disease, in which cognitive deficits result. To date, this has not been reported.

Special Diagnostic Considerations

Ataxic and hypokinetic dysarthria are not associated with KD. If the individual presents with only spastic dysarthria, KD would not be in the differential. If the individual presents with a mixed dysarthria (flaccid/spastic), ALS is a more probable diagnosis.

Treatment

Treatment for the dysarthria accompanying progressive degenerative neurological disease such as KD involves incorporating different strategies at various points in time during the disease process (Yorkston, Beukelman, Strand, & Bell, 1999). In the early stages of KD, the clinician may work with the individual to maximize intelligibility by increasing the individual's awareness of the increased background of physiological effort. This can improve respiratory support, increase subglottal air pressure, and improve the strength of articulatory movements, increasing the precision of articulatory contacts. As the disease progresses and the weakness makes speech less intelligible, treatment focuses on comprehensibility (Yorkston, Miller, & Strand, 2004), which facilitates more effective communication by teaching both the speaker and the listeners simple strategies for optimizing the communication environment and developing effective communication interaction strategies. Aids such as alphabet boards, on which patients point to the first letter of each word as they say it, can facilitate verbal communication even when the acoustic signal is degraded. Finally, if speech becomes too difficult to understand, alternative and augmentative communication (AAC) is initiated.

References

Fischer, D., Wullner, U., Klockgether, T., Schroder, R., & Wilhelm, K. (2001). Cervical spondylotic myelopathy and Kennedy syndrome mimicking amyotrophic lateral sclerosis. *Journal of Neurology Neurosurgery and Psychiatry, 71,* 414

Greenland, K.J. & Zajac, J.D. (2004). Kennedy's disease: pathogenesis and clinical approaches. *Internal Medicine Journal, 34,* 279–286

Kennedy, W.R., Alter, S., & Sung, J.H. (1968). Progressive proximal spinal and bulbar muscular atrophy of late onset. A sex-linked recessive trait. *Neurology, 18,* 671–680

La Spada, A.R., Wilson, E., Lubahn, D., Harding, A., & Fischbeck, K. (1991). Androgen receptor gene mutations in X-linked spinal and bulbar muscular atrophy. *Nature, 352,* 77–79

Windebank, A.J. (2003). Motor neuron diseases. In: J.H. Noseworthy (Ed.), *Neurological Therapeutics: Principles and Practice* (pp. 2214–2222). London and New York: Martin Dunitz

Yorkston, K., Beukelman, D., Strand, E., & Bell, K. (1999). *Management of Motor Speech Disorders in Children and Adults.* Austin, TX: Pro-Ed.

Yorkston, K., Miller, R., & Strand, E. (2004). *Management of Speech and Swallowing in Degenerative Disease,* 2nd ed. Austin TX: Pro-Ed.

Additional Readings

Figlewicz, D.A. & Orrell, R.W. (2003). The genetics of motor neuron diseases. *Amyotrophic Lateral Sclerosis & Other Motor Neuron Disorders, 4,* 225–231

Gallo, J.M. (2001). Kennedy's disease: a triplet repeat disorder or a motor neuron disease? *Brain Research Bulletin, 56,* 209–214

Ogino, S. & Wilson, R. (2002). Genetic testing and risk assessment for spinal muscular atrophy. *Human Genetics, 111,* 477–500

Zitzmann, M. & Eberhard, N. (2003). The CAG repeat polymorphism within the androgen receptor gene and maleness. *International Journal of Andrology, 26,* 76–83

Chapter 35

Klippel-Feil Syndrome

Joan C. Arvedson

◆ General Information on Disorder

Klippel-Feil syndrome (KFS) is characterized by fusion of the cervical vertebrae. A classic clinical triad first described by Klippel and Feil in 1912 includes short neck, low posterior hairline, and reduced neck movement. Four different KFS classes have been described on the basis of varied positions of vertebral fusions in the cervical spine (Clarke, Catalan, Diwan, & Kearsley, 1998). Hemivertebrae and other vertebral defects, such as sacral agenesis, may be present. Associated anomalies may include neck webbing, Sprengel shoulder (congenital elevation of the scapula), torticollis, scoliosis, cardiac and renal anomalies, developmental delay, cleft palate, and facial asymmetry. Hearing impairment may be sensorineural, conductive, or mixed type (McGaughran, Kuna, & Das, 1998).

Klippel-Feil syndrome can be part of Wildervanck syndrome described in 1952. This syndrome has the KF anomalad (cervico-), Duane-Stilling-Turk phenomenon with bilateral abducens palsy (oculo-), and deafness (acoustic) (Wildervanck, 1978). Congenital heart disease has been described (Gupte, Mahajan, Shreenivas, Kher, & Bharucha, 1992). Multiple cranial nerve deficits are not unexpected.

Diagnostic Signs and Symptoms

The complex interrelationships of speech-motor and swallowing issues have been attributed to multiple cranial nerve abnormalities (McGaughran et al, 1998) and craniofacial anomalies (Ozdiler, Akcam, & Sayin, 2000). The diagnosis of KFS is based on a primary finding of fusion of the cervical vertebrae, not on associated features.

Neuropathology

Neurological complications with cervical spine abnormalities include abnormalities of the medulla, spinal instability, narrowing of the cervical canal, and vascular dysfunction (Rouvreau, Glorion, Langlais, Noury, & Pouliquen, 1998). The more numerous the occipito-C1 abnormalities, the more significant the neurological risk.

Epidemiology

The incidence of KFS is reported to be approximately 1 in 40,000 births (Gorlin, Cohen, & Levin, 1990), with 65% being female, usually as a sporadic genetic occurrence. Risk factors related to hypermobility of the upper cervical segment are associated with neurological sequelae, whereas those with alteration in motion of the lower cervical segment are predisposed to degenerative disease (Pizzutillo, Woods, Nicholson, & MacEwen, 1994).

Genetics

Autosomal dominant and recessive inheritance patterns have been described in some families (Thompson, Haan, & Sheffield, 1998). A dominant inheritance associated with malformation of laryngeal cartilages and mild-to-severe vocal impairment appears related to pericentric inversion on chromosome 8 (q22.2q23.3) (Clarke, Singh, McKenzie, Kearsley, & Yip, 1995). Mutations in the *PAX1* gene may have a role in the pathogenesis of KFS (McGaughran, Oates, Donnai, Read, & Tassabehji, 2003).

◆ Speech Impairment Associated with Disorder

Speech production skills are directly affected by the specific associated cranial nerve deficits and may reflect characteristics of hearing impairment. Ataxic dysarthria resulting from cerebellar hypoplasia may be present. Flaccid dysarthria with velopharyngeal incompetence is not uncommon with a cleft palate (Thompson et al, 1998). Reduced intelligibility of speech would be expected with both dysarthria types. Upper esophageal sphincter (UES) dysfunction, reduced pharyngeal contractions, and brainstem and cerebellar hypoplasia, with magnetic resonance imaging (MRI) that revealed a cleft in the cervical spinal cord, are likely to be major contributing factors for the speech-motor and swallowing deficits (Arvedson, Rudolph, & Kerschner, 2004).

Diagnostic Signs and Symptoms

Speech production and swallowing skills of persons with KFS can be variable depending on specific signs and symptoms, for example, the presence or absence of cleft palate, degree of hearing loss, and pharyngeal/esophageal function. Ataxic dysarthria and limb ataxia may be seen with cerebellar hypoplasia. Velopharyngeal insufficiency may relate to specific cranial nerve damage or to a short soft palate. One would expect a stable neurological status with anticipated developmental gains. Clinical signs may include, but are not limited to, reduced hearing levels, drooling, reduced respiratory support with cardiac components, risks for aspiration noted by gurgly voice quality, and asymmetric facial features in some children.

Etiology

Speech and swallowing deficits in KFS result from brain damage that affects the brainstem and cerebellum. Both cortical and subcortical structures can be affected.

Neuropathology

Neuropathological changes in KFS are part of a spectrum of associated anomalies, and not KFS in its "pure" form. Hearing loss is a common association. Damage to the brainstem and cerebellum produces changes in strength, coordination, range of movement, and overall motor control.

Associated Cognitive, Linguistic, and Communicative Signs and Symptoms

Patients with neurological complications commonly demonstrate motor-based speech and swallowing problems. Mental deficiency is reported to be one of several defects that may occur in a nonrandom association with KFS (Jones, 1997).

Special Diagnostic Considerations

There are no specific diagnostic considerations for evaluation of speech and swallowing in KFS. A high degree of suspicion is needed for UES deficits.

Treatment

Medical/surgical intervention may be needed with UES problems, for example, dilatation of the UES (Muraji, Takamizawa, Satoh, et al, 2002), botulinum toxin injection of the cricopharyngeus muscle (Ahsan, Meleca, & Dworkin, 2000), and cricopharyngeal myotomy. Cervical discectomy may be used with cervical cord compression (Allsopp, Griffiths, & Sgouros, 2001).

Intervention by speech-language pathologists, audiologists, and other clinicians should aid in maximizing cognitive skills, facilitating optimal hearing, improving speech intelligibility, improving gross and fine motor coordination and strength, and increasing oral feeding capabilities. Research is needed to determine whether some interventions that have been reported in adults may be applicable to children with cervical vertebrae deficits (e.g., Shaker, Easterling, Kern, et al, 2002).

References

Ahsan, S.F., Meleca, R.J., & Dworkin, J.P. (2000). Botulinum toxin injection of the cricopharyngeus muscle for the treatment of dysphagia. *Otolaryngology: Head and Neck Surgery, 122*, 691–695

Allsopp, G.M., Griffiths, S., & Sgouros, S. (2001). Cervical disc prolapse in childhood associated with Klippel-Feil syndrome. *Childs Nervous System, 17*, 69–70

Arvedson, J.C., Rudolph, C.D., & Kerschner, J.E. (2004). Klippel-Feil syndrome with multiple cranial nerve deficits: impact on swallowing and speech. *Journal of Medical Speech-Language Pathology, 12*, xxxix–xlvi.

Clarke, R.A., Catalan, G., Diwan, A.D., & Kearsley, J.H. (1998). Heterogeneity in Klippel-Feil syndrome: a new classification. *Pediatric Radiology, 28*, 967–974

Clarke, R.A., Singh, S., McKenzie, H., Kearsley, J.H., & Yip, M.-Y. (1995). Familial Klippel-Feil syndrome and paracentric inversion inv(8)(q22.2q23.3). *American Journal of Human Genetics, 57*, 1364–1370

Gorlin, R.J., Cohen, M.M., & Levin, S.L. (1990). Klippel-Feil anomaly. In: R.J. Gorlin, M.M. Cohen, & S.L. Levin (Eds.), *Syndromes of the Head and Neck* (pp. 886–889). New York: Oxford University Press

Gupte, G., Mahajan, P., Shreenivas, V.K., Kher, A., & Bharucha, B.A. 1992. Wildervanck syndrome (cervico-oculo-acoustic syndrome). *Journal of Postgraduate Medicine, 38*, 180–182

Jones, K.L. (1997). Klippel-Feil Sequence. In: K.L. Jones (Ed.), *Smith's Recognizable Patterns of Human Malformations*, 5th ed. (p. 618). Philadelphia: W.B. Saunders

Klippel, M., & Feil, A. (1912). Un cas d/absence des vertebras cervicales, avec cage thoracique remontant jusqu'a la base du crane (cage thoracique cervicale), *Nouvelle Iconographic Salpetriere, 25*, 223

McGaughran, J.M., Kuna, P., & Das, V. (1998). Audiological abnormalities in the Klippel-Feil syndrome. *Archives of the Disabled Child, 79*, 352–355

McGaughran, J.M., Oates, A., Donnai, D., Read, A.P., & Tassabehji, M. (2003). Mutations in PAX1 may be associated with Klippel-Feil syndrome. *European Journal of Human Genetics, 11*, 468–474

Muraji, T., Takamizawa, S., Satoh, S., Nishijima, E., Tsugawa, C., Tamura, A., & Shimizu, N. (2002). Congenital cricopharyngeal achalasia: diagnosis and surgical management. *Journal of Pediatric* Surgery, 37, E12

Ozdiler, E., Akcam, M.O., & Sayin, M.O. (2000). Craniofacial characteristics of Klippel-Feil syndrome in an eight year old female. *Journal of Clinical Pediatric Dentistry, 24*, 249–254

Pizzutillo, P.D., Woods, M., Nicholson, L., & MacEwen, G.D. (1994). Risk factors in Klippel Feil syndrome. *Spine, 19*, 2110–2116

Rouvreau, P., Glorion, C., Langlais, J., Noury, H., & Pouliquen, J.C. (1998). Assessment and neurologic involvement of patients with cervical spine congenital synostosis as in Klippel-Feil syndrome: Study of 19 cases. *Journal of Pediatric Orthopedics [B], 7*, 179–185

Shaker, R., Easterling, C., Kern, M., et al. (2002). Rehabilitation of swallowing by exercise in tube-fed patients with pharyngeal dysphagia secondary to abnormal UES opening. *Gastroenterology, 122*, 1314–1321

Thompson, E., Haan, E., & Sheffield, L. (1998). Autosomal dominant Klippel-Feil anomaly with cleft palate. *Clinical Dysmorphology, 7*, 11–15

Wildervanck, L.S. (1978). The cervico-oculo-acousticus syndrome. In: P.J. Vinken, G.W. Bruyn, & N.C. Myrianthopoulous (Eds.), *Handbook of Clinical Neurology*, vol. 32 (pp. 123–130). New York: North Holland

Chapter 36

Landau-Kleffner Syndrome

Richard K. Peach

◆ General Information on Disorder

Landau-Kleffner syndrome (LKS) (acquired epileptic aphasia, acquired aphasia with convulsive disorder) arises in children approximately between the ages of 2 to 3 and 8 years in a context of epilepsy with severe, characteristic electroencephalographic (EEG) abnormality and speech disturbances. It is one of the epileptic syndromes in childhood that also include benign childhood epilepsy with centrotemporal spikes (BCECTS) and the syndrome of continuous spikes and waves during slow wave sleep.

Diagnostic Signs and Symptoms

Children with LKS show severe deterioration of receptive language that may extend to a total loss of auditory/verbal comprehension and expression. Nonverbal cognitive abilities are usually spared. Behavioral problems include hyperactivity, inattentiveness, and withdrawal (Robinson, Baird, Robinson, & Simonoff, 2001). The seizures can be focal clonic, generalized tonic-clonic, or complex partial (Camfield & Camfield, 2002). Simple partial motor or atypical absences have also been observed that may consist simply of eye blinking or ocular deviation, head drops, and minor automatisms. The EEG shows predominately bilateral spikes or spike-wave discharges over the posterior temporal and parietal regions during slow-wave sleep that decrease or even vanish during rapid eye movement sleep (Smith & Hoeppner, 2003).

Neuropathology

Any pathology capable of producing an epileptic condition can cause LKS (Smith & Hoeppner, 2003). Cole et al (1988) found mild subpial gliosis with white matter gliosis and occasional fibrous astrocytes throughout the gray matter of the cortex in one patient. Pathological abnormalities found in a series examined by Smith et al (1992) included subcortical astrocytosis, perivascular lymphocytosis, and microglial nodule formation suggestive of encephalitis; cryptic arteriovenous malformation; and excessive ectopic neurons, suggesting migration disorder. Despite these findings, a normal neuropathological exam is not unusual. LKS is not associated with any demonstrable structural abnormality (Sobel, Aung, Otsubo, & Smith, 2000). Volumetric reductions in bilateral auditory association cortex have been demonstrated recently, suggesting focal atrophy (Takeoka et al, 2004).

Epidemiology

The incidence and prevalence of LKS are low. Current estimates suggest that a little more than 300 cases have been reported in the literature since the disorder was first described in 1957 (Camfield & Camfield, 2002).

Genetics

Although much progress has been made in understanding the basis of other epileptic syndromes in childhood (Ottman, 2001), little has been published regarding a possible genetic basis for LKS. In a series of patients identified with BCECTS, a syndrome with a known genetic linkage, three of 26 cases evolved into LKS (Fejerman, Caraballo, & Tenembaum, 2000). Such findings raise questions whether LKS is one point on a spectrum of disorders caused by the same genetic susceptibility (Singh, Kalita, & Misra, 2002).

The similarities between the language loss and epileptiform EEG in children with autistic regression and LKS are also great enough to question whether children with autistic regression and LKS represent a single syndrome (Lewine et al, 1999; Stefanatos, Kinsbourne, & Wasserstein, 2002). Although no such link has been reported, autism associated with epilepsy and language regression may result from common genetic factors that give rise to LKS (Tuchman & Rapin, 2002).

◆ Speech Impairment Associated with Disorder

Diagnostic Signs and Symptoms

Because LKS shares many of the features of BCECTS (Deonna, Roulet, Fontan, & Marcoz, 1993; Roulet, Deonna, & Despland, 1989; Shafrir & Prensky, 1995), such as onset of speech, language, and related oral deficits associated with epileptiform activity, and may therefore be confused with one another, it is worth noting the characteristics of each syndrome. In BCECTS, word-finding difficulties, poor articulation, reduced speech rate, poor prosody, phonological errors, dysfluency, and speech arrest have been reported (Deonna et al, 1993). In the most severe form of BCECTS, these problems may be accompanied by dysphagia, drooling, dysarthria, and oral apraxia, and constitute the anterior opercular syndrome (Shafir & Prensky, 1995). Language comprehension is nonetheless preserved. Some authors, therefore, have considered this an "expressive variant" of LKS (Deonna et al, 1993). A few children with BCECTS may subsequently acquire comprehension deficits thus evolving into the syndrome of LKS. These children demonstrate the characteristic speech deficits associated with BCECTS: reduced fluency, dysarthria, and difficulty with articulation and pronunciation, along with a severe disturbance of receptive language (Fejerman et al, 2000; Kramer, Ben-Zeev, Harel, & Kivity, 2001).

Landau-Kleffner syndrome is more frequently characterized by verbal output containing paraphasias and phonological errors regressing to single words and subsequently mutism in severe cases accompanied by poor listening comprehension (Eslava-Cobos & Mejia, 1997; Robinson et al, 2001; Smith & Hoeppner, 2003). These characteristics are not, of course, of the same sensorimotor nature as those observed in BCECTS. However, one case with left temporal discharges on EEG demonstrated isolated prosodic changes characterized by slow speech with increased syllable lengths and pausing, monotony, decreased initiative, and occasional consonant and vowel imprecision in the initial position of words in the context of normal sentence comprehension and production (Deonna, Chevrie, & Hornung, 1987). Because responses to environmental sounds are relatively normal, at least initially, the disorder is thought to represent an auditory verbal agnosia (Korkman, Granström, Appelqvist, & Liukkonen, 1998).

Neuropathology

Localized, paroxysmal epileptic activity in the developing temporoparietal cortex is thought to disrupt synaptogenesis of the language cortex during a critical stage. The paroxysmal activity reinforces synaptic contacts that otherwise would be pruned, thus promoting abnormal language behavior. The activity must have bilateral effects to prevent assumption of function by the contralateral homotopic cortex (Morrell et al, 1995).

Associated Cognitive, Linguistic, and Communicative Signs and Symptoms

Children demonstrating LKS syndrome have normal intelligence and speech development until the time of onset. Long-term outcome is generally characterized by abnormal language, poor short-term memory, and normal nonverbal skills (Robinson et al, 2001).

Special Diagnostic Considerations

Documentation concerning a child's cognitive, behavioral, and academic history should be obtained in children suspected of having LKS. Neuropsychological testing should be performed by a team experienced in both linguistic and nonlinguistic evaluation. For a diagnosis of LKS, it is important to establish that the cognitive deficits are relatively restricted to the linguistic domain (Smith & Hoeppner, 2003).

Treatment

The seizures are amenable to treatment and usually respond well to anticonvulsant medications, although some variants of LKS do not (Otsubo et al, 2001). Corticosteroids should be administered if the seizures do not respond to anticonvulsants (Smith & Hoeppner, 2003). Multiple subpial transection may be used to treat the disorder in carefully selected cases. Although all of these treatments can result in dramatic improvements in seizure control and behavior, the effects on language performance are variable at best (Camfield & Camfield, 2002; Grote, Van Slyke, & Hoeppner, 1999; Irwin et al, 2001), suggesting that some children may require years of language therapy to treat the disorder.

References

Camfield, P. & Camfield, C. (2002). Epileptic syndromes in childhood: clinical features, outcomes, and treatments. *Epilepsia, 43*(suppl 3), 27–32

Cole, A.J., Andermann, F., Taylor, L., Olivier, A., Rasmussen, T., Robitaille, Y., et al. (1988). The Landau-Kleffner syndrome of acquired epileptic aphasia: unusual clinical outcome, surgical experience, and absence of encephalitis. *Neurology, 38*(1), 31–38

Deonna, T., Chevrie, C., & Hornung, E. (1987). Childhood epileptic speech disorder: prolonged, isolated deficit of prosodic features. *Developmental Medicine and Child Neurology, 29,* 96–109

Deonna T.W., Roulet, E., Fontan, D., & Marcoz, J.P. (1993). Speech and oromotor deficits of epileptic origin in benign partial epilepsy of childhood with rolandic spikes (BPERS). Relationship to the acquired aphasia-epilepsy syndrome. *Neuropediatrics, 24,* 83–87

Eslava-Cobos, J., & Mejia, L. (1997). Landau-Kleffner syndrome: much more than aphasia and epilepsy. *Brain and Language, 57,* 215–224

Fejerman, N., Caraballo, R., & Tenembaum, S.N. (2000). Atypical evolutions of benign localization-related epilepsies in children: are they predictable? *Epilepsia, 41,* 380–390

Grote, C.L., Van Slyke, P., & Hoeppner, J.A. (1999). Language outcome following multiple subpial transaction for Landau-Kleffner syndrome. *Brain, 122,* 561–566

Irwin, K., Birch, V., Lees, J., Polkey, C., Alarcon, G., Binnie, C., Smedley, M., Baird, G., & Robinson, R.O. (2001). Multiple subpial transection in Landau-Kleffner syndrome. *Developmental Medicine & Child Neurology, 43,* 248–252

Korkman, M., Granström, M., Appelqvist, K., & Liukkonen, E. (1998). Neuropsychological characteristics of five children with the Landau-Kleffner syndrome: dissociation of auditory and phonological discrimination. *Journal of the International Neuropsychological Society, 4,* 566–575

Kramer, U., Ben-Zeev B, Harel, S., & Kivity, S. (2001). Transient oromotor deficits in children with benign childhood epilepsy with central temporal spikes. *Epilepsia, 42*(5), 616–620

Lewine, J.D., Andrews, R., Chez, M., Patil, A., Devinsky, O., Smith, M., et al. (1999). Magnetoencephalographic patterns of epileptiform activity in children with regressive autism spectrum disorders. *Pediatrics, 104*(3 pt 1), 405–418

Morrell, F., Whisler, W.W., Smith, M.C., Hoeppner, T.J., de Toledo-Morrell, L., Pierre-Louis, S.I.C, et al. (1995). Landau-Kleffner syndrome: treatment with subpial intracortical transection. *Brain, 118,* 1529–1546

Otsubo, H., Chitoku, S., Ochi, A., Jay, V., Rutka, J.T., Smith, M.L., et al. (2001). Malignant rolandic-sylvian epilepsy in children: diagnosis, treatment, and outcomes. *Neurology, 57,* 590–596

Ottman, R. (2001). Progress in the genetics of the partial epilepsies. *Epilepsia, 42*(suppl 5), 24–30

Robinson, R.O., Baird, G., Robinson, B., & Simonoff, E. (2001). Landau-Kleffner syndrome: course and correlates with outcome. *Developmental Medicine and Child Neurology, 43,* 243–247

Roulet, E., Deonna, T., & Despland, P.A. (1989). Prolonged intermittent drooling and oromotor dyspraxia in benign childhood epilepsy with centrotemporal spikes. *Epilepsia, 30,* 564–568

Shafrir, Y. & Prensky, A.L. (1995). Acquired epileptiform opercular syndrome: a second case report, review of the literature, and comparison to the Landau-Kleffner syndrome. *Epilepsia, 36,* 1050–1057

Singh, M.B., Kalita, J., & Misra, U.K. (2002). Landau Kleffner syndrome: electro-clinical and etiopathogenic heterogeneity. *Neurology India, 50,* 417–423

Smith, M.C. & Hoeppner, T.J. (2003). Epileptic encephalopathy of late childhood Landau-Kleffner syndrome and the syndrome of continuous spikes and waves during slow-wave sleep. *Journal of Clinical Neurophysiology, 20,* 462–472

Smith, M.C., Pierre-Louis, S.J.C., Kanner, A.M., Morrell, F., Chez, M., Hasegawa, H., et al. (1992). Pathological spectrum of acquired epileptic aphasia of childhood. *Epilepsia,* 33(suppl), 115

Sobel, D.F., Aung, M., Otsubo, H., & Smith, M.C. (2000). Magnetoencephalography in children with Landau-Kleffner syndrome and acquired epileptic aphasia. *American Journal of Neuroradiology, 21,* 301–307

Stefanatos G.A., Kinsbourne M., & Wasserstein J. (2002). Acquired epileptiform aphasia: a dimensional view of Landau-Kleffner syndrome and the relation to regressive autistic spectrum disorders. *Child Neuropsychology (Neuropsychology, Development and Cognition: Section C), 8,* 195–228

Takeoka, M., Riviello, J.J., Jr., Duffy, F.H., Kim, F., Kennedy, D.N., Makris, N., et al. (2004). Bilateral volume reduction of the superior temporal areas in Landau–Kleffner syndrome. *Neurology, 63,* 1289–1292

Tuchman, R., & Rapin, I. (2002). Epilepsy in autism. *Lancet Neurology, 1,* 352–358

Chapter 37

Möbius Syndrome

Pam Enderby

◆ General Information on Disorder

Möbius syndrome (MS) is a congenital disorder that produces weakness of the facial muscles and bilateral failure of the eyes to abduct. The syndrome is caused by a congenital abnormality in the sixth and seventh cranial nerve nuclei in the brainstem. It is an idiopathic, nonprogressive hereditary condition. There may be other associated symptomatology such as clubfeet, delayed general development, and hypotonicity.

Diagnostic Signs and Symptoms

Although a range of unique symptoms are reported in the literature, the most common and unifying one in this syndrome is related to the lack of development of the sixth and seventh cranial nerves, which results in paralysis of the eye and facial muscles. The sixth cranial nerve (abducens nerve) controls lateral eye movements and blinking. The seventh cranial nerve (the facial nerve) controls not only the muscles of facial expression but also serves the taste buds on the front two thirds of the tongue. The lack of sensation as well as the paralysis and associated reduction in muscle bulk lead to a variety of problems, including the inability to smile, the absence of lateral eye movements and blinking, strabismus, swallowing and chewing problems, speech impairments, and dental abnormalities. As the syndrome is extremely rare, children frequently go undiagnosed for many months, and sometimes years, after birth. Diagnosis may occur later when treatment for various other symptoms are sought. Abramson, Cohen, and Mulliken (1998) undertook a retrospective analysis of 27 patients and found a broad range of additional cranial nerve deficits and musculoskeletal abnormalities of the face, limbs, and trunk. They developed a grading system to classify the different groups of patients with MS. These authors report that a complete facial nerve paralysis was documented in 11 patients and facial paresis in 16. Sixth nerve paralysis was present in 23 of the 27 patients, and other cranial nerves were affected in eight of them. Lower limb deficits were involved in 10 patients and upper limbs in seven. Chest wall deformities including scoliosis and hyperplasia of the breast were found in eight of the 27 patients.

Neuropathology

A magnetic resonance imaging (MRI) finding of three patients with MS demonstrated brainstem hyperplasia with straightening of the fourth ventricle floor, indicating an absence of the facial colliculus (Pedraza et al, 2000).

Epidemiology

Reliable population studies of the incidence or prevalence of this disorder have not been conducted, but it is frequently referred to as an extremely rare condition.

Genetics

The cause of MS is still unclear. Although it appears to be genetic, there are also other suggestions for its underlying cause, including substances or other events that may affect perinatal growth. MacDermot, Winter, Taylor, and Baraitser (1991) reviewed 26 cases within the heterogeneous Möbius spectrum of defects. These authors suggest that when cranial nerve palsies were associated with other defects, such as skeletal abnormalities, familial transmission was not found. However, family connections indicating genetic causes were found in those with MS restricted to abnormalities of the sixth and seventh nerve paralysis. Pregnancy histories of MS patients ($n = 25$) with additional problems did not identify any common etiological cause in a study in Sweden. However, bleeding during pregnancy was noted in eight and spontaneous abortion in seven cases (Stromland et al, 2002).

◆ Speech Impairment Associated with Disorder

The facial nerve enables one to wrinkle the forehead, close eyes tightly, produce a lip seal, pull back the corners of the mouth for a grimace or a smile, and tense the cheek and neck muscles. It guards the middle ear as well as innervates the stapedius muscles, which act to dampen excessive movement of the ossicles when loud noises occur. In patients with MS it may not be necessary to do formal testing of facial expression such as asking patients to wrinkle their forehead or purse their mouth, as flaccidity may be clear from general observation. Some individuals with MS may have some retained ability in some portion of one side of the face, but more frequently the problems are bilateral.

Diagnostic Signs and Symptoms

The most obvious and common diagnostic signs are associated with facial paralysis caused by a lack of development of the facial nerve (cranial nerve VII). This gives rise to flaccid dysarthria, fasciculation of anterior portion of tongue, and absence of facial expression.

Etiology

The etiology of the speech associated with MS is lower motor neuron dysfunction particularly of cranial nerve VII, causing a profound localized flaccid dysarthria.

Neuropathology

The facial nerve is a complex nerve made up of three nuclei. Some patients with MS have more deficits in one of these nuclei than others. This nerve is extremely complex and affects many structures of interest for speech production. Some fibers are distributed to the taste buds of the anterior two thirds of the tongue and others terminate in the taste buds in the hard and soft palate. The facial nerve travels through the tympanic cavity, innervating the stapedius muscle (affecting hearing). The parasympathetic nuclei also supply the superior salivatory and lacrimal nuclei, thus having an effect on production of saliva (volume and flow) as well as production of tears. The motor nucleus gives the face expression by innervation of the various facial muscles: the orbicularis oculi, zygomatic, buccinator, orbicularis oris, and labial muscles. Other muscles innervated are the platysma, stylohyoid, stapedius, and a portion of the digastric (Love & Webb, 1992).

Associated Cognitive, Linguistic, and Communicative Signs and Symptoms

Möbius syndrome has been associated with an increased presentation of autistic symptoms. The prevalence of autistic disorder was analyzed in 25 individuals with MS in a study in Sweden. This was a nationwide call and it is difficult to identify the incidence from the cohort. However, of the 18 males and seven females, 10 individuals had autistic spectrum disorder, with six meeting all diagnostic criteria. Additionally eight had learning disability and six individuals were functioning in the normal but subaverage range. Thus Johansson et al (2001) concluded that autistic spectrum disorder and learning disability occur in more than a third of the patients with MS, but they do caution that as this was a selected sample, the findings may be overestimates.

Special Diagnostic Considerations

Speech, communication, and swallowing are all major problems for children with MS, particularly in early development. With the inability to close the lips and form negative intraoral pressure, babies are unable to suckle, and frequently need alternative feeding. Some find that the use of an enlarged teat or specially adapted bottle, as is used with cleft palate children, is appropriate and successful. Those patients who have good tongue movement will learn with time to compensate for their suckling by additional elevation of the tip of the tongue and a good seal produced by the lateral edges.

The development of a smile in an infant is important in the bonding experience with parents. Parents may find it problematic to establish good communication with their child with the apparent lack of responsivity. However, many children learn to indicate pleasure by using vocal tone and other nonverbal expressions. The lack of lip movements cause particular difficulty in the development of sounds that are frequently learned early, for example "p," "b," "m," "w," "sh," "f," and "v." The child may learn to substitute other articulatory gestures to approximate these sounds in an intelligible way, and many will communicate clearly and effectively with time, but the development of intelligible speech is slow and needs particular attention and encouragement. Drooling is a further problem that can be socially harmful. Again, many persons with MS learn to adapt their swallow style to control salivary flow, for example by using a head jerk and tongue thrust to channel saliva.

Different surgical approaches to improving the appearance and function of the face of children with MS are reported. One study (Goldberg, DeLorie, Zuker, & Manktelow, 2003) reports the outcome of a bilateral gracilis muscle transplant enervation by the masseteric nerve. They report the outcome of 12 children who showed improved intelligibility of speech with a reduction in the compensatory phonemes.

Treatment

Although persons with MS have many severe problems, they are frequently able to adapt their speech using approximations, vocalizations, and intonation to compensate, and, although speech is abnormal, particularly for the bilabial sounds, there will be the ability to develop many effective compensatory communicative gestures.

References

Abramson, D.L., Cohen, M.M., Jr., & Mulliken, J.B. (1998). Mobius syndrome: classification and grading system. *Plastic and Reconstructive Surgery, 102,* 961–967

Goldberg, C., DeLorie, R., Zuker, R.M., & Manktelow, R.T. (2003). The effects of gracilis muscle transplantation on speech in children with Moebius syndrome. *Journal of Craniofacial Surgery, 14,* 687–690

Johansson, M., Wentz, E., Fernell, E., Stromland, K., Miller, M.T., & Gillberg, C. (2001). Autistic spectrum disorders in Mobius sequence: a comprehensive study of 25 individuals. *Developmental Medicine & Child Neurology, 43,* 338–345

Love, R.J., & Webb, W.G. (1992). *Neurology for Speech and Language Pathologists* (p. 119). Stoneham, MA: Butterworth-Heinemann

MacDermot, K.D., Winter, R.M., Taylor, D., & Baraitser, M. (1991). Oculofacialbulbar palsy in mother and son: review of 26 reports of familial transmission within the "Mobius spectrum of defects." *Journal of Medical Genetics, 28,* 18–26

Pedraza, S., Gamez, J., Rovira, A., Zamora, A., Grieve, E., Raguer, N., & Ruscalleda, J. (2000). MRI findings in Mobius syndrome: correlation with clinical features. *Neurology, 55,* 1058–1060

Stromland, K., Sjogreen, L., Miller, M., Gillbert, C., Wentz, E., Johansson, M., Nylen, O., Danielsson, A., Jacobsson, C., Andersson, J., & Fernell E. Mobius sequence—a Swedish multidisciplinary study. *European Journal of Paediatric Neurology, 6,* 35–45

Chapter 38

Moyamoya

Pam Enderby

◆ General Information on Disorder

Moyamoya disease is a chronic cerebrovascular occlusive disease that was first reported by Japanese surgeons in 1957. The term *moyamoya* is Japanese for "puff of smoke" and describes the haze of vascularization at the base of the brain that occurs following the narrowing or stenosis of the internal carotid and proximal portions of the anterior and middle cerebral arteries. Symptoms associated with neurovascular problems of this disease are often demonstrated in childhood (up to the age of 10). Another peak of onset is in early adult life (30 to 40 years). The symptomatology is associated with either ischemic attacks or cerebral infarction, often giving rise to transient ischemic attacks (Gosalakkal, 2002).

Diagnostic Signs and Symptoms

Children present most frequently with transient ischemic attacks or ischemic strokes presenting as acute onset of speech, language disorders, or hemiplegia. Some complain of headaches and demonstrate involuntary movements, seizures, and other motor disturbances. Episodic symptoms are frequently described. Intracranial hemorrhage is more common in adults with the disease, but occasionally has been reported in children. This can be associated with hypertension and aneurysms. Thus the signs and symptoms of both children and adults with moyamoya disease are similar to any patient suffering a transient ischemic attack or stroke (Fukui, Kono, Sueishi, & Ikezaki, 2000).

Neuropathology

Moyamoya disease is a condition characterized by chronic occlusion of the circle of Willis with the subsequent development of fine vascular networks in the ganglionic region of the brain. This abnormal development of circulation is thought to be a compensatory development for the unilateral or bilateral stenosis or occlusion of the internal carotid artery at the level of its terminal bifurcation along with associated abnormalities of the anterior and middle cerebral arteries. Pathological studies have indicated intimal thickening and excessive infolding in the internal elastic lamina (Shoskes & Novick, 1995).

Epidemiology

Moyamoya disease has a higher incidence in Japanese and other Asians populations than in Caucasians, with a familial occurrence of 10% in Japan and Korea. Although the etiology of the disease is still unknown, there is an indication that the pathogenesis varies between races (Fukui, 1997). In Japan there is a female dominance, with a 1:1.7 male-to-female ratio.

Genetics

Multifactorial inheritance and predispositions are considered possible because of the higher incidence of the disease across races. Recent genetic studies suggest some responsible genetic foci in chromosomes 3, 6, and 17 (Fukui, 2000).

◆ Speech Impairment Associated with Disorder

The symptoms associated with moyamoya disease are as varied as those associated with any vascular disturbance of the brain. Thus patients may present with dysarthria of any classification, as well as the frequent stroke-induced concomitants of dysphasia, dysphagia, apraxia of speech, and so on. Many children and adults have unstable symptomatology that is often associated with the varying blood flow and triggers that affect vascular efficiency and the viability of cell function.

Diagnostic Signs and Symptoms

Speech and language may vary in production and function, and many cases have been misdiagnosed as being functional or psychiatric conditions in the first instance.

Etiology

The etiology of the speech and language behaviors noted in moyamoya is associated with the cerebral functioning as affected by the vascular efficiency.

Neuropathology

The speech and language neuropathology mirrors that stated earlier. Vascular compensation may lead to variation in the symptoms and abilities displayed over time.

Associated Cognitive, Linguistic, and Communicative Signs and Symptoms

There have been some reports suggesting a decline in the IQ of children with symptomatic moyamoya. This is one of the reasons for advocating early surgery. Some studies have shown an improvement in IQ after surgery (Imaizumi, Imaizumi, & Osawa, 1999).

Special Diagnostic Considerations

Hartman, Vishwanat, and Heun (2000) alert speech-language pathologists to be aware of unusual and atypical conditions that can result in strange presentations of disorders of communication requiring inventive assessment and treatment by a multidisciplinary team.

Treatment

Several different medical and surgical approaches to the management of moyamoya have been described in the literature (see Gosalakkal, 2002, for a review). The surgical procedures aim to revascularize the ischemic areas, whereas medical treatments target vasodilatation or agents to reduce the viscosity of the blood (e.g., aspirin), or the stenosis (e.g., corticosteroids).

The condition is rare and the symptoms are heterogeneous. The speech-language pathologist has to provide a detailed assessment of the speech, language, and associated deficits to the multidisciplinary team. This can assist with team decision making regarding surgical or medical intervention. Many cases reported in the literature "indicate the varying nature of the symptomatology." Accurate assessment can indicate the progress of the disorder and its response to treatments (de Borchgrave, Saussu, Depre, & de Barsy, 2002; Ikezaki, 2000; Kawamoto, Inagawa, Ikawa, & Sakode, 2001). In spite of the paucity of literature on the speech production of moyamoya disease, the clinical experience of the author provides some insight into the disease. A young Asian woman presented with aphasia, muteness, and an inability to communicate either verbally or nonverbally. However, following revascularization, she regained nearly all her language abilities and functions. Interestingly, she reported that prior to diagnosis she had frequent periods of becoming mute, which were diagnosed initially as a psychiatric disorder. Furthermore, she explained that during these mute periods she felt that she was able to communicate and had no insight into her difficulties. She said that she felt that she had access to her language internally.

It is interesting that her recovery was good, suggesting that the collateral vascularization was maintaining cell life while being inadequate for cell function.

References

Achilli, M.A., Longoni, E., Milani, O., Spreafico, W., & Zamperini, E. (2001). The moyamoya syndrome: a case study on its clinical manifestations. *Iassistenza Infermineristica e Ricerca, 20,* 11–16

de Borchgrave, V., Saussu, F., Depre, A., & de Barsy, T. (2002). Moyamoya disease and Down syndrome: case report and review of the literature. *Acta Neurologica Belgica, 102,* 63–66

Fukui, M. (1997). Current state of study on moyamoya disease in Japan. *Surgical Neurology, 47,* 138–143

Fukui, M., Kono, S., Sueishi, K., & Ikezaki, K. (2000). Moyamoya disease. *Neuropathology, 20* (suppl), S61–64

Gosalakkal, J.A. (2002). Moyamoya disease: a review. *Neurology India, 50,* 6–10

Hartman, D.E., Vishwanat, B., & Heun, R. (2000). Cases of atypical neurovascular disease, stroke and aphasia. *Journal of Medical Speech-Language Pathology, 8,* 53–65

Ikezaki, K. (2000). Rational approach to treatment of moyamoya disease in childhood. *Journal of Child Neurology, 15,* 350–356

Imaizumi, C., Imaizumi,T., & Osawa, M.(1999). Serial intelligence test scores in pediatric moyamoya disease. *Neuropediatrics, 30,* 294–299

Kawamoto, H., Inagawa, T., Ikawa, F., & Sakode, E. (2001). A modified burr-hole method in galeoduroencephalosynangiosis for an adult patient with probably moyamoya disease—case report and review of the literature. *Neurosurgical Review, 24,* 147–150

Setzen, G., Cacace, A.T., Eames, F., Riback, P., Lava, N., McFarland, D.J., Artino, L.M., & Kerwood, J.A. (1999). Central deafness in a young child with moyamoya disease: paternal linkage in a Caucasian family: two case reports and a review of the literature. *International Journal of Paediatric Otorhinolaryngology, 48,* 53–76

Shoskes, D.A. & Novick, A.C. (1995). Surgical treatment of renovascular hypertension in moyamoya disease: case report and review of the literature. *Journal of Urology, 153,* 450–452

Chapter 39

Multiple Sclerosis

James L. Coyle

◆ General Information on Disorder

Multiple sclerosis (MS) is a neurodegenerative condition with either a variable relapsing-remitting course with brief to long-term remissions, or a variable progressive course without clinically detectable remission. Secondary progressive MS may follow a relapsing-remitting course. MS is characterized by demyelination and subsequent scarring (sclerosis) of central nervous system (CNS) white matter. It affects sensory, motor, cerebellar, autonomic, and cognitive domains of CNS function, and is relatively unselective in terms of lesion sites, though enhancing subcortical areas of plaque are seen with magnetic resonance imaging (MRI), most commonly in periventricular white matter, corpus callosum, and areas of white matter–gray matter interface. The most common clinical outcome of MS is caregiver dependence for basic needs.

Diagnostic Signs and Symptoms

Axial and appendicular sensorimotor signs are observed concurrently, with spasticity, tremor, loss of vibratory sense, ophthalmoplegia, loss of visual acuity, nystagmus, ataxia, and cognitive impairments predominating. Tremor and fatigue are common. Symptoms include cognitive complaints, weakness, incoordination, cramping, diplopia, dysphagia and dysarthria, diminished sensory detection, paresthesia, pain, limb and gait ataxia, and bowel and bladder abnormalities.

Neuropathology

Destruction of the myelin protein surrounding myelinated axons predominates the neuropathology of MS, resulting in slowed to absent neural conduction. Axonal transection and destruction are common in unabated exacerbation and in later stages of progressive MS (Trapp et al, 1998). Autoimmune mechanisms producing inflammation and destruction of myelin are believed to be triggered by causative agent exposure, though the etiology of MS remains unknown (Sorensen, 2005). Emotional stress has been suggested as a potential predisposing event (Ackerman et al, 2002).

Genetics

MS is thought to be a genetically transmitted condition. Linkage and association studies have attempted to identify specific genetic abnormalities responsible for MS. Results have been reported from studies investigating the *CTLA-4* gene and its effects on autoimmune disorders, though no consensus exists (Kantarci et al, 2003). Efforts to elucidate the underlying predisposing genetic anomaly, as well as to determine causative genetic alterations, are attempting to identify potential regenerative methods that may prevent or treat MS.

◆ Speech Impairment Associated with Disorder

Diagnostic Signs and Symptoms

All speech subsystems exhibit impairment, including both spasticity and ataxia (Hartelius, Runmarker, & Andersen, 2000). Speech characterized by abnormally equalized syllable duration and stressing is common. Interutterance syllabic variability and paradoxical syllabic variability within utterance interact with abnormally increased syllabic and phonemic duration and variability of interstress intervals in the speech of many MS patients. Disruptions of anticipatory coarticulation have also been reported (Tjaden, 2003). Temporal errors of linguapalatal contact during speech have been reported and may explain the perceptually abnormal and variable speech production observed in MS (Murdoch, Gardiner, & Theodoros, 2000). The prevalence of dysphonia is reportedly 2.5 times greater in MS than in normal control subjects, with higher fundamental frequency of phonation in MS patients and fewer phonatory abnormalities in females with MS than in males (Feijo et al, 2004). Phonatory instability is significantly more prevalent in MS compared with normal subjects (Hartelius, Buder, & Strand, 1997).

Etiology

Muscles containing spindles (tongue, mandibular and velar elevators, vocal fold adductors) exhibit spastic paresis (Katto, Okamura, & Yanagihara, 1987; Kubota, Negishi, & Masegi, 1975). Ataxia or dysmetria is caused by demyelination of cerebellar white matter and peduncles. Motor innervation redundancy in the trigeminal, vagal, and upper facial nerve fields mitigates motor asymmetry in these areas; however, unilateral corticobulbar lesions can cause contralesional lower facial and genioglossus weakness. Facial and oral paresthesias and altered salivary flow may also be observed due to damaged inputs to salivatory nuclei in the medulla pons.

Associated Cognitive, Linguistic, and Communicative Signs and Symptoms

Cognitive, language, and neuropsychological manifestations of MS include a variety of disorders of language and neuropsychological function and depression (Crayton, Heyman, & Rossman, 2004). Brain volume loss has been shown to correlate positively with cognitive deterioration in MS (Amato et al, 2004).

Special Diagnostic Considerations

Cognitive and linguistic testing and thorough sensorimotor oral-facial examination of fields innervated by cranial nerves V, VII, and IX through XII should be performed, and should not exclude assessment of the respiratory pump as the power source for speech production and airway protection. Cognitive and neuropsychological evaluations may elucidate the viability of behavioral motor speech compensatory interventions, assistive devices, and safety.

Treatment

Augmentation of axonal sodium channel physiology has been investigated as potential therapeutic target, in response to observations of adaptive axonal changes, and on the tendency of myelin to adapt to ischemia (Graumann, Reynolds, Steck, & Schaeren-Wiemers, 2003). Therapy to reduce inflammation, mitigating the extent of subsequent myelin and axonal damage during exacerbations, is the current primary therapeutic objective (Trapp et al, 1998). Research into medical therapies designed to reduce autoimmune reactivity to myelin is in its infancy, with limited effectiveness, adverse events, and toxicity reported. Interferonβ(appears to be of value in changing the course of the disease when combined with other agents (Polman & Uitdehaag, 2003). Stereotactic neurosurgery has been reported as somewhat effective in reducing tremor and subsequent motor disability (Alusi et al, 2001).

Behavioral intervention depends in part on the patient's cognitive and affective status. Decreasing the rate and increasing the loudness of speech production has been investigated in dysarthric speakers with MS and Parkinson's disease and normal subjects. Both dysarthric and normal speakers have been shown to produce more distinct consonants when employing increased loudness of speech, and perceptually greater vowel acoustic distinctiveness when employing reduced speed of production. Stereotactic neurosurgery has controlled tremor in some MS patients, but upper aerodigestive tract functions (speech, swallowing) and cognitive status seemed to be postoperatively unchanged in their severity and course (Alusi et al, 2001).

References

Ackerman, K.D., Heyman, R., Rabin, B.S., Anderson, B.P., Houck, P.R., Frank, E., et al. (2002). Stressful life events precede exacerbations of multiple sclerosis. *Psychosomatic Medicine, 64*, 916–920

Alusi, S.H., Aziz, T.Z., Glickman, S., Jahanshahi, M., Stein, J. F., & Bain, P.G. (2001). Stereotactic lesional surgery for the treatment of tremor in multiple sclerosis: a prospective case-controlled study. *Brain, 124*, 1576–1589

Amato, M.P., Bartolozzi, M.L., Zipoli, V., Portaccio, E., Mortilla, M., Guidi, L., et al. (2004). Neocortical volume decrease in relapsing-remitting MS patients with mild cognitive impairment. *Neurology, 63*, 89–93

Crayton, H., Heyman, R.A., & Rossman, H.S. (2004). A multimodal approach to managing the symptoms of multiple sclerosis. *Neurology, 63*, S12–S18

Feijo, A.V., Parente, M.A., Behlau, M., Haussen, S., De Veccino, M.C., & Faria Martignago, B.C. (2004). Acoustic analysis of voice in multiple sclerosis patients. *Journal of Voice, 18*, 341–347

Graumann, U., Reynolds, R., Steck, A.J., & Schaeren-Wiemers, N. (2003). Molecular changes in normal appearing white matter in multiple sclerosis are characteristic of neuroprotective mechanisms against hypoxic insult. *Brain Pathology, 13*, 554–573

Hartelius, L., Buder, E.H., & Strand, E.A. (1997). Long-term phonatory instability in individuals with multiple sclerosis. *Journal of Speech Language & Hearing Research, 40*, 1056–1072

Hartelius, L., Runmarker, B., & Andersen, O. (2000). Prevalence and characteristics of dysarthria in a multiple-sclerosis incidence cohort: relation to neurological data. *Folia Phoniatrica et Logopedica, 52*, 160–177

Kantarci, O.H., Hebrink, D.D., Achenbach, S.J., Atkinson, E.J., Waliszewska, A., Buckle, G., et al. (2003). CTLA4 is associated with susceptibility to multiple sclerosis. *Journal of Neuroimmunology, 134*, 133–141

Katto, Y., Okamura, H., & Yanagihara, N. (1987). Electron microscopic study of muscle spindle in human interarytenoid muscle. *Acta Oto-Laryngologica, 104*, 561–567

Kubota, K., Negishi, T., & Masegi, T. (1975). Topological distribution of muscle spindles in the human tongue and its significance in proprioception. *Bulletin of Tokyo Medical & Dental University, 22*, 235–242

Murdoch, B.E., Gardiner, F., & Theodoros, D.G. (2000). Electropalatographic assessment of articulatory dysfunction in multiple sclerosis: a case study. *Journal of Medical Speech-Language Pathology, 8*, 359–364

Polman, C.H. & Uitdehaag, B. M. (2003). New and emerging treatment options for multiple sclerosis. *The Lancet Neurology, 2*, 563–566

Sorensen, P.S. (2005). Multiple sclerosis: pathophysiology revisited. *Lancet Neurology, 4*, 9–10

Tjaden, K. (2003). Anticipatory coarticulation in multiple sclerosis and Parkinson's disease. *Journal of Speech Language & Hearing Research, 46*, 990–1008

Trapp, B.D., Peterson, J., Ransohoff, R.M., Rudick, R., Mork, S., & Bo, L. (1998). Axonal transection in the lesions of multiple sclerosis. *New England Journal of Medicine, 338*, 278–285

Chapter 40

Multiple System Atrophy and Shy-Drager Syndrome

Scott G. Adams and Mary E. Jenkins

◆ General Information on Disorder

Multiple system atrophy (MSA) is a sporadic neurodegenerative disorder that is characterized by various combinations of parkinsonian, cerebellar ataxia, pyramidal signs (spastic), and autonomic dysfunction. Historically, multiple system atrophy has been classified as three distinct syndromes: striatonigral degeneration (SND), olivopontocerebellar atrophy (OPCA), and Shy-Drager syndrome. Over the past 10 years this classification was reconsidered and finally revised in an MSA consensus statement in 1999 (Gilman, Low, Quinn, et al, 1999). The new MSA classification has two rather than three subtype designations. The first, MSA-P is applied if parkinsonian symptoms predominate and is similar to the previously used term SND. The second, MSA-C is applied if cerebellar symptoms predominate and is similar to the previously used term OPCA. The old subtype of Shy-Drager, which used to refer to MSA in which autonomic dysfunction predominates, has been deleted from the new MSA classification system. The primary reason for removing Shy-Drager syndrome from the MSA classification system appears to be because autonomic dysfunction is a common problem that will eventually develop in almost all forms of MSA including MSA-P and MSA-C. Thus, autonomic dysfunction is not a distinctive feature of just one subtype of MSA. Based on this new MSA classification system, a retrospective evaluation of patients diagnosed as Shy-Drager would require each patient to be changed to either MSA-P or MSA-C depending on the predominance of either parkinsonian or cerebellar features.

Diagnostic Signs and Symptoms

The diagnosis of MSA-P is based on the predominance of parkinsonian signs and symptoms (particularly those related to akinesia and rigidity) with additional, less predominant, ataxic or spastic signs and symptoms. Autonomic dysfunction may be present to varying degrees. In the early stages, MSA-P may be difficult to distinguish from idiopathic Parkinson's disease. MSA-P patients generally show a poor response to chronic dopamine-related antiparkinsonian drug therapy (although as many as one third of MSA-Ps may show a brief, initial, moderate response to levodopa) (Geser & Wenning, 2005; Wenning, Geser, & Stampfer-Kountchev, 2003).

The diagnosis of MSA-C is based on the predominance of cerebellar ataxic signs and symptoms with additional, more minor parkinsonian or spastic (pyramidal) signs and symptoms. Autonomic dysfunction is likely to be present to varying degrees. Autonomic dysfunction in both MSA-P and MSA-C is usually characterized by urinary incontinence (70% of the cases) or retention (30% of cases), orthostatic hypotension (a 15 to 30 mm Hg drop in blood pressure as the patient goes from supine to upright) and erectile dysfunction in males (Vidailhet, Bourdain, & Trocello, 2005). Of potential diagnostic importance is the finding that cognitive problems are limited or fairly mild in MSA. One study of 203 MSA patients found only 3% had moderate or severe dementia (Aarsland, Ehrt, & Ballard, 2005). It has been suggested that the relative lack of dementia throughout the course of the disease may be a useful diagnostic feature for distinguishing MSA from other forms of parkinsonism including idiopathic Parkinson's disease (Nichelli & Magherini, 2005).

Neuropathology

In MSA-P (formerly SND) the structures that are usually affected include the substantia nigra, putamen, caudate, and globus pallidus. In MSA-C (formerly OPCA) the cerebellum, inferior olivary nucleus, and pons are most affected (Mackenzie, 2005; Ozawa et al, 2004). Microscopically, the involved gray matter structures show neuronal loss and reactive gliosis, whereas the associated white matter tracts show loss of myelin (Mackenzie, 2005). The histopathological changes that characterize MSA include the presence of small "flame" or "sickle-shaped" structures in the cytoplasm of oligodendrocytes (referred to as glial cytoplasmic inclusions) (Mackenzie 2005). These glial inclusions have fairly specific staining properties because they have been found to be strongly immunoreactive for α-synuclein (Mackenzie, 2005). The presence of these α-synuclein–positive glial inclusions is considered necessary for a definite diagnosis of MSA (Geser 2005).

Epidemiology and Genetics

Multiple system atrophy is the second most common parkinsonism syndrome after idiopathic PD (Gesser, 2005). Based on North American and European studies, the prevalence of MSA is approximately 4 cases per 100,000 (Zermansky & Ben-Shlomo, 2005). The incidence of MSA is estimated to be approximately 0.6 per 100,000. When the greater than

50-year-old population is examined, the incidence rises to 3 cases per 100,000 (Geser, 2005). Age of onset is usually in the fifth decade, with a median age of onset at 53 years (Geser, 2005). The median survival time is approximately 9 years (Frattali & Duffy, 2005). MSA is believed to be linked to a combination of environmental factors and genetic factors, but the relevant evidence is very limited (Zermansky & Ben-Shlomo, 2005).

◆ Speech Impairment Associated with Disorder

Most individuals with MSA develop dysarthria fairly early in the progression of the disease. In the Kluin, Gilman, Lohman, and Junck (1996) study of 46 cases of MSA, 100% of the cases were found to have dysarthria. In these cases, the median onset of dysarthria was within 2 years of the onset of the general nonspeech MSA symptoms. It has also been reported that a severe speech impairment was present in 60% of individuals with MSA who were in the final stage of the disease (Muller, Wenning, Verny, et al, 2001).

A mixed type of dysarthria involving hypokinetic, ataxic, or spastic dysarthria is usually associated with MSA. In the Kluin et al (1996) study, 70% of individuals with MSA had a three-way mixed dysarthria that included a combination of hypokinetic, ataxic, and spastic characteristics. The hypokinetic speech symptoms predominated in 48% of the MSA cases, whereas ataxic symptoms predominated in 35% of the MSA cases. In 11% of the MSA cases, spastic speech symptoms predominated. In another, relatively large, study of 80 individuals with MSA (all originally diagnosed as Shy-Drager), a slightly different proportion of dysarthria types was reported (Linebaugh, 1979). Ataxic dysarthria was predominant in 43% of MSA cases, and hypokinetic dysarthria was predominant in 31% of MSA cases. Taken together, these studies suggest that the mixed dysarthrias of MSA will be predominated by either hypokinetic or ataxic dysarthria in approximately 30 to 40% of cases.

Usually, the predominant speech symptoms closely correspond to the generalized nonspeech neuromotor signs and symptoms. Thus, MSA-P would be expected to demonstrate a mixed dysarthria with predominant hypokinetic features, and MSA-C would be expected to show a mixed dysarthria with predominant ataxic features. Unfortunately, the speech characteristics corresponding to MSA-P and MSA-C have not been well described in previous group studies.

Of potential diagnostic importance is the report that as many as one third of MSA cases demonstrate inhalatory stridor (also referred to as laryngeal stridor) (Bower, 2000). Inhalatory stridor is characterized by phonation on inhalation. It often co-occurs with audible inspiration, which is characterized by an excessive fricative-like noise of the larynx during inhalation. It is of potential diagnostic importance because laryngeal stridor has rarely been reported in other of parkinsonian, ataxic, or spastic disorders. The cause of stridor in MSA is not known. Stridor can occur in flaccid dysarthria but MSA is not typically associated with flaccid, lower motor neuron signs and symptoms. As a possible explanation, it is suggested that laryngeal stridor in MSA may be related to the fairly unique combined effects of parkinsonism and cerebellar dysfunction on the laryngeal system. In particular, stridor may be related to the combined effects of parkinsonian vocal fold bowing (possibly the result of laryngeal rigidity) and an ataxic-related hypotonia of the vocal folds and related laryngeal muscles.

Treatment

Speech treatment studies of MSA are required. It is anticipated that speech treatments that focus on the individual's predominant dysarthria type will be most effective. For example, if hypokinetic dysarthria predominates, then treatments developed for hypokinetic dysarthria (i.e., Lee Silverman Voice Treatment for hypophonia) will probably be most beneficial (Fox, Morrison, Ramig, & Sapir, 2002). In addition, the mixed dysarthrias of MSA will likely benefit from combinations of dysarthria-specific treatment procedures (see Chapters 9, 11, and 12).

References

Aarsland, D., Ehrt, U., & Ballard, C. (2005). Role of neuropsychiatric assessment in diagnosis and research. In: Litvan, I. (Ed.), *Atypical Parkinsonian Disorders: Clinical and Research Aspects.* Totowa, NJ: Humana Press

Bower, J.H. (2000). Multiple system atrophy. In: Adler, C.H., Ahlskog, J.E. (Eds.), *Parkinson's Disease and Movement Disorders: Diagnosis and Treatment Guidelines for the Practicing Physician.* Totowa, NJ: Humana Press

Fox, C.M, Morrison, C.E., Ramig, L.O., & Sapir, S. (2002). Current perspectives on the Lee Silverman Voice Treatment (LSVT) for individuals with idiopathic Parkinson's disease. *American Journal of Speech Language Pathology, 11,* 111-123

Frattali, C. & Duffy, J.R. (2005). Characterizing and assessing speech and language disturbances. In: Litvan, I. (Ed.), *Atypical Parkinsonian Disorders: Clinical and Research Aspects.* Totowa, NJ: Humana Press.

Geser, F. & Wenning, G.K. (2005). Multiple system atrophy. In: Litvan, I. (Ed.), *Atypical Parkinsonian Disorders: Clinical and Research Aspects.* Totowa, NJ: Humana Press

Gilman, S., Low, P.A., Quinn, N., et al. (1999). Consensus statement on the diagnosis of multiple system atrophy. *Journal of Neurological Science, 163,* 94-98

Kluin, K.J., Gilman, S., Lohman, M., & Junck, L. (1996). Characteristics of the dysarthria of multiple system atrophy. *Archives of Neurology, 53,* 545-548

Linebaugh, C. (1979). The dysarthria of Shy-Drager syndrome. *Journal of Speech and hearing Disorders, 44,* 55-60

Mackenzie, I.R.A. (2005). Neuropathology of atypical Parkinsonian disorders. In: Litvan, I. (Ed.), *Atypical Parkinsonian Disorders: Clinical and Research Aspects.* Totowa, NJ: Humana Press

Muller, J., Wenning, G.K., Verny, M., et al. (2001). Progression of dysarthria and dysphasia in postmortem-confirmed parkinsonian disorders. *Archives of Neurology, 58,* 259-264

Nichelli, P. & Magherini, A. (2005). Role of visuospatial cognition assessment in the diagnosis and research of atypical Parkinsonian disorders.

In: Litvan, I. (Ed.) *Atypical Parkinsonian Disorders: Clinical and Research Aspects.* Totowa, NJ: Humana Press

Ozawa, T, Paviour, D., Quinn, N.P., Josephs, K.A., Sangha, H., Kilford, L., Healy, D.G., Wood, N.W., Lees, A.J., Holton, J.L., & Revesz, T. (2004). The spectrum of pathological involvement of striatonigral and olivoponto-cerebellar systems in multiple system atrophy: clinicopathological correlations. *Brain, 127,* 2657-2671

Vidailhet, M., Bourdain, F. & Trocello, J. (2005). Medical history and physical examination in Parkinsonian syndromes. In: Litvan, I. (Ed.), *Atypical Parkinsonian Disorders: Clinical and Research Aspects.* Totowa, NJ: Humana Press

Wenning, G.K., Geser, F., & Stampfer-Kountchev, M. (2003). Multiple system atrophy: an update. *Movement Disorders, 18,* S34-S42

Zermansky, A. & Ben-Shlomo, Y. (2005). Epidemiology of progressive supranuclear palsy and multiple system atrophy. In: Litvan, I. (Ed.), *Atypical Parkinsonian Disorders: Clinical and Research Aspects.* Totowa, NJ: Humana Press

Additional Reading

Litvan, I. (2005). *Atypical Parkinsonian Disorders: Clinical and Research Aspects.* Totowa, NJ: Humana Press

This edited text contains many chapters related to MSA including a chapter on speech and language disturbances (see Fratelli & Duffy, 2005). This text also comes with a companion DVD that includes video and audio samples of MSA cases.

Chapter 41

Myasthenia Gravis

Pam Enderby

◆ General Information on Disorder

Myasthenia gravis (MG) is an autoimmune disease that affects the neuromuscular junctions and leads to increasing weakness with movement. Neuromuscular transmission appears to fail after continuous muscle contraction as the result of reduced availability of acetylcholine at the myoneural junction.

Diagnostic Signs and Symptoms

Myasthenia gravis frequently occurs in young women in their childbearing years, with the most common presenting symptoms being ocular. The disease remains isolated to these muscles in up to 20% of patients. However, the majority of patients have more generalized symptoms associated with fatigue of the muscles of the head and neck and the proximal limbs. It can be associated with poor movements of the jaw, tongue, palate, pharynx, face, and the suprahyoid musculature as well as the neck extensors. Fatigue is particularly noticeable in patients with myasthenia with rapid deterioration in repeated movements. Temperature also affects performance, with heat exacerbating weakness and cooling improving the strength in muscles (Palace, Vincent, & Beeson, 2001).

Neuropathology

The etiology is heterogeneous, divided between those with rare congenital myasthenic syndromes that are genetic, and the bulk of affected persons with MG who have an acquired autoimmune condition. This autoimmune condition may be divided between those who posses serum acetylcholine receptor (AChR) antibodies and a smaller group that does not (Keesey 2004). In approximately 10% of cases thymoma is associated with MG.

The underlying pathological disruption is related to antibodies affecting calcium channels at the motor nerve synapse (either presynaptic or postsynaptic). The inflow of calcium into the nerve end plate induces the release of acetylcholine from the nerve terminal. Reduction in this causes potential to be reduced progressively during the impulses of a muscle contraction.

Epidemiology

Myasthenia gravis is reported to affect all races, with a prevalence of 5 to 10 per 100,000 (Cumming, 1998). There is thought to be a delay in diagnosis of 1 to 2 years, causing problems with identifying the incidence, which is estimated to be 1 in 10,000 (Armstrong & Schumann, 2003; Phillips, 2004). It is suggested that, as the population ages, an increasing number of individuals with MG can be expected, but the clinical pattern may be different (Phillips 2004).

Genetics

The pattern of inheritance for autoimmune conditions such as MG is complex and debated in the literature (Kristiansen, Larsen, & Pociot, 2000). The major histocompatibility complex (MHC) has been implicated. Giraud et al (2004) suggest three genetic loci giving rise to the variations in causes and presentations of MG.

◆ Speech Impairment Associated with Disorder

Diagnostic Signs and Symptoms

The signs and symptoms for speech mirror those described earlier for the general condition. A key diagnostic feature is that muscle weakness worsens with use and improves with rest. For example, speech may deteriorate when counting from 1 to 20, the speech may become more hypernasal on prolonged vocalization, intelligibility may deteriorate later in the day, and diadokokinetic tasks deteriorate. In addition to the very obvious ocular muscle involvement causing diplopia and ptosis, bulbar muscles are almost always involved, resulting in a lower motor neuron type of dysarthria, dysphagia, and poor respiratory support for speech. The involvement of head and jaw musculature may lead to abnormal posture and open mouth position. Speech can be hypernasal with low pitch, hoarseness, and imprecise articulation. Intelligibility frequently deteriorates over time, and the patient and family may report periods of totally normal speech, for example talking normally in one's sleep or after rest. A key diagnostic feature is that the muscle weakness worsens with use and improves with rest. For example, speech may deteriorate when counting from 1 to 20.

Etiology

The neural synapse is a juncture at which electrical impulses are transmitted from the nerve to the muscle, or other neuron. This electrical transmission requires the release of biochemical transmitters; for example, peripheral neuromuscular synapses require acetylcholine, which facilitates excitation and inhibition of impulses. Within MG, antibodies interfere with the transmission of acetylcholine.

Neuropathology

The neuropathology of the speech disorder is included in the earlier descriptions. However, it is of interest that the larynx and palate are frequently first to be affected by this disease. It is unclear why this is the case. It is possible that the continuous movements of these structures in speech lead to an early reflection of transmission disorders.

Associated Cognitive, Linguistic, and Communicative Signs and Symptoms

Many individuals with MG complain of cognitive impairments, such as mild memory disorders and difficulties with concentration. A review by Paul, Cohen, Zawacki, Gilchrist, and Aloia (2001) found that most studies had shortcomings; thus, issues with regard to cognitive involvement remain unclear.

Treatment

Speech-language pathologists can assist the multidisciplinary team in the management of this disorder. Methods of conserving speech to reduce effort will help with intelligibility. As patients are likely to increase both their dysarthria and their dysphagia with fatigue, it is important that they structure their life accordingly; for example, foods that require chewing may be managed earlier in the day when fatigue and hence dysphagia may be less problematic. Also, small frequent meals may be more tolerable than regular meals. Speech may be more effective if the context and content words are given earlier in the sentence, when articulation may be more precise and voice stronger. Management is generally recognized as requiring a graded approach, beginning with cholinesterase inhibitors for mild symptoms and advancing to immunomodulating medications for more severe weakness (Saperstein & Barohn, 2004). There is debate regarding the effectiveness of thymectomy in the treatment of patients having thymoma as the cause of their MG. However, some improvements have been reported (Jaretzki, Steinglass, & Sonett, 2004).

References

Armstrong, S.M. & Schumann, L. (2003). Myasthenia gravis: diagnosis and treatment. *Journal of American Academy of Nurse Practitioners, 15,* 72–78

Cumming, W.J. (1998). Myasthenic syndromes. In: R.C. Tallis, H.M. Fillit, & J.C. Brocklehurst (Eds.), *Textbook of Geriatric Medicine and Gerontology,* 5th ed. (pp. 611–613). London: Churchill Livingstone

Giraud, M., Beauraiu, G., Eymard, B., Tranchant, C., Gajdos, P., & Garchon, H.J. (2004). Genetic control of autoantibody expression in autoimmune Myasthenia gravis. *Genes and Immunology, 5,* 398–404

Jaretzki, A., Steinglass, K.M., & Sonett, J.R. (2004). Thymectomy in the management of myasthenia gravis. *Seminars in Neurology, 24,* 49–62

Keesey, J.C. (2004). Clinical evaluation and management of myasthenia gravis. *Muscle & Nerve, 29,* 484–505

Kristiansen, O.P., Larsen, Z.M., & Pociot, F. (2000). CTLA-4 in autoimmune disease—a general susceptibility gene to autoimmunity? *Genes and Immunology, 1,* 170–184

Paul, R.H., Cohen, R.A., Zawacki, T., Gilchrist, J.M., & Aloia, M.S. (2001). What have we learned about cognition in myasthenia gravis? A review of methods and results. *Neuroscience & Biobehavioral Reviews, 25,* 75–81

Palace, J., Vincent, A., & Beeson, D. (2001). Myasthenia gravis: diagnostic and management dilemmas. *Current Opinion in Neurology, 14,* 583–589

Phillips, L.H. (2004). The epidemiology of myasthenia gravis. *Seminars In Neurology, 24,* 17–20

Saperstein, D.S. & Barohn, R.J. (2004). Management of myasthenia gravis. *Seminars in Neurology, 24,* 41–48

Chapter 42

Neurofibromatosis Type 1

Jared Bennett and Julie L. Wambaugh

♦ General Information on Disorder

Neurofibromatosis type 1 (NF1) is a common genetic disorder that can involve multiple organ systems, including the central and peripheral nervous systems (Barton & North, 2004; Ozonoff, 1999). NF1 is extremely variable in terms of expressivity (Billingsley, Schrimsher, Jackson, Slopis, & Moore, 2002), with the most common clinical symptoms of NF1 being café-au-lait spots, neurofibromas, axillary or inguinal freckling, and Lisch nodules (Cnossen et al, 1998). Additional frequent manifestations and complications include macrocephaly, short stature, scoliosis, plexiform neurofibromas, headache, optic gliomas, learning disabilities, and cognitive impairments (North, Hyman, & Barton, 2002).

Diagnostic Signs and Symptoms

The National Institutes of Health Consensus Development Conference on Neurofibromatosis established diagnostic criteria for NF1 (Stumpf et al, 1988), with diagnosis being dependent on an individual demonstrating at least two of the following features: (1) six or more café-au-lait spots of specified size and number, (2) two or more neurofibromas of any type or one plexiform neurofibroma, (3) freckling in the axillary or inguinal regions, (4) optic glioma, (5) two or more Lisch nodules (iris hamartomas), (6) a distinctive osseous lesion such as sphenoid dysplasia or thinning of the long bone cortex, and (7) a first-degree relative diagnosed with NF1 by the above criteria.

Neuropathology

Neurofibromas are benign tumors of nerve sheaths for which the mechanisms of formation are unclear. However, it appears likely that the product of the intact *NF1* gene, neurofibrin, plays a role. Neuropathological studies have shown that some patients with NF1 may demonstrate disordered cortical architecture, particularly with respect to glial cells (e.g., atypical glial infiltrate, gliofibrillary nodules, increased number and size of astrocytes) (North et al, 2002). Neuroimaging studies have revealed that brain morphology may vary in some individuals with NF1. Individuals with NF1 have presented with increased volume laterally of the supratentorial compartment and an increasing velocity of brainstem growth with age (DiMario, Ramsby, & Burleson, 1999). Differences in perisylvian morphological features have also been identified (Billingsley et al, 2002).

Magnetic resonance imaging (MRI), utilizing T2-weighted protocols, have identified areas of abnormal, high signal intensity in approximately 70% of children with NF1 (Billingsley et al, 2002). These areas have most often been observed in the brainstem, cerebellum, basal ganglia, thalamus, and subcortical white matter. DiMario and Ramsby (1998) reported a decrease in total number of lesions and size over time, but noted region-specific effects; hemispheric and cerebellar lesions were more likely to resolve, whereas brainstem lesions were more likely to increase in number and size. High-intensity areas are not considered to be true masses, and their nature remains unclear. It has been suggested that they are regions of dysplasia, heterotopia, abnormal myelin, or low-grade glioma (North et al, 2002).

Epidemiology

NF1 has an estimated birth incidence of 1 in 3000 to 1 in 4000, with males and females affected at approximately equal rates (Stumpf et al, 1988).

Genetics

NF1 is an autosomal dominant genetic disorder with approximately 50% of cases being new mutations. The locus of the *NF1* gene has been determined to be on chromosome 17 (Barker et al, 1987). The *NF1* gene is typically classified as a tumor suppressor gene (North et al, 2002). Consequently, a disruption in its function may result in abnormal cell growth and differentiation.

♦ Speech Impairment Associated with Disorder

Speech has received little attention in the study of NF1. Johnson, Saal, Lovell, and Schorry (1999) reported that 60% of children with NF1 had speech problems in comparison to 5% of unaffected siblings. Cnossen et al (1998) found similar rates of occurrence of loosely defined speech abnormalities in their investigation of a cohort of 150 children with NF1. Only two investigations were identified in which speech production skills in NF1 were examined directly (Lorch, Ferner, Golding, & Whurr, 1999; Robin & Eliason, 1991).

Robin and Eliason (1991) assessed speech and prosody in seven children with NF1. They evaluated articulation, speech intelligibility, nasality, diadokokinetic rates, F_0, F_0 range, and voice quality. They also examined production of intonation and stress patterns. Their findings revealed "symptoms consistent with a diagnosis of dysarthria" (p. 141). Specifically, they found that all of the children produced imprecise consonants and that diadokokinetic rates were slower than normal. All of the children had pronounced vocal tremor, four had a hoarse voice quality, three were judged to have hypernasality, and six demonstrated decreased pitch range. The children were found to be impaired in their ability to use/demonstrate stress. Speech intelligibility was judged to be 80% or greater in all cases.

Lorch et al (1999) examined the speech characteristics of 30 adults with NF1 and reported rates of speech disorders in spontaneous speech as follows: hypernasality (37%), mild articulation difficulties (17%), atypically fast rate of speech (40%), and atypical volume (27%).

Diagnostic Signs and Symptoms

To date, there are no specific signs or symptoms that may be considered to typify speech production in NF1.

Etiology

The etiology of the speech disturbances observed in NF1 is not known. Central nervous system involvement would appear to be likely, especially given the high prevalence of learning disability in this population (see below). Tumors affecting any part of the sensorimotor speech system are a possibility with NF1.

Neuropathology

There have been no investigations focused on the neuropathology of speech disorders in NF1. In addition to tumors, it is possible that there may be a defect in neuronal functioning that impacts the sensorimotor speech system. In particular, the areas of abnormal signal intensity identified on MRI may be related to abnormal neuronal functioning and are considered to have some association with cognitive deficits in NF1 (North et al, 2002). Although these areas of high signal intensity appear to have a proclivity for critical areas of the sensorimotor speech system (see above), their relationship to speech is unknown.

Associated Cognitive, Linguistic, and Communicative Signs and Symptoms

Learning disabilities in individuals with NF1 have been identified at rates varying between 30% and 65% (North et al, 1997). These learning disabilities have been shown to be both nonverbal and verbal in nature, with expressive and receptive language disorders reported (Ozonoff, 1999). Mental retardation occurs at a slightly higher rate in NF1 than in the general population; estimates range from 4 to 8% (North et al, 2002). Fine and gross motor problems have been reported in individuals with NF1 (Ozonoff, 1999). Children with NF1 may also be at risk for social problems, particularly if they also present with attention-deficit hyperactivity disorder (Barton & North, 2004).

Special Diagnostic Considerations

Tumors or nervous system deficits may be present that affect speech production. Lesions may evolve over time with or without medical intervention, and repeated evaluations over time may be necessary. Evaluation of prosody should be considered.

Treatment

Any one or all of the speech subsystems may be impacted and targeted for treatment. Lesion resolution/progression may occur over time so that considerations should be made for the potentially nonstatic course of the disorder. Treatment of prosodic difficulties may be warranted.

References

Barker, D., Wright, E., Nguyen, K., Cannon, L., Fain, P., Goldgar, D., et al. (1987). Gene for von Recklinghausen neurofibromatosis is in the pericentromeric region of chromosome 17. *Science, 236,* 1100–1102

Barton, B. & North, K. (2004). Social skills of children with neurofibromatosis type 1. *Developmental Medicine and Child Neurology, 46,* 553–563

Billingsley, R.L., Schrimsher, G.W., Jackson, E.F., Slopis, J.M., & Moore, B.D. (2002). Significance of planum temporale and planum parietale morphologic features in neurofibromatosis type 1. *Archives of Neurology, 59,* 616–622

Cnossen, M.H., Goede-Bolder, A.D., van den Broek, K.M., Waasdrop, C.M.E., Oranje, A.P., Stroink H., et al. (1998). A prospective 10 year follow up study of patients with neurofibromatosis type 1. *Archives of Disease in Childhood, 78,* 408–412

DiMario, F.J. & Ramsby, G.R. (1998). Magnetic resonance imaging lesion analysis in neurofibromatosis type 1. *Archives of Neurology, 55,* 500–505

DiMario, F.J., Ramsby, G.R., & Burleson, J.A. (1999). Brain morphometric analysis in neurofibromatosis 1. *Archives of Neurology, 56,* 1343–1346

Johnson, N.S., Saal, H.M., Lovell, A.M., & Schorry, E.K. (1999). Social and emotional problems in children with neurofibromatosis type 1: evidence and proposed interventions. *Journal of Pediatrics, 134,* 767–772

Lorch, M., Ferner, R., Golding, J., & Whurr, R. (1999). The nature of speech and language impairment in adults with neurofibromatosis 1. *Journal of Neurolinguistics, 12,* 157–165

North, K., Hyman, S., & Barton, B. (2002). Cognitive deficits in neurofibromatosis 1. *Journal of Child Neurology, 17,* 605–612

North K. N., Riccardi, V., Samango-Sprouse, C., Ferner, R., Moore, B., Legius, E., et al. (1997). Cognitive function and academic performance in neurofibromatosis. 1. Consensus statement from the NF1 Cognitive Disorders Task Force. *Neurology, 48,* 1121–1127

Ozonoff, S. (1999). Cognitive impairment in neurofibromatosis type 1. *American Journal of Medical Genetics, 89,* 45–52

Robin, D.A., & Eliason, M.J. (1991). Speech and prosodic problems in children with neurofibromatosis. In: C.A. Moore, K.M. Yorkston, & D.R. Beukelman (Eds.), *Dysarthria and Apraxia of Speech: Perspectives on Management* (pp. 137–144). Baltimore: Paul H. Brookes

Stumpf, D.A., Alksne, J.F., Annegers, J.F., Brown, S.S., Conneally, M., Housman, D., et al. (1988). Neurofibromatosis conference statement. *Archives of Neurology, 45,* 575–578

Additional Reading

Maria, B.L. (Ed.) (2002). Neurobiology of disease in children: neurofibromatosis 1 [special issue]. *Journal of Child Neurology, 17*

Chapter 43

Neurofibromatosis Type 2

Skott E. Freedman, Edwin Maas, and Donald A. Robin

◆ General Information on Disorder

Neurofibromatosis type 2 (NF2), the less common form of the genetic neurofibromatoses (see Chapter 41 for a discussion of the more common form), results in the development of neural growths throughout the central (CNS) and peripheral nervous systems (PNS). Formerly known as bilateral acoustic neurofibromatosis (BAN), this chronic progressive disease is characterized by bilateral tumors on the cranial and spinal nerves, and it particularly affects the auditory and vestibular nerve branches of cranial nerve VIII.

Diagnostic Signs and Symptoms

The most common symptom associated with NF2 is progressive hearing loss (National Institutes of Health, 1988). Specific criteria differentiate NF2 from the more regularly occurring NF1. Some of the diagnostic markers for NF2 include the presence of bilateral vestibular tumors and additional CNS tumors such as meningiomas, astrocytomas, and ependymomas (Gutmann et al, 1997; Kanter & Eldridge, 1980; Martuza & Eldridge, 1988). Less common but still prevalent tumors of the peripheral nerves and cutaneous tumors may also be observed (Gutmann et al, 1997; Kanter & Eldridge, 1980; Martuza & Eldridge, 1988).

Neuropathology

As in NF1, most complications in conjunction with NF2 appear at the onset of puberty and early adulthood. The auditory nerve is consistently involved in NF2, which may result in hearing loss, audible ringing in the ears (tinnitus), and problems with balance (related to vestibular nerve compression). Other symptoms include facial weakness, visional changes, and headache due to tumor growths (NIH, 1988).

In addition to tumors on cranial nerve VIII, tumors often develop on other nerves. Termed *schwannomas*, the origin of these growths is believed to be Schwann cells found in the PNS. As these *schwannomas* continue to grow, they may eventually affect peripheral nerves and result in muscular weakness. In the event that a schwannoma continuously applies pressure to a vital structure such as the brainstem, the disorder may become life-threatening (NIH, 1988).

Epidemiology

NF2 equally affects both genders with an estimated incidence rate of 1 in 40,000 individuals (NIH, 1988).

Genetics

A disease with an autosomal dominant inheritance, NF2 is an inherited neurological disorder caused by a single genetic mutation on chromosome 22 (Rouleau et al, 1993; Trofatter et al, 1993). The NF2 gene product is a protein called merlin, responsible for tumor suppression in healthy individuals (Xiao, Chernoff, & Testa, 2003). In NF2, this function is considered to be impaired, which results in an uncontrollable spread of tumors throughout the CNS and notably the auditory nerve. Children of an affected parent have a 50% chance of inheriting the NF2 gene (NIH, 1988).

◆ Speech Impairment Associated with Disorder

Because the auditory nerve in NF2 is continuously subjected to bilateral tumor growth and accompanying pressure, speech and language are inevitably affected due to a progressive loss in hearing. Perkell et al (1997, 2000) suggested the important role of auditory feedback in accurate speech production. According to Perkell et al, auditory feedback enables an individual to maintain "phonemic settings" and distinguish speech sounds during production. Without this important auditory feedback, as in NF2 when hearing is compromised, articulation and prosody may suffer without sufficient self-monitoring skills (see Chapter 13). In addition, given that the distribution of lesions can affect cranial nerves other than the auditory nerve and spinal nerves, there is a possibility of the presence of flaccid dysarthria in people who suffer from NF2.

Auditory brainstem implants (ABIs) are often used in NF2 to restimulate the cochlear nucleus (Schwartz, Otto, Brackmann, Hitselberger, & Shannon, 2003). These implants have shown significant improvement in auditory comprehension (Schwartz et al, 2003).

Diagnostic Signs and Symptoms

No particular speech impairments have been documented as being exclusive to NF2.

However, as noted above, it is likely that any motor speech deficits would result in flaccid dysarthria.

Etiology

No known cause has been identified for speech impairments occurring in conjunction with NF2. Possible causes of speech complications in NF2 include CNS and PNS tumors, specifically on or around the auditory and vestibular branches of the auditory nerve.

Neuropathology

No investigations to date have considered the neuropathology behind speech disturbances observed in NF2. The most probable source is the presence of neural growths throughout the CNS and PNS that affect various speech subsystems.

Associated Cognitive, Linguistic, and Communicative Signs and Symptoms

Research on specific disabilities occurring with NF2 is scarce. Schautzer, Hamilton, Kalla, Strupp, and Brandt (2003) reported spatial learning and memory deficits in individuals with NF2, relative to controls. One proposed cause of these impairments is a chronic insufficient amount of vestibular input, a direct consequence of bilateral vestibular schwannomas (Schautzer et al, 2003). Hippocampal deficits are thus thought to ensue in NF2, caused by a lack of imperative vestibular input (Schautzer et al, 2003).

Special Diagnostic Considerations

Due to tumor growths on and around the CNS and PNS, speech production may be impaired in the areas of respiration, phonation, resonation, articulation, and prosody. Also, considering the high prevalence of bilateral tumors on the auditory nerve in NF2, hearing status should be evaluated as soon as possible and on a regular basis.

Treatment

Neurofibromatosis type 2 is highly sporadic and unpredictable, indicating a need for constant reevaluation to address new deficit areas or changes in impairment. Targeted speech subsystems in treatment may include respiration, phonation, resonation, and articulation.

References

Gutmann, D.H., Aylsworth, A., Carey, J.C., Korf, B., Marks, J., Pyeritz, E.E., Rubenstein, A., & Viskochil, D.T. (1997). The diagnostic evaluation and multidisciplinary management of neurofibromatosis 1 and neurofibromatosis 2 *J. of the American Medical Association, 278*, 51–57

Kanter, W.R., Eldridge, R., Fabricant, R., Allen, J.C., & Koerber, T. (1980). Central neurofibromatosis with bilateral acoustic neuroma: genetic, clinical and biochemical distinctions from peripheral neurofibromatosis. *Neurology, 30*, 851–859

Martuza, R.L. & Eldridge, R. (1988). Neurofibromatosis 2 (bilateral acoustic neurofibromatosis). *New England Journal of Medicine, 318*, 684–688

National Institutes of Health (NIH). (1988). National Institutes of Health Consensus Development Conference. Neurofibromatosis Conference Statement. *Archives of Neurology, 45*, 575–578

Perkell, J., Matthies, M., Lane, H., Guenther, F., Wilhelms-Tricarico, R., Wozniak, J., & Guiod, P. (1997). Speech motor control: acoustic goals, saturation effects, auditory feedback, and internal models. *Speech Communication, 22*, 227–250

Perkell, J.S., Guenther, F.H., Lane, H., Matthies, M.L., Perrier, P., Vick, J., Wilhelms-Tricarico, R., & Zandipour, M. (2000). A theory of speech motor control and supporting data from speakers with normal hearing and with profound hearing loss. *Journal of Phonetics, 28*, 233–272

Rouleau, G.A., Merel, P., Lutchman, M., Sanson, M., Zucman, J., Marineau, C., Hoang-Xuan, K., Demczuk, S., Desmaze, C., Plougstel, B., Pulst, S.M., Lenoir, G., Bijlsma, E., Fashold, R., Dumanski, J., de Jong, P., Parry, D., Eldridge, R., Aurias, A., Delattre, O., & Thomas, G. (1993). Alteration in a new gene encoding a putative membrane-organizing protein causes neuro-fibromatosis type 2. *Nature, 363*, 515–521

Schautzer, F., Hamilton, D., Kalla, R., Strupp, M., & Brandt, T. (2003). Spatial memory deficits in patients with chronic bilateral vestibular failure. *Annals of the New York Academy of Sciences, 1004*, 316–324

Schwartz, M.S., Otto, S.R., Brackmann, D.E., Hitselberger, W.E., & Shannon, R.V. (2003). Operative techniques in otolaryngology. *Head and Neck Surgery, 14*, 282–287

Trofatter, J.A., MacCollin, M.M., Rutter, J.L., Murrell, J.R., Duyao, M.P., Parry, D.M., Eldridge, R., Kley, N., Menon, A.G., Pulaski, K., Haase,V.H., Ambrose, C.M., Munroe, D., Bove, C., Haines, J.L., Martuza, R.L., MacDonald, M.E., Seizinger, B.R., Short, M.P., Buckler, A.J., & Gusella, J.F. (1993) A novel moesin-, ezrin-, radixin-like gene is a candidate for the neurofibromatosis 2 tumor suppressor. *Cell, 72*, 791–800

Xiao, G.H., Chernoff, J., & Testa, J.R. (2003). NF2: the wizardry of merlin. *Genes, chromosomes, and Cancer, 38*, 389–399

Chapter 44

Opercular Syndrome (Foix-Chavany-Marie Syndrome)

Chris Code

♦ General Information on Disorder

The opercular syndrome (OS) results from left to right cortical atrophy of the posterior inferior frontal lobe, notably the operculum. However, the specific term *Foix-Chavany-Marie syndrome* (FCMS) (Foix, Chavany, & Marie, 1926) describes a speech impairment from a facio-linguovelo-pharyngeo-masticatory diplegic paralysis resulting most often from bilateral opercular lesions with an automatic-voluntary dissociation (Weller, 1993). The term *operculum* means "lid," and these lids are formed where the cortex dips into the fissures of the brain. The frontal operculum is contiguous with the foot of the frontal motor cortex at areas 44 (pars triangularis) and 45 (pars opercularis), which make up most of Broca's area. Damage to the frontal operculum is common in severe and lasting forms of Broca's aphasia, within, as it is, the supply of the upper division of the middle cerebral artery. Broussolle et al (1996) reported a longitudinal study of eight patients with progressive conditions, most presenting initially with FCMS. With deterioration there was spastic, hypokinetic, or hyperkinetic dysarthria, apraxia of speech, buccofacial apraxia, dysphagia, and frontal signs ending in mutism.

Diagnostic Signs and Symptoms

The classic distinguishing signs of FCMS are bilateral facio-linguovelo-pharyngeo-masticatory paresis with a dissociation of automatic and voluntary control of the craniofacial muscles for facial expression (Weller, 1993).

Neuropathology

Bilateral opercular lesions often involving the rolandic operculum are usually required for diagnosis; however, cases with unilateral lesions have been described (Mao, Coull, Golper, & Rau, 1989; Weller, 1993). Magnetic resonance imaging (MRI) and computed tomography (CT) show predominantly left frontal atrophy in the progressive form, and positron emission tomography (PET) and single photon emission computed tomography (SPECT) show asymmetric blood flow with metabolic decrement primarily affecting the left inferior-posterior frontal gyri (Broussolle et al, 1996). In the most advanced cases the right operculum is affected. Pathological investigation showed predominantly left opercular spongiform changes in layers II and III with mild neuronal loss and astrogliosis.

Epidemiology

Pure FCMS is a rare condition and there are no incidence or prevalence figures available.

Genetics

Little or nothing is known about the genetics of the FCMS.

♦ Speech Impairment Associated with Disorder

Speech impairments can include signs akin to apraxia of speech (often called *anarthria*, but terminology is an unreliable guide in this area of the literature, and the term *aphemia* is sometimes used) and pyramidal (spastic) and extrapyramidal (hypokinetic and hyperkinetic) dysarthrias with substantive prosodic problems. Buccofacial apraxia is usually present with facial weakness, drooling, dysphagia, masticatory problems, and jaw jerks. For many, the speech impairment is dysarthric and not apraxic (Weller, 1993).

Etiology

Etiology of FCMS varies. Weller (1993) reviewed 62 published cases and identified five clinical types: (1) the classic and common form resulting from cerebrovascular disease, (2) a subacute type caused by central nervous system (CNS) infections, (3) a developmental form caused most commonly by neuronal migration disorders, (4) a reversible type in children with epilepsy (see Chapter 36), and (5) a rare progressive type. Speech production impairments result most commonly from bilateral damage to the frontal operculum and surrounding and connecting areas with the opercular region most affected, bilaterally in severest cases and with progressive conditions, then a range of dysarthric conditions with dysphagia and apraxia of speech can occur in a variety of combinations.

Associated Cognitive, Linguistic, and Communicative Signs and Symptoms

In its pure form FCMS is a motor disorder without language or other cognitive deficits. Broussolle et al (1996), however, report that individuals with the progressive form fail heavily on frontal tests including slowness in actions, distractibility, and perseveration in graphic and motor sequences.

Special Diagnostic Considerations

The diagnosis of FCMS requires clear automatic-voluntary dissociation in the control of craniofacial muscles, and tasks designed to elicit this feature are essential for its confirmation.

Treatment

No specific treatment is recommended for FCMS, although treatment for apraxia of speech, dysarthria, and dysphagia, if present, will take their usual forms depending on their combination and presentation.

References

Broussolle, E., Bakchine, S., Tommasi, M., Laurent, B., Bazin, B., Cinotti, L., Cohen, L. & Chazot, G. (1996). Slowly progressive anarthria with late anterior opercular syndrome: a variant form of frontal cortical atrophy syndromes. *Journal of the Neurological Sciences 144*, 44–58

Foix, C., Chavany, J.A. & Marie J. (1926) Diplégie facio-linguo-masticatrice d'origine sous-corticale sans paralysie des membres (contribution à l'étude de la localisation des centres de la face du membre supérieur). *Revue Neurologique, 33*, 214–219

Mao, C.-C., Coull, B.M., Golper, L.A.C., & Rau, M.T. (1989) Anterior opercular syndrome. *Neurology, 39*, 1169–1172

Weller, M. (1993) Anterior opercular cortex lesions cause dissociated lower cranial nerve palsies and anarthria but no aphasia: Foix-Chavany-Marie syndrome and "automatic voluntary dissociation" revisited. *Journal of Neurology, 240*, 199–208

Additional Reading

Lang, A.E. (1992) Cortical basal ganglionic degeneration presenting with 'progressive loss of speech output and orofacial dyspraxia. *Journal of Neurology, Neurosurgery, and Psychiatry, 55*, 1101

Lang, C., Reichwein, J., Ire, H. & Treig, T. (1989) Foix-Chavany-Marie syndrome: neurological, neuropsychological, CT, MRI, and SPECT findings in a case progressive for more than 10 years. *European Archives of Psychiatry and Neurological Science, 239*, 188–193

Chapter 45

Oromandibular Dystonia

Allyson Dykstra and Scott G. Adams

◆ General Information on Disorder

Dystonia is a slow hyperkinetic movement disorder characterized by sustained or tonic muscle contractions. These tonic muscle contractions are frequently associated with abnormal and sometimes painful posturing and positioning, twisting, and repetitive movements (Duffy, 1995; Fahn, Marsden, & Calne, 1987). Because dystonia is a heterogeneous disorder, it has been classified according to age of onset, distribution, and etiology. Etiology also can be classified according to whether or not the dystonia is primary (when dystonia is the only or primary symptom), or secondary, implying that the dystonia is one of several symptoms resulting from another condition. These conditions include, but are not limited to, tumors, focal cerebrovascular accidents (CVAs) of the basal ganglia, traumatic brain injury, or carbon monoxide poisoning (Freed, 2000). Classifying dystonias according to the above parameters can assist with accurate diagnosis, appropriate approaches to management and therapy, and prognostic factors.

Diagnostic Signs and Symptoms

Oromandibular dystonia (OMD) is a focal dystonia manifested by excessive muscle contractions or abnormal postures of the jaw and lower facial and lingual muscles. It can be characterized as jaw opening, jaw closing, jaw deviation, jaw retraction, lip dystonia, tongue dystonia, or mixed type (Tan & Jankovic, 2000; Yoshida, Kaji, Shibasaki, & Iizuka, 2002). When OMD is associated with blepharospasm, the condition is known as Meige's syndrome. The dystonic movements associated with OMD can cause facial grimacing and involuntary tongue and jaw movements and postures (Yoshida et al, 2002). As a result, dysphagia and dysarthria are often present (Blitzer, Brin, & Fahn, 1991). When OMD involves the tongue, there can be significant effects on swallowing and speech intelligibility (Dykstra, Adams, & Jog, 2007).

Epidemiology

It is estimated that the prevalence of all focal dystonias is approximately 300 cases/million persons (Brin & Comella, 2004). The prevalence of OMD has been estimated at 68.9 cases/million persons (Nutt, Muenter, Aronson, Kurland, & Melton, 1988), and the incidence has been estimated to be 3.3 cases/million persons (Nutt et al, 1988). The average age of onset of OMD is estimated to be 66 years (range 40 to 86 years), with more women affected than men by a ratio of 4:1 (Nutt et al, 1988).

Genetics

Thirteen different forms of dystonia have been distinguished genetically. They are designated DYT 1–13 (Klein & Ozelius, 2002). Chromosomal locations have been identified for eight of the 13 types, and specific genes have been identified for three forms (DYT 1, 5, and 11) (Klein & Ozelius, 2002). Evidence that suggests a possible genetic cause for OMD was demonstrated in a case study by Steinberger, Topka, Fischer, and Muller (1999), who reported a mutation of the *GCH1* gene located on chromosome 14 in an individual with adult-onset OMD. Although it appears that some individuals with OMD may have a genetic predisposition, most forms of OMD, however, appear to be sporadic in nature (Steinberger et al., 1999; Tan, 2004).

◆ Speech Impairment Associated with Syndrome

As a result of dystonic movements or postures of the orofacial structures, individuals with OMD often present with dysarthria and speech intelligibility deficits. In 1969, Darley, Aronson, and Brown studied 30 patients with hyperkinetic dysarthria associated with dystonia. These researchers established the most deviant speech dimensions of dystonia from most to least severe to be imprecise consonant articulation, vowel distortion, harsh voice, irregular articulatory breakdown, strained-strangled voice quality, monopitch, and monoloudness. Speech rate in dystonia also was found to be generally slow, with abnormal direction and rhythm of movement. It should be noted, however, that Darley, Aronson, and Brown's 30 subjects with dystonia included individuals with OMD and individuals with laryngeal dystonia (spasmodic dysphonia).

Etiology

The etiology of OMD is largely unknown and often is idiopathic in nature (Tan, 2004). However, possible etiological factors identified can include neuroleptic exposure, central nervous system (CNS)/head trauma, hypoxia, metabolic disorders, demyelinating lesions in the upper brainstem, neurodegenerative diseases, or diencephalitic stroke (Dworkin, 1996; Sankhla, Lai, & Jankovic, 1998; Tan & Jankovic, 2000).

Neuropathology

Although the neuropathological mechanisms contributing to OMD are poorly understood, the underlying site(s) of lesion in OMD are thought to involve lesions of the basal ganglia. In addition, a neurochemical imbalance in dopaminergic and cholinergic activity has been suggested in OMD (Duffy, 1995; Dworkin, 1996).

Treatment

There is no cure for OMD or any dystonia. The principal goals of therapy focus on reducing painful spasms or abnormal postures of the jaw, lower face, tongue, and oral muscles; improving orofacial aesthetics; and ultimately restoring functional speech and masticatory and swallowing capabilities. The current literature reviewing therapeutic options report that pharmacotherapy, dental appliances (i.e., bite-block therapy), chemodenervation, and neurosurgery have been used with various success rates in the treatment of OMD.

The traditional treatment of OMD has included a variety of systemic pharmacological agents, including anticholinergics (trihexyphenidyl, benztropine), benzodiazepines (clonazepam, lorazepam, diazepam), baclofen, and drugs that deplete dopamine (tetrabenazine) (Klein & Ozelius, 2002; Tan 2004; Tinter & Jankovic, 2002). Frequent side effects and poor to modest therapeutic improvement suggest that pharmacotherapy with these agents is largely unsatisfactory for patients with OMD (Charles, Davis, Shannon, Hook, & Warner, 1997; Dworkin, 1996; Tinter & Jankovic, 2002).

Bite-block therapy was demonstrated to improve the speech intelligibility and orofacial postural control in two patients with Meige's syndrome (Dworkin, 1996). Results from this study revealed that when a bite-block was placed between the teeth of each of the two patients with dystonia, there was improvement in facial appearance, articulatory precision, and hyperactive oromandibular movements (Dworkin, 1996). The dramatic improvement in articulatory precision evidenced when the bite block was in place was suggested to be primarily related to stabilization of the jaw (Dworkin, 1996). These benefits may be directly related to a reduction in dystonic jaw movements. It also is possible that jaw stabilization helps to reduce the disruptive effects of dystonic jaw movements on normal lip and tongue movements. In addition, jaw stabilization may also allow for improved control of dystonic lip and tongue movements by providing a more consistent platform or framework for these abnormal speech movements. A final consideration is that a bite block may provide a novel type of sensory stimulation that acts to reduce the dystonic oral movements (see below for more information on sensory tricks in dystonia).

The most contemporary management of OMD and other focal dystonias is achieved site-specifically by chemodenervation with botulinum toxin. Botulinum toxin is derived from *Clostridium botulinum* and exists as eight antigenically distinct serotypes, designated A, B, C1, C2, D, E, F, and G

(Blitzer & Sulica, 2001). In the United States and Canada, serotype A (BtA) (Botox®, Allergan Ltd., Buckinghamshire, England) is most commonly used for clinical use. Botulinum toxin works by blocking the presynaptic release of acetylcholine into the neuromuscular junction. This results in chemical denervation and a flaccid paralysis/weakness of the muscle(s) (Goldman & Comella, 2003). Botulinum toxin is injected locally into the symptomatic muscle(s). Dosing is highly individualized and is based on the mass of the muscle being injected and individual characteristics of the patient such as body mass and any preexisting weakness (Munchau & Bhatia, 2000). The weakness induced by injection with BtA typically does not appear for 1 to 3 days. By 2 weeks, a marked effect is present and the effects last for approximately 3 months (Blitzer & Sulica, 2001). Side effects of BtA are usually well tolerated but can include mild dysarthria, difficulty chewing, and mild dysphagia (Goldman & Comella, 2003; Munchau & Bhatia, 2000).

A less common treatment for OMD is neurosurgery. Deep brain stimulation (DBS) of the globus pallidus internus (GPi) has been performed typically for very severe forms of generalized dystonia that are unresponsive to more conventional treatment options (Ondo & Krauss, 2004). There is a growing body of literature suggesting that DBS of the GPi may be of therapeutic benefit for certain focal dystonias such as Meige's syndrome (Hans-Holger, Weigel & Krauss, 2003). Hans-Holger et al (2003) performed bilateral pallidal DBS surgery for a case of blepharospasm-oromandibular dystonia (Meige's syndrome). They reported that OMD and blepharospasm improved, but only a minimal improvement in swallowing function was achieved following DBS of the GPi. Despite a limited empirical database, this case report supports further exploration of neurosurgical techniques as a treatment for severe, medication-resistant forms of focal dystonias.

One final and poorly understood phenomenon unique to the dystonias is sensory tricks. A sensory trick, also known as a *geste antagoniste,* is a specific movement or action an individual with dystonia can make to temporarily inhibit dystonic postures or movements. The physiological mechanism of sensory tricks remains unknown (Duffy, 2005). However, sensory tricks such as touching the hand to the chin or jaw to achieve jaw closure or touching the hand to the lips to relieve jaw spasms can be facilitory in reducing dystonic posturing in some individuals with OMD (Brin & Comella, 2004; Duffy, 2005). Other sensory tricks that have been reported in the literature to alleviate dystonic symptoms include singing, humming, sleeping, and relaxing (Tan, 2004).

Quality of Life

The social, emotional, and vocational consequences of OMD can be profoundly disabling in those affected. Decreased speech intelligibility, difficulty managing oral intake of food and liquids, dysphagia, and altered orofacial aesthetics are likely sequelae of a diagnosis of OMD. Because treatment is not curative but rather to manage symptomatology, many individuals with OMD feel a sense of helplessness over their condition and can become depressed and socially isolated

(Charles et al, 1997). Obtaining quality of life (QoL) measures can provide important information regarding the impact of the speech disorder associated with OMD on an individual's daily functions in the context of his or her personal, social, and environmental milieu (Ma & Yiu, 2001). The Voice Activity and Participation Profile (VAPP) (Ma & Yiu, 2001) is an assessment tool developed to assess an individual's perception of his/her voice problem, activity limitation, and participation restrictions using the International Classification of Impairments, Disabilities and Handicaps–2 (ICIDH-2) (World Health Organization, 1997). Dykstra et al (2007) modified the VAPP by replacing the word *voice* with *speech* to assess the impact of reduced speech intelligibility

on the activity limitations and participation restrictions on an individual with lingual dystonia. Results of this qualitative assessment revealed poignantly that only a mild to moderate reduction in speech intelligibility was required to negatively impact the individual's activity and participation scores, and hence, QoL. This example emphasizes the importance of gathering subjective information in addition to traditional objective assessment measures as it can help clinicians establish a more comprehensive view of the communication disorder. Additionally, understanding patients' perception of disablement with regard to their activity and participation restrictions may serve as a good prognostic indicator for intervention (Ma & Yiu, 2001).

References

Blitzer, A., Brin, M.F., & Fahn, S. (1991). Botulinum toxin injections for lingual dystonia. *Laryngoscope, 101,* 799

Blitzer, A., & Sulica, L. (2001). Botulinum toxin: basic science and clinical uses in otolaryngology. *Laryngoscope, 111,* 218–226

Brin, M.F., & Comella, C.L. (2004). Pathophysiology of dystonia. In: M.F. Brin, C.L. Comella, & J. Jankovic (Eds.) *Dystonia: Etiology, Clinical Features, and Treatment* (pp. 5–10). Philadelphia: Lippincott Williams & Wilkins

Charles, P.D., Davis, T.L., Shannon, K.M., Hook, M.A., & Warner, J.S. (1997). Tongue protrusion dystonia: treatment with botulinum toxin. *Southern Medical Journal, 90,* 522–525

Darley, F.L., Aronson, A.E., & Brown, J.R. (1969). Clusters of deviant speech dimensions in the dysarthrias. *Journal of Speech and Hearing Research 12,* 462–496

Duffy, J.R. (1995). *Motor Speech Disorders: Substrates, Differential Diagnosis, and Management* (pp. 189–221). Toronto: Mosby

Duffy, J.R. (2005). *Motor Speech Disorders: Substrates, Differential Diagnosis, and Management,* 2nd ed. (p. 227). St. Louis: Elsevier Mosby

Dworkin, J.P. (1996). Bite-block therapy for oromandibular dystonia. *Journal of Medical Speech-Language Pathology, 4,* 47–56

Dykstra, A.D., Adams, S.G., & Jog, M. (2007). The effect of botulinum toxin type A on speech intelligibility in lingual dystonia. *Journal of Medical Speech-Language Pathology, 15,* 173–186

Fahn, S., Marsden, C.D., & Calne, D.B. (1987). Classification and investigation of dystonia. In: C. D. Marsden & S. Fahn (Eds.) *Movement Disorders 2* (pp. 332–358). London: Butterworths

Freed, D. (2000). *Motor Speech Disorders: Diagnosis and Treatment* (pp. 229–255). San Diego, CA: Singular

Goldman, J.G., & Comella, C.L. (2003). Treatment of dystonia. *Clinical Neuropharmacology, 26,* 102–108

Capelle, H.H., Weigel, R., & Krauss, J.K. (2003). Bilateral pallidal stimulation for blepharospasm-oromandibular dystonia (Meige syndrome). *Neurology, 60,* 2017–2018

Klein, C., & Ozelius, L.J. (2002). Dystonia: clinical features, genetics and treatment. *Current Opinion in Neurology, 15,* 491–497

Ma, E.P., & Yiu, E. (2001). Voice activity and participation profile: assessing the impact of voice disorders on daily activities. *Journal of Speech, Language, and Hearing Research, 44,* 511–524

Munchau, A., & Bhatia, K.P. (2000). Uses of botulinum toxin injection in medicine today. *British Medical Journal, 320,* 161–165

Nutt, J.G., Muenter, M.D., Aronson, A., Kurland, L.T., & Melton, L.J. (1988). Epidemiology of focal and generalized dystonia in Rochester, Minnesota. *Movement Disorders, 3,* 188–194

Ondo, W.G., & Krauss, J.K. (2004). Surgical therapies for dystonia. In: M.F. Brin, C.L. Comella, & J. Jankovic (Eds.) *Dystonia: Etiology, Clinical Features, and Treatment* (pp. 125–147). Philadelphia: Lippincott Williams & Wilkins

Sankhla, C., Lai, E.C., & Jankovic, J. (1998). Peripherally induced oromandibular dystonia. *Journal of Neurology, Neurosurgery, and Psychiatry, 65,* 722–728

Steinberger, D., Topka, H., Fischer, D., & Muller, U. (1999). GCH1 mutation in a patient with adult-onset oromandibular dystonia. *Neurology, 52,* 877–879

Tan, E.-K. (2004). Oromandibular dystonia. In: M.F. Brin, C.L. Comella, & J. Jankovic (Eds.) *Dystonia: Etiology, Clinical Features, and Treatment* (pp. 167–174). Philadelphia: Lippincott Williams & Wilkins

Tan, E.-K., & Jankovic, J. (2000). Tardive and idiopathic oromandibular dystonia: a clinical comparison. *Journal of Neurology, Neurosurgery, and Psychiatry, 68,* 186–190

Tinter, R., & Jankovic, J. (2002). Botulinum toxin type A in the management of oromandibular dystonia and bruxism. In: M.F. Brin, M. Hallet, & J. Jankovic (Eds.) *Scientific and Therapeutic Aspects of Botulinum Toxin* (pp. 1–12). Philadelphia: Lippincott Williams & Wilkins

World Health Organization. (1997). ICIDH-2: international classification of impairment, disability and handicap–2. Geneva, Switzerland: WHO

Yoshida, K., Kaji, R., Shibasaki, H., & Iizuka, T. (2002). Factors influencing the therapeutic effect of muscle afferent block for oromandibular dystonia and dyskinesia: implications for their distinct pathophysiology. *International Journal of Oral and Maxillofacial Surgery, 31,* 499–505

Additional Reading

Brin, M.F., Comella, C.L., & Jankovic, J. (Eds.) (2004). *Dystonia: Etiology, Clinical Features, and Treatment.* Philadelphia: Lippincott Williams & Wilkins

Chapter 46

Pallidotomy and Deep Brain Stimulation in Parkinson's Disease

Steven M. Barlow and Michael J. Hammer

Parkinson's disease (PD) is a common neurodegenerative disorder affecting more than one million people in the United States, with more than 50,000 new cases diagnosed each year. Initially described as "shaking palsy" in 1817 by a British physician, James Parkinson (essay reprinted as Parkinson, 2002), PD results primarily from the progressive death of dopaminergic neurons in the substantia nigra pars compacta in the midbrain, and the striatum. Most reported cases are in patients over 50 years of age, predominantly male, but early-onset or juvenile PD appears in people in their 20s and 30s.

A constellation of sensorimotor impairments accompany PD, including resting tremor, akinesia, bradykinesia, disturbances in gait (festination) and posture, dysphagia, anosmia, dystonia, hypophonia, dysarthria, masked face, micrographia, muscle rigidity, and disturbances to somatosensory and proprioceptive function. At high levodopa blood levels in patients with advanced PD, involuntary nonpurposive movements (dyskinesias) of the extremities, trunk, neck, and face may occur.

Two of the most widely used neurosurgical methods for the treatment of advanced idiopathic PD include pallidotomy and deep brain stimulation (DBS) of the subthalamic nucleus (STN) or globus pallidus interna (GPI). Pallidotomy involves the placement of a thermolesion on one or both sides of the GPI to ameliorate the motor symptoms of PD, whereas DBS involves the placement of a four-channel depth electrode in the region of the STN or GPI for delivery of therapeutic electric field stimulation by an implantable pulse generator (pacemaker).

◆ Pallidotomy

A stereotactic neurosurgical treatment for PD known as posteroventral pallidotomy (PVP) was introduced in 1956 by Dr. Lars Leksell in Sweden after the serendipitous discovery that lesions of the globus pallidus ameliorated parkinsonian features (Laitinen, 2000). Functional stereotactic neurosurgery went into a hiatus after the discovery of the drug levodopa (L-dopa) in 1968, which rapidly became the primary pharmacological treatment for relieving the motor symptoms of PD. Administration of other antiparkinson medications like dopamine agonists often results in improvement of motor fluctuations and dyskinesias. The PVP reemerged in the 1990s, as some of the long-term limitations of levodopa treatment became more apparent, coupled with advances in stereotactic surgery and neuroimaging.

Pallidotomy has been reported to be effective for the treatment of tremor, rigidity, bradykinesia, and drug-induced dyskinesia among limb muscle systems in PD (Laitenen, Bergenheim, & Hariz, 1992; Svennilson, Torvik, Lowe, & Leksell, 1960). Speech loudness also improved in most patients. Laitenen et al hypothesized that PVP interrupts hyperactive striopallidal or subthalamopallidal pathways, which ultimately helps to reestablish more normal motor functioning in PD patients.

Significant reductions in akinetic symptoms including freezing and arising from a chair, along with improvements in posture, gait, postural instability, and bradykinesia, are reported following PVP for patients with idiopathic PD (Iacono et al, 1994). These positive changes are thought to result from the interruption of amplified collateral inhibitory output from the pallidum to brainstem locomotor centers such as the pedunculopontine nucleus (PPN), whereas interruption of collaterals to ventral lateral thalamus by PVP may account for the elimination of hyperkinesia.

◆ Deep Brain Stimulation

An early observation with ablative neurosurgery was that electrical stimulation of the anatomical targets resulted in similar clinical effects as lesioning. Chronic high-frequency stimulation of the globus pallidus or STN using an implanted electrode in patients with PD produced significant improvement in all subscales of the Unified Parkinson Disease Rating Scale (UPDRS) without the adverse effects often associated with pallidotomy (Limousin et al, 1998; Pahwa et al, 1997). Over the past 10 years, DBS of the STN has rapidly emerged as a routine method for the treatment of advanced idiopathic PD producing remarkable improvements in motor function and quality of life (Breit, Schulz, & Benabid, 2004). However, the effects of electrode location and parameters of deep brain stimulation on speech, vocalization, and other skills involving the coordination of respiratory and vocal tract muscle systems are not well understood.

◆ Speech Function Following Posteroventral Pallidotomy

Experimental observations of the effects of unilateral pallidotomy on speech (vowels, syllables, reading, picture description) have shown that PD patients subjectively rated as having mild dysarthria exhibited improvements in sound pressure level (SPL), whereas those rated as having moderate dysarthria exhibited negative changes in SPL (Schulz, Greer, & Friedman, 2000). Left-side PVP resulted in negative changes in SPL, whereas right-sided PVP resulted in negligible changes in speech SPL. The authors concluded that PVP may provide greater benefit to participants with mild dysarthria due to less basal ganglia pathophysiology, and that the side of lesion is important to consider due to the possible influence on speech.

Bilateral PVP completed in a consecutive series of 11 patients with advanced idiopathic PD revealed remarkable improvement on posture, gait, locomotion, and axial and limb (appendicular) muscle systems (Barlow, Iacono, Paseman, Biswas, & D'Antonio, 1998). However, only half of these PD patients exhibited significant changes in lip contractile instability, peak rate of lip force recruitment, average rate of lip force recruitment, and lip compression reaction time. Overall, perioral force recruitment trajectories were down-scaled following pallidotomy, resulting in a perioral muscle system that is slower in force generation but significantly more stable. Laryngeal airway resistance, chest wall driving pressures, speech rate control, timing of voice onset, and the dynamics of burst-release and laryngeal engagement were also significantly reorganized following PVP.

◆ Speech Function Following Subthalamic Nucleus Deep Brain Stimulation

Recently the effects of unilateral STN DBS on speech production were examined in right-handed participants who received unilateral STN DBS (three right DBS, three left DBS) (Wang, Metman, Bakay, Arzbaecher, & Bernard, 2003). Although significant improvements on the UPDRS were observed for all six participants, only right STN DBS patients exhibited improved speech measures, whereas patients with left STN DBS exhibited further deterioration in these measures. These data indicate that the influence of STN DBS on measures of speech function may depend on the hemisphere stimulated.

Some studies have reported improvements in speech acoustics following bilateral STN DBS. For example, Gentil, Chauvin, Pinto, Pollak, and Benabid (2001) reported that a group of 26 PD subjects with STN DBS exhibited between 57% and 59% improvements in UPDRS scores, and improvement from a group mean of 2 to 1 on the speech item of the UPDRS. These participants also exhibited significant improvements on select acoustic measures (voice fundamental frequency, maximum vowel duration) during speech production.

Significant improvements in force recruitment, timing, and precision were found for upper lip, lower lip, and tongue among 10 PD participants with STN DBS (Gentil, Garcia-Ruiz, Pollak, & Benabid, 1999). Long-term improvements through 5 years post-STN DBS have been observed for measures of lip and tongue force control (Pinto, Gentil, Fraix, Benabid, & Pollak, 2003). Although these sustained improvements reflect isometric force control in isolated muscle groups, the collective subsystems contributing to dysarthria worsened for the participants over the course of the follow-up study based on the UPDRS.

A series of studies conducted in 18 patients with idiopathic PD and bilateral STN DBS demonstrated that all participants exhibited significant improvements in limb function as indicated by the UPDRS, but only a subset of these patients exhibited significant changes on measures of speech aerodynamics, including estimates of subglottal pressure, translaryngeal air flow, and laryngeal airway resistance (Barlow, Hammer, Pahwa, & Seibel, 2003). Significant "on" versus "off" changes in speech aerodynamics were found in 39 to 56% of participants. A related experiment (Hammer, Barlow, & Pahwa, 2004), used ensemble averaging techniques to model the pressure-flow dynamics of laryngeal engagement (LE) following burst (plosive) release. Significant changes in LE were found among 89% of the PD participants. The sensitivity of LE as an objective measure of laryngeal control in PD following DBS is most likely related to differences in electrode location proximal to the STN, parameter settings, electric field properties of the active DBS contact, disease progression, and postsurgical reduction of antiparkinson medications.

◆ Posteroventral Pallidotomy versus Deep Brain Stimulation

Deep brain stimulation has almost completely replaced lesioning procedures. DBS does not require deliberate ablation of brain tissue, and because it is reversible, DBS does not preclude future therapies. DBS parameters can be tuned postoperatively over time to improve outcome efficacy and reduce adverse effects. DBS surgery can be safely performed bilaterally (Breit et al, 2004). STN DBS is currently considered superior to GPI DBS because the anti-akinetic effect appears more pronounced with a more marked reduction of antiparkinsonian medication, and requires less stimulation energy (Volkmann, 2004). Additional research is needed to provide a more complete definition of factors that impact the neural and behavioral responses to DBS, including the reorganization of neuromotor systems underlying speech and voice production.

References

Barlow, S.M., Iacono, R.P., Paseman, L.A., Biswas, A., & D'Antonio, L.D. (1998). The effects of experimental posteroventral pallidotomy on force and speech aerodynamics in Parkinson's disease. In: M.P. Cannito, K.M. Yorkston, & D.R. Beukelman (Eds.), *Speech Motor Control* (pp. 117-156). Baltimore: Paul H. Brookes

Barlow, S.M., Hammer, M.J., Pahwa, R., & Seibel, L. (2003). The effects of subthalamic nucleus deep brain stimulation on vocal tract dynamics in Parkinson's disease. *55th Annual Meeting of the American Academy of Neurology*, 2146

Breit, S., Schulz, J.B., & Benabid, A.-L. (2004). Deep brain stimulation. *Cell Tissue Research, 318*, 275-288

Gentil, M., Chauvin, P., Pinto, S., Pollak, P., & Benabid, A.L. (2001). Effect of bilateral stimulation of the subthalamic nucleus on parkinsonian voice. *Brain and Language*, 78, 233-240

Gentil, M., Garcia-Ruiz, P., Pollak, P., & Benabid, A.L. (1999). Effect of stimulation of the subthalamic nucleus on oral control of patients with parkinsonism. *Journal of Neurology, Neurosurgery and Psychiatry, 67*, 329-333

Hammer, M.J., Barlow, S.M., & Pahwa, R. (2004). Laryngeal Engagement Following Bilateral Deep Brain Stimulation in Parkinson's Disease. 12th Biennial Speech Motor Control Conference, Albuquerque, NM

Iacono, R.P., Lonser, R.R., Mandybur, G., Morenski, J.D., Yamada, S., & Shima, F. (1994). Stereotactic pallidotomy results for Parkinson's exceed those of fetal graft. The *American Surgeon, 60*, 777-782

Laitinen, L.V. (2000). Leksell's unpublished pallidotomies of the 1958-1962. *Stereotactic and Functional Neurosurgery, 74*, 1-10

Laitinen, L.V., Bergenheim, A.T., & Hariz, M.I. (1992). Leksell's posteroventral pallidotomy in the treatment of Parkinson's disease. *Journal of Neurosurgery, 76*, 53-61

Limousin, P., Krack, P., Pollak, P., Benazzouz, A., Ardouin, C., Hoffmann, D., & Benabid, A.L. (1998). Electrical stimulation of the subthalamic nucleus in advanced Parkinson's disease. *New England Journal of Medicine*, 339, 1105-1111

Pahwa, R., Wilkinson, S., Smith, D., Lyons, K., Miyawaki, E., & Koller, W.C. (1997). High-frequency stimulation of the globus pallidus for the treatment of Parkinson's disease. *Neurology*, 49, 249-253

Parkinson, J. (2002). An essay on the shaking palsy. Originally published in 1817 as a monograph (London). *Journal of Neuropsychiatry and Clinical Neuroscience, 14*, 223-236

Pinto, S., Gentil, M., Fraix, V., Benabid, A.L., & Pollak, P. (2003). Bilateral subthalamic stimulation effects on oral force control in Parkinson's disease. *Journal of Neurology*, 250, 179-187

Schulz, G.M., Greer, M., & Friedman, W. (2000). Changes in vocal intensity in Parkinson's disease following pallidotomy surgery. *Journal of Voice, 14*, 589-606

Svennilson, E., Torvik, A., Lowe, R., & Leksell, L. (1960). Treatment of parkinsonism by stereotactic thermolesions in the pallidal region. A clinical evaluation of 81 cases. *Acta Psychiatrica Scandinavica, 35*, 358-377

Volkmann, J. (2004). Deep brain stimulation for the treatment of Parkinson's disease. *Journal of Clinical Neurophysiology*, 21, 6-17

Wang, E., Metman, L.V., Bakay, R., Arzbaecher, J., & Bernard, B. (2003). The effect of unilateral electrostimulation of the subthalamic nucleus on respiratory/phonatory subsystems of speech production in Parkinson's disease—a preliminary report. *Clinical Linguistics & Phonetics, 17*, 283-289

Additional Reading

Breit, S., Schulz, J.B., & Benabid, A.-L. (2004). Deep brain stimulation. *Cell tissue Research, 318*, 275-288

Deep-Brain Stimulation for Parkinson's Disease Study Group. (2001). Deep-brain stimulation of the subthalamic nucleus or the pars interna of the globus pallidus in Parkinson's disease. *New England Journal Medicine, 345*, 956-963

Jenkinson, N., Nandi, D., Aziz, T.Z., & Stein, J.F. (2005). Pedunculopontine nucleus: a new target for deep brain stimulation for akinesia. *Neuroreport, 16*, 1875-1876

Laitinen, L.V. (2004). Personal memoires of the history of stereotactic neurosurgery. *Neurosurgery*, 55, 1420-1429

Chapter 47

Parkinson's Disease

Scott G. Adams and Mandar Jog

◆ General Information on Disorder

Diagnostic Signs and Symptoms

In 1817, James Parkinson first described the major clinical features of a progressive neurological disorder that is now referred to as Parkinson's disease (PD) (Parkinson, 1817). Currently, a neurologist's diagnosis of PD is based on the presence of four major signs: tremor, rigidity, akinesia, and postural instability. Tremor typically occurs at rest and at a frequency of approximately 4 to 7 Hz. Rigidity is characterized by an involuntary resistance to passive movement that may be released momentarily during testing (cogwheel rigidity). Akinesia refers to a reduction in the range, complexity, and speed of movement. Reduced movement speed, referred to as bradykinesia, is an important component of akinesia. Postural instability is reflected in the PD patient's unsteady gait and the reduced ability to compensate for being pushed off balance. Other secondary signs of PD include stooped posture, reduced arm swing, micrographia, reduced facial expression, and difficulties initiating movement. The speech signs and symptoms of PD are discussed in Chapter 11.

The typical profile of a patient with PD in the early stages of the disease (1 to 5 years) includes a unilateral resting tremor, usually involving the hand, complaints of a loss of dexterity for fine movements (i.e., manipulating of small objects), and handwriting that has become small (micrographia) and difficult to decipher. In addition, the patient may have mild complaints of stiffness, slowness, or a lack of power in one limb. There also may be a reduction in facial expression, a reduction in arm swing during walking, and a slightly stooped and asymmetrical posture.

In the later stages of the disease (+15 years), the early symptoms become progressively more severe. The resting tremor usually becomes bilateral and extends to all limbs, as well as the trunk, neck, and jaw. The stiffness, slowness, and loss of coordination and power expand to include a wider range of movements. The patient often cannot perform most fairly simple skilled movements. Periods of immobility, in which the patient appears to be frozen, become more frequent and prolonged. Immobile periods are often separated by periods of hyperactivity involving uncontrolled, rapid movements of the limbs, trunk, and head. These so-called dyskinesias resemble the hyperkinetic movements of patients with Huntington's disease, and are associated with the higher doses of levodopa medication required to overcome the severe immobility that can occur in the later stages of PD. It has been estimated that 80 to 90% of PD patients develop dyskinesias within the first 5 to 10 years after diagnosis (Weiner & Lang, 1989). Because some of these dyskinesias can involve the speech mechanism, there is the potential for a certain number of patients with PD to develop both hyperkinetic and hypokinetic dysarthria. The percentage of patients with PD who demonstrate a mixed hypo-hyperkinetic dysarthria is not known but it is estimated to be in the range of 10 to 20%. In most cases, the hypokinetic symptoms are much more severe than the hyperkinetic symptoms. Dementia, memory loss, language impairment, and depression may also become apparent in the later stages of PD (Aarsland, Andersen, Larsen, et al, 2003; Grossman, Lee, Morris, et al, 2002).

Epidemiology and Genetics

The prevalence of PD in the general population has been estimated to be between 1 and 2 cases per 1000 (Weiner & Lang, 1989). However, in the segment of the population that is 65 years or older, the prevalence of PD rises to approximately 10 in 1000 (Tanner & Goldman, 1996). Annually, 60,000 new cases of PD are diagnosed in the United States each year. The average age of onset is approximately 60 years, with approximately 10% of PD patients exhibiting symptoms before 40 years of age (young-onset PD). The cause of PD is not known, and genetic studies have been fairly inconclusive. The current consensus appears to be that PD involves a genetic susceptibility in combination with certain undetermined environmental factor(s) (Guttman, Kish, & Furukawa, 2003; Mouradian, 2002). Genetic mapping has identified several genes (*Park1* to *Park11*) that are associated with PD (Mark, 2005). Although these PD genes have very limited diagnostic value, they may lead to the development of important new drug therapies.

Neuropathology

Lesions in the part of the basal ganglia referred to as the substantia nigra, and the associated loss of the dopaminergic nigrastriatal pathways, have generally been accepted as the primary explanations for most of the motor symptoms observed in PD (Weiner & Lang, 1989). It should be noted that research emphasizes the potential importance of additional brain regions and pathways (Braak, Del Tredici, Rub, et al, 2003). Some of these newly identified regions of brain pathology, such as the dorsomotor nuclei of the glossopharyngeal and vagus nerves, may have important implications for our understanding of the progression of speech and swallowing symptoms in PD (Braak et al, 2003).

In the 1960s, the recognition of the role of the nigrostriatal dopaminergic pathways in PD led to the discovery that levodopa medication could reduce many of the major symptoms of PD (Cotzias, Papauasiliou, & Gellene, 1969). Ongoing pharmaceutical research has led to numerous refinements in levodopa therapy (i.e., carbidopa/levodopa, controlled release levodopa), and the development of several dopamine-enhancing medications (i.e., dopamine-receptor agonists, monoamine oxidase inhibitors) (see Schapira, 2005, for details). Prior to levodopa therapy, approximately 50% of patients with PD became severely disabled or died within the first 10 years after diagnosis (Weiner & Lang, 1989). Since the introduction of levodopa, the mortality rate among patients with PD has decreased to approximately that of the normal population. Furthermore, levodopa therapy has been shown to significantly delay the development of major disabilities in PD (Weiner & Lang, 1989).

◆ Speech Impairment Associated with Syndrome

The reader is referred to Chapter 11 for a detailed discussion of speech symptoms, abnormal acoustic and physiological findings, cognitive and linguistic features, and behavioral speech treatments for PD. The following sections focus on pharmacological and surgical treatments and their effect on speech in PD.

Pharmacological Treatment

During the early 1970s, when many individuals with PD were beginning to receive levodopa medication for the first time, several speech studies reported on the beneficial effects of introducing levodopa medication (see Adams, 1997, for a review). Across these early studies, levodopa medication was associated with initial improvements in intelligibility, fluency, voice quality, pitch variation, and vocal intensity. More recently, several studies have examined the effects of levodopa on the speech and voice characteristics of PD subjects who have been on continuous dopamine therapy for several years. These studies involve having PD subjects stop their medication for approximately 12 hours and then comparing their off-medication speech to their on-medication speech. In these on- versus off-levodopa studies, improvements have been noted for the following measures: vocal jitter (Sanabria, Ruiz, & Gutierrez, 2001), shimmer (Jiang, Lin, Wang, & Hanson, 1999), single word intelligibility (De Letter, Santens, & Van Borsel, 2005), and vocal tremor (Jiang et al, 1999; Sanabria et al, 2001). On the other hand, several studies have failed to show improvements on the following measures: vocal jitter and shimmer (Winkel & Adams, 1992), speech dysfluency (Goberman & Blomgren, 2003), maximum phonation time, sound pressure level, intelligibility, rate of speech (Kompoliti, Wang, Goetz, Leurgans,

& Raman, 2000), vowel formants and duration (Poluha, Teulings, & Brookshire, 1998), standard deviation of fundamental frequency, and intensity range (Goberman, Coelho, & Robb, 2002). Overall, these results suggest that dopamine-related improvements in speech are fairly small, inconsistent across studies, and highly variable across individual subjects with PD.

Interestingly, several studies also have suggested that, for patients who have had PD for more than 10 years, speech symptoms can begin to show a selective resistance to levodopa medication (Bonnet, Loria, Saint-Hilaire, 1987; Klawans, 1986). It has been suggested that the relatively inconsistent and increasingly poor response to levodopa is because speech symptoms are predominantly linked to the loss of nondopaminergic pathways in PD (Bonnet et al, 1987; Rascol, Payoux, Ory, Ferreira, Brefel-Courbon, & Montastruc, 2003; Schapira, 2005). Several other PD symptoms that are thought to be nondopaminergic include gait and balance disturbances, cognitive impairments, depression, hallucinations, pain, sleep disorders, and fatigue (Schapira, 2005). As the disease progresses, these nondopaminergic symptoms generally become the most troubling for patients and have a significant impact on quality of life (Hely, Morris, & Reid, 2005; Schapira, 2005). The finding that speech shows an inconsistent and increasingly poor response to dopamine medication underscores the potential importance of behavioral and instrumental treatments of hypokinetic dysarthria in PD.

Surgical Treatment

Surgical procedures are considered in a small proportion of patients with PD whose symptoms are poorly controlled by medications or behavioral therapies. Several neurosurgical procedures have been used in the treatment of PD. These include thalamotomy, pallidotomy, and deep brain stimulation of the globus pallidus or subthalamic nucleus. These procedures are used to treat the major nonspeech symptoms of PD. None of these procedures are used specifically to treat speech symptoms; however, changes in speech symptoms often occur. These speech changes can be both positive and negative. Thalamotomy, which involves the placement of a lesion in the region of the ventrolateral thalamus, was regularly used in the 1960s and 1970s as one of the first neurosurgical procedures for PD. Unfortunately, several studies reported significant speech impairments in patients with PD following both unilateral and bilateral thalamotomy (Bell, 1968; Jenkins, 1968; Laitinen, 1972). Pallidotomy, which involves placing a lesion in the posteroventral region of the globus pallidus interna, has had inconsistent effects on speech and nonspeech oral performance ranging from a worsening of dysarthria in some individuals and an improvement in dysarthria in others (Barlow, Iacono, Paseman, Biswas, & D'Antonio, 1998; Schultz, Peterson, Sapienza, Greer, & Friedman, 1999; Theodoros, Ward, Murdoch, Silburn, & Lethlean, 2000).

Over the past 10 years a procedure called deep brain stimulation (DBS) has been developed as an alternative to ablation procedures such as pallidotomy and thalamotomy (Pollock, Benabid, Limousin, & Benazzouz, 1997). It involves implanting a permanent pulse generator (pacemaker) that applies a continuous high-frequency stimulation (+100 Hz) to the target brain areas to block or reduce neural activity. Stimulation of the globus pallidus internus or pallidal DBS has been shown to benefit many of the limb symptoms of PD, but the effects on speech have been variable across studies and include reports of worsening (Scott, Gregory, Hines, Carroll, Hyman, & Papanasstasiou, 1998), minimal change (Bejjani, Gervais, Arnulf, Papadopoulos, & Bonnet, 2000; Gross, Rougier, Guehl, Boraud, Julien, & Bioulac, 1997), or positive changes for only a small proportion of patients (Maruska, Smit, Koller, & Garcia, 2000; Solomon, McKee, Larson, Nawrocki, Tuite, & Eriksen, 2000). More recently, subthalamic nucleus (STN) DBS has come to be preferred over pallidal DBS in many centers because it is reported to be technically simpler and allows for greater reduction in medication (Hamani, Richter, Schwalb, & Lozano, 2005). Effects of STN-DBS on speech also have been inconsistent across studies. Improvements have been noted for some speech and oral measures (Gentil, Chauvin, Pinto, Pollak & Benabid, 2001; Gentil, Garcia-Ruiz, Pollak,

& Benabid, 1999). On the other hand several studies have failed to observe improvements on many of these same measures (Farrell, Theodoros, Ward, Hall & Silburn, 2005; Dromey, Kumar, Lang, & Lozano, 2000; Wang, Verhagen Metman, Bakay, Arzbaecher, & Bernard, 2003). In general, these findings suggest that DBS effects on speech can be highly variable across facilities, measures, and patients.

In summary, Parkinson's disease is an idiopathic neurodegenerative disease caused by damage to specific basal ganglia subsystems and their associated sensorimotor processes. A variety of neurosurgical and dopamine-related drug therapies have been developed to treat the major limb symptoms of Parkinson's disease. These medical therapies have been found to have limited or inconsistent effects on speech in PD. These findings emphasize the potential importance of behavioral and instrumental treatments for hypokinetic dysarthria in PD. Fortunately, there is growing evidence that several behavioral programs, instrumental procedures, and assistive devices are relatively effective in the treatment of hypokinetic dysarthria in PD.

References

Aarsland, D., Andersen, K., Larsen, J.P., Lolk, A., & Kragh-Sorensen, P. (2003). Prevalence and characteristics of dementia in Parkinson's disease: an 8-year prospective study. *Archives of Neurology, 60,* 387–392

Adams, S.G. (1997). Hypokinetic dysarthria in Parkinson's disease. In: M.R. McNeil (Ed.), *Clinical Management of Sensorimotor Speech Disorders.* New York: Thieme

Barlow, S.M., Iacono, R.P., Paseman, L.A., Biswas, A., & D'Antonio, L. (1998). The effects of postventral pallidotomy on force and speech aerodynamics in Parkinson's disease. In: M. Cannito, K.M. Yorkston, & D. Beukelman (Eds.), *Neuromotor Speech Disorders: Nature, Assessment, and Management* (pp. 117–155). Baltimore: Brookes

Bejjani, B.P., Gervais, D., Arnulf, I., Papadopoulos, S., & Bonnet, A.M. (2000). Axial parkinsonian symptoms can be improved: the role of levodopa and bilateral subthalamic stimulation. *Journal of Neurology, Neurosurgery, and Psychiatry, 68,* 595–600

Bell, D.S. (1968). Speech functions of the thalamus inferred from effects of thalamotomy. *Brain, 91,* 619–638

Bonnet, A.M., Loria, Y., Saint-Hilaire, M.H., et al. (1987). Does long-term aggravation of Parkinson's disease result from nondopaminergic lesions? *Neurology, 37,* 1539–1542

Braak, H., Del Tredici, K., Rub, U., de Vos, R.A.I., Jansen Steur, E.N.H., & Braak, E. (2003). Staging of brain pathology related to sporadic Parkinson's disease. *Neurobiology of Aging, 24,* 197–211

Cotzias, G.C., Papauasiliou, P.S., & Gellene, R. (1969). Modification of parkinsonism—chronic treatment with l-dopa. *New England Journal of Medicine, 280,* 337–345

De Letter, M., Santens, P., & Van Borsel, J. (2005). The effects of levodopa on word intelligibility in Parkinson's disease. *Journal of Communication Disorders, 38,* 187–196

Dromey, C., Kumar, R., Lang, A.E., & Lozano, A.M. (2000). An investigation of the effects of subthalamic nucleus stimulation on acoustic measures of voice. *Movement Disorders, 15,* 1132–1138

Farrell, A., Theodoros, D., Ward, E., Hall, B., & Silburn, P. (2005). Effects of neurosurgical management of Parkinson's disease on speech characteristics and oromotor function. *Journal of Speech, Language, and Hearing Research, 48,* 5–20.

Gentil, M., Chauvin, P., Pimnto, S., Pollak, P., & Benabid, A.L. (2001). Effect of bilateral stimulation of the subthalamic nucleus on parkinsonian voice. *Brain and Language, 78,* 233–240

Gentil, M., Garcia-Ruiz, P., Pollak, P., & Benabid, A.L. (1999). Effect of stimulation of the subthalamic nucleus on oral control of patients with Parkinsonism. *Journal of Neurology, Neurosurgery, and Psychiatry, 67,* 329–333

Goberman, A., & Blomgren, M. (2003). Parkinsonian speech disfluencies: effects of L-dopa-related fluctuations. *Journal of Fluency Disorders, 28,* 55–70

Goberman, A., Coelho, C., & Robb, M. (2002). Phonatory characteristics of Parkinsonian speech before and after morning medication: the ON and OFF states. *Journal of Communication Disorders, 35,* 217–239

Gross, C., Rougier, A., Guehl, D., Boraud, T., Julien, J., & Bioulac, B. (1997). High-frequency stimulation of the globus pallidus internalis in Parkinson's disease: a study of seven cases. *Journal of Neurosurgery, 87,* 491–498

Grossman, M., Lee, C., Morris, J., Stern, M.B., & Hurtig, H.I. (2002). Assessing resource demands during sentence processing in Parkinson's disease. *Brain and Language, 80,* 603–616

Guttman, M., Kish, S.J., & Furukawa, Y. (2003). Current concepts in the diagnosis and management of Parkinson's disease. *Canadian Medical Association Journal, 168,* 293–301

Hamani, C., Richter, E., Schwalb, J.M., Lozano, A.M. (2005). Bilateral subthalamic nucleus stimulation for Parkinson's disease: a systematic review of the clinical literature. *Neurosurgery, 56,* 1313–1324

Hely, M.A., Morris, J.G., & Reid, W.G. (2005). Sydney multicenter study of Parkinson's disease: non-L-dopa-responsive problems dominate at 15 years. *Movement Disorders, 20,* 190–192

Jenkins, A. (1968). Speech following stereotaxic operations for the relief of tremor and rigidity in parkinsonism. *Medical Journal of Australia, 7,* 585–588

Jiang, J., Lin, E., Wang, J., & Hanson, D.G. (1999). Glottographic measures before and after Levodopa treatment in Parkinson's disease. *Laryngoscope, 109,* 1287–1294

Klawans, H.L. (1986). Individual manifestations of Parkinson's disease after ten or more years of levodopa. *Movement Disorders, 1,* 187–192

Kompoliti, K., Wang, Q.E., Goetz, C.G., Leurgans, S., & Raman, R. (2000). Effects of central dopaminergic stimulation by apomorphine on speech in Parkinson's disease. *American Academy of Neurology, 54,* 458–462

Laitinen, L. (1972). Surgical treatment, past and present in Parkinson's disease. *Acta Neurological Scandinavica Supplementum, 51,* 43–58

Mark, M.H. (2005). Parkinson's disease: pathogenesis, diagnosis, and treatment. *Primary Psychiatry, 12,* 36–41

Maruska, K.G., Smit, A.B., Koller, W.C., & Garcia, J.M. (2000). Sentence production in Parkinson disease treated with deep brain stimulation and medication. *Journal of Medical Speech-Language and Pathology, 8,* 265–270

Mouradian, M.M. (2002). Recent advances in the genetics and pathogenesis of Parkinson disease. *Neurology, 22,* 179–185

Parkinson, J. (1817). *An Essay on the Shaking Palsy.* London: Sherwood, Neely, and Jones

Pollock, P., Benabid, A.L., Limousin, P., & Benazzouz, A. (1997). Chronic intracerebral stimulation in Parkinson's disease. *Advances in Neurology, 74,* 213–220

Poluha, P.C., Teulings, H.L., & Brookshire, R.H. (1998). Handwriting and speech changes across the levodopa cycle in Parkinson's disease. *Acta Psychologica (Amsterdam), 100,* 71–84

Rascol, O., Payoux, P., Ory, F., Ferreira, J.J., Brefel-Courbon, C., Montastruc, J.L. (2003). Limitations of current Parkinson's disease therapy. *Annals of Neurology, 53,* S3–S15

Sanabria, J., Ruiz, P.G., Gutierrez, R., et al. (2001). The effect of Levodopa on vocal function in Parkinson's disease. *Clinical Neuropharmacology, 24,* 99–102

Schapira, A.H.V. (2005). Present and future drug treatment for Parkinson's disease. *Journal of Neurology, Neurosurgery, and Psychiatry, 76,* 1472–1478

Schultz, G.M., Peterson, T., Sapienza, C.M., Greer, M., & Friedman, W. (1999). Voice and speech characteristics of persons with Parkinson's disease pre- and post-pallidotomy surgery: preliminary findings. *Journal of Speech, Language, and Hearing Research, 42,* 1176–1194

Scott, R., Gregory, R., Hines, N., Carroll, C., Hyman, N., & Papanasstasiou, V. (1998). Neuropsychological, neurological and functional outcome following pallidotomy for Parkinson's disease. *Brain, 121,* 656–675

Solomon, N.P., McKee, A.S., Larson, K.J., Nawrocki, M.D., Tuite, P.J., & Eriksen, S. (2000). Effects of pallidal stimulation on speech in 3 men with severe Parkinson's disease. *American Journal of Speech and Language Pathology, 9,* 241–256

Tanner, C.M., & Goldman, S.M. (1996). Epidemiology of Parkinson's disease. *Neurology Clinics, 14,* 317–335

Theodoros, D.G., Ward, E.C., Murdoch, B.E., Silburn, P., & Lethlean, J. (2000). The impact of pallidotomy on motor speech function in Parkinson disease. *Journal of Medical Speech-Language and Pathology, 8,* 315–322

Wang, E., Verhagen Metman, L., Bakay, R., Arzbaecher, J., & Bernard, B. (2003). The effect of unilateral electrostimulation of the subthalamic nucleus on respiratory/phonatory subsystems of speech production in Parkinson's disease—a preliminary report. *Clinical Linguistics and Phonetics, 17,* 283–289

Weiner, W.J., & Lang, A.E. (1989). *Movement Disorders: A Comprehensive Survey.* Mount Kisko, NY: Futura

Winckel, J., & Adams, S.G. (1992). Drug-cycle related voice changes in parkinsonian patients. Journal of the American Speech and Hearing Association, 34, 158

Additional Reading

Ackermann, H., Ziegler, W., & Oertel, W.H. (1989). Palilalia as a symptom of levodopa induced hyperkinesia in Parkinson's disease. *Journal of Neurology, Neurosurgery, and Psychiatry, 52,* 805–807

Gamboa, J., Jimenez-Jimenez, F.J., Nieto, A., Montojo, J., Orti-Pareja, M., Molina, J.A., Garcia-Albea, E., & Cobeta, I. (1997). Acoustic voice analysis in patients with Parkinson's disease treated with dopaminergic drugs. *Journal of the Voice, 11,* 314–320

Gentil, M., Pinto, S., Pollak, P., & Benabid, A.L. (2003). Effect of bilateral stimulation of the subthalamic nucleus on Parkinsonian dysarthria. *Brain and Language, 85,* 190–196

Chapter 48

Pick's Disease

Richard I. Zraick

◆ General Information on Disorder

Pick's disease, first described in a seminal case study, "On the Relationship Between Aphasia and Senile Atrophy of the Brain" (Pick, 1892), is a slowly progressive atrophic disease of the frontal and temporal lobes that results in dementia. Over the past century the concept of Pick's disease has been expanded, with the disease now considered by some to be part of a complex of neurodegenerative disorders with similar or related histopathological and clinical features (McKhann, Albert, & Grossman, 2001). Most commonly these disorders are classified under the umbrella term *frontotemporal lobar degeneration* (Kertesz, 2003).

Diagnostic Signs and Symptoms

In contrast to Alzheimer's disease, in which early memory loss predominates, the first symptoms of Pick's disease are often personality changes and a decline in function at work and home. Personality changes may take the form of apathy and indifference toward customary interests, or of disregard for social decorum and for the feelings of others. Poor social judgment, inappropriate sexual advances, or a coarse and jocular demeanor may be seen. Function declines because the patient simply does very little, or displays confusion and poor judgment. Often the patient performs well when directed to do something, but cannot undertake the very same thing independently. What is lost is the ability to initiate, organize, and follow through on even very simple plans and familiar activities.

As the illness advances, difficulties with language become common. Patients become unusually quiet, and when they do speak it may be slowly and in brief sentences. They may labor to articulate and their speech may sound distorted. Some patients become extremely apathetic; they may sit for hours doing nothing at all unless prompted to do something. Other patients become extraordinarily restless and may pace unceasingly. Some patients are hypersexual, and some, like a small child, may place anything they pick up in their mouths. Gluttonous eating occurs in some cases. Attention span is poor and patients seem to be distracted instantly by anything that they hear or see. Later in the disease, patients usually become mute. Restlessness gives way to profound apathy, and the patient may not respond at all to the surrounding world. Eventually, they enter a terminal vegetative state.

Neuropathology

Histopathologically, there is extensive neuronal loss concentrated in the outer third of the cerebral cortex. *Pick bodies*, abnormal cytoplasmic inclusions, are seen in the cortex. In addition to Pick bodies, the cortex may contain *Pick cells*, "ballooned" cytoplasm that represents deafferented neurons. Computed tomography (CT) and magnetic resonance imaging (MRI) are useful in identifying shrinkage of cortex and low density of the white matter in the involved lobes. Brain single photon emission computed tomography (SPECT) imaging shows greatly decreased or absent perfusion to the affected lobes. Gross pathological changes are so severe that the diagnosis can easily be made by visual inspection. There is a sharp line of demarcation between the affected portions and the remaining brain. It is rare to see unilateral involvement.

Epidemiology

Of individuals with dementia, 10 to 15% exhibit clinical characteristics suggestive of Pick's disease. It is the third most common neurodegenerative cortical dementia after Alzheimer's disease (AD) and diffuse Lewy body disease and the fourth most common if vascular dementia is included (Neary, Snowden, & Gustafson, 1998). Pick's disease occurs in a younger age group than dementia of the Alzheimer's type: peak incidence occurs in individuals aged 55 to 65 years, and more men than women may be affected (Ratnavalli, Brayne, Dawson, & Hodges, 2002).

Genetics

Mutations in the *tau* gene, which codes for tau, a protein that is associated with microtubules, can be found in Pick's disease. This mutation can be sporadic, familial, or hereditary, but in the majority of the cases it develops by chance rather than being inherited. Approximately 20 to 50% of patients have a positive family history for Pick's disease or a related neurodegenerative condition, and 5 to 10% of patients have a family history that suggests a hereditary condition with an autosomal dominant pattern of inheritance (Raux et al, 2000).

◆ Speech Impairment Associated with Disorder

As noted by Duffy (2005), some primary dementing illnesses can be associated with parkinsonian signs. As such, hypokinesia may result, the effects of which can be perceived during speech, seen during speech and oral mechanism examination, measured physiologically, and inferred from acoustic measurements. As reported by Darley, Aronson, and Brown (1969), the eight most prominent auditory-perceptual features of hypokinetic dysarthria were monopitch, reduced stress, monoloudness, imprecise consonants, inappropriate silences, short rushes of speech, harsh voice quality, and breathy voice. Collectively these features reflect prosodic insufficiency (see Chapter 11).

In addition to hypokinetic dysarthria, patients with Pick's disease and other dementing illnesses may also exhibit *echolalia* (unsolicited repetition of another's utterances) (Shimomura & Mori, 1998). As described by Duffy (2005), repetition may be complete (i.e., automatic, effortless, compulsive, and parrot-like in quality) without comprehension of meaning, or partial (i.e., less automatic and more incomplete) with the repetition perhaps serving as an aid to comprehension.

Etiology and Neuropathology

Although not usually associated with motor or sensory deficits, Pick's disease can be associated with parkinsonian signs (Kertesz, 2003). As such, the dysarthria resulting from Pick's disease can be characterized as a type of hypokinetic dysarthria, a label that suggests a primary underlying etiology of hypokinesia.

Associated Cognitive, Linguistic, and Communicative Signs and Symptoms

Less is known about the cognitive and linguistic signs and symptoms associated with frontotemporal dementia than that of dementia of the Alzheimer's type, and even less is known about these signs and symptoms specifically in Pick's disease. The terms *primary nonfluent progressive aphasia* and *semantic dementia* are often used to characterize

the cognitive-language deficits in such patients (McKhann et al, 2001). Perseveration (cognitive and motor) may be noted, and patients may have relatively preserved visuospatial and visual orientation skills.

Special Diagnostic Considerations

The increasing awareness of Alzheimer's disease, both to clinicians and laypersons, poses a challenge to the accurate diagnosis of Pick's disease because of the risk of assigning a diagnosis of AD to any older person presenting with cognitive impairment. Because there are many potential non-AD causes of dementia, the assessment of a patient suspected of having Pick's disease should be conducted by an experienced multidisciplinary team. Another challenge to accurate diagnosis is the sometimes confusing nomenclature associated with the diseases of frontotemporal degeneration. Although the histological changes with each disease are fairly well described, their clinical correlation with patient behavior is less well understood. Recent diagnostic advances include the development of comprehensive caregiver-based neuropsychiatric instruments, neurological tasks sensitive to semantic memory and other key cognitive impairments, and functional and structural brain imaging techniques.

Treatment

Unfortunately, no available drugs arrest or reverse Pick's disease. Currently, clinicians use a combination of neuroprotective and symptomatic therapies. These may include nonsteroidal antiinflammatory drugs, vitamins, antidepressants, cholinergic agents, hormones, and dopaminergic agents. Nondrug therapies may also improve behavior and mood problems and relieve other symptoms. For example, a speech-language pathologist may be able to help patients improve their ability to communicate. The usual support services for caregivers of persons with other types of dementia may also be of benefit to those caring for the person with Pick's disease.

References

Darley, F.L., Aronson, A., & Brown, J. (1969). Clusters of deviant speech dimensions in the dysarthrias. *Journal of Speech and Hearing Research, 12,* 462–496

Duffy, J.R. (2005). *Motor Speech Disorders—Substrates, Differential Diagnosis, and Management,* 2nd ed. (pp. 353–379). St. Louis: Elsevier Mosby.

Kertesz, A. (2003). Pick Complex: an integrative approach to frontotemporal dementia: primary progressive aphasia, corticobasal degeneration, and progressive supranuclear palsy. *Neurologist, 9,* 311–317

McKhann, G.M., Albert, M.S., Grossman, M., et al. (2001). Clinical and pathological diagnosis of frontotemporal dementia: report of the work group on frontotemporal dementia and Pick's disease. *Archives of Neurology, 58,* 1803–1809

Neary D., Snowden, J.S., & Gustafson, L. (1998). Frontotemporal lobar degeneration: q consensus on clinical diagnostic criteria. *Neurology, 51,* 1546–1554

Pick, A. (1892). Ueber die beziehungen der senilen hirnatrophie zur aphasie pragmatische [On the relationship between aphasia and senile atrophy of the brain]. *Medizinsche Wehnschrift, 17,* 165–167

Ratnavalli, E., Brayne, C., Dawson, K., & Hodges, J.R. (2002). The prevalence of frontotemporal dementia. *Neurology, 58,* 1615–1621

Raux, G., Gantier, R., Thomas-Anterion, C., et al. (2000). Dementia with prominent frontotemporal features associated with L113P presenilin 1 mutation. *Neurology, 55,* 1577–1578

Shimomura, T. & Mori, E. (1998). Obstinate imitation behavior in differentiation of frontotemporal dementia from Alzheimer's disease. *Lancet, 352,* 623–624

Additional Reading

Pick's disease. http://www.emedicine.com/NEURO/topic311.htm#section~bibliography

Pick's disease. http://www.emedicinehealth.com/articles/39623–1.asp

Chapter 49

Postpolio Syndrome

Shannon Cook Mauszycki and Julie L. Wambaugh

◆ General Information on Disorder

Postpolio syndrome (PPS) is a slowly progressive motor neuron disorder, characterized by a collection of symptoms that develop in individuals who had contracted poliomyelitis many years earlier (Halstead, 1998; Nollet & de Visser, 2004). Polio is a viral disease that involved epidemics in the first half of the 20th century in the United States and other parts of the world prior to the development of the polio vaccine in 1955. Polio is a communicable disease transmitted through contaminated food or water. In more than 95% of cases, polio involved an infection with no symptoms or influenza-like symptoms with rapid and complete recovery in a matter of days (Saxon, 2001). In 1% of cases, the effects of the virus were paralytic (Saxon, 2001). In such cases, the virus crossed into the central nervous system, attacking the motor neurons of the spinal cord or brainstem, causing muscle weakness or paralysis (Halstead, 1998; Saxon, 2001). The trunk and extremities were commonly affected, and when the brainstem was implicated, paralysis or weakness also occurred in the musculature for respiration, swallowing, and speech. Eighty percent of paralytic polio survivors regained muscle strength and function within 6 months (Saxon, 2001).

In the late 1970s, numerous individuals who had suffered an acute paralytic episode of polio many years earlier reported experiencing a cluster of symptoms, which was eventually termed PPS (Halstead, 1998). The average onset of PPS has been 35 years after the acute episode, with a range of 8 to 71 years (Jubelt & Agre, 2000). The development of PPS has been associated with age of acute attack, with a higher incidence in those who acquired the virus as an adult or adolescent (Jubelt & Agre, 2000). Although individuals who experienced paralysis as a result of polio may be at greatest risk for development of PPS, individuals who had negligible effects of polio may also develop PPS (Halstead, 1998; Saxon, 2001). The onset of symptoms of PPS tends to be gradual and progresses slowly with an estimated 1 to 2% loss of muscle strength per year (Jubelt & Agre, 2000).

Diagnostic Signs and Symptoms

Clinical features of PPS include debilitating fatigue, muscle and joint pain, and new muscle weakness. Weakness typically occurs in previously affected muscles involved in acute poliomyelitis, but can also occur in unaffected muscles (Jubelt & Agre, 2000). Other signs and symptoms of PPS include muscle atrophy, respiratory problems, speech problems, swallowing difficulty, and cold intolerance (Jubelt & Agre, 2000; Silver & Aiello, 2002).

The diagnosis of PPS is based on the following diagnostic criteria: (1) a prior episode of poliomyelitis with residual motor loss confirmed by history, neurological examination, or electromyography; (2) a period of neurologic recovery and functional stability typically greater than 15 years; (3) gradual or rarely, abrupt onset of new weakness or abnormal muscle fatigue, muscle atrophy, or generalized fatigue; (4) exclusion of other conditions that may be responsible for the above-listed symptoms (Jubelt & Agre, 2000; Silver & Aiello, 2002).

There are no definitive diagnostic tools for PPS. Many diagnostic tests often reveal the same abnormalities in polio survivors with or without PPS. However, diagnostic tests are useful for identifying and excluding other disease or conditions (Jubelt & Agre, 2000).

Neuropathology

Microscopically, there is a slow degeneration of the terminal axon sprouts that innervate muscle fibers responsible for muscle contraction (Halstead, 1998). The cause of the degeneration remains unknown. The most widely accepted hypothesis proposes that after several years, the motor neurons that survived the initial polio episode are enlarged due to excessive sprouting compensating for lost motor neurons. The remaining motor neurons must work harder to perform activities of daily living (Jubelt & Agre, 2000). Eventually, these overused motor neurons become metabolically exhausted, resulting in muscle denervation (Nollet & de Visser, 2004). The consequence of muscle denervation is the loss or reduction of muscle contraction resulting in weakness or paralysis. Hypotonia, reduced reflexes, and atrophy may be seen in the affected muscles, and fasciculation and fibrillations may or may not be present (Duffy, 1995).

Epidemiology

As of the end of 2003, poliomyelitis had been eradicated from all but six countries in the world (World Health Organization, 2003). Although polio no longer represents a significant health care challenge, the sequelae of polio may impact millions of survivors worldwide (Farbu, Rekand, & Gilhus, 2003). A 1987 survey by the National Center for Health Statistics indicated that there were more than 1.6 million polio survivors in the United States (641,000 of those were diagnosed with paralytic polio) (Jubelt & Agre, 2000). Studies have indicated that the prevalence of PPS may range from 29 to 64% (Halstead, 1998).

Genetics

There is no genetic component to polio or PPS.

◆ Speech Impairment Associated with Disorder

PPS involves degeneration of the terminal axonal sprouts in the lower motor neuron system, resulting in flaccid dysarthria when speech production is affected. Speech characteristics of flaccid dysarthria can impact all speech subsystems due to diffuse bulbar damage or may be limited to one subsystem with focal damage to cranial or spinal nerves resulting in unilateral or bilateral weakness. Respiration, laryngeal function, and resonance are commonly affected because of the predilection in the initial attack for cranial nerves IX and X (Duffy, 1995). Speech production deficits may progress or evolve over time due to the slowly progressive nature of PPS (Jubelt & Agre, 2000). Disturbances in speech production, however, are not common in PPS. For example, in a survey of a cohort of 551 polio survivors, Ramlow, Alexander, LaPorte, Kaufmann, and Kuller (1992) reported that "voice changes" were noted by 2.6% and 7.4% of nonparalytic and paralytic respondents, respectively. Because of the apparently low prevalence of speech disruptions in PPS, there is limited description of speech signs or symptoms in the literature. Deviant speech characteristics that have been reported include hypernasality, aphonia, hoarseness, reduced pitch range, decreased voice intensity, and poor breath support for speech (Abaza, Hawkshaw, Mandel, & Sataloff, 2001; Driscoll et al, 1995; Robinson, Hillel, & Waugh, 1998).

Diagnostic Signs and Symptoms

There are no specific speech signs or symptoms that define PPS.

Etiology

Speech disturbances in PPS result from degeneration of axonal sprouts in the lower motor neuron system. Specifically, cranial or spinal nerve involvement is implicated.

Neuropathology

Speech disorders in PPS are associated primarily with neuropathology of the bulbar nerves, with cranial nerves IX and X being most often affected (Duffy, 1995). These changes result in diminished motor control, with reductions in muscle strength and tone as well as fatigue.

Associated Cognitive, Linguistic, and Communicative Signs and Symptoms

A common complaint of individuals with PPS is mental fatigue, including difficulty with attention and memory (Hazendonk & Crowe, 2000). However, deficits in cognitive functioning have not been clearly identified and reported problems may be associated with the physical or psychological aspects of the disease (Hazendonk & Crowe, 2000).

Special Diagnostic Considerations

Due to the infrequency of speech disturbances and the varying site and severity of the neuropathology among people with PPS it is unlikely that differential diagnosis of PPS would be based solely on speech signs or symptoms. Frequently, individuals with speech disturbances were found to have laryngeal abnormalities or pathologies and many also had complaints of dysphagia or dyspnea (Abaza et al, 2001; Driscoll et al, 1995; Robinson et al, 1998). These disorders may require instrumental evaluation to specify muscle involvement and degree of weakness as part of the process of selecting the appropriate treatment approach or medical intervention. The progressive nature of the disorder necessitates ongoing assessment to make modifications in treatment, medical management, or compensatory strategies.

Treatment

There are no specific treatment approaches for speech disorders associated with PPS. Treatment should be dependent on assessment findings and should be consistent with approaches utilized with flaccid dysarthria. The clinician should consider the fatigue and weakness that accompanies PPS. Research findings involving physical exercise in this population has revealed that nonfatiguing exercise, including strengthening, may have beneficial effects in terms of improvement in muscle strength (Chan, Amirjani, Sumrain, Clarke, & Strohschein, 2003). Exercise is recommended every other day to avoid fatigue and allow for recovery (Jubelt & Agre, 2000). Energy conservation strategies were also found to be advantageous (Jubelt & Agre, 2000). These treatment principles could be incorporated into speech therapy to maximize treatment effectiveness and to avoid detrimental treatment effects.

Dysphagia is more prevalent than speech disturbances in PPS (Halstead & Grimby, 1995). This population may require further evaluation and treatment for swallowing problems.

References

Abaza, M.M., Hawkshaw, M.J., Mandel, S., & Sataloff, R.T. (2001). Laryngeal manifestations of postpoliomyelitis syndrome. *Journal of Voice, 15,* 291–294

Chan, K.M., Amirjani, N., Sumrain, M., Clarke, A., & Strohschein, F.J. (2003). Randomized controlled trial of strength training in post-polio patients. *Muscle & Nerve, 27,* 332–338

Driscoll, B.P., Gracco, C., Coelho, C., Goldstein, J., Oshima, K., Tierney, E., & Sasaki, C.T. (1995). Laryngeal function in postpolio patients. *Laryngoscope, 105*, 35–41

Duffy, J.R. (1995). *Motor Speech Disorders*. St. Louis: Mosby-Yearbook

Farbu, E., Rekand, T., & Gilhus, N.E. (2003). Post-polio syndrome and total health status in a prospective hospital study. *European Journal of Neurology, 10*, 407–413

Halstead, L.S. (1998). Post-polio syndrome. *Scientific American, 278*, 42–47

Halstead, L.S., & Grimby, G. (1995). *Post-polio syndrome*. Philadelphia: Hanley & Belfus

Hazendonk, K.M. & Crowe, S.F. (2000). A neuropsychological study of the postpolio syndrome. *Neuropsychiatry, Neuropsychology, and Behavioral Neurology, 13*, 112–118

Jubelt, B. & Agre, J.C. (2000). Characteristics and management of postpolio syndrome. *Journal of the American Medical Association, 284*, 412–414

Nollet, F. & de Visser, M. (2004). Postpolio syndrome. *Archives of Neurology, 61*, 1142–1144

Ramlow, J., Alexander, M., LaPorte, R., Kaufmann, C., & Kuller, L. (1992). Epidemiology of the post-polio syndrome. *American Journal of Epidemiology, 136*, 769–786

Robinson, L.R., Hillel, A.D., & Waugh, P. (1998). New laryngeal muscle weakness in post-polio syndrome. *Laryngoscope, 108*, 732–734

Saxon, D.F. (2001). Another look at polio & postpolio syndrome. *Orthopaedic Nursing, 20*, 17–26

Silver, J.K., & Aiello, D. D. (2002). What internists need to know about postpolio syndrome. *Cleveland Clinic Journal of Medicine, 69*, 704–712

World Health Organization. (2003). *Global Polio Eradication Initiative Strategic Plan*. Geneva, Switzerland: WHO Library Cataloguing-in-Publication Data

Additional Reading

Hollingsworth, L., Didelot, M.J., & Levington, C. (2002). Post-polio syndrome: psychological adjustment to disability. *Issues in Mental Health Nursing, 23*, 135–156

Chapter 50

Primary Lateral Sclerosis

Shannon N. Austermann Hula and Nayan P. Desai

◆ General Information on Disorder

Primary lateral sclerosis (PLS) is a neurodegenerative disorder involving the upper motor neuron (UMN) system (Pringle, Hudson, Munoz, Kiernan, Brown, & Ebers, 1992; Stark & Moersch, 1945; Younger, Chou, & Hays, 1988). There is gradually progressive irreversible loss of UMNs, leading to increasing motor deficits. It is clinically characterized by weakness and stiffness, balance problems, and dysarthria. This disorder is a subtype of motor neuron disease in which there is typically no clinical or electrophysiological evidence of lower motor neuron (LMN) involvement, and thus is different from amyotrophic lateral sclerosis (ALS), although the exact nosology has been disputed (see LeForestier, Maisonobe, Piquard, et al, 2001a). The prognosis for life is much better for PLS compared with ALS. PLS is sporadic, although an autosomal recessive childhood-onset form has been described (Gascon, Chavis, Yaghmour, et al, 1995). It typically occurs in adults in the age range of 35 to 65 (median 51 years) and usually progresses very gradually over 15 to 20 years, with increasing disability.

Symptoms typically begin in the legs, but may start in the hands or tongue. Weakness and stiffness lead to difficulty walking or clumsiness. Ocular muscles are typically spared, but spastic dysarthria and dysphagia commonly develop. Motor examination is notable for spasticity and weakness, mainly of the shoulder abductors, hip flexors, ankle dorsiflexors, and elbow, wrist, finger, and knee extensors. Sensory examination is normal if there are no other comorbidities such as diabetes. Muscle stretch reflexes are hyperactive, and there may be spontaneous clonus. Bilateral Babinski signs and abnormal oral reflexes are present. Coordination is typically normal, with no truncal or appendicular ataxia. Gait is slow and stiff, with scissoring noted in advanced spasticity. A small proportion of patients, if followed for 10 to 15 years, may reveal clinical evidence of LMN involvement (atrophy, muscle fasciculations), changing the diagnosis to ALS.

Epidemiology

Primary lateral sclerosis is rare, and exact incidence and prevalence are unknown. Estimated incidence is 1 per 10 million and prevalence is 2 per million (Armon, 2003).

Diagnostic Signs and Symptoms

PLS is a diagnosis of exclusion, and the differential diagnosis includes cervical spondylotic myelopathy, ALS, hereditary spastic paraparesis, subacute combined degeneration of the spinal cord, primary progressive multiple sclerosis, and the recently described neuronal intermediate filament inclusion disease (NIFID) (Cairns, Grossman, Arnold, et al, 2004). Laboratory testing includes magnetic resonance imaging (MRI) of the brain and spinal cord to exclude intrinsic lesions and extrinsic cervical cord compression by osteoarthritic changes of the spine. An electromyogram (EMG) helps in excluding electrophysiological evidence of progressive LMN degeneration; however, minor nonprogressive EMG abnormalities (fibrillation potentials in distal muscles) may be noted in PLS. Motor evoked potentials are delayed or absent in PLS.

Pathogenesis

The triggers and mechanisms of motor neuron cell death in PLS are unknown. It is unclear if some of the hypotheses that apply to ALS (glutamate excitotoxicity, mitochondrial dysfunction, calcium-mediated toxicity or a combination of all these) can be applied to PLS.

Neuropathology

Autopsy findings reveal motor neuron cell degeneration of the upper motor neurons. Loss of Betz cells has been noted in the precentral gyrus.

Genetics

There is no genetic component to adult-onset PLS. An autosomal recessive, childhood-onset form has been described.

◆ Speech Impairment Associated with Disorder

Spastic dysarthria of gradually increasing severity, often accompanied by dysphagia, is commonly observed in PLS. Slurred speech or difficulty swallowing may be the first presenting complaint of the motor neuron disease (Kuipers-Upmeijer, deJager, Hew, et al, 2001; Pringle et al, 1992; Swash, Desai, & Misra, 1999), or may develop following many years of progressing limb involvement. One case report (Pringle et al) describes a patient who did not develop symptoms of dysarthria until more than a decade after initial limb symptoms presented. Slow and monotone speech, often accompanied by strained vocal quality, is the most salient feature of the spastic dysarthria observed in PLS (LeForestier et al, 2001a). Progression to profound dysarthria may render individuals unintelligible or anarthric after several years (Pringle et al, 1992).

Diagnostic Signs and Symptoms

Although specific diagnostic signs and symptoms of the motor speech impairment in PLS have not been established per se, the isolated corticobulbospinal neuropathology in this disorder indicates that the resultant dysarthria type is spastic. Clinical findings described in case reports (Kuipers-Upmeijer et al, 2001; LeForestier, Masinobe, Piquard, et al, 2001a; Le Forestier, Maisonobe, Spelle, et al, 2001b; Pringle et al, 1992; Swash et al, 1999), including positive signs of spasticity and hyperreflexia in the absence of sensory and LMN involvement, are consistent with this classification. Pathological oral reflexes documented in PLS include pout and palmomental reflexes, masseter hyperreflexia, and abnormally brisk gag reflex. Other abnormalities affecting speech musculature include reduced amplitude and speed of lingual and buccolingual movements, slow lip and palatal movements, and labial, laryngeal, and mandibular stiffness. Dysphonia characterized by strained and hypernasal voice has also been observed in PLS. The severity of the spastic dysarthria gradually worsens over time with progression of the disease. The presence of dysphagia has been reported in between 11 and 78% of PLS cases.

Etiology

The etiology of the pseudobulbar syndrome observed in PLS is the progressive symmetric spinobulbar spasticity resulting from motor cortex degeneration (Pringle et al, 1992).

Neuropathology

Pathological changes in the cerebral cortex producing spasticity and movement abnormalities in PLS include selective loss of Betz cells and degeneration of precentral pyramidal neurons. Lower motor neurons are spared.

Associated Cognitive, Linguistic, and Communicative Signs and Symptoms

Although most case reports cite intact mental status (Pringle et al, 1992; Swash et al, 1999), mild subclinical frontal lobe-related cognitive deficits have been documented in many patients with PLS upon administration of sensitive neuropsychological tests (Caselli, Smith, & Osborne, 1995). Frank dementia is not associated with the disease.

Pseudobulbar affect, although not as prevalent as in ALS, is a relatively prominent feature in PLS (LeForestier et al, 2001a; Pringle et al, 1992), and can impact speech intelligibility, communicative effectiveness, and ability to participate in therapy (Duffy, 1995).

Special Diagnostic Considerations

Primary lateral sclerosis is a rare disease with controversial nosology, and careful assessment of oral-motor symptomatology may be important for distinguishing it from other varieties of motor neuron disease. For example, patients with heredity spastic paraparesis typically do not exhibit a significant degree of oral-motor involvement, whereas patients with PLS do tend to develop dysarthria and dysphagia (Pascuzzi, 2002). Furthermore, the clinical discrimination between the spastic dysarthria in PLS and the mixed spastic-flaccid dysarthria observed in ALS may facilitate differential diagnosis of these two motor neuron diseases and serve as an important prognostic indicator of life span (Duffy, 1995).

Treatment

There is no medication that can prevent or reverse the continued loss of motor neurons. Riluzole is the only Food and Drug Administration (FDA)-approved medication that may slow down the rate of motor neuron death in ALS. The efficacy of riluzole in PLS is unknown, but it has been empirically used. The drug is expensive (around $10,000 per year), and requires periodic monitoring of liver function tests and complete blood counts. Symptomatic treatment in PLS includes amitriptyline for control of pseudobulbar features and baclofen, tizanidine, and benzodiazepines for the management of spasticity. Intrathecal baclofen pumps are used for severe spasticity. Ongoing speech, physical, and occupational therapy and a supportive relationship with a multidisciplinary clinic team can be very helpful to provide a better quality of life for affected individuals.

Although speech treatment specific to PLS has not been addressed in the literature, it may be hypothesized that general treatment principles employed with spastic dysarthria may be effectively applied to this disorder, particularly in cases of mild severity or slow progression. However, because PLS is a progressively degenerative disease frequently associated with development of profound dysarthria, application of alternative and augmentative communication (AAC) techniques should be an early consideration in the planning of communication intervention. Patient and caregiver counseling emphasizing communication-oriented strategies to maximize efficiency and intelligibility of messages should also be an important component of treatment.

References

Armon, C. (2003). Primary lateral sclerosis. In: e-medicine.com:www.emedicine.com/Neuro/topic324.htm

Cairns, N.J., Grossman, M., Arnold, S.E., et al. (2004). Clinical and neuropathologic variation in neuronal intermediate filament inclusion disease. *Neurology, 63*, 1376–1384

Caselli, R.J., Smith B.E., & Osborne, D. (1995). Primary lateral sclerosis: a neuropsychological study. *Neurology, 45*, 2005–2009

Gascon, G.G., Chavis, P., Yaghmour, A., et al (1995). Familial childhood primary lateral sclerosis with associated gaze paresis. *Neuropediatrics, 26*, 313–319

Kuipers-Upmeijer, J., deJager, A.E.J., Hew, J.M., Snoek, J.W., & van Weerden, T.W. (2001). Primary lateral sclerosis: clinical, neurophysiological, and magnetic resonance findings. *J Neurol Neurosurg Psychiatry, 71,* 615–620

Le Forestier, N., Maisonobe, T., Piquard, A., et al. (2001a). Does primary lateral sclerosis exist? A study of 20 patients and a review of the literature. *Brain, 124,* 1989–1999

Le Forestier, N., Maisonobe, T., Spelle, L., et al. (2001b). Primary lateral sclerosis: Further clarification. *Journal of the Neurological Sciences, 185,* 95–100

Pascuzzi, R.M. (2002). ALS, motor neuron disease, and related disorders: a personal approach to diagnosis and management. *Seminars in Neurology, 22,* 75–88

Pringle, C.E., Hudson, A.J., Munoz, D.G., Kiernan, J.A., Brown, W.F., & Ebers, G.C. (1992). Primary lateral sclerosis: clinical features, neuropathology and diagnostic criteria. *Brain, 115,* 495–520

Stark, F.M. & Moersch, F.P. (1945). Primary lateral sclerosis: a distinct clinical entity. *Journal of Nervous and Mental Disease, 102,* 332–337

Swash, M., Desai, J., & Misra, V.P. (1999). What is primary lateral sclerosis? *Journal of the Neurological Sciences, 170,* 5–10

Younger, D.S., Chou, S. & Hays, A.P. (1988). Primary lateral sclerosis: a clinical diagnosis reemerges. *Archives of Neurology, 45,* 1304–1307

Chapter 51

Progressive Apraxia of Speech

Harrison N. Jones

◆ General Information on Disorder

Apraxia of speech (AOS) has been defined by McNeil, Robin, and Schmidt (1997) as a phonetic-motoric disorder of speech production caused by inefficiencies in the translation of a well-formed and filled phonological frame to previously learned kinematic parameters assembled for carrying out the intended movements, resulting in intra- and interarticulator temporal and spatial segmental and prosodic distortions.

Typical etiologies for AOS include stroke, tumor, and trauma (Duffy, 1995). Progressive apraxia of speech (PAOS) is a neurodegenerative disorder with the primary symptom of a slowly progressive AOS of insidious onset and prolonged course. Cognitive and language function may initially remain intact (McNeil & Duffy, 2001). In contrast to AOS, PAOS is not related to a specific lesion in the central nervous system but rather a focal degenerative process likely localized in the anterior portion of the left cerebral hemisphere. Some authors have reported that AOS may be the only sign of a neurodegenerative process (McNeil et al, 1997) and have suggested the terminology primary progressive apraxia of speech (McNeil et al, 1997; Duffy, 1995; McNeil & Duffy, 2001; Rosenbek, 2004). Other terms that may be synonymous with PAOS that have appeared internationally include slowly progressive anarthria (Fukui, Sugita, Kawamura, Shiota, & Nakano, 1996), primary progressive anarthria (Broussolle et al, 1996), and pure progressive aphemia (Silveri, Cappa, & Salvigni, 2003). Onset of PAOS is usually reported to occur in the sixth decade of life (Broussolle et al, 1996; Cohen, Benoit, Van Beckhout, Ducarne, & Brunet, 1993; Didic, Ceccaldi, & Poncet, 1998; Fukui et al, 1996; Silveri et al, 2003), although it has been described in patients from 48 (Cohen et al, 1993) to 81 (Silveri et al, 2003) years of age. Over time, more pervasive behavioral and cognitive-linguistic decline consistent with more widespread frontal lobe damage has been reported.

Diagnostic Signs and Symptoms

A slowly progressive AOS is the presenting symptom of neurological disease in patients with PAOS. PAOS may often be accompanied by dysarthria (Broussolle et al, 1996; Chapman, Rosenberg, Weiner & Shobe, 1997; Cohen et al, 1993), orofacial apraxia (Broussolle et al, 1996; Chapman et al, 1997; Cohen et al, 1993; Didic et al, 1998; Fukui et al, 1996; Silveri et al, 2003), and limb apraxia (Cohen et al,

1993; Didic et al, 1998). Impairments in speech production gradually become more severe with disease progression (Broussolle et al, 1996; Chapman et al, 1997; Cohen et al, 1993; Didic et al, 1998; Fukui et al, 1996; Silveri et al, 2003), including the development of mutism (Didic et al, 1998; Fukui et al, 1996; Rosenbek, 2004; Silveri et al, 2003). A variety of other neuropsychological symptoms may also develop. Frontal lobe cognitive deficits have often been reported to occur approximately 5 years after onset, including "major slowness, difficulties in elaboration strategies, distractibility, and frequent perseverative errors" (Broussolle et al, 1996, p.53). Widespread cognitive decline with impaired response inhibition has also been reported in this population by other researchers (Didic et al, 1998). Additionally, neurological signs have been discovered after 5 years or longer of illness, including pyramidal signs "usually restricted to brisk deep tendon and jaw reflexes" (Broussolle et al, 1996, p. 53). Late progression of the disease may be associated with dementia and changes in personality (Fukui et al, 1996). However, some patients with PAOS have been reported to have isolated speech difficulties without cognitive-linguistic decline 6 years after onset (Chapman et al, 1997).

In the early stage of PAOS, cerebral metabolism studies (single photon emission computed tomography [SPECT] or positron emission tomography [PET]) have shown decreased cerebral blood flow in the left frontal lobe, even in the absence of abnormality on brain imaging studies (computed tomography [CT] or magnetic resonance imaging [MRI]) (Broussolle et al, 1996; Chapman et al, 1997; Cohen et al, 1993; Didic et al, 1998). With disease progression, CT or MRI often reveals cortical atrophy, particularly in the left frontal cortex, as well as the left parietal and temporal lobes (Broussolle et al, 1996; Chapman et al, 1997; Fukui et al, 1996; Silveri et al, 2003).

Neuropathology

The neuropathology of PAOS at the time of onset is unknown and difficult to determine due to its progressive neurodegenerative nature. However, some patients with initial PAOS and subsequent further neuropsychological decline indicative of disease progression have gone to autopsy. Neuropathological evaluations at that time have found the presence of Pick bodies (Fukui et al, 1996), spongiform changes with mild neuronal loss and astrogliosis, an unspecified degenerative process accompanied by severe neuronal loss (Broussolle et al, 1996), and other nonspecific changes (Silveri et al, 2003).

Epidemiology

The incidence and prevalence of PAOS is unknown, but it should be considered a rare disorder. PAOS may be under-diagnosed due to the difficulty in distinguishing between disorders of speech, as seen in PAOS, and disorders of language, such as with primary progressive aphasia (PPA) (Chapman et al, 1997; McNeil, Pratt, & Fossett, 2004).

Genetics

Little is known about the role of genetics in PAOS. One report describes a single patient with progressive decline of motor-speech function (with elements of dysarthria and AOS), intact cognitive-linguistic function, and a familial history positive for similar disorders. This family history was notable for comparable motor-speech disorders affecting his mother, his maternal aunt, and his sister (Chapman et al, 1997).

◆ Speech Impairment Associated with Disorder

As previously described, a slowly progressive AOS is the presenting sign of neurogenic disease in patients with PAOS, though the speech of these patients has not been detailed extensively. The subsequent development of dysarthria (Broussolle et al, 1996), unintelligible speech, and mutism has been reported (Cohen et al, 1993; Didic et al, 1998; Fukui et al, 1996; Rosenbek, 2004).

Diagnostic Signs and Symptoms

Patients with PAOS describe a history of a slowly progressive decline in speech abilities (Chapman et al, 1997), rather than the acute onset of speech problems as seen in traditional AOS (Duffy, 1995). The perceptual speech features of patients with AOS include an overall slowed rate, distorted speech, prosodic abnormalities, trial-and-error struggle behavior, audible and visible groping and searching, increased effort, and increased errors with increased speech demands (McNeil et al, 2004). However, it must be recognized that the speech characteristics of patients with AOS have not been formally determined to be the same as in patients with PAOS.

Etiology

The etiology of the changes in speech in patients with PAOS may be due to neurodegenerative changes in the left frontal, parietal, and temporal lobes (Broussolle et al, 1996; Chapman et al, 1997; Fukui et al, 1996; Silveri et al, 2003). More specific lesion sites have been reported in patients with traditional AOS, including the primary motor cortex (Brodmann area [BA] 4), the premotor cortex (BA 6), pars opercularis (BA 44), the supplementary motor cortex (BA 6), the insula, the parietal lobe, and the lenticular zone (Square, Roy, & Martin, 1997).

Neuropathology

As previously described, patients with initial PAOS and subsequent neuropsychological decline have shown neuropathological findings remarkable for the presence of Pick bodies (Fukui et al, 1996), spongiform changes, astrogliosis, neuronal loss (Broussolle et al, 1996), and other nonspecific changes (Broussolle et al, 1996; Didic et al, 1998).

Associated Cognitive, Linguistic, and Communicative Signs and Symptoms

Upon onset, patients with PAOS may have an isolated AOS without cognitive-linguistic deficits. However, with disease progression a decline in cognitive-linguistic functioning may occur.

Special Diagnostic Considerations

Differential diagnosis of PAOS is confounded by the challenges in distinguishing between apraxia of speech and aphasia. For example, several of the perceptual features of the speech in patients with AOS are also seen in patients who make phonemic paraphasic errors. These frequently co-occurring characteristics include trial-and-error struggle behavior, audible and visible groping and searching, increased effort, and increased errors with increased speech demands (McNeil et al, 2004).

Treatment

Little to no information is available regarding treatments for PAOS from a speech-language pathology perspective. However, PAOS may be amenable to treatment strategies applied in traditional AOS. Furthermore, some concepts from approaches used to treat PPA may also be applicable, including patient and family education regarding the progressive nature of the disorder, an emphasis on enhancing communication in a setting of progressive disease, involvement of the family and/or other appropriate individuals, and the possible early introduction of augmentative and alternative communication (McNeil & Duffy, 2001).

References

Broussolle, E., Bakchine, S., Tommasi, M., Laurent, B., Bazin, B., Cinotti, L., Cohen, L., & Chazot, G. (1996). Slowly progressive anarthria with late anterior opercular syndrome: a variant form of frontal cortical atrophy syndromes. *Journal of the Neurological Sciences, 144,* 44–58

Chapman, S.B., Rosenberg, R.N., Weiner, M.F., & Shobe, A. (1997). Autosomal dominant progressive syndrome of motor-speech loss without dementia. *Neurology, 49,* 1298–1306

Cohen, L., Benoit, N., Van Beckhout, P., Ducarne, B., & Brunet, P. (1993). Pure progressive aphemia. *Journal of Neurology, Neurosurgery and Psychiatry, 56,* 923–924

Didic, M., Ceccaldi, M., & Poncet, M. (1998). Progressive loss of speech: a neuropsychological profile of premotor dysfunction. *European Neurology, 39,* 90–96

Duffy, J.R. (1995). *Motor Speech Disorders.* St. Louis: Mosby

Fukui, T., Sugita, K., Kawamura, M., Shiota, J., & Nakano, I. (1996). Primary progressive apraxia in Pick's disease: a clinicopathologic study. *Neurology, 47,* 467–473

McNeil, M.R., & Duffy, J.R. (2001). Primary progressive aphasia. In: R. Chapey (Ed.), *Language Intervention Strategies in Adult Aphasia* (pp. 472–486). Baltimore: Lippincott Williams & Wilkins

McNeil, M.R., Pratt, S.R., & Fossett, T.R.D. (2004). The differential diagnosis of apraxia of speech. In: B. Maassen, R. Kent, H. Peters, P. van Lieshout, & W. Hulstijn (Eds.), *Speech Motor Control in Normal and Disordered Speech* (pp. 389–413). Oxford, England: Oxford University Press

McNeil, M.R., Robin, D.A., & Schmidt, R.A. (1997). Apraxia of speech: definition, differentiation, and treatment. In: M.R. McNeil (Ed.), Clinical Management of Sensorimotor Speech Disorders (pp. 311–344). New York: Thieme

Rosenbek, J.C. (2004). Mutism, neurogenic. In: K.D. Kent (Ed.), *The MIT Encyclopedia of Communication Disorders* (pp. 145–147). Cambridge, MA: MIT Press

Silveri, M.C., Cappa, A., & Salvigni, B.L. (2003). Speech and language in primary progressive anarthria. *Neurocase, 9,* 213–220

Square, P.A., Roy, E.A., & Martin, R.E. (1997). Apraxia of speech: another form of praxis disruption. In: L.J. Rothi & K.M. Heilman (Eds.), *Apraxia: The Neuropsychology of Action* (pp. 173–206). East Sussex, UK: Psychology Press

Chapter 52

Progressive Bulbar Palsy (PBP)

Justine V. Goozée and Bruce E. Murdoch

◆ General Information on Disorder

Progressive bulbar palsy (PBP) is a condition caused by degeneration of the motor neurons supplying the bulbar muscles (i.e., tongue, palate, pharynx, larynx, face, and mastication), resulting in the dominant features of progressively worsening dysarthria and dysphagia (Carrow, Riviera, Maulding, & Shamblin, 1974; Chancellor, Slattery, Fraser, Swingler, Holloway, & Warlow, 1993). PBP is a subtype of the progressive neurodegenerative condition known as motor neuron disease (MND). Other MND subtypes include amyotrophic lateral sclerosis (ALS), progressive spinal muscular atrophy (PMA), and primary lateral sclerosis (PLS). PBP differs from these other subtypes in that its presentation is restricted to the bulbar muscles only. Some believe, however, that the diagnosis of PBP simply indicates a bulbar onset of ALS, with signs expected to develop in other parts of the body with progression of the disease (Beresford, 1995; Chancellor et al, 1993; Norris et al, 1993). Of all of the subtypes of MND, PBP demonstrates the poorest prognosis, with death typically occurring less than 3 years post-onset due to life-threatening muscle weakness occurring in structures crucial for breathing and swallowing (Beresford, 1995; Carrow et al, 1974; Cerero Lapiedra, Moreno Lopez, & Esparza Gomez, 2002).

Diagnostic Signs and Symptoms

The dominant features of PBP are progressively worsening dysarthria and dysphagia, with involvement restricted to the bulbar musculature including the muscles of the tongue, palate, pharynx, and larynx (Norris et al, 1993). The muscles of the face and shoulder girdle may also be affected (Beresford, 1995). These muscles can be affected by both upper motor neuron and lower motor neuron degeneration with features including weakness, denervation atrophy, spasticity, fasciculations (twitching caused by muscle motor unit contractions), and abnormal corticobulbar reflexes such as brisk jaw jerk (Carrow et al, 1974; Cerero Lapiedra et al, 2002; Evans & Shaw, 2001). Oromotor examinations reveal reductions in tongue movement, palate elevation, and mastication (Cerero Lapiedra et al, 2002; Evans & Shaw, 2001). Electrophysiological procedures (e.g., electromyogram [EMG]) and transcranial magnetic stimulation (TMS) can be used to support the clinical findings of lower and upper motor neuron involvement.

Important negative features for diagnosis of PBP include no disturbances in walking or other limb movements, and a lack of sensory and eye movement disturbances, the presence of which could be indicative of other diseases or other subtypes of MND (Beresford, 1995; Cerero Lapiedra et al, 2002; Evans & Shaw, 2001).

Neuropathology

PBP results from degeneration or atrophy of the cranial motor neurons and nuclei in the brainstem (lower motor neurons), which supply the pharynx, palate, larynx, tongue, face, and muscles of mastication (i.e., cranial nerves V, VII, IX, X, XI, XII), with degeneration of corticobulbar fibers (upper motor neurons) also typical (Carrow et al, 1974; Norris et al, 1993; Poungvarin & Viriyavejakul, 1991).

Epidemiology

An increased frequency of occurrence of PBP has been observed in older adults and in women compared with men (Chancellor et al, 1993). In a study conducted at a Mexico City referral hospital, the mean age of onset of PBP was reported to be 60.4 years (standard deviation [SD] 9.8; 65.2 years for males and 56.3 years for females; Otero-Siliceo, Arriada-Mendicoa, & Corona-Vazquez, 1997). A slightly greater proportion of females (53% females versus 47% males) was found to exhibit PBP (Otero-Siliceo et al, 1997).

PBP as a pure form of MND is considered to be rare and is often regarded to be simply the initial presentation in some cases of ALS (Norris et al, 1993). The percentage of MND cases diagnosed specifically with PBP ranges from 0 to 34% (Norris et al, 1993; Otero-Siliceo et al, 1997; Poungvarin & Viriyavejakul, 1991). As an indication of the incidence of PBP, the annual incidence rate of ALS in developed countries has been estimated to be only 0.4 to 2.4 per 100,000 individuals (Mayeux, 2003).

Genetics

Motor neuron disease presents in sporadic and familial (4 to 5% of cases; inherited as an autosomal dominant trait) forms. In at least some cases, the MND is likely due to a genetic deficit of neuronal enzymes (Carrow et al, 1974; Evans & Shaw, 2001).

◆ Speech Impairment Associated with Disorder

Limited detailed reports of the speech features exhibited in PBP are available. Given that both upper and lower motor neurons may be affected in PBP, the resulting dysarthria can be a mixed form of spastic and flaccid dysarthria. Reports of the deviant speech features exhibited in ALS with bulbar involvement indicate the types of speech features expected in PBP. These features include effortful, slow productions, short phrases, inappropriate pauses, imprecise consonants and vowels, hypernasality, nasal emission, strain-strangled voice, harshness, breathiness, tremor, continuous voicing, and a decreased pitch and loudness range (Carrow et al, 1974; Watts & Vanryckeghem, 2001). If corticobulbar involvement predominates, the vocal cords may be hyperadducted, whereas if lower motor neuron involvement is dominant, then hypoadduction of the vocal cords may be exhibited (Watts & Vanryckeghem, 2001).

Diagnostic Signs and Symptoms

Bulbar signs and symptoms (i.e., dysarthria, dysphagia) without motor dysfunction in the trunk, limbs, or eyes, together with a lack of sensory deficits would be suggestive of PBP.

A range of diagnostic electrophysiological (i.e., EMG and nerve conduction), neural imaging (e.g., magnetic resonance imaging [MRI], computed tomography [CT]) of the brain and spine, identification of biochemical markers in the blood and cerebrospinal fluid, muscle and nerve biopsies, and genetic testing would be required, however, to support a diagnosis of PBP and to rule out other diseases/disorders that could be causing the apparent bulbar symptoms (Cerero Lapiedra et al, 2002).

Etiology

The etiology of MND, including its subtype, PBP, is largely unknown. Various hypotheses have been proposed including a chronic slow virus infection of the central nervous system (CNS), biomechanical or metabolic abnormalities of the neurons, immunological disturbances, toxins, aging, trauma, genetic factors, oxidative stress or free-radical oxidative damage of neurons, and glutamatergic toxicity, which could lead to damage of critical target proteins (e.g., neurofilaments) and organelles (e.g., mitochondria) resulting in motor neuron injury and death (Carrow et al, 1974; Cerero Lapiedra et al, 2002; Evans & Shaw, 2001; Poungvarin & Viriyavejakul, 1991). Apoptosis, or an "intracellular suicide program" has also been proposed (Evans & Shaw, 2001).

Neuropathology

The sites of neuronal degeneration can occur within the corticobulbar tracts or the cranial motor neurons and nuclei within the brainstem, resulting in upper or lower motor neuron signs, respectively. The bulbar muscles may be affected then by weakness, abnormal tone (e.g., spasticity), fasciculations, and abnormal reflexes.

Associated Cognitive, Linguistic, and Communicative Signs and Symptoms

In the past it was presumed that intellect was preserved in MND (Poungvarin & Viriyavejakul, 1991). More sophisticated testing has revealed, however, that subtle cognitive impairments reflective of frontal lobe disturbances are exhibited by the majority of patients with MND (Bak & Hodges, 1999). Approximately 3 to 5% of patients with MND demonstrate frontotemporal dementia (FTD) or aphasia (Bak & Hodges, 1999; Evans & Shaw, 2001). The language deficits encompass impaired language comprehension and expression, and particularly impairments of syntax and verbs (with relative preservation of nouns), indicative of frontal and frontostriatal damage (Bak & Hodges, 1999; Doran, Xuareb, & Hodges, 1995). Cognitive signs specific to PBP have not been reported.

Special Diagnostic Considerations

Upper and lower motor neuron signs may be exhibited in the bulbar musculature of persons with PBP. The bulbar disturbances (e.g., dysarthria, dysphagia) that are observed at onset progressively worsen over the course of the disease.

Treatment

With no known cure or disease modifying medication currently available, treatment for PBP is symptomatic, palliative, and multidisciplinary (Poungvarin & Viriyavejakul, 1991). Given the progressive nature of the disease, the needs and disabilities of a patient with PBP should be regularly monitored, and treatment aids and plans modified accordingly.

In the treatment of dysarthria and dysphonia in MND, rapidly progressive cases have been found to be difficult to treat using behavioral techniques (Watts & Vanryckeghem, 2001). Augmentative and alternative communication aids may be needed to provide a means of communication. Effective dysphagia management is critical to prevent aspiration, choking, malnutrition, and dehydration, and may include altering the consistency of the diet to assist bolus control, compensatory swallowing strategies, and changes in eating habits (e.g., smaller portions, increased chewing time). A percutaneous endoscopic gastrostomy needs to be considered early, and particularly before excess weight loss or aphagia develops (Watts & Vanryckeghem, 2001).

References

Bak, T.H. & Hodges, J.R. (1999). Cognition, language and behaviour in motor neurone disease: evidence of frontotemporal dysfunction. *Dementia and Geriatric Cognitive Disorders, 10* (suppl 1), 29–32

Beresford, S. (1995). *Motor Neurone Disease.* London: Chapman & Hall

Carrow, E., Riviera, V., Maulding, M., & Shamblin, L. (1974). Deviant speech characteristics in motor neuron disease. *Archives of Otolaryngology, 100,* 212–218

Cerero Lapiedra, R., Moreno Lopez, L.A., & Esparza Gomez, G.C. (2002). Progressive bulbar palsy: a case report diagnosed by lingual symptoms. *Journal of Oral Pathology and Medicine, 31,* 277–279

Chancellor, A.M., Slattery, J.M., Fraser, H., Swingler, R.J., Holloway, S.M., & Warlow, C.P. (1993). The prognosis of adult-onset motor neuron disease: a prospective study based on the Scottish Motor Neuron Disease Register. *Journal of Neurology, 240,* 339–346

Doran, M., Xuareb, J., & Hodges, J.R. (1995). Rapidly progressive aphasia with bulbar motor neurone disease: a clinical and neuropsychological study. *Behavioral Neurology, 8,* 169–180

Evans, J. & Shaw, P.J. (2001). Motor neurone disease: (1) clinical features and pathogenesis. *The Pharmaceutical Journal, 267,* 681–684

Mayeux, R. (2003). Epidemiology of neurodegeneration. *Annual Review of Neuroscience, 26,* 81–104.

Norris, F., Shepherd, R., Denys, E., Mukai, E., Elias, L., Holden, D., & Norris, H. (1993). Onset, natural history and outcome in idiopathic adult motor neuron disease. *Journal of Neurological Science, 118,* 48–55

Otero-Siliceo, E., Arriada-Mendicoa, N., & Corona-Vazquez, T. (1997). Frequency of motor neuron diseases in a Mexico City referral center. *Revista de Investigacion Clinica, 49,* 445–448

Poungvarin, N. & Viriyavejakul, A. (1991). Motor neurone disease in Thailand: the clinical aspects of 77 patients. *Journal of the Medical Association of Thailand, 74,* 181–186

Watts, C.R. & Vanryckeghem, M. (2001). Laryngeal dysfunction in amyotrophic lateral sclerosis: a review and case report. *BMC Ear, Nose, and Throat Disorders, 1*(1), 1.

Additional Reading

Howard, R.S. & Orrell, R.W. (2002). Management of motor neurone disease. *Postgraduate Medical Journal, 78,* 736–741

Talbot, K. (2002). Motor neurone disease. *Postgraduate Medical Journal, 78,* 513–519

Chapter 53

Progressive Multifocal Leukoencephalopathy

Brooke-Mai Whelan and Bruce E. Murdoch

◆ General Information on Disorder

Progressive multifocal leukoencephalopathy (PML) is a fatal demyelinating disease of the central nervous system (CNS), commonly occurring in immunosuppressed populations (Koralnik, 2004). PML develops as a consequence of polyomavirus JC activation (Koralnik, 2004). In a nonimmunosuppressed state, the virus is ubiquitous, remaining dormant within the kidney epithelium (Huang, Skolasky, Dal Pan, Royal, & McArthur, 1998).

Diagnostic Signs and Symptoms

In immunocompromised hosts, however, viral reactivation may result in a neurological assault, causing symptoms such as hemiparesis, hemianopia, aphasia, ataxia, dysarthria, and mental deterioration (Colucci et al, 2004).

Neuropathology

PML has been described as a multiple sclerosis (MS)-like disease, typically involving either a relapse-remitting course or more commonly, fatal progression (Corral et al, 2004). The JC virus primarily infects oligodendrocytes, resulting in demyelination of the CNS (Portegies et al, 2004).

Epidemiology

AIDS has been held accountable for up to 85% of PML cases (Major, Amemiya, Tornatore, Houff, & Berger, 1992). A male-to-female incidence ratio of 7.6:1.0 has been highlighted, with the highest incidence of occurrence between the ages of 25 and 50 years (Berger, Pall, Lanska, & Whiteman, 1998).

◆ Speech Impairment Associated with Disorder

Diagnostic Signs and Symptoms

Speech disturbances represent one of the most common initial symptoms reported by PML patients (i.e., up to 40% of cases) (Berger et al, 1998). Reports of facial paralysis (Factor, Troche-Panetto, & Weaver, 2003; Langford-Kuntz, Reichart, & Pohle, 1988), facial numbness (Langford-Kuntz et al, 1988),

lack of facial expression, dysphonia (de Toffol et al, 1994), and articulatory imprecision (Arai et al, 2002) have been highlighted in the literature. The dysarthria of PML has been comprehensively described in a single case (Lethlean & Murdoch, 1993). Severe speech deficits characterized by imprecise articulation, incoordinated speech respiration, reduced breath support for speech, reduced laryngeal control, hypernasality, and significantly reduced speech intelligibility (Lethlean & Murdoch, 1993) were reported.

Etiology

Acute HIV-associated neuropathy, including PML, may present forms of craniofacial nerve dysfunction, typically involving the facial (cranial nerve VII), trigeminal (V), and vestibulocochlear nerves (VIII) (Langford-Kuntz et al, 1988). This profile suggests specific implications for the articulators; however, the particular motor speech profile presented may vary greatly from patient to patient, dependent on the areas of demyelination involved.

Neuropathology

JC virus infection results in multiple areas of demyelination, which may produce focal or global neurological impairments. The most common type of PML is reportedly cerebral; however, cerebellar and brainstem involvement have also been reported (Arai et al, 2002).

Associated Cognitive, Linguistic, and Communicative Signs and Symptoms

Deterioration in mental functions has been reported to occur in the majority of PML cases (Major et al, 1992), including confusion, emotional lability, and dementia (Hou & Major, 2000). Of note, language difficulties have been described as one of the most common complaints relating to mental deterioration (Karahalios, Breit, Dal Canto, & Levy, 1992). Both general and higher-level linguistic impairments have been described in PML cases in the literature (Hseuh & Reyes, 1988; Lethlean & Murdoch, 1993).

Special Diagnostic Considerations

Conventionally, neurological disorders affecting the white matter pathways of the brain have been thought to primarily produce deficits in motor function (Filley et al, 1999). Contemporary literature, however, highlights that cognition may also be affected by such disorders, including language processing

(Lethlean & Murdoch, 1993). This evidence, in combination with the fact that orofacial neural lesions may possibly represent early manifestations of HIV infection (Langford-Kuntz et al, 1988), suggests that speech-language pathologists may play a role in contributing to the definitive diagnosis of PML.

Treatment

No effective therapy is currently available for PML; however, patients on highly active antiretroviral therapy (HAART) may have a prolonged clinical course of up to years (Goodkin et al, 2001). Active speech pathology intervention may be sought for PML patients in maximizing communication skills during the course of disease progression or remission. Traditional behavioral, functional, or augmentative therapeutic strategies may be employed. As per other demyelinating diseases (e.g., MS), all treatment approaches must be considered within the context of potential fatigue effects (Freal, Kraft, & Coryell, 1984).

References

Arai, Y., Tsutsui, Y., Nagashima, K., Shinmura, Y., Kosugi, T., Wakai, M., Nishikage, H., & Yamamoto, J. (2002). Autopsy case of the cerebellar form of progressive multifocal leukoencephalopathy without immunodeficiency. *Neuropathology, 22,* 48–56

Berger, J.R., Pall, L., Lanska, D., & Whiteman, M. (1998). Progressive multifocal leukoencephalopathy in patients with HIV infection. *Journal of Neurovirology, 4,* 59–68

Colucci, M., Cocito, L., Capello, E., Mancardi, G.L., Serrati, C., Cinque, P., & Schenone, A. (2004). Progressive multifocal leukoencephalopathy in an adult patient with ICF syndrome. *Journal of Neurological Sciences, 217,* 107–110

Corral, I., Quereda, C., Garcia-Villanueva, M., Casado, J. L., Perez-Elias, M.J., Navas, E., Ariza, A., & Moreno, S. (2004). Focal monophasic demyelinating leukoencephalopathy in advanced HIV infection. *European Neurology, 52,* 36–41

de Toffol, B., Vidailhet, M., Gray, F., Besnier, J.M., Menage, P., Lescs, M.C., Choutet, P., & Autret, A. (1994). Isolated motor control dysfunction related to progressive multifocal leukoencephalopathy during AIDS with normal MRI. *Neurology, 44,* 2352–2355

Factor, S.A., Troche-Panetto, M., & Weaver, S.A. (2003). Dystonia in AIDS: report of four cases. *Movement Disorders, 18,* 1492–1498

Filley, C.M., Thompson, L.L., Sze, C.I., Simon, J.A., Paskavitz, J.F., & Kleinschmidt-DeMasters, B.K. (1999). White matter dementia in CADASIL. *Journal of Neurological Sciences, 163,* 163–167

Freal, J.E., Kraft, G.H., & Coryell, J.K. (1984). Symptomatic fatigue in multiple sclerosis. *Archives of Physical Medicine and Rehabilitation, 65,* 135–138

Goodkin, K., Wilkie, F.L., Concha, M., Hinkin, C.H., Symes, S., Baldewicz, T.T., Asthana, D., Fujimura, R.K., Lee, D., van Zuilen, M.H., Khamis, I., Shapshak, P., & Eisdorfer, C. (2001). Aging and neuro-AIDS conditions and the changing spectrum of HIV-1–associated morbidity and mortality. *Journal of Clinical Epidemiology, 54*(suppl 1), S35–43

Hou, J. & Major, E.O. (2000). Progressive multifocal leukoencephalopathy: JC virus induced demyelination in the immune compromised host. *Journal of Neurovirology, 6* (suppl 2), S98–S100

Hseuh, C. & Reyes, C. V. (1988). Progressive multifocal leukoencephalopathy. *American Family Physician, 37,* 129–132

Huang, S.S., Skolasky, R.L., Dal Pan, G.J., Royal, W. 3rd, & McArthur, J.C. (1998). Survival prolongation in HIV-associated progressive multifocal leukoencephalopathy treated with alpha-interferon: an observational study. *Journal of Neurovirology, 4,* 324–332

Karahalios, D., Breit, R., Dal Canto, M.C., & Levy, R.M. (1992). Progressive multifocal leukoencephalopathy in patients with HIV infection: lack of impact of early diagnosis by stereotactic brain biopsy. *Journal of Acquired Immune Deficiency Syndrome, 5,* 1030–1038

Koralnik, I.J. (2004). New insights into progressive multifocal leukoencephalopathy. *Current Opinion in Neurology, 17,* 365–370

Langford-Kuntz, A., Reichart, P., & Pohle, H.D. (1988). Impairment of cranio-facial nerves due to AIDS. Report of 2 cases. *International Journal of Oral Maxillofacial Surgery, 17,* 227–229

Lethlean, J.B. & Murdoch, B.E. (1993). Language dysfunction in progressive multifocal leukoencephalopathy: a case study. *Journal of Medical Speech Language Pathology, 1,* 27–34

Major, E.O., Amemiya, E.E., Tornatore, C.S., Houff, S.A., & Berger, J.R. (1992). Pathogenesis and molecular biology of progressive multifocal leukoencephalopathy, the JV virus-induced demyelinating disease of the human brain. *Clinical Microbiological Reviews, 5,* 49–73

Portegies, P., Solod, L., Cinque, P., Chaudhuri, A., Begovac, J., Everall, I., Weber, T., Bojar, M., Martinez-Martin, P., & Kennedy, P.G. (2004). Guidelines for the diagnosis and management of neurological complications of HIV infection. *European Journal of Neurology, 11,* 297–304

Additional Reading

Murdoch, B.E., & Theodoros, D.G. (2000). *Speech and Language Disorders in Multiple Sclerosis.* London: Whurr

Chapter 54

Progressive Supranuclear Palsy

Christine T. Matthews

♦ General Information on Disorder

Progressive supranuclear palsy (PSP) is a neurodegenerative disease of unknown etiology that produces an akinetic-rigid form of parkinsonism. It is generally not responsive to drug therapies used in Parkinson's disease, likely due to numerous neurotransmitter pathway deficiencies and widespread neuropathology (Muller et al, 2001; Rajput & Rajput, 2001). PSP was first described in the 1960s and is typically marked initially by ophthalmoplegia (inability to suppress the horizontal vestibule-ocular reflex and impaired downward saccades), with eventual rigidity of the trunk, pseudobulbar palsy, and mild dementia (Steele, Richardson, & Olszewski, 1964; Yorkston, Beukelman, Strand, & Bell, 1999). Accurate diagnosis requires both clinical and pathological information to differentiate it from its closest clinical neighbors. Early diagnosis is difficult in PSP because of the variability of symptom onset and similarity to other neurodegenerative diseases including Parkinson's disease (PD), corticobasal degeneration (see Chapter 23), multiple system atrophy (MSA) of the parkinsonian type, and Pick's disease (Rajput & Rajput, 2001; Tolosa, Vallderliola, & Marti, 1994).

Diagnostic Signs and Symptoms

The classic initial diagnostic sign of PSP is supranuclear ophthalmoplegia. In contrast to PD, where rigidity primarily affects the limbs, PSP includes postural instability and axial rigidity resulting in frequent falls (Duffy, 1995; Rajput & Rajput, 2001; Yorkston et al, 1999). Nonspecific dizziness, generalized motor slowing, personality changes, dystonia, and resting tremor can also be observed. Cognitive impairments are evident in most patients. Palilalia and movement perseverations are also common (Duffy, 1995; Rajput & Rajput, 2001). Additional signs and symptoms may include erect posture, blepharospasm, bulbar symptoms including dysphagia and dysarthria, and sleep difficulties (Golbe, 1997; Rajput & Rajput, 2001). Neuroimaging markers of the disease include MRI-observed atrophy in the putamen and midbrain as well as third ventricle enlargement (Price et al, 2004).

Neuropathology

PSP is characterized by tau-positive neurofibrillary tangles, neuropil threads, tufted astrocytes, and oligodendroglial coiled bodies (Verny, Duyckaerts, Agid, & Hauw, 1996). These pathological abnormalities are often widespread and are typically observed in the globus pallidus, substantia nigra, subthalamic nucleus, locus ceruleus, periaqueductal gray matter, midbrain tectum, and pontine nuclei. Less often, the caudate, putamen, and cerebral cortex are involved, and occasionally the Purkinje cells of the cerebellum. Several neurotransmitter systems including dopaminergic, cholinergic, γ-aminobutyric acid (GABA)-ergic, serotonergic, and adrenergic may also be affected in PSP secondary to the multiple sites of pathology (Kluin et al, 2001; Rajput & Rajput, 2001).

Epidemiology

The incidence of PSP has been estimated to be 5.3 cases per 100,000 people aged 50 to 99 years. The true incidence of the disease may be higher than reported, due to the difficult nature of definitive diagnosis. More men are affected, and the average age of onset is 63 years, with mean disease duration of 9 years from symptom onset to death (Rajput & Rajput, 2001). Epidemiological data do not support the notion that PSP results from any known toxin exposure (Golbe, Rubin, & Cody, 1996).

Genetics

There are reported cases of familial PSP, but this is rare, and therefore a positive family history is not considered to be a risk factor for developing PSP (de Yebenes, Sarasa, & Daniel, 1995).

♦ Speech Impairment Associated with Disorder

The dysarthria of PSP is often mixed with hypokinetic, spastic, and ataxic components (Duffy, 1995; Kluin, Gilman, Berent, & Gilman, 1993). The speech clinical picture is likely to change as the disease progresses. An analysis of 44 patients with PSP revealed that although ataxic signs are often present early in the disease, they become overshadowed by the spastic and hypokinetic components of the dysarthria (Kluin et al, 2001). Dysarthria evolving to anarthria (defined as the complete loss of speech motor control) has been described to reflect the severity of the advanced neuropathological and motor speech changes from initial diagnosis to death (Kluin et al, 1993).

Diagnostic Signs and Symptoms

Hypokinetic dysarthria is a prominent dysarthria type in PSP due to neuronal loss and other neuropathological changes in the substantia nigra, globus pallidus, subthalamic nucleus, periaqueductal gray, caudate nucleus, and putamen. Changes in regions of corticobulbar pathways, specifically diffuse changes in the frontal cortex, can account for the spastic signs, and changes in the cerebellum and related structures such as the dentate nuclei, inferior olives, and red nuclei can account for the presence of ataxic signs (Kluin et al, 2001; Rajput & Rajput, 2001). Forty percent of persons with PSP exhibit speech production behaviors consistent with two of the three dysarthria types, and the remainder exhibit all three (Kluin et al, 1993). It is most common for patients with PSP to exhibit a mixed hypokinetic-spastic dysarthria (Duffy, 1995; Kluin et al, 1993). Clinical signs might include various confirmatory signs present in hypokinetic, spastic, and ataxic dysarthria, including bradykinesia, rigidity, and the presence of pathological reflexes. Monopitch, hoarseness, nasal emission, excess and equal stress, hypernasality, imprecise articulation, and slow rate occur more frequently in PSP than in PD, and vocal flutter, reduced loudness, reduced stress, tremor, breathiness, and rapid rate occur more frequently in PD than in PSP (Yorkston et al, 1999).

Etiology

Although the etiology of the disease is largely unknown, the motor speech deficits in PSP reflect damage to the extrapyramidal, pyramidal, and cerebellar systems. They are derived from impairment of multiple cortical and subcortical structures and neurotransmitter systems important for speech motor control.

Neuropathology

Postmortem examination of neuropathological changes in the extrapyramidal pathways has revealed a significant positive correlation between the severity of the hypokinetic component of the dysarthria and the amount of atrophy

and neurofibrillary tangles in the substantia nigra (Kluin et al, 2001). Damage to these structures and others of the basal ganglia, cerebellum, and frontal lobes produce changes in speed, strength, tone, range of motion, force, timing, and overall motor control (Duffy, 1995).

Associated Cognitive, Linguistic, and Communicative Signs and Symptoms

Dementia has been reported as a common concomitant feature of PSP (Steele et al, 1964). Rajput and Rajput (2001) reported evidence of cognitive impairment in 62.5% of their patients with PSP, including deficits associated with frontal lobe dysfunction. Additionally, palilalia has been reported as a prevalent sign (Lapointe & Horner, 1981; Metter & Hanson, 1991).

◆ Special Diagnostic Considerations

Sensorimotor speech evaluation should focus on the presence of more than one type of dysarthria. Specifically, hypokinetic plus spastic or ataxic speech symptoms suggests that the observed motor speech impairment is not due to PD. Additionally, dysarthria has been reported to be one of the first symptoms in PSP; however, in PD, dysarthria is not frequently reported as an early symptom (Yorkston et al, 1999).

◆ Treatment

Reports of pharmacological treatments have been less than encouraging (Rajput & Rajput, 2001), and reports of direct speech treatment are sparse (Yorkston et al, 1999). Caregiver-focused communication strategies can aid in facilitating successful communicative interactions. Persons who develop severe dysarthria but who have sufficient cognition may benefit from alternative and augmentative communication (AAC) as a means to supplement or replace verbal communication.

References

de Yebenes, J.G., Sarasa, J.L., & Daniel, S.E. (1995). Familial progressive supranuclear palsy: Description of a pedigree and review of the literature. *Brain, 118,* 1095–1103

Duffy, J.R. (1995). *Motor Speech Disorders: Substrates, Differential Diagnosis, and Management,* 1st ed. St. Louis: Mosby

Golbe, L.I. (1997). Progressive supranuclear palsy. In: R.L. Watts & W.C. Koller (Eds.), *Movement Disorders: Neurological Principles and Practice* (pp. 279–295). New York: McGraw-Hill

Golbe, L.I., Rubin, S.I., & Cody, R.P. (1996). Follow-up study of risk factors in progressive supranuclear palsy. *Neurology, 47,* 148–154

Kluin, K.J., Gilman, S., Berent, S., & Gilman, S. (1993). Perceptual analysis of speech disorders in progressive supranuclear palsy. *Neurology, 43,* 563–566

Kluin, K., Gilman, S., Foster, N.L., Siman, A.A.F., D'Amato, C.J., Bruch, L.A. et al. (2001). Neuropathological correlates of dysarthria in progressive supranuclear palsy. *Archives of Neurology, 58,* 265–269

Lapointe, L.L. & Horner, J. (1981). Palilalia: a descriptive study of pathological reiterative utterances. *Journal of Speech and Hearing Disorders, 46,* 34–38

Metter, E.J. & Hanson, W.R. (1991). Dysarthria in progressive supranuclear palsy. In: C. Moore, K. Yorkston, & D. Beukelman (Eds.), *Dysarthria and*

Apraxia of Speech: Perspective on Management (pp. 127–136). Baltimore: Paul H. Brookes

Muller, J., Wennings, G.K., Verny, M., McKee, A., Chaudhuri, K.R., Jellinger, K. et al. (2001). Progression of dysarthria and dysphagia in post-mortem-confirmed parkinsonian disorders. *Archives of Neurology, 58,* 259–264

Price, S., Paviour, D., Scahill, R., Stevens, J., Rossor, M., Lees, A., et al. (2004). Voxel-based morphometry detects patterns of atrophy that help differentiate progressive supranuclear palsy and Parkinson's disease. *NeuroImage, 23,* 663–669

Rajput, A. & Rajput, A.H. (2001). Progressive supranuclear palsy: clinical features, pathophysiology and management. *Drugs and Aging, 18,* 913–925

Steele, J.C., Richardson, J.C., & Olszewski, J. (1964). Progressive supra-nuclear palsy: a heterogeneous degeneration involving the brain stem, ganglia and cerebellum with vertical gaze and pseudobulbar palsy, nuchal dystonia and dementia. *Archives of Neurology, 10,* 333–359

Tolosa, E., Vallderliola, F., & Marti, M.J. (1994). Clinical diagnosis and diagnostic criteria of progressive supranuclear palsy (Steele-Richardson-Olszewski syndrome). *Journal of Neural Transmission Supplement, 42,* 15–31

Verny, M., Duyckaerts, C., Agid, Y., & Hauw, J.J. (1996). The significance of cortical pathology in progressive supranuclear palsy: clinico-pathological data in 10 cases. *Brain, 119,* 1123–1136

Yorkston, K., Beukelman, D., Strand, E., & Bell, K.R. (1999). Dysarthria in degenerative diseases. In: C. Olson (Ed.), *Management of Motor Speech Disorders in Children and Adults,* 2nd ed. (pp. 115–190). Austin: Pro-Ed

Chapter 55

Rett Syndrome

Gail Woodyatt

◆ General Information on Syndrome

Rett syndrome (RTT), a neurodevelopmental disorder affecting mainly females, has been linked to mutations in the *MECP2* gene (Amir et al, 1999). Development seems normal for the first 6 to 30 months, and then motor, communication, and cognitive skills regress to profound levels of disability in the majority of those affected (Rett Syndrome Diagnostic Criteria Work Group, 1988). It is a progressive but not degenerative disorder (Kerr & Ravine, 2003).

Diagnostic Signs and Symptoms

Diagnosis for classic RTT is largely determined by criteria established by the Rett Syndrome Diagnostic Criteria Work Group (1988). Symptoms are consistent across the population of RTT, but the degree of severity varies from mild to severe expression (Kerr & Ravine, 2003). Loss of purposeful hand use and the presentation of unusual hand wringing and hand mouthing are distinctive features of the disorder. The phenotypic spectrum of RTT, however, is now broader than previously considered, particularly for the mild variants (Huppke, Held, Laccone, & Hanefeld, 2003). Laboratory confirmation of the *MECP2* gene in children with other syndromes and disorders no longer precludes the diagnosis of RTT (Leonard et al, 2004).

Neuropathology

No gross cerebral malformations have been identified in RTT, although brain volume is reduced for age and height of the individual (Armstrong, 2002; Jellinger, 2003). The neurons are smaller with increased density of packing in the cerebral cortex, thalamus, basal ganglia, amygdala, and hippocampus (Bauman, Kemper, & Arin, 1995); dendritic trees are small particularly in frontal, motor, and temporal lobes; and a reduction in and changing receptivity of neurotransmitters have been noted (Armstrong, 2002; Jellinger, 2003). Decreased neuromelanin content in the substantia nigra is a consistent neuropathological finding (Armstrong, 1992; Jellinger, 2003; Jellinger & Seitelberger, 1986).

Epidemiology

Estimated prevalence is from a weighted prevalence of 3.8:10,000 in a United Kingdom study (Fombonne, Simmons, Ford, Meltzer, & Goodman, 2001) to 1:22,800 females in the Texas Rett Syndrome Registry (Kozinetz et al, 1993). Thus RTT may be second only to Down syndrome as a cause of intellectual disability in females and twice as prevalent as phenylketonuria (Jellinger, 2003).

Genetics

Most cases of RTT are sporadic except in rare familial cases (Jellinger, 2003). Mutations of the *MECP2* gene related to the Xq28 locus have been identified in almost 80% of those with classic RTT and almost 50% of those with atypical presentation of the disorder, including some males (Amir et al, 1999; Shahbazian & Zoghbi, 2002).

◆ Speech Impairment Associated with Syndrome

Few authors have commented on the quality of the speech in RTT. Kerr, Belichenko, Woodcock, and Woodcock (2001), however, reported clear speech in 6% of their group of 265 British girls and women. More commonly, grunts, vowel-like sounds of normal pitch and tonal quality, syllable repetitions, and strings of variegated babble with a variety of intonation patterns have been reported in those individuals with classic RTT (Bashina, Simashkova, Grachev, & Gorbachevskaya, 2002; Garber & Veydt, 1992; Lewis & Wilson, 1998; Woodyatt & Ozanne, 1994).

Diagnostic Signs and Symptoms

No specific diagnostic signs or symptoms have been identified, although dyspraxia has been suggested for those girls with classic RTT (Hunter, 1999; Woodyatt & Ozanne, 1994). No paralysis indicative of a dysarthria was reported in a group of 50 girls with RTT (Bashina et al, 2002), although changes over time, from hypotonicity of cheeks, lips, and tongue to hypertonicity, have been noted (Budden, Meek, & Henighan, 1990). Though undescribed to date, dysarthria would be expected with these neurological signs in these articulatory structures.

Etiology

No specific etiology as been identified for the speech problems of RTT. Belichenko (2001) hypothesized that the profound motor disturbances of people with RTT "interfere with speech processing" (p. 285) affecting motor speech production. However, consistent with the distribution on central nervous system (CNS) pathology in the cortex, thalamus, and basal ganglia, mixed spastic, hypokinetic, or hyperkinetic dysarthria would be a likely possibility.

Neuropathology of Speech

Neuronal size in motor speech areas in the brains of 14 individuals with RTT was less than those of controls, with a possible decrease in the number of synaptic sites in the speech areas (Armstrong & Kinney, 2001; Belichenko, 2001). Aspects of impaired speech production are likely to be associated with the global neuropathological features described for the syndrome.

Associated Cognitive, Linguistic, and Communicative Signs and Symptoms

Cognitive and linguistic functioning for most individuals seems to be at preintentional levels (Sandberg, Ehlers, Hagberg, & Gillberg, 2000; Woodyatt & Ozanne, 1992, 1994), although skills may be underestimated due to impaired oral and motor behaviors (Woodyatt & Ozanne, 1994). Most individuals develop only single words before regression and no new words are acquired following regression (Coleman, Brubaker, Hunter, & Smith, 1988; Kerr & Ravine, 2003).

Treatment

No speech treatments have been identified for RTT. Rather, speech therapy has focused on the facilitation of communicative interactions using eye gaze and alternative and augmentative communication (AAC), and the functional use of retained words and phrases in those individuals with preserved speech (Hunter, 1999; Jellinger, 2003; Koppenhaver et al, 2001).

References

Amir, R.E., Van den Veyver, I.B., Wan, M., Tran, C.Q., Francke, U., Zoghbi, H.Y. (1999). Rett syndrome is caused by mutations in X-linked MECP2, encoding methyl-CpG-binding protein 2. *Nature Genetics, 23,* 185–188

Armstrong, D.D. (2002). Neuropathology of Rett syndrome. *Mental Retardation and Developmental Disabilities Research Reviews, 8,* 72–76

Armstrong, D.D. & Kinney, H.C. (2001). The neuropathology of the Rett disorder. In: A. Kerr & I. Witt Engerstrom (Eds.), *Rett Disorder and the Developing Brain* (pp. 57–84). Oxford, UK: Oxford University Press

Bashina, V.M., Simashkova, N.V., Grachev, V.V., & Gorbachevskaya, N.L. (2002). Speech and motor disturbances in Rett syndrome. *Neurosciences and Behavioral Physiology, 32,* 323–327

Bauman, M.L., Kemper, T.L., & Arin, D.M. (1995). Pervasive neuroanatomical abnormalities of the brain in three cases of Rett's syndrome. *Neurology, 45,* 1581–1586

Belichenko, P.V. (2001). The morphological substrate for communication. In A. Kerr & I. Witt Engerstrom (Eds.), *Rett Disorder and the Developing Brain* (pp. 277–301). Oxford, UK: Oxford University Press

Budden, S., Meek, M., & Henighan, C. (1990). Communication and oral-motor function in Rett syndrome. *Developmental Medicine and Child Neurology, 32,* 51–55

Coleman, M., Brubaker, J., Hunter, K., & Smith, G. (1988). Rett syndrome: a survey of North American patients. *Journal of Mental Deficiency Research, 32,* 117–124

Fombonne, E., Simmons, H., Ford, T., Meltzer, H., & Goodman, R. (2001). Prevalence of pervasive developmental disorders in the British survey of child mental health. *Journal of the American Academy of Child and Adolescent Psychiatry, 40,* 820–827

Garber, N., & Veydt, N. (1992). Speech and language development in Rett syndrome: literature review and case study. *Australian Journal of Human Communication Disorders, 20,* 49– 62

Hunter, K. (1999). *The Rett Syndrome Handbook.* Clinton, MD: International Rett Syndrome Association

Huppke, P., Held, M., Laccone, F., & Hanefeld, F. (2003). The spectrum of phenotypes in females with Rett syndrome. *Brain and Development, 25,* 346–351

Jellinger, K.A. (2003). Rett syndrome—an update. *Journal of Neural Transmission, 110,* 681–701

Jellinger, K.A., & Seitelberger, F. (1986). Neuropathology of Rett syndrome. *American Journal of Medical Genetics, 24,* 259–288

Kerr, A.M., Belichenko, P., Woodcock, T., Woodcock, M. (2001). Mind and brain in Rett disorder. *Brain and Development, 23,* S44–S49

Kerr, A.M., & Ravine, D. (2003). Review article: breaking new ground in Rett syndrome. *Journal of Intellectual Disability Research, 47,* 580–587

Koppenhaver, D.A., Erikson, K.A., Harris, B., McLellan, J., Skotko, B.G., & Newton, R.A. (2001). Storybook-based communication intervention for girls with Rett syndrome and their mothers. *Disability and Rehabilitation, 23,* 149–159

Kozinetz, C.A., Skender, M.L., MacNaughton, N., Almes, M.J., Schultz, R.J., Percy, A.K., & Glaze, D.G. (1993). Epidemiology of Rett syndrome: a population based registry. *Pediatrics, 91,* 445–450

Leonard, H., Weaving, L., Eastaugh, P., Smith, L., Delatycki, M., Witt Engerstrom, I., & Christadoulou, J. (2004). Trisomy 21 and Rett syndrome: a double burden. *Journal of Paediatrics and Child Health, 40,* 406–409

Lewis, J., & Wilson, D. (1998). *Pathways to Learning in Rett Syndrome.* London, UK: David Fulton

Rett Syndrome Diagnostic Criteria Work Group. (1988). Diagnostic criteria for Rett syndrome. *Annals of Neurology, 23,* 425–428

Sandberg, A.D., Ehlers, S., Hagberg, B., & Gillberg, C. (2000). The Rett syndrome complex: communicative functions in relation to developmental level and autistic features. *Autism, 4,* 249–267

Shahbazian, M.D., & Zoghbi, H.Y. (2002). Rett syndrome and MeCP2: linking epigenetics and neuronal function. *American Journal of Human Genetics, 71,* 1259–1272

Woodyatt, G., & Ozanne, A. (1992). Communication abilities and Rett syndrome. *Journal of Autism and Developmental Disorders, 22,* 155–173

Woodyatt, G. & Ozanne, A. (1994). Intentionality and communication in four cases of children with Rett syndrome. *Australia and New Zealand Journal of Developmental Disabilities, 19,* 173–183

Additional Reading

Kerr, A., & Witt Engerstrom, I. (Eds.). (2001). *Rett Disorder and the Developing Brain.* Oxford, UK: Oxford University Press.

von Tetzchner, S. (1997). Communication skills among children with Rett syndrome. *European Child and Adolescent Psychiatry, 6* (suppl 1), 33–37.

Chapter 56

Spastic Cerebral Palsy

Tara L. Whitehill

◆ General Information on Disorder

Cerebral palsy is a nonprogressive condition that occurs as a result of neurological damage prenatally, perinatally, or during the first 2 years of life. It is primarily a disorder of movement and postural control. Although nonprogressive, deterioration in symptoms may occur over time. Spasticity refers to excessive muscle tone and hyperactive reflexes (Yorkston, Beukelman, Strand, & Bell, 1999). Spastic cerebral palsy is classified topologically according to limb involvement: hemiplegia (affecting upper and lower limb ipsilaterally, and accounting for approximately 20%), diplegia (affecting lower limbs more than upper limbs, approximately 20%), and quadriplegia (affecting all four limbs, approximately 30%) (Eicher & Batshaw, 1993). In addition to the primary motor impairment, individuals with spastic cerebral palsy may have cognitive impairments, seizure disorders, and impairments in hearing, vision, speech, language, feeding, and swallowing.

Diagnostic Signs and Symptoms

The diagnosis of spastic cerebral palsy is based on history and neurological examination. It is usually made on the basis of abnormal motor movements, failure to reach developmental motor milestones, or persistence of primitive reflexes (Ashwal et al, 2004; Hodge & Wellman, 1999; Yorkston et al, 1999). A progressive disorder needs to be ruled out and is usually done so on the basis of medical history (Ashwal et al, 2004). Neuroimaging is recommended to establish timing of etiology (i.e., whether neurological injury was prenatal, perinatal, or postnatal), with magnetic resonance imaging (MRI) preferred to computed tomography (CT) (Ashwal et al, 2004). Electroencephalogram (EEG) is recommended only when clinical features suggest epilepsy (Ashwal et al, 2004).

Neuropathology

Spastic cerebral palsy is associated with lesions in the upper motor neuron system. The most common neuropathologies are periventricular leukomalacia and periventricular-intraventricular hemorrhage (Hoon, Belsito, & Negae-Poetscher, 2003; Love, 2000). Findings may differ for preterm versus full-term infants, and according to type of spastic cerebral palsy (Hoon et al, 2003; Koman, Smith, & Shilt, 2004).

Epidemiology

Cerebral palsy affects approximately 2 to 3 per 1000 live births (Winter, Autry, Boyle, & Yeargin-Allsopp, 2002). Spastic cerebral palsy is the most common subtype, accounting for approximately 75% of cases. Prevalence rates for all types of cerebral palsy are higher for babies born preterm or at very low birth weight. Prevalence trends are complex as they are affected by improved maternal health, advances in neonatal care, and improved documentation and national registries (Koman et al, 2004).

Genetics

The true incidence of genetic causes of cerebral palsy is unknown, due to a lack of prospective studies (Ashwal et al, 2004). However, current evidence suggests that metabolic or genetic causes account for less than 5% of cases; genetic studies, therefore, are not routinely recommended (Ashwal et al, 2004).

◆ Speech Impairment Associated with Disorder

The most common speech disorder in cerebral palsy is dysarthria, which occurs in an estimated 31 to 88% of the population (Yorkston et al, 1999). A recent review reported 38% of children with cerebral palsy have articulation disorders and impaired intelligibility (Ashwal et al, 2004). Spastic cerebral palsy is most commonly associated with spastic dysarthria. There is some difficulty with this characterization, which is based on models of acquired disorder in adults, as well as on trunk and limb involvement, which may differ from speech system impairment (Love, 2000). Nevertheless, this terminology is commonly used. The presence and severity of dysarthria, which may range from very mild to complete anarthria, varies according to type of spastic cerebral palsy. For example, spastic diplegia is rarely associated with speech disorder; spastic quadriplegia commonly is. There may be disruptions in any of the speech subsystems: respiratory, laryngeal, velopharyngeal, articulatory, and prosodic (Hardy, 1983; Love, 2000). Murdoch and Horton (1998) characterized children with spastic cerebral palsy as having "imprecise consonants, reduced rate, low pitch, harsh voice, strained-strangled phonation"

(p. 376). There have been several attempts to differentiate spastic and athetoid cerebral palsy on the basis of speech symptoms. Most studies have found no significant differences in type of errors, although speakers with athetosis are frequently more severely affected (but see Workinger & Kent, 1991). The type of dysarthria may be mixed (for example, spastic plus ataxic), and may change over time (Hardy, 1983).

Diagnostic Signs and Symptoms

As noted earlier, a diagnosis of spastic cerebral palsy is normally based on abnormal motor movements. Persistence of infant reflexes, feeding difficulties, and dysfunction in other nonspeech activities may be early signs of dysarthria (Hodge, 2004).

Etiology

Causes of cerebral palsy are classified as prenatal, natal, or postnatal, with postnatal causes accounting for the smallest percentage (Ashwal et al, 2004). Common prenatal causes include intrauterine infection, stroke, toxemia, and placental abruption. Common perinatal etiologies include hypoxic ischemic encephalopathy, kernicterus, and trauma. The most common etiologies for postnatal onset include infection, trauma, and progressive hydrocephalus (Ashwal et al, 2004). Etiological patterns differ for preterm and full-term babies (Ashwal et al, 2004). The precise cause of cerebral palsy is unknown in approximately 50% of cases (Erenberg, 1984).

Neuropathology

Dysarthria in individuals with spastic cerebral palsy can be broadly linked to upper motor neuron damage and the resulting impairment in neuromuscular control of the speech mechanism. More precise correspondence between neuropathology and speech symptoms usually is not possible.

Associated Cognitive, Linguistic, and Communicative Signs and Symptoms

As noted earlier, individuals with spastic cerebral palsy may have cognitive impairment, language delay, or language disorder. A passive communication style may occur as a result of motor limitations or reduced social interactions. Drooling may interfere with acceptance of the individual as a communicative partner (Hodge, 2004).

Special Diagnostic Considerations

Conditions that may complicate speech diagnosis include visual, hearing, or cognitive impairment, and the effect of antiepilepsy medication. Seating posture should be maximized during assessment. Although many individuals with a diagnosis of spastic cerebral palsy exhibit spastic dysarthria, mixed dysarthrias may occur, and apraxia may co-occur (Hodge, 2004).

Treatment

The goal of treatment is to assist the individual to communicate as successfully and independently as possible (Hodge, 2004). Treatment is best delivered in a multidisciplinary context, working closely with professionals such as physical and occupational therapists, and involving family members. Early intervention is recommended, although efficacy is not well demonstrated (Love, 2000). Treatment for individuals with spastic cerebral palsy may focus on language and feeding as well as speech and effective communication strategies. A subsystems approach has been most widely advocated to address dysarthria (Hardy, 1983; Hodge & Wellman, 1999; Love, 2000). Alternative and augmentative communication should be considered for individuals who might benefit from these approaches. Seating and positioning for speech production should be maximized (Love, 2000). There is a need for well-designed efficacy studies for speech and language therapy with this population (Pennington, Goldbart, & Marshall, 2004).

References

Ashwal, S., Russman, B.S., Blasco, P.A., Miller, G., Sandler, A., Shevell, M., & Stevenson, R. (2004). Practice parameter: diagnostic assessment of the child with cerebral palsy: Report of the Quality Standards Subcommittee of the American Academy of Neurology and the Practice Committee of the Child Neurology Society. *Neurology, 62*, 851–863

Eicher, P.S. & Batshaw, M.L. (1993). Cerebral palsy. *Pediatric Clinics of North America, 40*, 537–551

Erenberg, G. (1984). Cerebral palsy. *Postgraduate Medicine, 75*, 87–93

Hardy, J.C. (1983). *Cerebral Palsy*. Englewood Cliffs, NJ: Prentice-Hall

Hodge, M. (2004). Childhood motor speech disorders (known origin). In: R.D. Kent (Ed.), *The MIT Encyclopedia of Communication Disorders* (pp. 200–204). Philadelphia: P.M. Gordon Associates

Hodge, M.M. & Wellman, L. (1999). Management of children with dysarthria. In: A.J. Caruso & E.A. Strand (Eds.), *Clinical Management*

of Motor Speech Disorders in Children (pp. 209–280). New York: Thieme

Hoon, A.H., Belsito, K.M., & Nagae-Poetscher, L.M. (2003). Neuroimaging in spasticity and movement disorders. *Journal of Child Neurology, 18*, S25–39

Koman, L.A., Smith, B.P., & Shilt, J.S. (2004). Cerebral palsy. *Lancet, 363*, 1619–1631

Love, R.J. (2000). *Childhood Motor Speech Disability,* 2nd ed. Boston: Allyn & Bacon

Murdoch, B.E. & Horton, S.K. (1998). Acquired and developmental dysarthria in childhood. In: B.E. Murdoch (Ed.), *Dysarthria: A Physiological Approach to Assessment and Treatment* (pp. 373–427). Cheltenham, UK: Stanley Thornes

Pennington, L., Goldbart, J., & Marshall, J. (2004). Speech and language therapy to improve the communication skills of children with cerebral palsy (Cochrane Review). In: The Cochrane Library, Issue 4. Chichester, UK: John Wiley & Sons

Winter, S., Autry, A., Boyle, C., & Yeargin-Allsopp, M. (2002). Trends in the prevalence of cerebral palsy in a population-based study. *Pediatrics, 110,* 1220–1225

Workinger, M.S. & Kent, R.D. (1991). Perceptual analysis of the dysarthria in children with athetoid and spastic cerebral palsy. In: C.A. Moore, K.M. Yorkston, & D.R. Beukelman (Eds.), *Dysarthria and Apraxia of Speech: Perspectives on Management* (pp. 109–126). Baltimore: Paul H. Brookes

Yorkston, K.M., Beukelman, D.R., Strand, E.A., & Bell, K.R. (1999). *Management of Motor Speech Disorders in Children and Adults,* 2nd ed. Austin, TX: Pro-Ed.

Chapter 57

Systemic Lupus Erythematosus

Ryan C. Branski and Amy H. Kao

◆ General Information on Disorder

Systemic lupus erythematosus (SLE) is an autoimmune inflammatory disease that can affect multiple organ systems. The various clinical manifestations of SLE are a consequence of tissue injury caused by the production of autoantibodies and the formation of complement-fixing immune complexes (Steinberg et al, 1991). The most common clinical features are polyarthritis and dermatitis (Pistiner, Wallace, Nessim, Metzger, & Klinenberg, 1991). Patients with SLE may experience a myriad of symptoms including photosensitivity, oral ulcers, renal diseases, hematological disorders, immunological disorders, and fatigue. Neurological or psychiatric manifestations occur in approximately two thirds of patients (Cook, Wedgwood, Craig, Hartmann, & Janeway, 1960; Iverson, 1993; Madden, 1932).

Diagnostic Signs and Symptoms

The diagnosis of SLE is based primarily on the clinical manifestations of the disease as described by the American College of Rheumatology (Hochberg, 1997). In addition, the analysis of antinuclear antibodies (ANAs) is often used as a screening tool. ANAs occur in over 95% of patients, making their detection a sensitive but not specific screening test for SLE (Hochberg, 1990).

Neuropathology

The neurological sequelae of SLE can affect any part of the nervous system and have been documented in up to 70% of patients (Bruyn, 1995; Hay et al, 1992; Iverson, 1993; Sibley, Olszynski, Decoteau, & Sundaram, 1992). The most common central nervous system (CNS) findings associated with SLE are small vessel ischemic changes and microfocal scarring primarily of the subcortical white matter due to intimal changes in small arterioles (Hanly, Walsh, & Sanglang, 1992). However, stroke or intracranial hemorrhage secondary to arteritis of larger cerebral vessels has also been reported, although infrequently (Weiner & Allen, 1991). Furthermore, inflammatory disease-related damage to the basal ganglia control circuit is implicated in dysarthria associated with SLE. However, movement disorders are relatively rare sequelae of SLE.

Epidemiology

In North America, the prevalence of SLE is approximately 40 per 100,000 persons (Hochberg, 1990). Prevalence and incidence rates are higher in women than in men, and higher in African-Americans, Afro-Caribbeans, Hispanics, and Asians than in Caucasians. Although historically considered fatal, SLE mortality rates have significantly diminished over the past half-century. The estimated 5-year survival of SLE patients has increased from less than 50% to greater than 95% (Borchers, Keen, Shoenfeld, & Gershwin, 2004).

Genetics

The concordance rate in dizygotic twins or siblings is 2 to 5%, six to eight times greater than that for unrelated persons. In monozygotic twins, it is 24 to 58%, about 10 times the rate of dizygotic twins or in siblings (Reichlin, Harley, & Lockshin, 1992).

◆ Speech Impairment Associated with Disorder

The broad scope of pathogenesis associated with SLE may alter speech production on many levels. Vocal fold inflammation or nodular vocal fold lesions have been reported (Burge, Frith, Juniper, & Wojnarowska, 1989; Hosako-Naito et al, 1999; Murano et al, 2001). Respiratory compromise may also limit communicative effectiveness. Dysarthria, characterized by chorea or Parkinson-like manifestations, suggestive of basal ganglia involvement, has been reported (Garcia-Moreno & Chacon, 2002; Olfat, Al-Mayouf, & Muzaffer, 2004). The prevalence of peripheral neuropathy is less common and often subclinical. Most frequently, bilateral polyneuropathy with both motor and sensory involvement is seen (Campello, Almarcegui, Velilla, Hortells, & Oliveros, 2001).

Diagnostic Signs and Symptoms

Compared with the CNS, the peripheral nervous system (PNS) is clinically less affected. Manifestation of systemic autoimmune disease may include choreiform movements resembling Sydenham's or Huntington's chorea. In addition, Parkinson-like manifestations of juvenile SLE including hypophonia have been reported.

Etiology

The manifestations of SLE are related to the inflammatory process associated with the disease. Mucosal inflammatory disease can cause dysphonia. This dysphonia may be exacerbated by arthritic conditions of the cricoarytenoid joint (Curley, Byron, & Bates, 1986; Karim, Ahmed, Siddiqui, Marder, & Mattana, 2002; Nossent & Berend, 1998). Cognitively based communication deficits are likely attributable to transient ischemic attacks or ischemic stroke (Esdaile et al, 2001; Manzi et al, 1997; Roman et al, 2003; Ward, 1999). Communication deficits in patients with SLE may be associated with the distribution of the CNS and PNS pathology throughout which SLE expresses itself.

Neuropathology

The neuropathology of disordered speech production resulting from SLE is directly related to the disease process.

Associated Cognitive, Linguistic, and Communicative Signs and Symptoms

The pathogenesis of cognitive dysfunction is likely multifactorial, accounting for the broad range of deficits. Transient ischemic attacks and ischemic stroke may account for the deficits. However, the majority of patients SLE present wih cognitive-linguistic deficits without evidence of cerebrovascular events. Neuropsychometric testing typically reveals diminished performance on attention, memory, language, and psychomotor speed tasks (Sanna, Bertolaccini, & Mathieu, 2003). The diffuse nature of neurological involvement associated with the cerebrovascular sequelae of SLE may yield a myriad of cognitive or language deficits. In addition, one fourth of patients with SLE experience sensorineural hearing loss (Kastanioudakis et al, 2002). Swallowing disorders may be secondary to neuropathy or psychiatric manifestations of the disease.

Special Diagnostic Considerations

Assessment of the speech production system in SLE does not require special procedures beyond those of the typical motor speech examination. However, because the course of the disease may change over time or with treatment, frequent periodic evaluations are indicated.

Treatment

Treatment of patients with SLE varies greatly depending on the presentation and severity of symptoms associated with the disease. Because speech, voice, and cognitive function may be affected in patients with SLE, treatment should be tailored to each individual. Regardless of the deficit, compensatory strategies should be employed to maximize communication. For patients with more advanced neurological disease with resultant limitations in communicative abilities, treatment should include counseling the caregiver on strategies to facilitate communicative interaction and in some cases alternative and augmentative communication (AAC) may be appropriate. From a medical standpoint, the primary treatment is immunosuppressive therapy including steroids. In addition, emerging data may suggest a role for intravenous immunoglobulin (Milstone, Meyers, & Elia, 2005).

References

Borchers, A.T., Keen, C.L., Shoenfeld, Y., & Gershwin, M.E. (2004). Surviving the butterfly and the wolf: mortality trends in systemic lupus erythematosus. *Autoimmunity Reviews, 3,* 423–453

Bruyn, G.A. (1995). Controversies in lupus: nervous system involvement. *Annals of the Rheumatic Diseases, 54,* 159–167

Burge, S.M., Frith, P.A., Juniper, R.P., & Wojnarowska, F. (1989). Mucosal involvement in systemic and chronic cutaneous lupus erythematosus. *British Journal of Dermatology, 121,* 727–741

Campello, I., Almarcegui, C., Velilla, J., Hortells, J.L., & Oliveros, A. (2001). Peripheral neuropathy in systemic lupus erythematosus. *Revue Neurologique, 33,* 27–30

Cook, C.D., Wedgwood, R.J., Craig, J.M., Hartmann, J.R., & Janeway, C.A. (1960). Systemic lupus erythematosus. Description of 37 cases in children and a discussion of endocrine therapy in 32 of the cases. *Pediatrics, 26,* 570–585

Curley, J.W., Byron, M.A., & Bates, G.J. (1986). Crico-arytenoid joint involvement in acute systemic lupus erythematosus. *Journal of Laryngology and Otology, 100,* 727–732

Esdaile J.M., Abrahamowicz M, Grodzicky T, Li Y, Panaritis C, du Berger R, Cote R, Grover S.A., Fortin PR, Clarke, A.E. & Senecal J.L. (2001). Traditional Framinghan risk factors fail to fully account for accelerated atherosclerosis in systemic lupus erythematosus. Arthritis Rheum. 44(10);2331–7.

Garcia-Moreno, J.M. & Chacon, J. (2002). Juvenile parkinsonism as a manifestation of systemic lupus erythematosus: case report and review of the literature. *Movement Disorders, 17*(6), 1329–1335

Hanly, J.G., Walsh, N.M.G., & Sanglang, V. (1992). Brain pathology in systemic lupus erythematosus. *Journal of Rheumatology, 19,* 732–741

Hay, E.M., Black, D., Huddy, A., Creed, F., Tomenson, B., Bernstein, R.M., et al. (1992). Psychiatric disorder and cognitive impairment in systemic lupus erythematosus. *Arthritis and Rheumatism, 35,* 411–416

Hochberg, M. C. (1990). Systemic lupus erythematosus. *Rheumatic Disease Clinics of North America, 16,* 617–639

Hosako-Naito, Y., Tayama, N., Niimi, S., Aotsuka, S., Miyaji, M., Oka, T., et al. (1999). Diagnosis and physiopathology of laryngeal deposits in autoimmune disease. *ORL Journal of Otorhinolaryngol and Related Specialities, 61,* 151–157

Iverson, G.L. (1993). Psychopathology associated with systemic lupus erythematosus: a methodological review. *Seminars in Arthritis and Rheumatism, 22,* 242–251

Karim, A., Ahmed, S., Siddiqui, R., Marder, G.S., & Mattana, J. (2002). Severe upper airway obstruction from cricoarytenoiditis as the sole presenting manifestation of a systemic lupus erythematosus flare. *Chest, 121,* 990–993

Kastanioudakis, I., Ziavra, N., Voulgari, P.V., Exarchakos, G., Skevas, A., & Drosos, A.A. (2002). Ear involvement in systemic lupus erythematosus patients: a comparative study. *Journal of Laryngology and Otology, 116,* 103–107

Madden, J.F. (1932). Acute disseminated lupus erythematosus. *Archives of Dermatology and Syphilis, 25,* 854–875

Manzi S, Meilahn E.N., Rairie J.E., Conte C.G., Medsger T.A. Jr, Jansen-McWilliams L, D'Agostino R.B., & Kuller L.H. (1997). Age-specific incidence rates of myocardial infarction and angina in women with systemic lupus erythematosus: comparison with the Framingham Study. Am J Epidemiol 145(5);408–15.

Milstone, A.M., Meyers, K., & Elia, J. (2005). Treatment of acute neuropsychiatric lupus with intravenous immunoglobulin (IVIG): a case report and review of the literature. *Clinical Rheumatology, 24,* 394–397

Murano, E., Hosako-Naito, Y., Tayama, N., Oka, T., Miyaji, M., Kumada, M., et al. (2001). Bamboo node: primary vocal fold lesion as evidence autoimmune disease. *Journal of the Voice, 15*(3), 441–450

Nossent, J.C., & Berend, K. (1998). Cricoarytenoiditis in systemic lupus erythematosus. *Scandinavian Journal of Rheumatology, 27,* 237–238

Olfat, M.O., Al-Mayouf, S.M., & Muzaffer, M.A. (2004). Pattern of neuropsychiatric manifestations and outcome in juvenile systemic lupus erythematosus. *Clinical Rheumatology, 23,* 395–399

Pistiner, M., Wallace, D.J., Nessim, S., Metzger, A.L., & Klinenberg, J.R. (1991). Lupus erythematosus in the 1980s: a survey of 570 patients. *Seminars in Arthritis and Rheumatism, 21,* 55–64

Reichlin, M., Harley, J.B., & Lockshin, M.D. (1992). Serologic studies of monozygotic twins with systemic lupus erythematosus. *Arthritis and Rheumatism, 35,* 457–464

Roman M.J., Shanker B.A., Davis A, Locksin M.D., Sammaritano L, Simantov R, Crow M.K., Schwartz J.E., Paget S.A., Devereux R.B., & Salmon J.E. (2003). Prevalence and correlates of accelerated atherosclerosis in system lupus erythematous. N Engl J Med 349(25);2399–406.

Sanna, G., Bertolaccini, M.L., & Mathieu, A. (2003). Central nervous system lupus: a clinical approach to therapy. *Lupus, 12,* 935–942. ACR Ad Hoc Committee on Neuropsychiatric Lupus Nomenclature. The American College of Rheumatology nomenclature and case definitions for neuropsychiatric lupus syndromes (1999). *Arthritis and Rheumatism, 42,* 599–608

Sibley, J.T., Olszynski, W.P., Decoteau, W.E., & Sundaram, M.B. (1992). The incidence and prognosis of central nervous system disease in systemic lupus erythematosus. *Journal of Rheumatology, 19,* 47–52

Steinberg, A.D., Gourley, M.F., Klinman, D.M., Tsokos, G.C., Scott, D.E., & Kreig, A.M. (1991). Systemic lupus erythematosus. *Annals of Internal Medicine, 115,* 548–559

Ward M.M. (1999). Premature morbidity from cardiovascular and cerebrovascular diseases in women with systemic lupus ertythematosus. Arthritis Rheum 42(2);338–46.

Weiner, D.K. & Allen, N.B. (1991). Large vessel vasculitis of the central nervous system in systemic lupus erythematosus: report and review of the literature. *Journal of Rheumatology, 18,* 748–751

Chapter 58

Tardive Dyskinesia

Sakina S. Drummond

◆ General Information on Disorder

Tardive dyskinesia (TD) is a late-onset, acquired movement disorder resulting from adverse reaction to prolonged use of neuroleptic (antipsychotic) drugs. Although such drugs have been prescribed for psychiatric disorders since the 1930s, attention has been given to their adverse effects since the 1960s, when the term *tardive dyskinesia* was coined. Sometimes identified as Meige syndrome, TD is a form of focal dystonia involving the cranial-cervical region (Ferguson, 1992).

Diagnostic Signs and Symptoms

A history of neuroleptic treatment with acquired dystonia aids in the diagnosis of TD. Involuntary dyskinesic movements are commonly observed in the orofacial region involving the lips, tongue, face, palate, mandible, and pharynx, and are therefore also known as the buccolingual-masticatory syndrome. Related inconsistent, jerky movements are manifested as lip or tongue smacking, facial tics, or eye blinking behaviors. Approximately 78% of individuals with TD also exhibit some degree of limb dyskinesia seen as jerky finger and hand movements, ankle and feet rotation, or involuntary adduction and abduction of thighs. Occasionally, other dystonic movements such as tremor at rest, choreiform movements, or myoclonus are also been observed in TD. The dystonic symptoms are affected by attention, emotion, posture, and activity, and tend to worsen under anxiety-producing situations. The duration of dyskinesic episodes typically last for $1\frac{1}{2}$ to 2 seconds, and may cease during drowsiness and sleep. The onset of symptoms may progress from mild abnormal movements during the first year of neuroleptic treatment to a progressive increase in severity; the diagnosis of probable TD, however, may not be made until the end of the second year after the first sign is noted (Bell & Smith, 1978; Drummond & Fitzpatrick, 2004; Gerratt, Goetz, & Fisher, 1984).

Neuropathology

Macroscopically, TD is associated with psychosis. Microscopically, the dystonia results from increased dopaminergic and noradrenergic activity in the basal ganglia, specifically the postsynaptic receptors on the caudate and putamen. Superimposed lesion of the basal ganglia in these individuals has been shown to reduce the involuntary movements, which also implicates the involvement of the basal ganglia and the extrapyramidal system as the site of lesion for TD (Fabbrini, Barbanti, & Aurilia, 2001; Walters, Katchen, Fleishman, Chokroverty, & Duvoisin, 1986).

Epidemiology

An estimated 30% of individuals who take antipsychotic medication develop TD, and this number increases to 50% for individuals 65 years and older. The incidence and severity of TD is greater in women, and a linear correlation exists between age and severity of symptoms. The symptoms of TD appear earlier among older patients who are also less likely to show a reversal of symptoms following cessation of the neuroleptics. Prevalence data show a wide variation due to factors such as type, dose, and duration of neuroleptic treatment, and the population studied. Other risk factors include alcohol consumption, diabetes, and smoking (Brown & White, 1991; Fabbrini, et al, 2001).

Genetics

There is no genetic basis for the onset of TD because it is a drug-induced disorder.

◆ Speech Impairment Associated with Disorder

About one half of individuals with TD are diagnosed with mild to moderate dysarthria with symptoms dispersed across four of the five speech processes: respiration, articulation, phonation, and prosody. Reduced breath support and speech intelligibility, as well as abnormal vocal quality and dysprosodic speech, characterize their dysarthria (Drummond & Fitzpatrick, 2004; Ferguson, 1992; Gerratt et al, 1984; Khan, Jampala, Dong, Chandragupta, & Vedak, 1994; Laporta, Archambault, Ross-Chourinard, & Chourinard, 1990).

Diagnostic Signs and Symptoms

An assessment of the five speech processes helps identify the dysarthric symptoms. Respiratory insufficiency is reflected through reduced phonation time and vital capacity. Phonatory symptoms are perceived as intermittent pitch breaks, reduced pitch range, audible inspiration, strained-strangled and harsh vocal quality, and vocal tremor. Resonatory problems are infrequent, and if present, they are observed as reduced velar movement and hypernasality. Articulatory imprecision contribute to impaired speech intelligibility. Finally, impaired speech prosody is reflected through use of short phrases, slow speaking rate, and disrupted/dysfluent speech (Drummond & Fitzpatrick, 2004; Ferguson, 1992; Gerratt et al, 1984; Khan et al, 1994; Laporta et al, 1990).

Etiology

The dystonic movements occur inconsistently as momentary arrests of lower facial and mandibular muscles. These motor problems tend to exacerbate when performing voluntary oral movements and in connected speech.

Neuropathology

The focal dyskinesia involving vocal tract musculature interferes with efficient speech production. The fluctuation in observed dysarthric symptoms across multiple examinations implicates possible interactions between the underlying psychiatric disorder, its pharmacological intervention, and the resultant neuromotor problems (Drummond & Fitzpatrick, 2004).

Associated Cognitive, Linguistic, and Communicative Signs and Symptoms

Although there is no formal report linking TD to linguistic-cognitive communication problems, we observed two opposing affective reactions from the same individual when reading the "Grandfather" passage. During one reading, there was a progressive increase in severity and frequency of the dystonia leading to crying and refusal to complete the task; in a subsequent reading, however, the subject had no dystonic episodes and laughed when the reading the final sentence of the passage (Drummond & Fitzpatrick, 2004). Such inconsistent reactions may perhaps be a component of the primary psychiatric diagnosis and not a feature of the TD.

Special Diagnostic Considerations

Either mild or mild-to-moderate severe dysarthria with fluctuating problems for some measures within the four speech processes are possible across examinations. Of these, respiratory symptoms may stabilize and improve, whereas those for phonation, articulation, and prosody may persist. Speech symptoms are compounded in the presence of pain in the tongue, mandible, and temporomandibular joint. Although voluntary speech and nonspeech lingual and mandibular movements are frequently determined as "impaired," they do not adversely affect overall speech intelligibility or functional communication (Drummond & Fitzpatrick, 2004).

Treatment

Medical management via subcutaneous botulinum toxin injections into the superficial facial muscles has yielded temporary relief of the dystonia; however, its impact on speech is unknown. Because patients often need to continue to take neuroleptics, there may be little done to prevent the speech symptoms; however, there is some indication of improvement and stabilization of speech symptoms upon cessation of the neuroleptic treatment (Drummond & Fitzpatrick, 2004).

References

Bell, R.C. & Smith R. (1978). Tardive dyskinesia: characterization and prevalence in a statewide system. *Journal of Clinical Psychiatry, 39*, 39–47

Brown, K.W. & White T. (1991). The psychological consequences of tardive dyskinesia, the effect of drug induced parkinsonism and the topography of the dyskinetic movements. *British Journal of Psychiatry, 159*, 399–403

Drummond, S. & Fitzpatrick, A. (2004). Speech and swallowing performances in tardive dyskinesia: a case study. *Journal of Medical Speech Language Pathology, 12*, 9–19

Fabbrini, G., Barbanti, P., & Aurilia, C. (2001). Tardive dyskinesia in the elderly. *International Journal of Geriatric Psychiatry, 16*, S19–S23

Ferguson, A. (1992). Speech control in persistent tardive dyskinesia: a case study. *European Journal of Disorders of Communication, 27*, 89–93

Gerratt, B.R., Goetz, C., & Fisher, H. (1984). Speech abnormalities in tardive dyskinesia. *Archives of Neurology, 41*, 273–276

Khan, R., Jampala, V., Dong, K., & Vedak, C. (1994). Speech abnormalities in tardive dyskinesia. *American Journal of Psychiatry, 151*, 760–762

Laporta, M., Archambault, D., Ross-Chourinard, A., & Chourinard, G. (1990). Articulatory impairment associated with TD. *Journal of Nervous & Mental Disease, 178*, 660–662

Walters, A.S., Katchen, M., Fleishman, J., Chokroverty, S. & Duvoisin, R. (1987). Role of the basal ganglia and cerebral cortex in tardive dyskinesia: evidence from cerebrovascular accident. *Journal of Neurology, Neurosurgery, and Psychiatry, 50*, 367–368

Additional Reading

Sachdev, P.S. (2000). The current status of tardive dyskinesia. *Australian & New Zealand Journal of Psychiatry, 34*, 355–369

Chapter 59

Traumatic Brain Injury

Edwin Maas, Skott E. Freedman, and Donald A. Robin

◆ General Information on Disorder

Traumatic brain injury (TBI) is defined as brain damage resulting from sudden movement or trauma to the head (Kolb & Whishaw, 1990). TBI can result from closed-head injury (CHI) or open-head injury (OHI), and may cause a range of potentially long-lasting physical and cognitive impairments (Hammond, Hart, Bushnik, Corrigan, & Sasser, 2004), depending on the site, nature, and severity of the impact.

Diagnostic Signs and Symptoms

Signs and symptoms diagnostic of TBI may include loss of consciousness, headache, amnesia, anosognosia, aphasia, personality changes, depression, epilepsy, and sensory and motor disorders (Hammond et al, 2004; Kolb & Whishaw, 1990).

Neuropathology

CHI and OHI injury result in neurological damage in five distinct ways (Kolb & Whishaw, 1990). First, there is often focal damage where the brain impacts the cranium (at impact site and the opposite side). Second, diffuse cortical and subcortical damage occurs, including axon shearing (disrupting pathways such as the corpus callosum, basal ganglia control circuits) and cutting of cranial nerve fibers. Depending on which nerves are involved, a variety of dysarthric speech characteristics may be perceived. Third, ischemia or hemorrhage may disrupt blood supply. Fourth, pressure from hematomas, brain swelling, or edema may damage the brain. Fifth, in OHI, damage may also occur due to penetration of brain tissue and possible infection.

Epidemiology

Each year in the United States, 1.4 million people suffer a TBI, the majority of whom are male (Guerrero, Thurman, & Sniezek, 2000; National Institute of Neurological Disorders and Stroke, 2004). Although TBI can occur at any age, the incidence is highest among children, for whom falls are the most common cause of TBI, and individuals between 15 and 24, for whom the main causes are motor vehicle accidents and violence (Guerrero et al, 2000; National Institute of Neurological Disorders and Stroke, 2004). The leading causes for adults of ages 25 to 44 are motor vehicle accidents and intentional injuries; for persons 45 and over, falls are more frequently the cause of TBI (Guerrero et al, 2000).

Genetics

Because TBI results from trauma to the head, genetic factors play no direct role.

◆ Speech Impairment Associated with Disorder

Although clinicians tend to focus on language and social-pragmatic difficulties rather than motor speech impairments, approximately one third of all TBI victims suffer from motor speech disorders (Stierwalt & Robin, 1997). All types of motor speech disorders may occur as a result of TBI, affecting any of the speech subsystems depending on the area of damage (Wang, Kent, Duffy, Thomas, & Weismer, 2004). Dysarthrias occur more commonly than apraxia of speech (Duffy, 2005).

Diagnostic Signs and Symptoms

Perceptual studies of motor speech disorders in TBI often report overall reduced intelligibility (Cahill, Murdoch, & Theodoros, 2002; Wang et al, 2004), a slowed speech rate (Cahill et al, 2002; Campbell & Dollaghan, 1995; Wang et al, 2004), an increased speech rate (Wang et al, 2004), distortions of consonants and vowels (Cahill et al, 2002), voice quality changes (Cahill, Murdoch, & Theodoros, 2003; Wang et al, 2004), and hypernasality (Cahill et al, 2002). For example, when two clinicians rated the speech of 16 children with TBI and dysarthria on 33 dimensions (Cahill et al, 2002), the TBI group was judged to display abnormalities of prosody (rate, phrase length, pitch and loudness variation, stress patterns), respiration (reduced breath support for speech), resonation (hypernasality), articulation (phoneme distortions and prolongations), and intelligibility. Dysarthric speakers exhibited more glottal fry (low-pitched phonation with audible individual vocal fold vibrations) than controls.

Several studies supplemented perceptual observations with acoustic measures (Campbell & Dollaghan, 1995; Wang et al, 2004). The most detailed acoustic analysis to date of TBI-induced dysarthric speech was conducted by Wang et al (2004), who analyzed speech rate and quality in seven adults with TBI, using both conversational speech and alternating motion rates (AMRs). The TBI group demonstrated a reduced syllable rate (mostly due to increased syllable durations) and temporal irregularities, with a high correlation between syllable rate during AMRs and conversation. Qualitative acoustic analyses for each speaker revealed a variety of deviant speech characteristics (e.g., spirantization, altered voice quality, plosive abnormalities).

Physiological measures of nonspeech tasks have been used to relate performance on such tasks with speech characteristics, including intelligibility (McHenry, Minton, Wilson, & Post, 1994; Stierwalt et al, 1994). McHenry et al found no relation between intelligibility and maximum voluntary contraction, whereas Stierwalt et al found that articulatory precision was related to tongue endurance in a task requiring maintenance of 50% of a participant's maximal force. Cahill et al (2003) compared speech phonation in children with and without TBI using perceptual, and laryngeal aerodynamic measures. Laryngeal function was mostly normal, contrary to often reported voice abnormalities in adults with TBI (Wang et al, 2004). This discrepancy may be due to different etiologies or developmental changes (Cahill et al, 2003).

Kinematic analyses have also been used to examine speech production in children and adults with TBI. For example, Murdoch and Goozée (2003) studied four children with dysarthria secondary to TBI using electromagnetic articulography (EMA). All children exhibited reduced speech rate and phoneme prolongation, but it was difficult to determine perceptually which aspects of the speech movements were prolonged. Consistent with perceptual judgments, EMA analyses revealed increased word durations. Interestingly, two of the four children showed normal kinematic patterns for consonants (suggesting increased word durations resulted from vowel lengthening), and the other two showed abnormal consonant kinematics (suggesting difficulties with consonants). Furthermore, the latter two children showed different kinematic patterns (abnormal velocity or abnormal displacement), potentially indicating different impairments or compensatory strategies.

Etiology

Motor speech disorders resulting from TBI may be caused by focal cortical and subcortical lesions and diffuse axonal damage. Each etiology may lead to distinct speech characteristics depending on structures, circuits, and cranial nerves affected.

Neuropathology

Common lesion sites affecting speech involve the cerebellum, which may result in ataxic dysarthria (Wang et al, 2004), the basal ganglia, which may lead to hypokinetic dysarthria (Cahill et al, 2002; Wang et al, 2004), or hyperkinetic dysarthria. Spastic dysarthria can occur and any of the cranial nerves can be involved.

Associated Cognitive, Linguistic, and Communicative Signs and Symptoms

Due to the diverse nature of lesions in TBI, a wide spectrum of cognitive and linguistic symptoms may co-occur with a motor speech disorder.

Special Diagnostic Considerations

Concomitant impairments of cognition and language may interfere with testing, including deficits of memory, attention and executive functions, and socially inappropriate behavior.

Treatment

Despite a relative dearth of treatment studies for dysarthria in TBI, the entire range of interventions for motor speech disorders of other etiologies is in principle applicable (see Chapter 16). Rather than reiterate these interventions, several concomitant problems resulting from TBI require consideration in treatment of motor speech disorders in this population. Many patients with TBI have anosognosia (McHenry et al, 1994), which may negatively affect motivation. Patients with TBI also may display emotional-behavioral problems and may be socially inappropriate, aggressive, or depressed (Hammond et al, 2004). These emotional complications may interfere with establishing rapport and with treatment itself. Many patients with TBI have anterograde amnesia (Kolb & Whishaw, 1990), which may reduce the effectiveness of explicitly taught strategies. Patients with TBI often show reduced speed of cognitive processing (Campbell & Dollaghan, 1995), which can affect stimulus and feedback processing. Patients with TBI often exhibit deficits of attention and executive functions (Robin, Max, Stierwalt, Guenzer, & Lindgren, 1999), possibly affecting the structure and duration of treatment.

References

Cahill, L.M., Murdoch, B.E., & Theodoros, D.G. (2002). Perceptual analysis of speech following traumatic brain injury in childhood. *Brain Injury, 16,* 415–446

Cahill, L.M., Murdoch, B.E., & Theodoros, D.G. (2003). Perceptual and instrumental analysis of laryngeal function after traumatic brain injury in childhood. *Journal of Head Trauma Rehabilitation, 18,* 268–283

Campbell, T.F. & Dollaghan, C.A. (1995). Speaking rate, articulatory speed, and linguistic processing in children and adolescents with severe traumatic brain injury. *Journal of Speech and Hearing Research, 38,* 864–875

Duffy, J.R. (2005). *Motor Speech Disorders: Substrates, Differential Diagnosis, and Management,* 2nd ed. St. Louis: Mosby-Year Book

Guerrero, J.L., Thurman, D.J., & Sniezek, J.E. (2000). Emergency department visits associated with traumatic brain injury: United States, 1995–1996. *Brain Injury, 14,* 181–186

Hammond, F.M., Hart, T., Bushnik, T., Corrigan, J.D., & Sasser, H. (2004). Change and predictors of change in communication, cognition, and social function between 1 and 5 years after traumatic brain injury. *Journal of Head Trauma Rehabilitation, 19,* 314–328

Kolb, B. & Whishaw, I.Q. (1990). *Fundamentals of Human Neuropsychology,* 3rd ed. New York: W.H. Freeman

McHenry, M.A., Minton, J.T., Wilson, R.L., & Post, Y.V. (1994). Intelligibility and nonspeech orofacial strength and force control following traumatic brain injury. *Journal of Speech and Hearing Research, 37,* 1271–1283

Murdoch, B.E. & Goozée, J.V. (2003). EMA analysis of tongue function in children with dysarthria following traumatic brain injury. *Brain Injury, 17,* 79–93

National Institute of Neurological Disorders and Stroke. (2004). Traumatic Brain Injury. http://www.ninds.nih.gov/disorders/tbi/detail_tbi.htm

Robin, D.A., Max, J.E., Stierwalt, J.A.G., Guenzer, L.C., & Lindgren, S.D. (1999). Sustained attention in children and adolescents with traumatic brain injury. *Aphasiology, 13,* 701–708

Stierwalt, J.G., Robin, D.A., Solomon, N.P., Weiss, A.L., Max, J.E., & Luschei, E.S. (1994). Dysarthria following traumatic brain injury: strength, endurance and speech ability. Paper presented at the Conference on Motor Speech, Sedona, AZ

Stierwalt, J.A.G. & Robin, D.A. (1997). Predictors of outcome in TBI. Paper presented at the Clinical Aphasiology Conference, Bigfork, MT

Wang, Y.-T., Kent, R.D., Duffy, J.R., Thomas, J.E., & Weismer, G. (2004). Alternating motion rate as an index of speech motor disorder in traumatic brain injury. *Clinical Linguistics & Phonetics, 18,* 57–84

Chapter 60

Vascular Dementia

Bruce E. Murdoch and Brooke-Mai Whelan

◆ General Information on Disorder

Vascular dementia (VaD) is the second most common form of dementia after Alzheimer's disease (AD) (Jorm & Jolley, 1998) and is defined clinically by sudden onset of cognitive decline, stepwise deterioration, and focal neurological findings (Erkinjuntti & Rockwood, 2003). Although historically VaD was termed multiinfarct dementia (MID), more recently the concept of VaD has been extended beyond the original concept of MID as introduced by Hachinski, Lassen, and Marshall (1974) to include all forms of cognitive loss due to cerebrovascular disease. Consequently, VaD now encompasses a group of clinical syndromes related to different vascular mechanisms and changes in the brain, with different causes and clinical manifestations.

Neuropathology

VaD results from ischemic, hypoperfusive, or hemorrhagic brain lesions that are associated with numerous clinical syndromes. The major subcategories of ischemic VaD according to the current clinicopathological classification include large-vessel vascular dementia and subcortical ischemic vascular dementia (SIVD). Large-vessel VaD includes MID and strategic single-infarct dementia. The former is associated with multiple large complete infarcts occurring secondary to diseases of the extracranial arteries that can involve both cortical and subcortical structures, usually with perifocal incomplete infarction involving the cerebral white matter. Strategic single-infarct dementia, in contrast, involves a single infarct in functionally critical areas of the brain, such as the angular gyrus, thalamus, territory of the anterior cerebral artery, and others. SIVD involves small-vessel disease as the chief vascular etiology in which lacunar infarction and ischemic white matter lesions, particularly involving the periventricular white matter and frontal region, are the primary types of brain lesions and the primary location of lesions is subcortical. Two clinical syndromes related to SIVD are "lacunar state" and subcortical arteriosclerotic encephalopathy (Binswanger disease). The clinical manifestations of SIVD result from interruption of parallel circuits from the prefrontal cortex to the basal ganglia and corresponding thalamocortical connections by ischemic lesions.

Diagnostic Signs and Symptoms

The major clinical features of MID include an abrupt onset of focal neurological symptoms and signs, along with cortical cognitive impairments such as aphasia, apraxia, and agnosia. MID evolves slowly or in association with silent infarction, with long plateaus between events and day-to-day fluctuations in severity (Erkinjuntti, 1999). In contrast, the clinical features of strategic single-infarct dementia vary with the location of the lesion in cortical or subcortical regions. Memory impairment, impaired executive function, confusion, and fluctuating levels of consciousness may occur. Behavioral changes may include apathy, lack of spontaneity, and perseveration (Desmond et al, 1999).

The clinical manifestations of SIVD can be separated into two groups. In the first, symptomatic lacunes present with acute sensorimotor deficits (e.g., pure motor hemiplegia, pseudobulbar palsy, etc.). In the second, subacute manifestations, usually associated with lesions that injure specific prefrontal subcortical circuits, include cognitive impairment, personality and mood disorders, gait disturbances (small step gait), motor dysfunction (e.g., dysarthria, dysphagia, and mild focal motor deficits), and urinary symptoms. A prominent feature of the cognitive impairment is dysexecutive syndrome associated with impairment of goal formulation, initiation, planning, organizing, sequencing, executing, and abstracting.

A diagnosis of VaD can rarely be reached in the absence of vascular lesions (e.g., territorial infarcts, lacunes, and white matter changes) as demonstrated by brain imaging. Consequently a radiological examination is vital as a confirmatory test. Infarcts in specific arterial territories (as seen in large-vessel VaD), lacunar infarcts, and white matter disease (as seen in small-vessel VaD) can be detected by both computed tomography (CT) and magnetic resonance imaging (MRI) of the brain, but the two methods differ in sensitivity, with MRI having greater sensitivity for detection of white matter lesions.

Epidemiology

VaD is predominantly a disease of elderly people and is the second most common single cause of dementia, accounting for 10 to 50% of cases (Herbert & Brayne, 1995). According to Herbert and Brayne, the prevalence of VaD ranges from 1.2 to 4.2% in persons aged 65 years and older, whereas reports of the incidence of VaD vary from 6 to 12 cases per year per 1000 persons of ages 70 years and older. The incidence of VaD increases with increasing age, with men and women being equally affected.

Genetics

Although not all subtypes of VaD are inherited, genetic varieties do exist. The most common genetic form of VaD is a cerebral autosomal dominant arteriopathy with subcortical infarcts and leukoencephalopathy (CADSIL, or familial Binswanger disease). This autosomal dominant disorder of small cerebral vessels maps to chromosome 19q12 and is caused by mutations in the *Notch 3* gene.

◆ Speech Impairment Associated with Disorder

Although the presence of motor speech impairments has been noted in cases of VaD, they have only been superficially described. Powell, Cummings, Hill, and Benson (1988) reported that 14 of the 18 VaD subjects in their study exhibited some speech abnormality, with only four having normal articulation. All five of the dysarthria measures used by Powell et al together with phrase length and speech melody were abnormal to some degree. Given the reported diversity of lesion sites associated with VaD (e.g., periventricular white matter, cerebral cortex), the profile of deviant speech dimension exhibited by persons with VaD could be expected to vary from case to case but with a predominance of deviant speech features typically associated with spastic dysarthria as a result of involvement of the upper motor neuron pathways. It is noteworthy that pseudobulbar palsy has been reported to occur on occasion as part of the symptom complex of VaD.

Etiology

The etiology of the abnormal speech behaviors observed in VaD is damage secondary to vascular events to the upper motor neuron supply of the muscles of the speech production mechanism. The damage can occur at either the cortical or subcortical level of the cerebral hemispheres.

Neuropathology

Focal motor signs, including dysarthria in VaD, in some cases can be the result of territorial infarcts that involve the primary motor cortex. In the majority of cases, however, persistent dysarthria in VaD is most likely the outcome of bilateral damage to the corticobulbar tracts by lacunar infarcts in the subcortical frontal region or white matter lesions that interrupt pyramidal tract fibers in the periventricular white matter.

Associated Cognitive, Linguistic, and Communicative Signs and Symptoms

A stepwise decline in cognitive function is a major characteristic of VaD. Although overt aphasia is an uncommon clinical sign of VaD, individual cases may exhibit a range of "aphasic deficits" including word-finding difficulties, word fluency deficits, and high-level language dysfunction (Murdoch & Lethlean, 1996). These latter deficits may include problems with verbal explanation, verbal reasoning, reconstruction of sentences, the formation of inferences, and the interpretation of absurdities, ambiguities, and metaphors (Murdoch & Lethlean, 1996). Hier, Hagenlocker, and Shindler (1985) investigated patients with VaD and reported the presence of what they called a "brocoid" pattern of speech output characterized by a decrease in syntactic complexity (e.g., few subordinate clauses), shortened utterance length, diminished total and unique words, and increased sentence fragmentation.

Special Diagnostic Considerations

The presence of motor speech anomalies, especially articulatory deficits and abnormal speech melody, in VaD may aid in the differential diagnosis of this condition from dementia of the Alzheimer type (DAT) (Powell et al, 1988). Whereas the descending motor pathways, as evidenced by focal motor signs (e.g., dysarthria, pseudobulbar palsy, etc.) appear to be compromised at an early stage in VaD, they appear to be spared for most of the course of DAT. Conversely, although language impairments do occur in VaD, they may not be as marked as in DAT.

Treatment

VaD is eventually fatal. Currently there is no approved symptomatic pharmacological treatment of VaD despite numerous compounds having been purported to be useful in the symptomatic treatment of VaD, including antithrombotics, ergot alkaloids, nootropics, thyrotropin-releasing hormone analogue, gingko biloba extracts, plasma viscosity drugs, hyperbaric oxygen, antioxidants, and serotonin, among others. Other drugs that have been the subject of controlled clinical trials include central anticholinesterase inhibitors such as donepezil and galanthamine.

In the acute stages of VaD prior to significant cognitive decline, associated motor speech impairments can be treated using traditional methods for upper motor neuron dysarthria. However, as the decline in cognitive executive function proceeds, treatment goals need to focus on counseling for caregivers and procedures to prolong communicative function and to maximize any residual communicative abilities.

References

Desmond, D.W., Erkinjuntti, T., Sano, M., Cummings, J.L., Bowler, J.V., Pasquier, F., Moroney, J.T., Ferris, S.H., Stern, Y., Sachdev, P.S., & Hachinski, V. (1999). The cognitive syndrome of vascular dementia: implications for clinical trials. *Alzheimer Disease and Associated Disorders*, suppl 3, S21–S29

Erkinjuntti, T. (1999). Cerebrovascular dementia: pathophysiology, diagnosis and treatment. *CNS Drugs, 12*, 35–48

Erkinjuntti, T. & Rockwood, K. (2003). Vascular dementia. *Seminars in Clinical Neuropsychiatry, 8*, 37–45

Hachinski, V.C., Lassen, N.A., & Marshall, J. (1974). Multi-infarct dementia: a cause of mental deterioration in the elderly. *Lancet, 2,* 207–209

Hebert, R. & Brayne, C. (1995). Epidemiology of vascular dementia. *Neuroepidemiology, 14,* 240–257

Hier, D.B., Hagenlocker, K., & Shindler, A.G. (1985). Language disintegration in dementia: effects of etiology and severity. *Brain and Language, 25,* 117–133

Jorm, A.F. & Jolley, D. (1998). The incidence of dementia: a meta-analysis. *Neurology, 51,* 728–733

Murdoch, B.E. & Lethlean, J.B. (1996). Language dysfunction in subcortical arteriosclerotic encephalopathy (Binswanger disease). *Journal of Medical Speech-Language Pathology, 4,* 275–288

Powell, A.L., Cummings, J.L., Hill, A., & Benson, D.F. (1988). Speech and language alterations in multi-infarct dementia. *Neurology, 38,* 717–719

Additional Reading

Erkinjuntti, T., Roman, G., Gauthier, S., Feldman, H., & Rockwood, K. (2004). Emerging therapies for vascular dementia and vascular cognitive impairment. *Stroke, 35,* 1010–1017

Chapter 61

Wilson's Disease

Christine T. Matthews and Richard I. Zraick

♦ General Information on Disorder

Wilson's disease (WD) is a genetic disorder that affects the liver's ability to excrete copper, resulting in copper accumulation in the bloodstream and organs, eventually becoming toxic. Accumulation of excess copper results in oxidant damage to cells in the liver, brain, and other organs (Brewer, 2001). WD is also referred to as hepatolenticular degeneration because of the copper deposition in the liver and lenticular nucleus of the basal ganglia (Lauterbach, 2002). WD is present at birth; however, symptoms of the disease most often present in the second and third decades of life due to the slow accumulation of excess copper in the liver and spread to other organs. Early definitive diagnosis is not straightforward, because the initial clinical presentation varies and can even go misdiagnosed for years, resulting in progressive hepatic and neurological damage and premature death. With accurate diagnosis and treatment, persons with WD can experience significant recovery and lead a normal life (Brewer, 2001).

Diagnostic Signs and Symptoms

Symptom onset can occur anywhere between the first and fifth decades of life; however, the most common time is during the second and third decades (Brewer, 2001). WD has three dominant disease presentations: hepatic, neurological, and behavioral/psychiatric (Brewer, 2001; Keller, Torta, Lagget, Crasto, & Bergamasco, 1999; Lauterbach, 2002; Portala, Levander, Westermark, Ekselius, & von Knorring, 2001). Hepatic presentation typically occurs with an earlier symptom onset reflecting a more severe genetic mutation. The more severe case causes a greater degree of difficulty in excreting copper from the liver. Hepatitis may be the initial diagnosis, or, in more extreme cases, severe liver failure requiring organ transplantation (Lauterbach, 2002). Neurological and psychiatric presentations are more likely to occur in later disease presentations because of gradual buildup and deposition of copper in the brain and other organs via the bloodstream (Brewer, 2001). The neurological symptoms are confined to the motor system and commonly consist of a wing beating-like tremor with outstretched arms, trunkal rigidity, and slowed movement (Duffy, 1995). Other common neurological symptoms include chorea, ataxia, dysarthria, dysphagia, and drooling. Psychiatric symptoms include cognitive impairments, dementia, mental retardation, anxiety, depression, suicide, emotional lability, mania, schizophrenic-like states, behavioral abnormalities, personality disorders, criminality, and substance abuse. Accurate diagnose of WD requires clinical and biochemical data (Keller et al, 1999). Biochemical indicators include low blood ceruloplasmin, high urinary copper levels, and high hepatic copper levels obtained via liver biopsy (Lauterbach, 2002). Clinical data include abnormal magnetic resonance imaging (MRI) findings and the presence of Kayser-Fleisher rings, which are copper deposits surrounding the cornea of the eye. Not all persons with WD have these distinctive rings, however. Ninety-nine percent of persons with neurological or psychiatric presentations have the rings, whereas only approximately 15% of persons with hepatic presentations have them (Brewer, 2001; Lauterbach, 2002).

Neuropathology

Because the neurological presentation of WD involves damage to the structures of the basal ganglia, WD is often characterized by movement disorders. These extrapyramidal symptoms can be attributed to the toxic action of copper in the basal ganglia (Nicholl, Ferenci, Polli, Burdon, & Pall, 2001). MRI findings are characterized by reduced T1-weighted and increased T2-weighted images of the putamen, pars compacta of the substantia nigra, periaqueductal gray matter, pontine tegmentum, and thalamus (Keller et al, 1999). These findings in combination with basal ganglia hyperdensity, ventricular dilation, and atrophy of the cortex, brainstem, and cerebellum on computed tomography (CT) suggest widespread atrophy from the oxidative action of the copper toxicity. Severity of neurological symptoms has been correlated with reduced positron emission tomography (PET)-demonstrated glucose metabolism in the striatum, thalamus, cortex, and cerebellum (Lauterbach, 2002). Abnormal dopamine, noradrenaline, and serotonin neurotransmitter metabolism has also been reported in WD (Portala et al, 2001).

Epidemiology

The incidence of WD has been estimated to be between one and three cases per 100,000, although higher rates can be found and are attributed to greater consanguinity (Keller et al, 1999; Lauterbach, 2002). WD is a genetic disease and therefore does not result from any known external toxin exposure. The disease affects men and women equally, and the average length of disease duration may be as short as 6 months from symptom onset to death if left untreated.

Patients who receive early accurate diagnosis and treatment may have normal life spans (Lauterbach, 2002).

Genetics

WD is an autosomal recessive disorder resulting from mutations to the *ATP7B* gene on chromosome 13q14.3. Symptom onset depends on the severity of the gene mutation, with a more severe mutation resulting in earlier onset. Approximately 1% of the population carries the gene for WD, and because it is a recessive gene disorder, both parents must carry the defective allele in order for there to be a one in four chance that their offspring will develop the disease (Lauterbach, 2002).

◆ Speech Impairment Associated with Disorder

A mixed dysarthria with ataxic, hypokinetic, and spastic components can be observed in WD and has been reported to be a prominent neurological feature, and perhaps in its milder form, one of the earliest neurological signs of the disease. When left untreated, damage to the neurological system can lead to marked dysarthria and a masked open-mouthed expression (Berry, Darley, Aronson, & Goldstein, 1974) or perhaps deteriorate to the point of anarthria. Dysphagia and drooling are also often noted (Day & Parnell, 1987).

Diagnostic Signs and Symptoms

Berry, Aronson, and Goldstein (1974) examined and described the speech of 20 persons with WD before treatment and a subsample of 10 following drug and diet therapy. This is the largest endeavor to date to accurately describe and relate sensorimotor speech characteristics with neurological symptomatology. In doing so, Berry et al described the motor speech disorder as a mixed dysarthria due to the widespread neural involvement. The mixed components resemble the dysarthria types of patients with cerebellar disorders, parkinsonism, and pseudobulbar palsy resulting in ataxic, hypokinetic, and spastic components, respectively. They found that the severity and combination of features varied from patient to patient, but that in more advanced cases of WD, ataxic speech characteristics along with the prosodic features of hypokinetic and spastic dysarthria were more prominent. The majority of the abnormal speech characteristics are shared among the three dysarthria types. In addition to these shared symptoms are inappropriate silences, irregular articulatory breakdowns, hypernasality, short phrases with prolonged phonemes and intervals, and strained vocal quality that are also distinct features of each of these dysarthria types (Berry et al, 1974; Duffy, 1995).

Etiology

Motor speech production deficits arise from the widespread oxidative damage to various cortical and subcortical neural structures. The absence of bulbar signs indicates a sparing of the lower motor neuron pathways of the motor system (Berry et al, 1974). Damage to selected neurotransmitter systems also affects the motor speech disturbances observed in WD.

Neuropathology

The known neural structures affected by WD support the observed motor speech impairments in those affected by the disease. Damage to the basal ganglia structures is reflected in the hypokinetic features of the mixed dysarthria. The ataxic symptoms can be attributed to cerebellar damage, and spastic symptoms to damage in the frontal and parietal-subcortical pathways (Lauterbach, 2002; Portala et al, 2001). Damage to the basal ganglia, cerebellum, and cortex can produce the observed changes in speed, strength, tone, range of motion, force, timing, and overall motor control (Duffy, 1995).

Associated Cognitive, Linguistic, and Communicative Signs and Symptoms

The degree of cognitive impairment increases with disease duration and severity of neurological symptoms (Lauterbach, 2002). One study identified a pattern of neuropsychological deficits observed in WD, and these include impaired executive functions specifically in dividing attention and slowed speed of processing (Portala et al, 2001). Poor school performance has been reported in persons who develop symptoms during childhood and adolescence. Broad cognitive impairments and dementia have also been described, as well as short-term memory impairments (Keller et al, 1999; Portala et al, 2001).

Special Diagnostic Considerations

Psychiatric presentations of WD are often misdiagnosed as schizophrenic disorders and neurological presentation as movement or cognitive disorders, whereas hepatic presentations are diagnosed as hepatitis or liver failure without the diagnosis of WD (Brewer, 2001). So while the symptoms of WD are commonly shared with each of these diagnoses, all symptoms and biochemical data must be carefully considered for an accurate diagnosis (Keller et al, 1999).

Treatment

Accurate diagnosis of WD is imperative to early treatment and recovery. In the past, the most common treatment was to recommend a restricted copper diet and anticopper drug therapy, most commonly penicillamine (e.g., Day & Parnell, 1987). Currently, treatment still focuses on the use of anticopper drug therapy with the more successful zinc acetate, as this drug appears to be less toxic. Anticopper drug therapy is a lifelong treatment for the disease, and dietary restrictions are not nearly as strict as once thought necessary (Brewer, 2001).

References

Berry, W., Darley, F.L., Aronson, A.E., & Goldstein, N.P. (1974). Dysarthria in Wilson's disease. *Journal of Speech and Hearing Research, 17,* 165–168

Brewer, G.J. (2001). Overview of the disease for the clinician. In: *Wilson's Disease: A Clinician's Guide to Recognition, Diagnosis, and Management* (pp. 1–7). Boston: Kluwer Academic Publishers

Day, L.S. & Parnell, M.M. (1987). Ten-year study of a Wilson's disease dysarthric. *Journal of Communication Disorders, 20,* 207–218

Duffy, J.R. (1995). *Motor Speech Disorders: Substrates, Differential Diagnosis, and Management,* 1st ed. St. Louis: Mosby

Keller, R., Torta, R., Lagget, M., Crasto, S., & Bergamasco, B. (1999). Psychiatric symptoms as late onset of Wilson's disease: neuroradiological findings, clinical features and treatment. *Italian Journal of Neurological Sciences, 20,* 49–54

Lauterbach, E. C. (2002). Wilson's disease. *Psychiatric Annals, 32,* 114–120

Nicholl, D. J., Ferenci, P., Polli, C., Burdon, M. B., & Pall, H. S. (2001). Wilson's disease presenting in a family with an apparent dominant history of tremor. *Journal of Neurology, Neurosurgery, and Psychiatry, 70,* 514–515

Portala, K., Levander, S., Westermark, K., Ekselius, L., & von Knorring, L. (2001). Pattern of neuropsychological deficits in patients with treated Wilson's disease. *European Archives of Psychiatry and Clinical Neuroscience, 251,* 262–268

Chapter 62

Worster-Drought Syndrome

Anita van der Merwe

◆ General Information on Disorder

Congenital suprabulbar paresis was first described by Charles Worster-Drought (1956), and since then this disorder has been termed Worster-Drought syndrome (WDS). The syndrome is characterized by paresis of the lips (orbicularis oris), tongue, soft palate, pharynx, and laryngeal muscles either in combination or separately (Worster-Drought, 1956, 1968, 1974). Although it is classified by some authors as belonging to the cerebral palsies (Clark, Carr, Reilly, & Neville, 2000), there are usually no or only very mild signs of limb involvement. In some cases a mild tetraplegia or monoplegia may be present (Arbelaez, Castillo, & Tennison, 2000; Clark et al, 2000; Neville, 1997; van der Merwe, 1974; Worster-Drought, 1956, 1974).

The primary lesion or deficit is congenital, the localization is suprabulbar (upper motor neuron), and it affects the muscular structures that derive their nerve supply mainly through cranial nerves X (vagus) and XII (hypoglossal) (Worster-Drought, 1956, 1974). Worster-Drought (1956) preferred the term *paresis* to *paralysis,* and rejected the term *pseudobulbar* in the description of congenital suprabulbar paresis. The term *pseudobulbar* distinguishes a bilateral disorder of the upper motor neurons from disorders of the bulbar nuclei (e.g., motor neuron disease). Pseudobulbar palsy is usually associated with double spastic hemiplegia or diplegia, which does not occur in WDS (Worster-Drought, 1956, 1974).

Diagnostic Signs and Symptoms

The severity and extent of the paresis varies in different cases. Worster-Drought (1956, 1968, 1974) described the complete syndrome and the incomplete syndrome. In the *complete syndrome* the child is unable to round his lips due to paresis of the orbicularis oris, whereas the other facial muscles move normally. There is extreme weakness of the tongue, showing only minimal protrusion. The soft palate shows no movement during attempted speech and no reflexive lifting on stimulation. The pharyngeal and laryngeal muscles may also be affected in severe cases (Worster-Drought, 1956). These cases usually present with severe dysarthria, feeding disorders, hypernasality, and voice disorders. An increased jaw jerk, a positive snout reflex, an increased pharyngeal (gag) reflex, and infantile oral reflexes may be present (Arbelaez et al, 2000; Van der Merwe, 1974; Worster-Drought, 1956, 1968, 1974). In some cases sensitivity of the gums and buccal mucous membranes is impaired (Worster-Drought, 1974).

In milder cases, termed the *incomplete syndrome*, different combinations and degrees of paresis may occur. Weakness of the orbicularis oris and the tongue or of the tongue and the soft palate may be present. There may also be an isolated weakness of the lips, the tongue, or the soft palate. The most frequent single structure involvement is weakness of the soft palate. This weakness may be accompanied by an increased jaw jerk, but by no other manifestation of the syndrome (Worster-Drought, 1956, 1968, 1974). The paresis in both the complete and incomplete syndrome is bilateral, although the severity may differ between the two sides (Van der Merwe, 1974).

Important diagnostic signs of WDS are the presence of persistent drooling and early feeding problems (Worster-Drought, 1974). Problems with lip closure, sucking, chewing, or airway protection result in swallowing problems. From an early age, choking during feeding may occur. Recurrent episodes of bronchospasm, lower respiratory infection, asthma, wheezing, sleep disturbance, esophageal pain, vomiting, and early malnutrition may indicate aspiration (Clark et al, 2000; Neville, 1997).

Neuropathology

Static cerebral pathology of early onset is present in WDS (Neville, 1997). Worster-Drought (1956) ascribed the syndrome to agenesis or hypogenesis of the corticobulbar neurons. Arbelaez et al (2000) reported on a case in which magnetic resonance imaging (MRI) showed cortical dysplasia in the region of the sylvian fissures. The sylvian fissures extended more superiorly and posteriorly than normal. In a case study by Nevo, Segev, Gelman, Rieder-Grosswasser, and Harel (2001), MRI revealed perisylvian and frontal polymicrogyria. The bilateral perisylvian cortical dysplasia suggestive of polymicrogyria is also present in congenital bilateral perisylvian syndrome. The latter is described as a syndrome of childhood-onset epilepsy (Arbelaez et al, 2000; Clark et al, 2000). Nevo et al (2001) suggested a continuum between WDS and perisylvian syndrome.

Epidemiology

In 1974 Worster-Drought reported that he had studied 200 cases, 193 children and seven adults. Of the 200, 48 showed the complete syndrome and 152 the incomplete syndrome. Of the 152 incomplete cases, 68 presented with soft palate involvement only, 34 with palate and tongue involvement,

28 with tongue and orbicularis oris involvement, and 22 with soft palate and orbicularis oris involvement. According to Neville (1997), WDS is underdiagnosed, and therefore the prevalence of this disorder is unknown.

Genetics

Worster-Drought (1974) reported that the syndrome was familial in 12 of the 200 cases he assessed. Among these were three pairs of twins. Patton, Baraitser, and Brett (1986) described a three-generation family in which four members were found to present with WDS. The authors suggested that some cases of WDS are inherited as an autosomal dominant trait. In a study of 47 cases, Clark et al (2000) reported that six children had a family history of WDS. However, in many instances WDS seems to be sporadic (Arbelaez et al, 2000).

◆ Speech Impairment Associated with Disorder

In WDS there is bilateral suprabulbar paresis of the speech structures, and therefore these cases present with dysarthria. Immobility or reduced range of movement is present in the orbicularis oris muscle, the tongue, soft palate, pharynx, and the laryngeal muscles in the complete syndrome. The type of dysarthria may be classified as spastic dysarthria.

Diagnostic Signs and Symptoms

The diagnostic signs depend on the specific speech structures that are involved. An inability to round the lips but a normal smile due to normal movement of the risorius and other facial muscles is an important diagnostic sign. Drooling, and problems with chewing, sucking, and swallowing are indicators of motor execution problems. Weakness or immobility of the soft palate causes nasal speech. If the laryngeal muscles are affected, voice quality, pitch, and loudness are compromised. An inability to protrude the tongue or to move it laterally is an indication of the lingual paresis. Due to the labial and lingual weakness or immobility, bilabial and lingual sounds will be absent or distorted (Clark et al, 2000; van der Merwe, 1974; Worster-Drought 1956, 1968, 1974). Speech may be characterized by vowel production and articulation of consonant sounds such as the /n/, /k/, and /g/. These patients may use words such as /a a/ for /papa/ or /u a na/ for /juhana/. Intonation, rhythm, and stress may sound normal (van der Merwe, 1974). Worster-Drought (1956, 1974) suggested that speech might gradually improve as the child gets older.

Etiology

The suprabulbar disorder results in spasticity of those speech structures that are involved (Neville, 1997; Worster-Drought, 1956, 1968, 1974). The spasticity results in paresis, and all parameters of movement are affected. These parameters include the range, rate, and accuracy of movement. No atrophy or fasciculations are present, as the disorder is suprabulbar (Worster-Drought, 1974).

Neuropathology

In WDS there is involvement of the corticobulbar tract that runs from the motor area in the frontal lobe of the brain to the motor nuclei in the brainstem (Worster-Drought, 1956, 1968, 1974).

Associated Cognitive, Linguistic, and Communicative Signs and Symptoms

In its pure form, WDS is not associated with cognitive or language problems. However, congenital neurological disorders often cause associated cognitive and language problems. Clark et al (2000) found that 23 of the 47 children they studied had moderate learning difficulties and 15 had severe learning difficulties. Neville (1997) suggested that cognitive impairment varies widely, but that it is usually not severe. Young children and babies with WDS may be unhappy and irritable due to feeding problems and may show lack of social responsiveness (Neville, 1997). Other associated problems may be middle ear infection, sensorineural hearing loss, epilepsy, and behavior or psychiatric problems.

Special Diagnostic Considerations

Differential diagnosis between WDS and other speech disorders is important. An inability to move the tongue must be differentiated from a too short lingual frenulum. Unnecessary surgery can be avoided this way. A congenitally too short soft palate or a submucous cleft should be differentiated from an isolated paresis of the soft palate. Cranial nerve nuclear agenesis (the Möbius syndrome) should be differentiated from WDS. In the case of Möbius syndrome there may be wasting and fasciculation of the tongue (Worster-Drought 1956, 1974).

Differentiating between incomplete WDS and developmental apraxia of speech (DAS) may pose a problem. In WDS all movements of the affected structures are consistently compromised. In DAS there may be inconsistency with repeated attempts of the same movement. Consistent hypernasality can be expected in cases with WDS soft palate involvement, whereas a discrepancy between voluntary velar closure during speech and involuntary reflex movements can occur in DAS. Drooling, and problems with chewing, sucking, and swallowing indicate the presence of dysarthria. Dysarthria and DAS may co-occur in the same client. A comprehensive differential diagnosis is important, and a pediatric neurologist should be consulted.

Treatment

The early feeding problems should be managed by a specialist dysphagia team. Nasogastric or gastrostomy feeding can counteract aspiration, malnutrition, and esophageal reflux (Neville, 1997). Infantile reflexes and a hyperactive gag reflex can be desensitized and inhibited, velar lifting can be facilitated through direct stimulation, and swallowing can be facilitated and the frequency increased to decrease drooling. The articulation of sounds such as the /m/ both in isolation and in words can be facilitated. Icing, vibration, and assistance and resistance techniques can be used (Gangale, 2001). In two cases with WDS, these techniques reduced drooling and improved lip movement and production of /m/ in words (Van der Merwe, 1974). Surgery for the management of drooling and velar incompetence may be considered. Alternative and augmentative communication devices should be implemented if verbal communication is not possible.

References

Arbelaez, A., Castillo, M., & Tennison, M. (2000). MRI in a Patient with Worster-Drought Syndrome. *Neuroradiology, 42,* 403–405

Clark, M., Carr, L., Reilly, S. & Neville, B.G.R. (2000). Worster-Drought syndrome, a mild tetraplegic perisylvian cerebral palsy. *Brain, 123,* 2160–2170

Gangale, D.C. (2001). *The Source for Oral-Facial Exercises Updated and Expanded.* East Moline, IL: LinguiSystems

Neville, B. (1997). The Worster-Drought syndrome: a severe test of paediatric neurodisability services? *Developmental Medicine and Child Neurology, 39,* 782–784

Nevo, Y., Segev, Y., Gelman, Y., Rieder-Grosswasser, I. & Harel, S. (2001). Worster-Drought and congenital perisylvian syndromes—a continuum? *Pediatric Neurology, 24,* 153–155

Patton, M.A., Baraitser, M., & Brett, E.M. (1986). A family with congenital suprabulbar paresis (Worster-Drought syndrome). *Clinical Genetics, 29,* 147–150

Van der Merwe, A. (1974). Dysarthria: congenital suprabulbar paresis. *South African Speech and Hearing Association Newsletter, 179,* 7–11

Worster-Drought, C. (1956). Congenital suprabulbar paresis. *Journal of Laryngology and Otology, 70,* 453–463

Worster-Drought, C. (1968). Speech disorders in children. *Developmental Medicine and Child Neurology, 10,* 427–440.

Worster-Drought, C. (1974). Suprabulbar Paresis. Congenital supra bulbar paresis and its differential diagnosis, with special reference to acquired suprabulbar paresis. *Developmental Medicine and Child Neurology Suppl, 30,* 1–33.

Additional Reading

Christen, H.J., Hanefeld, F., Kruse, E., Imhauser, S., Ernst, J.P. & Finkenstaedt, M. (2000). Foix-Chavany-Marie (anterior operculum) syndrome in childhood: a reappraisal of Worster-Drought Syndrome. *Developmental Medicine and Child Neurology, 42,* 122–132

Crary, M.A. (1993). *Developmental Speech Disorders.* San Diego: Singular

Index

Note: Page numbers followed by *f* and *t* indicate figures and tables, respectively.

The Life and Work of...

Michelangelo Buonarroti

Richard Tames

Heinemann Library
Chicago, Illinois

© 2001 Reed Educational & Professional Publishing
Published by Heinemann Library,
an imprint of Reed Educational & Professional Publishing,
100 N. LaSalle, Suite 1010
Chicago, IL 60602
Customer Service 888-454-2279
Visit our website at www.heinemannlibrary.com

Designed by Celia Floyd
Illustrations by Sam Thompson
Originated by Dot Gradations
Printed in Hong Kong/China

05 04 03 02 01
10 9 8 7 6 5 4 3 2 1

Library of Congress Cataloging-in -Publication Data
Tames, Richard.
     Michelangelo Buonarotti / Richard Tames.
        p. cm. – (The Life and work of--)
     Includes bibliographical references and index.
     Summary: A biography of the Renaissance sculptor, painter, architect, and poet,
including a list of places where his art can be seen today.
     ISBN 1-57572-343-3
     1. Michelangelo Buonarotti, 1475-1564—Juvenile literature. 2.
Artists—Italy—Biography—Juvenile literature. [1. Michelangelo Buonarotti, 1475-1564.
2. Artists.] I. Title. II. Series.

N6923.B9 T36 2000
709'.2—dc21
[B]   00-025785

Acknowledgments
The Publishers would like to thank the following for permission to reproduce photographs:

Archivi Alinari, pp. 5, 9, 11, 13, 15, 21; Archivio Buonarroti, p. 27; Bridgeman Art Library/Casa Buonarroti, Florence, p. 7; Bridgeman Art Library/Vatican Museums and Galleries, Italy, p. 17; E. T. Archive, p. 28; J. Allan Cash, Ltd., p. 23; Photo RMN/R. G. Ojeda, p. 19; Robert Harding Picture Library/Simon Harris, p. 25; Scala, Museo dellí Opera del Duomo, p. 29

Cover photograph reproduced with permission of The Bridgeman Art Library

Every effort has been made to contact copyright holders of any material reproduced in this book. Any omissions will be rectified in subsequent printings if notice is given to the Publisher.

Some words are shown in bold, **like this.** You can find out what they mean by looking in the glossary.

Contents

Who Was Michelangelo?

Michelangelo was one of the greatest artists of all time. He lived during the **Renaissance**. He thought of himself as a **sculptor**. But he was also a painter, a poet, and an **architect**.

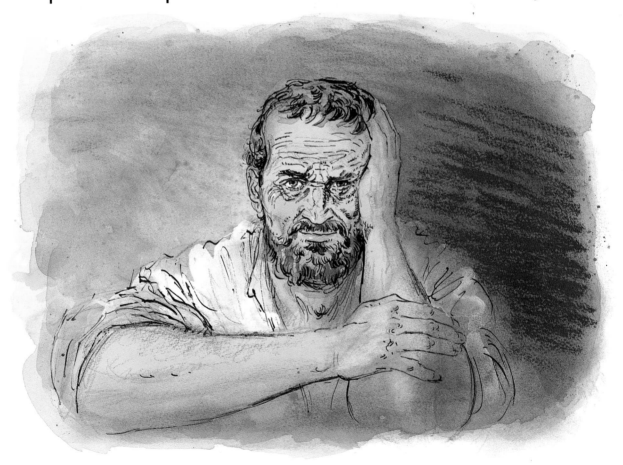

4

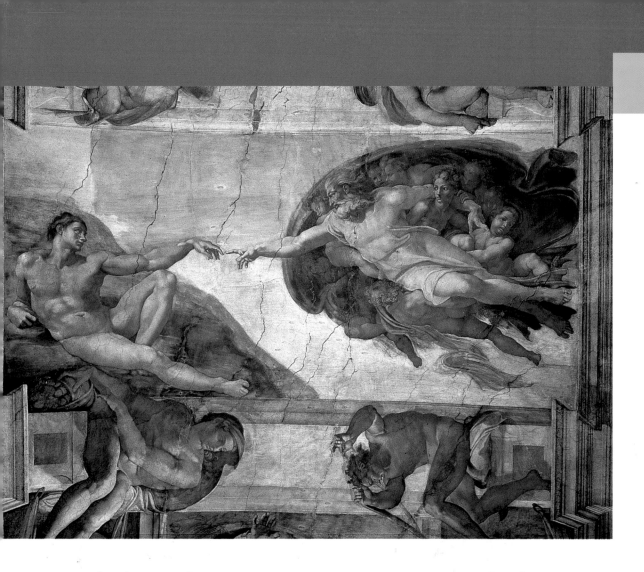

In Michelangelo's time, most art was made for churches. This painting shows God giving life to Adam. Michelangelo painted it on the ceiling of the Sistine **Chapel** in Rome, Italy.

The Pupil

Michelangelo was born in Italy on March 6, 1475. As a boy, he studied painting with Ghirlandaio, a respected artist. Later, he studied artworks owned by an important, powerful family—the Medici.

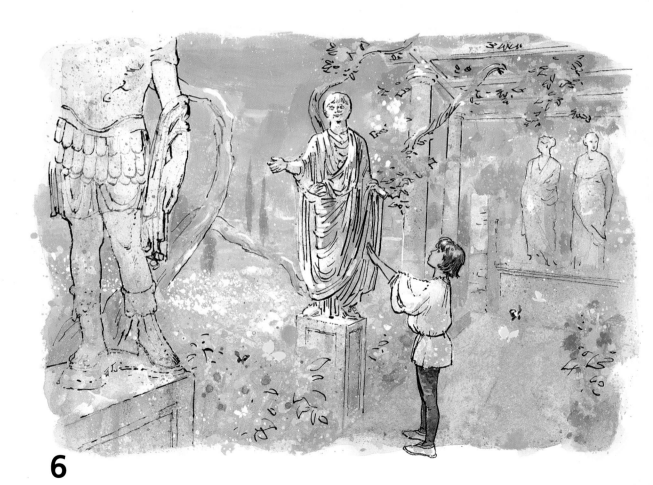

Soon Michelangelo became interested in **sculpture** as well as painting. He was only sixteen when he carved this sculpture of the baby Jesus with his mother, Mary.

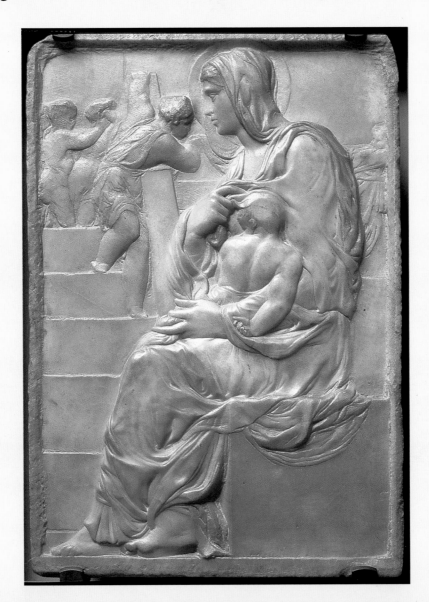

The Student

Michelangelo wanted to understand how the human body worked. He studied human bodies in a hospital in a city called Florence. This helped him make his paintings and **sculptures** look real.

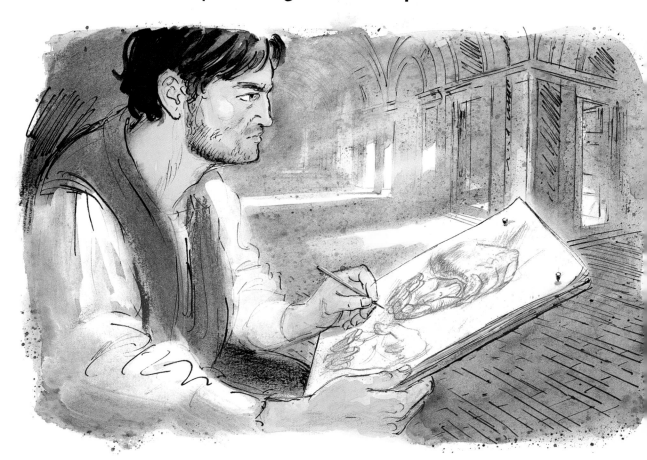

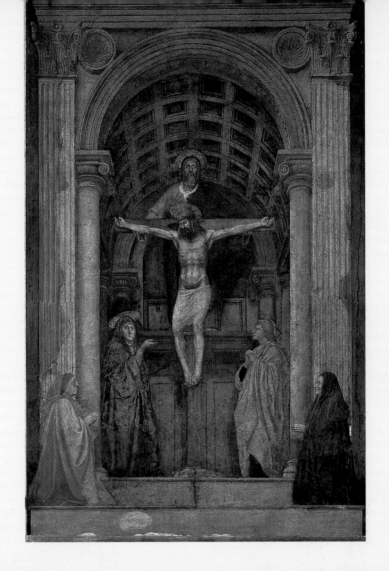

Michelangelo also studied the work of other artists. He made his own drawings of **frescoes** like this one, by Masaccio. This helped him learn about color and **perspective**.

Fame

Michelangelo moved to the city of Rome in 1496. There, he carved a famous **statue**. It shows Jesus lying in his mother's arms after he has died.

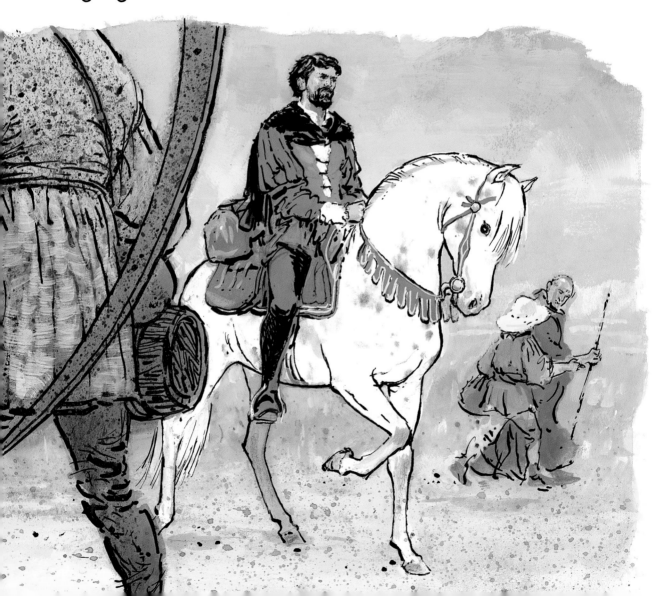

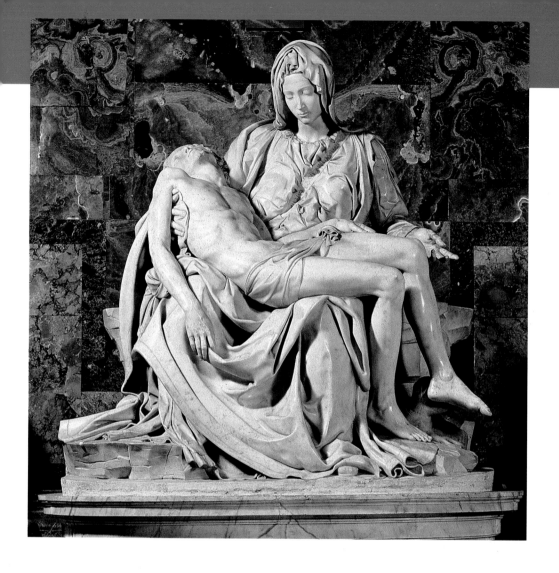

The statue is called the *Pietà*. Michelangelo used one piece of stone to make the two figures. It is very **realistic**. You can see the folds in the cloth of Mary's dress.

Working in Florence

In 1501, Michelangelo returned to Florence. He had been asked to make a **statue** of **David.** David was a hero and a leader. His life is described in the **Bible.**

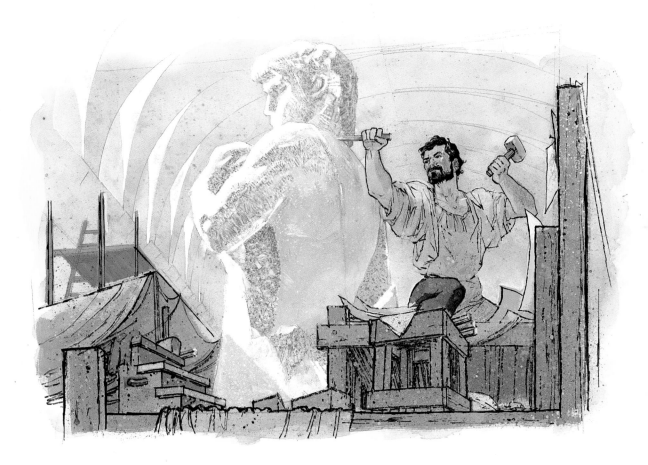

Michelangelo's statue of David was for the city's **cathedral**. The statue became famous. People thought it showed a perfect human being.

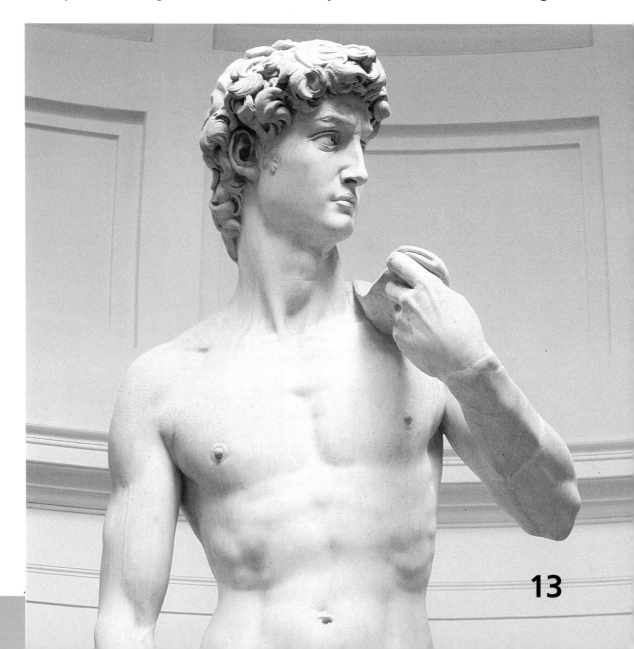

The Pope's Tomb

In 1505, Michelangelo was asked to plan a huge **tomb.** It would be for **Pope** Julius II. But Michelangelo had agreed to do too much work. He did not have time to finish the tomb.

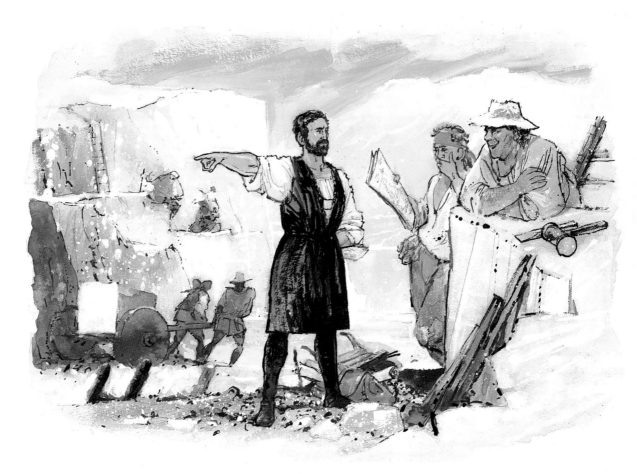

Over 40 **statues** were planned for the tomb. This famous statue of **Moses** was meant to be on the tomb.

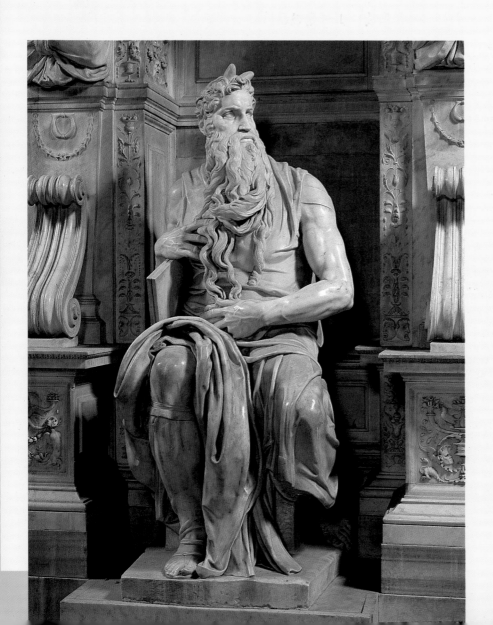

The Sistine Chapel

In 1508, **Pope** Julius II gave Michelangelo a special job. He asked Michelangelo to paint works of art. They would be painted on the ceiling of the Sistine **Chapel** in Rome.

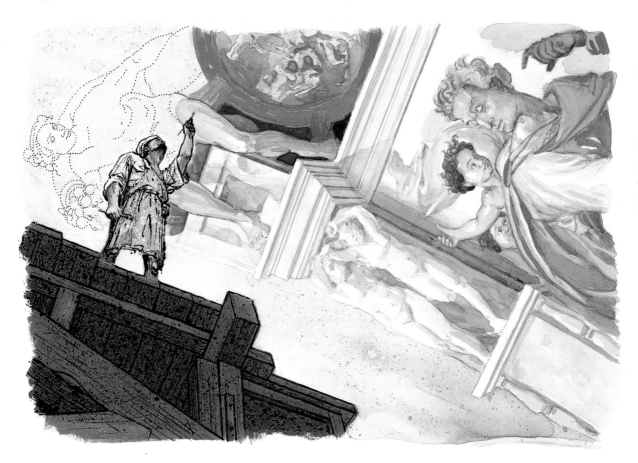

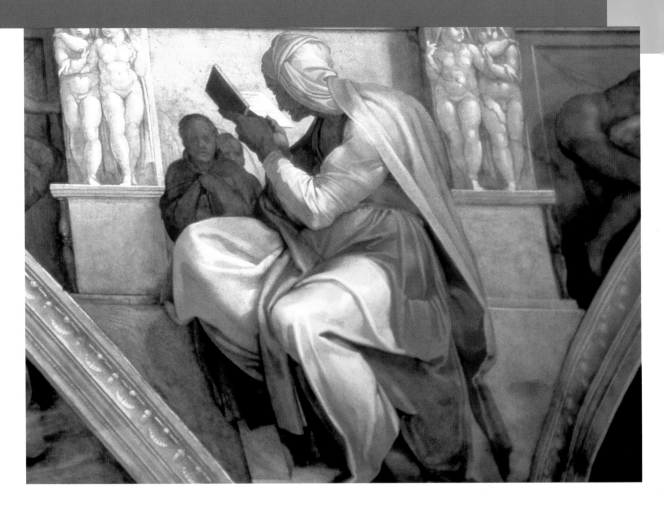

It took Michelangelo four years to paint the
ceiling. The paintings tell stories from the **Bible.**
They are among the most famous paintings in
the world.

Cities at War

Italy was often at war during Michelangelo's lifetime. Between 1528 and 1529, he worked on plans for buildings and walls to protect Florence during an attack.

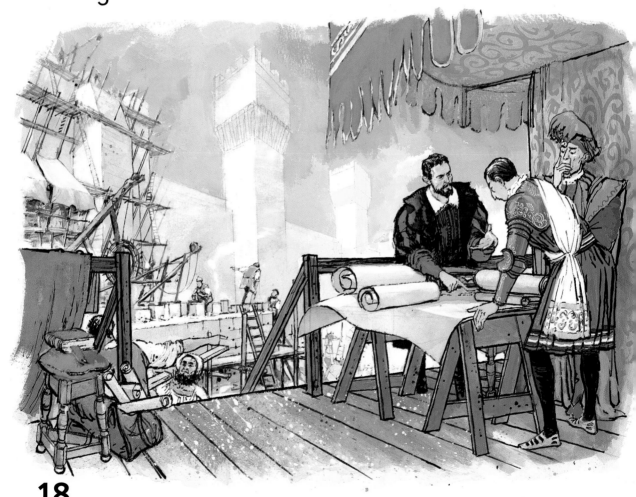

Michelangelo made this sketch in 1528. It shows his plans for the **defense** of Florence. He wanted ditches dug all around the city.

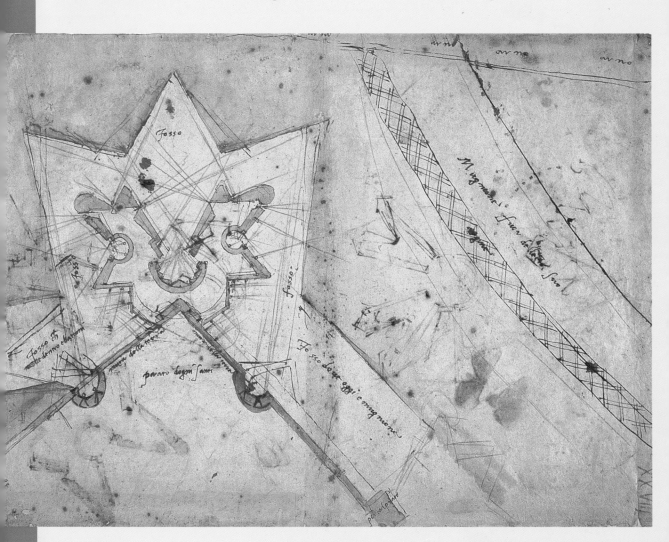

Working for the Medici

From 1515 until 1534, Michelangelo worked for the Medici family in Florence. He **designed** a **chapel**, a library, two **tombs,** and a grand house for them.

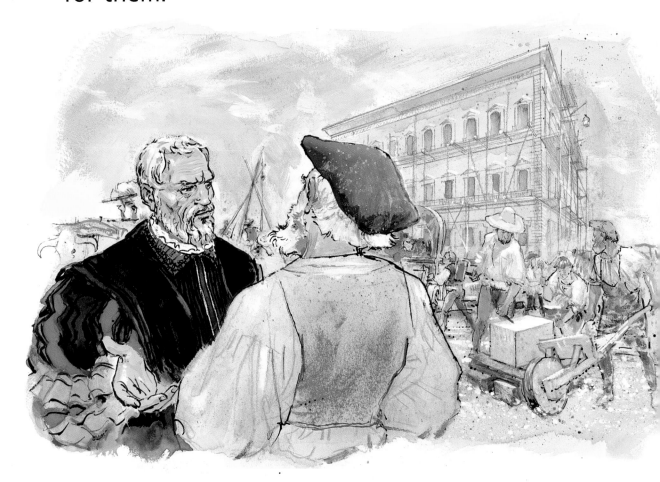

This is a tomb Michelangelo designed for the Medici family. The two figures at the front are meant to be Dawn and **Dusk**.

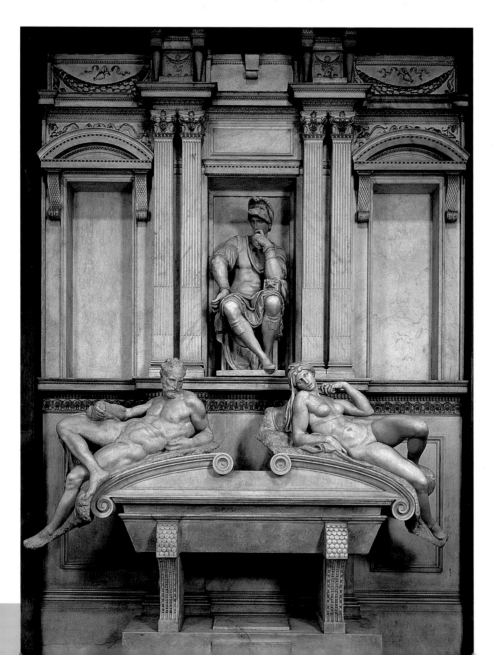

Back to Rome

From 1534 until he died, Michelangelo lived in Rome. He **designed** a new square for the center of the city.

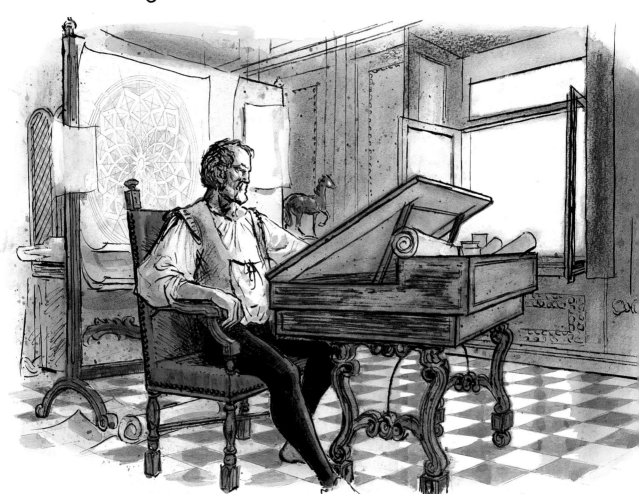

Michelangelo redesigned the old city hall on Capitolene Hill. He also created a floor design of oval patterns. He had a **statue** placed at the center of the pattern.

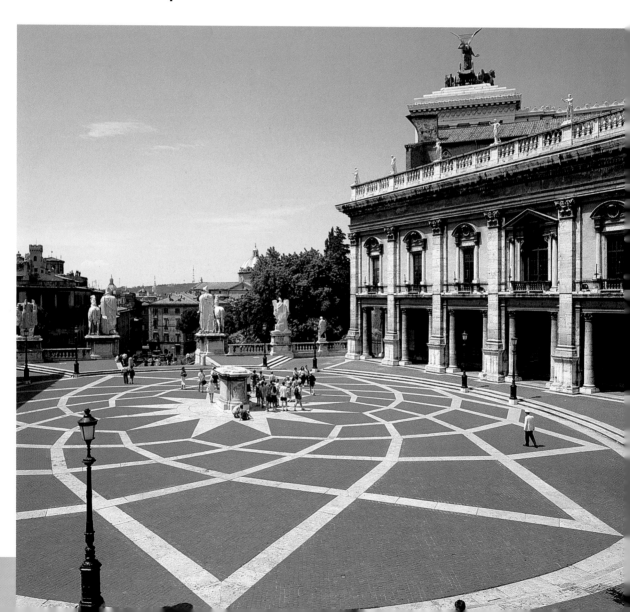

The Pope's Architect

In 1546, Michelangelo became the **pope's** main **architect**. He worked on the great church of St. Peter in Rome.

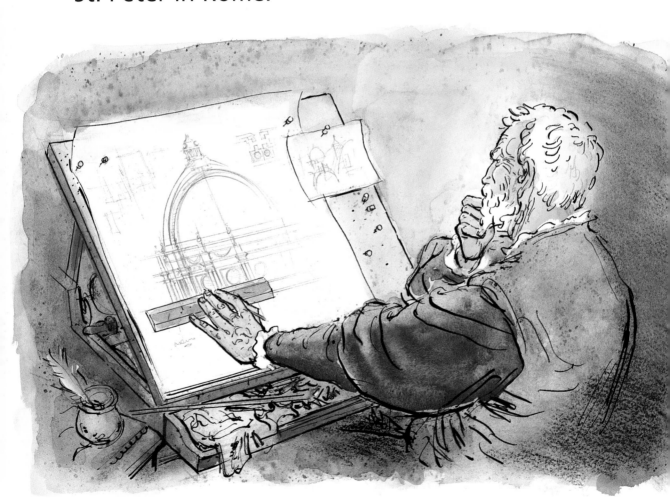

Michelangelo **designed** the **dome** of St. Peter's.
Sadly, he died before it was finished.

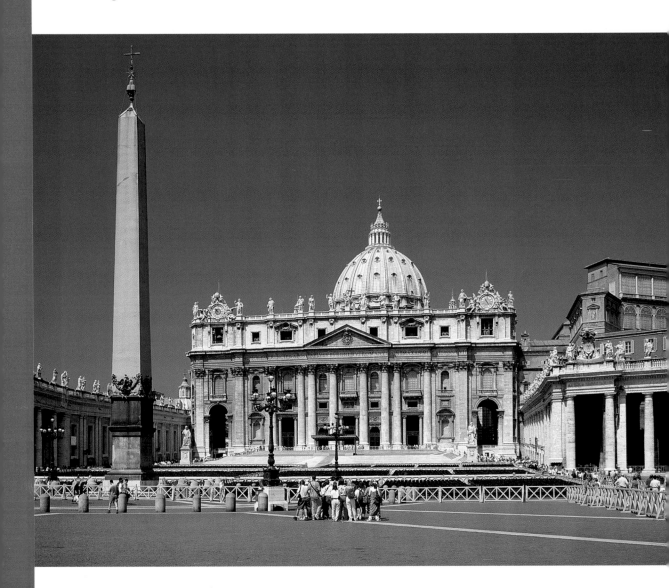

Last Years

From 1546 to 1547, Michelangelo **designed** a palace. It was for **Pope** Paul III's family. He also wrote many poems and letters to his friends and family.

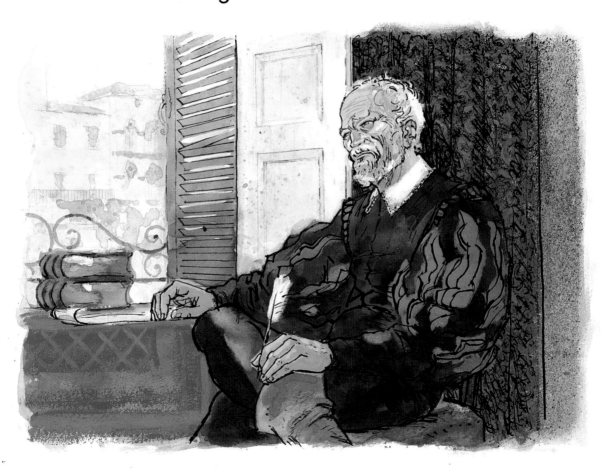

Michelangelo had beautiful handwriting. Many of his poems are about love. But he never married.

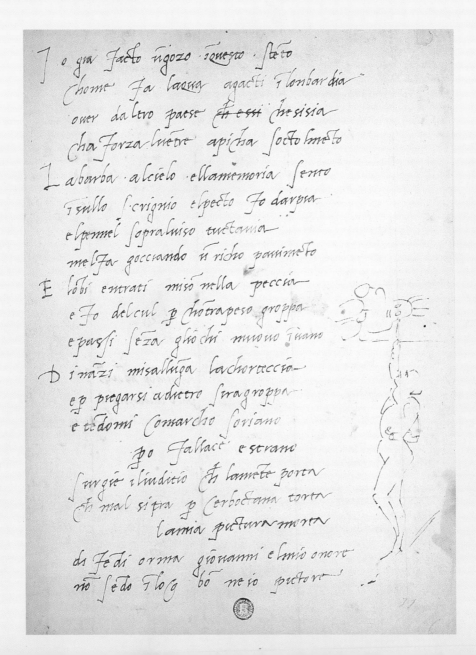

Michelangelo Dies

Michelangelo died on February 18, 1564. He was 88 years old. He was buried in Florence. His **tomb** was designed by one of his students, Giorgio Vasari.

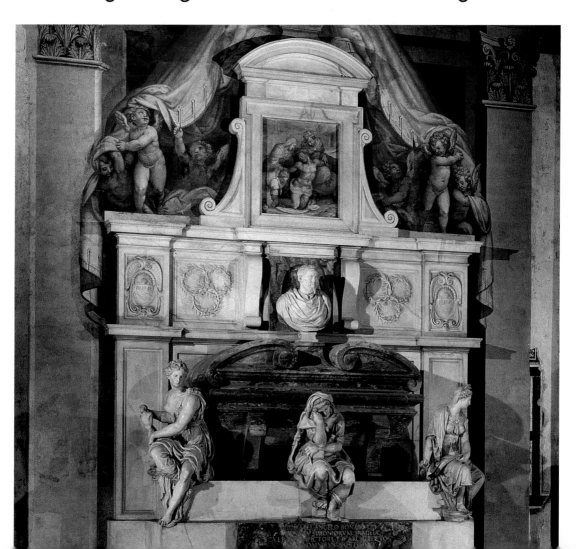

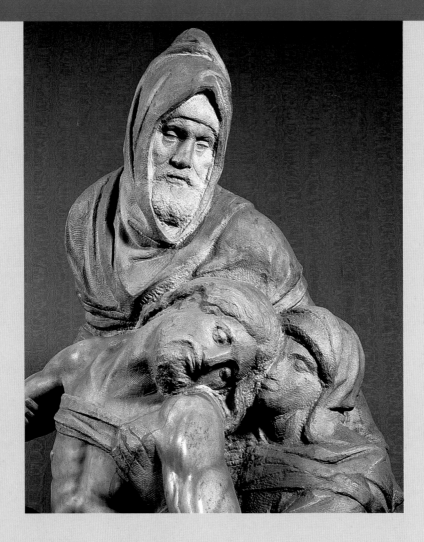

This is part of a **statue** Michelangelo was making
for his own tomb. But he never finished it.
It shows Michelangelo at the age of 75.

Timeline

1475	Michelangelo Buonarroti born in Caprese, Italy on March 6
1475	Family moves to Florence
1488	Trains with the artist Ghirlandaio
1490–1492	Lives in the Medici Palace and studies art
1496	Moves from Florence to Rome
1501–1504	Carves **statue** of **David**
1508–1512	Paints ceiling of Sistine **Chapel**
1528–1529	**Designs defenses** for Florence
1534	Last time Michelangelo leaves Florence
1534–1541	Michelangelo paints **fresco** (*The Last Judgment*) for Sistine Chapel
1546	Michelangelo becomes pope's chief **architect**
1564	Michelangelo dies, February 18

Glossary

architect person who designs buildings

Bible book of Christian holy writings, divided into the Old and the New Testaments

biography story of a person's life

cathedral large and important church

chapel small church or part of a bigger church or cathedral

David hero of the Old Testament and later King of Israel

defense something built to keep a city safe

design to make a plan

dome rounded roof

dusk evening

fresco painting done on wet plaster so the color soaks in

Moses Old Testament leader to whom God gave the Ten Commandments

perspective way of drawing to show distance

pope leader of the Roman Catholic Church

realistic lifelike

Renaissance the fourteenth through the seventeenth centuries in Europe, when there was great new interest in art and learning

sculptor person who makes statues or carvings

sculpture statue or carving

statue carved, molded, or sculptured figure

tomb burial place

More Books to Read

McLanathan, Richard B. *Michelangelo.* New York, Harry N. Abrams, Inc., 1993.

Venezia, Mike. *Michelangelo.* Danbury, Conn.: Children's Press, 1991.

More Artwork to See

Drawing for the *Libyan Sybil*, Metropolitan Museum of Art, New York, New York

Drawing for the *Holy Family with the Infant John the Baptist,* Getty Museum, Los Angeles, California

Index

3m